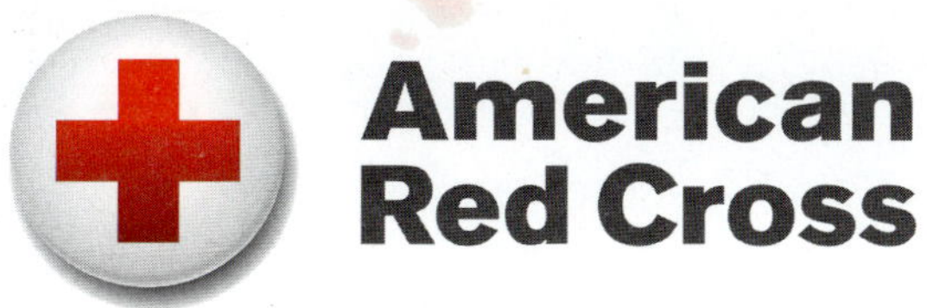

American Red Cross Nurse Assistant Training

Textbook

I worked hard!
I deserve this!
I will succeed!

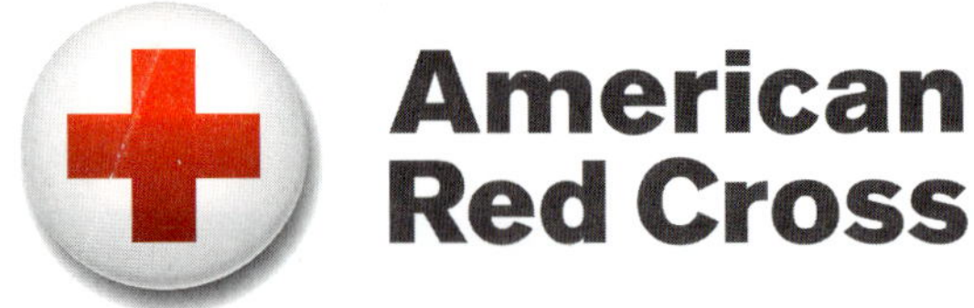

This textbook is part of the American Red Cross Nurse Assistant Training program. By itself, it does not constitute complete and comprehensive training. Visit redcross.org to learn more about this program.

The emergency care procedures outlined in this book reflect the standard of knowledge and accepted emergency practices in the United States at the time this book was published. It is the reader's responsibility to stay informed of changes in emergency care procedures.

The infection control procedures outlined in this book reflect the current standards and guidelines of the Centers for Disease Control (CDC) and Occupational Safety and Health Administration (OSHA) in the United States at the time this book was published. Because regulations influencing these standards and guidelines change frequently and because laws are redefined, it is the reader's responsibility to stay current with information such as infection control by attending in-service courses offered by employers or through other sources.

Published by Krames StayWell Strategic Partnerships Division

Printed in the United States of America

ISBN: 978-1-58480-568-7

This textbook is dedicated to the employees and volunteers of the American Red Cross who contribute their time and talent to supporting and teaching caregiving skills worldwide, and to the students who have decided to make a career out of helping others.

How far you go in life depends on your being tender with the young, compassionate with the aged, sympathetic with the striving, and tolerant of the weak and strong—because someday in life you will have been all of these.

—George Washington Carver

CONTENTS

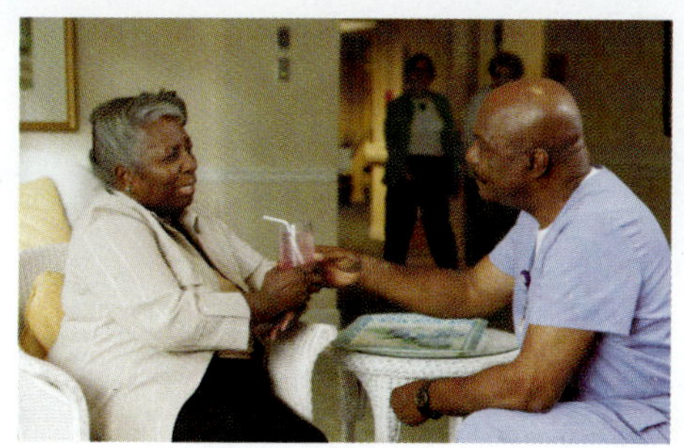
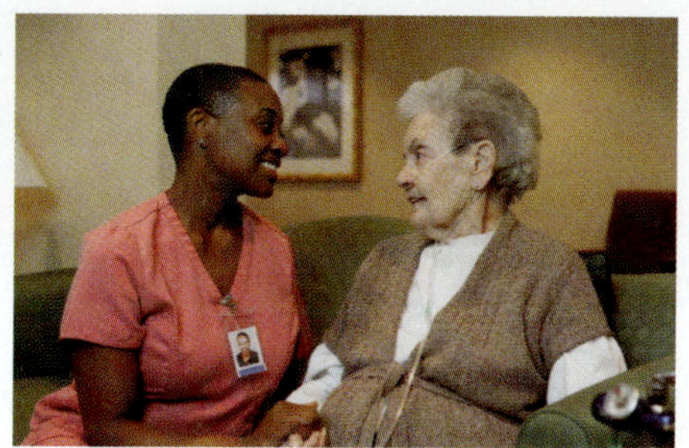
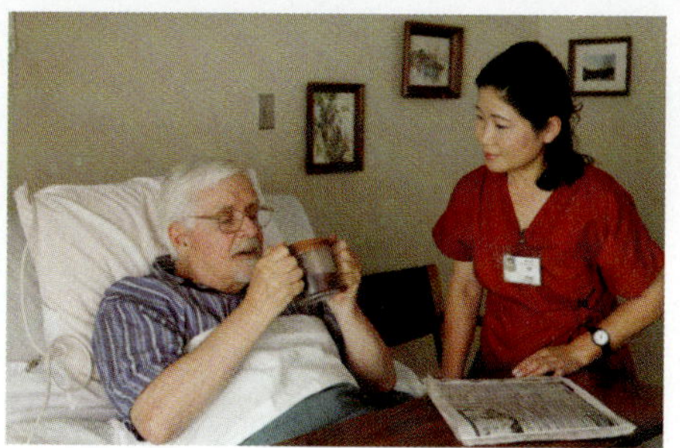

UNIT 4

SPECIAL CARE SITUATIONS 294

UNIT 5

TRANSITIONING FROM STUDENT TO EMPLOYEE 372

Appendices 400

ACKNOWLEDGMENTS

Many individuals shared in the development and revision process in various supportive, technical and creative ways. The American Red Cross Nurse Assistant Training textbook was developed through the dedication of both employees and volunteers. Their commitment to excellence made this manual possible.

The following members of the American Red Cross Scientific Advisory Council provided guidance and review:

Jean Johnson, PhD, RN, FAAN
Chair, Nursing and Caregiving Sub-Council
Dean, School of Nursing
The George Washington University
Washington, District of Columbia

Christy Blackstone, MSW, LCSW
Department of Veterans Affairs
VA Health Care System
Alexandria, Louisiana

Barbara J. Burgel, RN, ANP, PhD, FAAN
Professor of Nursing
University of California, San Francisco School of Nursing
San Francisco, California

Susan L. Carlson, MSN, APRN, ACNS-BC, GNP-BC, FNGNA
Neurology Nurse Practitioner
South Texas Veterans Health Care System
San Antonio, Texas

Marie Etienne, DNP, ARNP, PLNC
Professor
Miami Dade College, School of Nursing
Miami, Florida

Susan M. Heidrich, PhD, RN
Helen Denne Schulte Emeritus Professor
University of Wisconsin–Madison, School of Nursing Nurse Scientist
William S. Middleton Memorial Veterans Administration Hospital
Madison, Wisconsin

Deanna Colburn Hostler, DPT, PhD (ABD)
Senior Physical Therapist
Presbyterian Hospital, University of Pittsburgh Medical Center
Pittsburgh, Pennsylvania

Carla M. Tozer, MSN, APN/CPN, ACHPH, ANP-BC, GNP-BC
Visiting Nursing Practice Specialist
Visiting Clinical Instructor
University of Illinois–Chicago, College of Nursing
Chicago, Illinois

The following individuals also provided guidance and review throughout the manuscript development process:

Nelly Azizi, LVN
Instructor, Nurse Assistant Training Program
American Red Cross Southern California Territory
Commerce, California

Anika Bailey, MSN, MEd, RN
Health Care Training Programs Manager
American Red Cross of Southeastern Michigan
Detroit, Michigan

Melissa C. Beadle, MBA
Program Manager II, Nurse Assistant Training
American Red Cross Northern Ohio Territory
Cleveland, Ohio

Mary Jane Carpenter, RN
Instructor, Nurse Assistant Training Program
American Red Cross Northern Ohio Territory
Cleveland, Ohio

Linda Carter, RN
Instructor, Nurse Assistant Training Program
American Red Cross Northern Ohio Territory
Cleveland, Ohio

Nancy Daly, RN
Instructor, Nurse Assistant Training Program
American Red Cross of Eastern Massachusetts
Cambridge, Massachusetts

Abigail Filius, LVN
Instructor, Nurse Assistant Training Program
American Red Cross Southern California Territory
Commerce, California

Sharon Garwood, RN, BSN
Instructor, Nurse Assistant Training Program
American Red Cross of Southeastern Michigan
Detroit, Michigan

Jason Kang, LVN
Instructor, Nurse Assistant Training Program
American Red Cross Southern California Territory
Commerce, California

Jane Lash, RN
Instructor, Nurse Assistant Training Program
American Red Cross
Cambridge, Massachusetts

Agnes Liclican, RN
Interim Director of Nurses, Nurse Assistant Training Program
American Red Cross Southern California Territory
Commerce, California

Marianne Mastrangelo, BSN, RN
Director, Health Care Training
American Red Cross of Eastern Massachusetts
Cambridge, Massachusetts

Diane M. Minor, RN, BSN
Program Manger I, Nurse Assistant Training
American Red Cross Northern Ohio Territory
Cleveland, Ohio

Loralyn Penzella, MPA
Program Manager, Nurse Assistant Training/Competency
Evaluation Program Testing
American Red Cross Southern California Territory
Commerce, California

Marion Reed, RN
Instructor, Nurse Assistant Training Program
American Red Cross of Southeastern Michigan
Detroit, Michigan

Lula Robinson, RN
Instructor, Nurse Assistant Training Program
American Red Cross Northern Ohio Territory
Cleveland, Ohio

The following individuals assisted with the creation of the content by providing subject matter expertise:

Wanda Murray-Goldschmidt, RN, BSN, BC, MA
Clinical Faculty
Department of Nursing, Towson University
Towson, Maryland
Faculty
The Copper Ridge Institute
Eldersburg, Maryland

Theresa Kyle, RN, MSN, CPNP
Director of Nursing
El Camino College
Torrance, California

Ginger Schuerger-Davison, RNBC, LNHA
Long-Term Care Consultant
Ohio Health Care Association Member
Berea, Ohio

Sandra J. Soditch, RN
Long-Term Care Consultant
Centerville, Ohio

Diana F. Waugh, BSN, RN
Long-Term Care Consultant
Waugh Consulting
Waterville, Ohio

The American Red Cross also gives special thanks to the following organizations and individuals for their contributions to this project:

- The residents, staff and administrators at Roland Park Place in Baltimore, Maryland, for their assistance with the photography shoot
- The residents, staff and administrators at Stella Maris in Timonium, Maryland, for their assistance with the video shoot
- The staff of Portfolio Productions in Portland, Oregon, for their assistance with producing the photography and video assets
- The staff of Krames StayWell Strategic Partnerships Division, for their assistance with editing and producing the textbook

Photography credit: Chapter 21, page 338 © iStockPhoto.com/Juanmonino

PREFACE

Nurse assistants are key members of the health care team, providing care for patients, residents and clients in a variety of health care settings. The aging population, longer life spans, and changes in the way health care is provided and paid for are presenting many opportunities for people who want to train for a career in health care. During a time when employment opportunities are decreasing in many industries in the United States, employment opportunities in health care are increasing, and they are expected to continue to increase in the future. As a nation, we must maintain and continue to build a workforce prepared to meet the needs of the population.

The American Red Cross Nurse Assistant Training textbook and course are based on the belief that caregiving is an art. This textbook and course seek to train students in the art of caregiving, focusing on five principles of care that should inform every decision the caregiver makes and every action the caregiver takes: safety, privacy, dignity, independence and communication. In addition to learning the technical skills needed to provide competent care, students learn the principles and concepts necessary to provide compassionate, person-centered care.

Features

The American Red Cross Nurse Assistant Training textbook was developed to help students understand, remember and put into practice important concepts and skills. Features of the third edition that support student learning include a conversational, engaging writing style; a completely new art program; and a clean, open page design. In addition, the following pedagogical features were developed to aid students in acquiring the skills and knowledge they need to provide safe, competent, compassionate care:

- **Case studies.** Each chapter begins by introducing a recipient of health care and providing some basic information about the person and his or her situation. As students progress through the chapter, they are provided with more information about the person introduced in the case study, and they are given the opportunity to apply the concepts they have just read about. The case studies serve to personalize and enliven the reading, reinforce key concepts and promote critical thinking skills.
- **Nurse Assistant Do's and Don'ts.** These boxes summarize guidelines for providing safe, efficient, person-centered care.
- **Observations into Action.** A very important role of the nurse assistant is to function as the "eyes and ears" for the rest of the health care team. The "Observations into Action" feature highlights observations the nurse assistant may make that should be reported immediately.
- **Elder Care Notes.** Many of the people the nurse assistant will care for will be elderly. This feature draws the student's attention to special considerations that should be kept in mind when caring for an elderly person.
- **Skill Sheets.** The skill sheets walk the student through key nurse assistant skills step by step. Photographs and illustrations are provided to clarify written instructions and enhance understanding. Standard preparation and completion steps are included as part of every skill to help students learn and remember these very important actions. All skills emphasize the five principles of care: safety, privacy, dignity, independence and communication.
- **Goals.** Each chapter begins with a list of learning objectives or goals.
- **Key Terms** and **Glossary.** Important vocabulary words to learn and remember are listed at the beginning of each chapter and defined within the context of the chapter. A glossary, included at the end of the book, allows students to quickly look up definitions for the key terms highlighted throughout the book.
- **Check Your Understanding.** Each chapter concludes with **Questions for Review** (multiple-choice questions that allow students to assess their understanding of the chapter content) and **Questions to Ask Yourself** (short-answer, usually scenario-based questions designed to help students apply and think critically about the information they have just learned). The answers to the multiple-choice Questions for Review are provided in Appendix E.

Organization

The third edition of the American Red Cross Nurse Assistant Training textbook has been reorganized to facilitate logical progression from one topic to another and to allow students to build and expand on previously acquired knowledge. Chapters have been organized into thematic units.

Unit 1: The Art of Caregiving

In this unit, students are introduced to fundamental concepts that are essential to working in the health care field. Chapter 1, *Being a Nurse Assistant*, describes the nurse assistant's roles and responsibilities as a member of the health care team and the educational requirements necessary to become a nurse assistant, and it introduces the concept of professionalism. Chapter 2, *Working in the Health Care System*, provides an overview of the health care system. Settings where health care is delivered, methods of paying for health care, and legislation and organizations that serve to protect both the recipients and providers of health care are described. Chapter 3, *Understanding Legal and Ethical Aspects of Health Care*, seeks to give students a basic understanding of legal and ethical issues that can arise in health care, and it explains how to protect themselves from legal or ethical difficulties on the job. Chapter 4, *Understanding the People in Our Care,* reviews qualities and experiences that all human beings have in common. Chapter 5, *Communicating with People*, teaches students the skills they need in order to communicate effectively with those in their care, as well as with their co-workers.

Unit 2: Promoting Safety

This unit focuses on topics, skills and principles that are essential for ensuring the safety of everyone who lives or works in a health care setting. Chapter 6, *Controlling the Spread of Infection*, gives students a basic understanding of how infections can spread throughout a health care facility and the methods that are used to protect recipients of health care and health care workers from health care–associated infections. Chapter 7, *Preventing Injuries*, provides information about maintaining a safe workplace and living environment. Principles of body mechanics and safe lifting are reviewed, along with "no-lift" policies, which seek to limit on-the-job injuries. Factors that put recipients of health care at risk for injury, along with common injuries and their prevention, are reviewed, including expanded coverage of fall-prevention strategies. Chapter 7 also reviews the safe use of equipment, including issues related to the use of side rails and restraints. Chapter 8, *Responding to Emergencies*, gives students a brief overview of common medical emergencies, describes how to prevent and respond to fire emergencies and reviews basic principles of care in the event of common weather emergencies or disasters.

Unit 3: Providing Care

Unit 3 teaches the concepts and skills used to provide routine care to patients, residents and clients. The unit begins with Chapter 9, *Measuring Vital Signs, Weight and Height*. In this chapter, students learn the skills they need to obtain basic measurements accurately. Chapter 10, *Maintaining a Comfortable Environment*, teaches bedmaking skills and reviews environmental factors that can affect a person's comfort while in a health care facility. Chapter 11, *Providing Restorative Care,* introduces students to the important role nurse assistants play in helping those in their care maintain or regain function, and it reviews skills related to exercise and preventing complications of immobility. Chapter 12, *Assisting with Positioning and Transferring*, describes pressure ulcer prevention strategies and reviews the skills needed to safely assist with repositioning and transferring. Chapter 13, *Assisting with Personal Cleanliness and Grooming*, teaches personal care skills. Chapter 14, *Assisting with Meals and Fluids*, describes the concepts and skills needed to ensure adequate nutrition and hydration. Chapter 15, *Assisting with Elimination*, describes the skills needed to assist people with elimination and describes common problems with elimination. Chapter 16, *Promoting Comfort and Rest*, is new to this edition and discusses the nurse assistant's role in recognizing, reporting and managing pain and in promoting adequate rest and sleep. The unit concludes with Chapter 17, *Assisting with Admissions, Transfers and Discharges*, which describes the nurse assistant's responsibilities, including providing emotional support, during these times of transition.

Unit 4: Special Care Situations

This unit delves deeper into specific caregiving situations. The unit begins with Chapter 18, *Providing Care for People with Specific Illnesses*, which provides an overview of commonly encountered medical conditions and special considerations for the nurse assistant in caring for people with these conditions. Chapter 19, *Providing Care for People with Cognitive Changes and Dementia,* begins by reviewing common causes of cognitive changes, including normal age-related changes in cognition, as well as delirium and dementia. The rest of the chapter is devoted to helping students understand how a person with dementia experiences the world, and provides strategies for effectively communicating with and providing care for the person with dementia. Chapter 20, *Providing Care for People at the End of Life*, seeks to help students understand the very important role nurse assistants have in caring for people and their family members in the time leading up to and following a person's death.

Chapter 21, *Providing Care to Infants and Children*, provides a basic overview of care considerations for the pediatric population. Chapter 22, *Providing Care for People in Their Homes*, introduces the student to the unique aspects of working as a home health aide and providing care in the home.

Unit 5: Transitioning from Student to Employee

The final unit in the textbook gives students the skills they need to succeed in the workplace. Chapter 23, *Entering the Workforce*, provides basic information about identifying appropriate job opportunities, preparing a resume and reference list, writing cover letters and thank-you notes, and interviewing successfully. Chapter 24, *Enjoying Professional Success*, helps students acquire the skills and knowledge they need to stay healthy and happy on the job. Time-management strategies, interpersonal skills, self-care skills and opportunities for career advancement are reviewed.

Appendices and Glossary

The textbook concludes with five appendices and a glossary. Appendix A, *Medical Terminology and Abbreviations*, gives students tools they need to discern the meaning of unfamiliar medical words. A listing of commonly used abbreviations and acronyms in health care is also provided. Appendix B, *Body Basics*, reviews the structure and function of the ten organ systems and describes normal age-related changes for each. Appendix C, *Math and Measurements Review*, helps students refresh their skills related to mathematical calculations and units of measure. Appendix D, *Additional Skills*, provides skill sheets for skills related to measuring temperature with a glass thermometer and the one-step method of measuring blood pressure. Appendix E, *Answers to Questions for Review*, provides the answers to the multiple-choice questions in the text for student self-assessment. Finally, the glossary provides an alphabetized list of all of the key terms in the book and their definitions, for quick reference and review.

Instructor Support Materials

In addition to this textbook, several items have been developed to assist instructors in teaching the course and students in learning the content.

American Red Cross Nurse Assistant Training Videos. These brand-new training videos, developed in conjunction with the textbook, include step-by-step demonstrations of key nurse assistant skills. In addition to step-by-step demonstrations of skills, testimonial-based videos focusing on topics such as end-of-life care, dementia care and restorative care have been added to the series. The five principles of care—safety, privacy, dignity, independence and communication—are emphasized throughout.

American Red Cross Nurse Assistant Training Instructor's Manual. The Instructor's Manual provides lesson plans, classroom activities, tips for individualizing teaching methods to meet individual students' needs, and tools and forms for course management and administration.

Instructor's Corner. This website provides course updates, digital materials, teaching tools, course record forms and more.

DETAILED TABLE OF CONTENTS

UNIT 4: SPECIAL CARE SITUATIONS

UNIT 5: TRANSITIONING FROM STUDENT TO EMPLOYEE

APPENDICES

SKILLS

Skills are numbered according to chapter number and sequence within the chapter.

HOW TO USE THIS BOOK

The American Red Cross Nurse Assistant Training textbook is designed with you, the student, in mind. Let's look at some of the features that have been included to help you learn and retain key information and skills.

GOALS

The goals listed at the beginning of each chapter provide a road map for the chapter; they tell you which ideas are most important to learn. Before you begin reading, review the list of goals. This will give you an overview of the concepts and skills that will be covered in the chapter. After you finish reading the chapter, review the goals again. Can you meet each goal? If not, review the sections of the chapter where that information is covered.

Goals

After reading this chapter, you will have the information needed to:

- Plan a job search.
- Prepare a résumé, reference list and cover letter.
- Describe the job application process.
- Interview effectively.
- Accept or decline a job offer.
- Know what to expect during your first few days on the job.

KEY TERMS

At the beginning of each chapter, you will also find a list of key terms, or vocabulary words. These words are **boldfaced** and defined in the chapter. You can also look up the definitions of these words in the glossary that appears at the end of the textbook. Familiarize yourself with these words before you begin reading the chapter. When you are finished reading the chapter, review the list of key terms again. Can you define each one?

Key Terms:

laws
ethics
informed consent
advance directive
durable power of attorney for health care
living will
abuse
assault
battery
negligence
fraud
larceny
ethical dilemma
ethics committee

CASE STUDY

At the beginning of each chapter, you will be introduced to a person who is receiving care in a health care setting, and you will be given a little bit of information about the person and his or her situation. Throughout the chapter, you will be prompted to pause and think about how the concepts and skills you are learning would apply to the person you met. Take these opportunities to reflect on what you are learning, and think about how this knowledge could apply to situations you will encounter on the job.

In about half an hour, Mary finds you and says, "Mrs. Whitchurch's primary care provider has requested that we obtain a 'clean catch' urine sample because she suspects a urinary tract infection. Can you make sure to obtain this sample the next time Mrs. Whitchurch uses the commode? I explained to Mrs. Whitchurch that she will need to start the flow of urine, then stop it, and then collect the urine sample from the restarted flow, but she might forget, so be sure to remind her."

How will you use your communication skills to reinforce the information Mary has given Mrs. Whitchurch?

NURSE ASSISTANT DO'S AND DON'TS

Throughout the text, you will see boxes that summarize guidelines for key nurse assistant responsibilities. Learning and following these guidelines will help you provide safe, efficient, person-centered care.

Box 1-2 Nurse Assistant DO's and DON'Ts

Maintaining a Professional Appearance

DO wear a clean, pressed uniform; clean shoes; and your name badge in accordance with your employer's policies.

DO bathe or shower, shampoo your hair and brush your teeth regularly.

DO keep your nails short, filed smooth, free of polish, and clean. This helps to prevent accidental scratches when you are providing care, and is also important for infection control.

DO keep your hair neatly styled and pulled back from your face. If not secured, long hair can get tangled in equipment, or a confused person or a young child may pull it. Keeping hair off your face is also important for infection control; you do not want to be reaching up to move your hair out of the way with dirty hands or gloves.

DON'T wear dangly or excessive jewelry. A confused person or a child may pull necklaces, bracelets or dangly earrings. Wearing rings and bracelets makes it difficult to wash your hands properly. Although some employers permit employees to wear a plain wedding band, it is safest to avoid wearing rings while you are at work.

DON'T wear excessive make-up.

DON'T wear fragrance (for example, perfume or cologne).

DO keep facial hair trimmed and neat.

DO try to select a uniform style that will cover tattoos.

DO remove visible body piercings.

DON'T wear undergarments that show through your clothing (for example, avoid wearing dark-colored undergarments under a light-colored uniform).

OBSERVATIONS INTO ACTION

As a nurse assistant, you will get to know the people in your care well. Knowing what is "normal" for each of them gives you the ability to recognize changes in their condition. These boxes summarize changes in a person's condition that are important to report to the nurse.

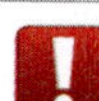

Observations Into Action!

When caring for a person who is receiving IV therapy, be sure to report any of the following observations to the nurse right away:

- **Disconnected IV line**
- **Empty fluid bag**
- **Pain, swelling or redness at the IV site**

ELDER CARE NOTES

Many of the people you will care for will be elderly. Elder Care Notes placed throughout the text raise your awareness of special considerations you must take into account when caring for people who are older.

ELDER CARE NOTE. It is important to remember that *all* people, young and old alike, have the need to think of themselves as sexual beings and engage in intimate relationships (which may or may not involve sexual activity).

SKILL SHEETS

At the end of each chapter that contains skills, you will find illustrated skill sheets. These skill sheets guide you step by step through the skills you must learn to be a nurse assistant. The skill sheets are divided into three parts. The first part, the **preparation** section, lists the steps you should follow before beginning any skill. Similarly, the last part, the **completion** section, lists the steps you should perform after finishing any skill. These preparation and completion steps emphasize the five principles of care—safety, privacy, dignity, independence and communication—and help to promote safe, efficient, person-centered care. In between, in the **procedure** section, you will find the steps you take that are specific to the particular skill.

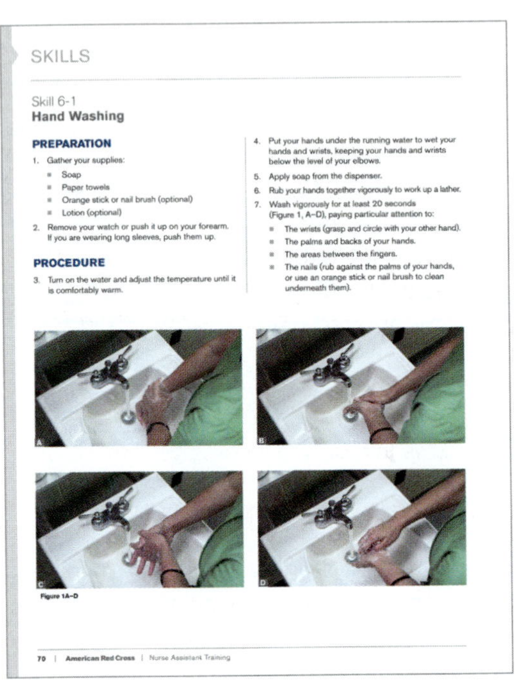

SKILLS

Skill 6-1
Hand Washing

PREPARATION

1. Gather your supplies:
   - Soap
   - Paper towels
   - Orange stick or nail brush (optional)
   - Lotion (optional)
2. Remove your watch or push it up on your forearm. If you are wearing long sleeves, push them up.

PROCEDURE

3. Turn on the water and adjust the temperature until it is comfortably warm.
4. Put your hands under the running water to wet your hands and wrists, keeping your hands and wrists below the level of your elbows.
5. Apply soap from the dispenser.
6. Rub your hands together vigorously to work up a lather.
7. Wash vigorously for at least 20 seconds (Figure 1, A–D), paying particular attention to:
   - The wrists (grasp and circle with your other hand).
   - The palms and backs of your hands.
   - The areas between the fingers.
   - The nails (rub against the palms of your hands, or use an orange stick or nail brush to clean underneath them).

Figure 1A–D

70 | American Red Cross | Nurse Assistant Training

CHECK YOUR UNDERSTANDING

The Check Your Understanding section at the end of each chapter gives you an opportunity to see how well you learned and understood the chapter content. **Questions for Review** are multiple-choice questions. Each has one best answer. Try answering these questions and then check the answers in Appendix E at the end of the book. If you answered any of the questions incorrectly, go back and review the appropriate sections of the chapter. The **Questions to Ask Yourself** section poses real-life situations that encourage you to apply your knowledge and decision-making skills. These questions may have several correct answers. Think about the situations posed in the questions and how you would respond. Because there may be many different ways to approach the situation, try discussing your answers with your instructor, your classmates or both.

CHECK YOUR UNDERSTANDING

Questions for Review

1. **Temperature, pulse, respirations and blood pressure usually are taken together and are referred to as:**
   a. Life measurements.
   b. Vital signs.
   c. Routine measurements.
   d. Monitoring.
2. **Mrs. Tyler has just been admitted to the nursing home. What measurements will you obtain?**
   a. Blood pressure, temperature, respiratory rate, pulse rate
   b. Height
   c. Weight
   d. All of the above
3. **What instrument is used to listen to sounds when obtaining a blood pressure or an apical pulse measurement?**
   a. Stethoscope
   b. Diaphragm
   c. Sphygmomanometer
   d. Thermometer
4. **Mr. Rollins is receiving oxygen therapy. You could use any of the following methods to take his temperature EXCEPT the:**
   a. Oral method
   b. Axillary method
   c. Rectal method
   d. Tympanic method
5. **Which of the following measurements is outside of the normal range for an adult?**
   a. Temperature, 99° F
   b. Respirations, 13 breaths/min
   c. Pulse, 63 beats/min
   d. Blood pressure, 107/70 mm Hg
6. **Where is the brachial pulse located?**
   a. The inside of the elbow
   b. At the top of the heart, just under the left nipple
   c. On the inside of the wrist at the base of the thumb
   d. On the inside of the groin where the thigh meets the hip
7. **What equipment is needed to evaluate a radial pulse?**
   a. Sphygmomanometer
   b. Stethoscope
   c. Watch with a second hand
   d. All of the above
8. **Mrs. Wilson's pulse is very weak. How would you describe her pulse?**
   a. Shallow
   b. Thready
   c. Bounding
   d. Irregular
9. **Which of the following factors can affect a person's vital sign measurements?**
   a. Illness
   b. Emotions
   c. The time of day
   d. All of the above
10. **The nurse has asked you to measure Mr. Simon's temperature rectally. What equipment will you use?**
    a. A tympanic thermometer
    b. An axillary thermometer
    c. An electronic thermometer with a blue probe
    d. An electronic thermometer with a red probe

Questions to Ask Yourself

1. *You are getting ready to assist Mrs. Perkins to the bathroom when she tells you that she feels very dizzy. You decide to take her vital sign measurements, which are as follows: temperature, 97° F (oral); pulse, 80 beats/min; respirations, 15 breaths/min; and blood pressure, 90/52 mm Hg. Which of these measurements is significant and why?*
2. *When you go into Mrs. Clement's room to take her oral temperature, you notice a cup of coffee on her over-bed table. What should you consider, and what should you do?*
3. *When you take Mr. Wilson's pulse at 8:00 a.m., the rate is 72 beats/min and the rhythm is regular. When you take it again at 9:00 a.m., the rate is 56 beats/min and irregular. What should you do?*
4. *Mrs. O'Neill wants to talk with you while you are trying to measure and record vital signs. How should you handle this situation? What should you say to her?*

Chapter 9 | Measuring Vital Signs, Weight and Height | 115

APPENDICES, GLOSSARY, RESOURCES AND INDEX

The appendices at the end of the book provide additional information that may be useful to you. Appendix A, *Medical Terminology*, will help you become familiar with the "language of caregiving." A listing of common abbreviations is also provided. Appendix B, *Body Basics*, gives you an overview of how the human body works, and changes that normally occur with aging. Appendix C, *Math and Measurements Review*, will help you refresh your skills related to mathematical calculations and units of measure. Appendix D, *Additional Skills*, provides skill sheets for skills that are taught in some states, but not all. Your instructor will tell you if you need to learn these skills. Appendix E, *Answers to Questions for Review*, provides the answers to the multiple-choice questions at the end of each chapter, so that you can check your understanding of what you have learned. Also at the end of the book, you will find a *Glossary*, which is an alphabetized list of the key terms in the book, with their definitions. You will also find *Resources*, which provides references for the information given in the text, and an *Index*, which you can use to find specific topics within the book quickly and easily.

UNIT 1

THE ART OF CAREGIVING

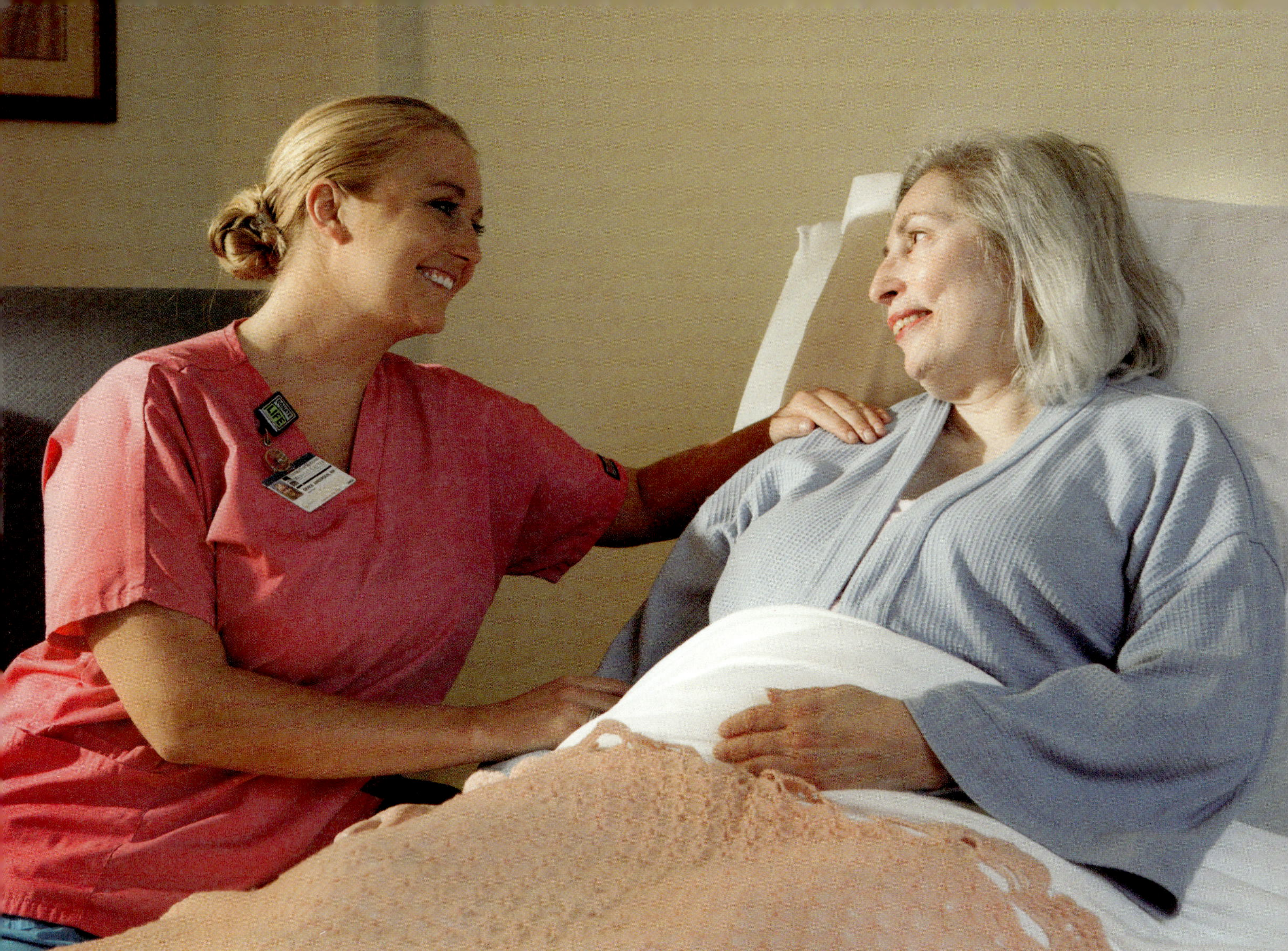

CHAPTER

1 Being a Nurse Assistant

Goals

After reading this chapter, you will have the information needed to:

- Describe the nurse assistant's responsibilities and the requirements that a person must meet in order to work as a nurse assistant.
- Describe how the nurse assistant functions as a member of the health care team and of the nursing team.
- Describe tasks that are usually outside of the nurse assistant's scope of practice.
- Explain how focusing on the person who is receiving care can lead to better care.
- List the five principles of care, and explain why each is important.
- Explain what it means to be a professional, and describe how a nurse assistant can display professionalism on the job.

Key Terms:

activities of daily living (ADLs)

health care team

nursing team

delegation

scope of practice

empathy

compassion

Angus McCarthy is a 78-year-old man who was admitted to Morningside Nursing Home yesterday after being discharged from the hospital with chronic heart failure. When you enter the room today to provide care, Mr. McCarthy's 75-year-old wife, Martha, is sitting with him. You introduce yourself and explain that you are there to help Mr. McCarthy with bathing and dressing. After talking with Mr. McCarthy and his wife for several minutes, you ask him about getting washed and dressed. He says, "Let me finish watching my favorite game show first, and then we can take care of business." You agree and ask if you can sit with him while he watches his show. He says, "Have a seat and I'll tell you why I like this show so much."

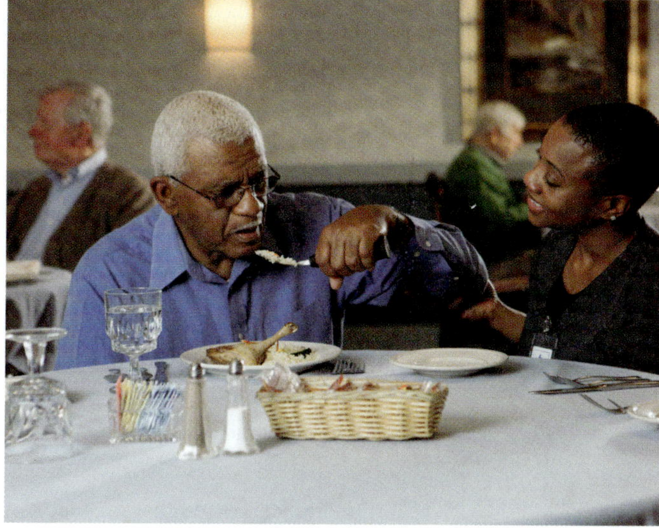

Figure 1-1 Many of the nurse assistant's responsibilities involve helping people with activities of daily living (ADLs).

NURSE ASSISTANT RESPONSIBILITIES AND TRAINING

The Nurse Assistant's Responsibilities

A nurse assistant works under the supervision of a licensed nurse (that is, a registered nurse [RN] or licensed practical nurse [LPN]) to provide basic nursing care to people who are ill, injured or disabled. Nursing care seeks to care for the whole person, meeting the person's physical *and* emotional needs.

As a nurse assistant, many of your responsibilities will have to do with helping the people in your care with **activities of daily living (ADLs)**, such as eating, bathing, dressing, grooming, using the toilet and moving (Figure 1-1). Nurse assistants are also responsible for obtaining routine measurements (such as vital signs, height and weight); assisting with admissions, transfers and discharges; and maintaining a safe and clean environment.

In addition to helping to meet the physical needs of the people in your care, you will help to meet their emotional needs. People who find themselves in need of health care, and their family members, are often frightened, worried and upset. They may feel lonely and isolated.

As a nurse assistant, you will have a great deal of daily contact with the people in your care and their family members. Getting to know the people in your care as individuals and taking a genuine interest in them are things you can do to support them emotionally. A smile, a pat on the shoulder, and a willingness to listen lets the person know that you care, and that she is not alone (Figure 1-2).

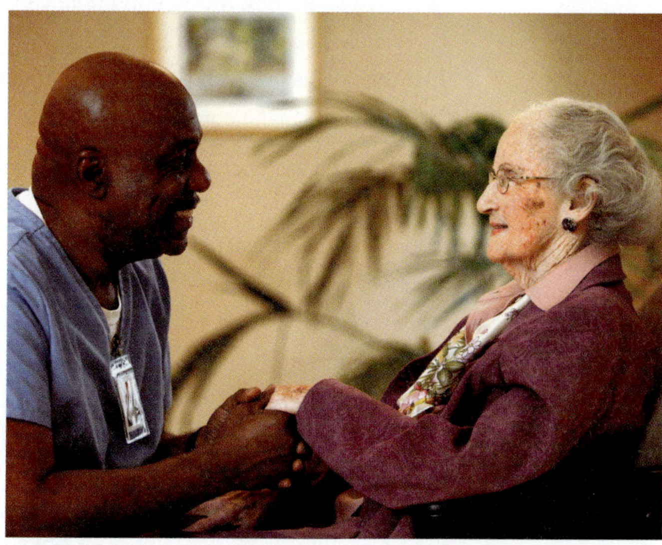

Figure 1-2 Providing emotional support is an important part of the nurse assistant's job too.

Because of the amount of time you will spend with the people in your care, you may be the first to recognize a change in the person's condition, or learn of a concern the person has. For example, you may notice that a person's appetite has decreased, or a person may mention to you that she is worried about a surgical procedure she is scheduled to have the next day.

When you share this type of information with the nurse, you promote quality care by helping to ensure that steps are taken to determine the cause of the change or to address the person's concerns.

A sample job description for a nurse assistant is shown in Figure 1-3.

Morningside Nursing Home
JOB DESCRIPTION
Certified Nurse Assistant (CNA)

Duties	1. Reports to work as scheduled and on time. 2. Attends shift report, organizes assignments and makes rounds on residents. 3. Delivers personal care and emotional support to those under his or her care. 4. Regards all residents as under his or her care when assistance or supervision is needed; answers all requests for help promptly within 5 minutes. 5. Provides care according to the resident's care plan in a manner that protects the resident's dignity and privacy. 6. Assists residents to maintain or regain their maximum level of independence. 7. Works to build relationships with residents and their family members that are warm, positive and supportive. 8. Reports to supervisor/charge nurse any observations or concerns about the resident's status in a timely fashion. 9. Documents the care provided and observations promptly and accurately. 10. Practices infection-control measures, including taking standard precautions, in accordance with facility policy and the resident's care plan. 11. Keeps work area and residents' environment neat, clean and orderly. 12. Measures and accurately reports and records vital signs, height and weight. 13. Monitors and records intake and output; assists in serving meals, meal supplements and fluids; assists residents with eating as necessary. 14. Assists residents with repositioning, transferring and exercise. 15. Assists residents with toileting, bathing and grooming. 16. Assists with admissions, transfers and discharges as necessary. 17. Takes initiative in delivery of services—sees what needs to be done and does it, within scope of practice. 18. Participates in providing end-of-life care to residents who are dying, and their family members. 19. Knows fire and disaster plans and personal duties in case of fire or disaster. 20. Participates in resident-care conferences. 21. Attends all mandatory in-service training sessions.
Job Requirements	* Must have a valid nurse assistant certification in good standing with the state * Must have current CPR certification * Must pass a criminal background check * Must complete a health screening and tuberculosis screening within 2 weeks of hire * Must pass a mandatory drug screening test within 90 days of hire * Must be able to lift, push and pull up to 30 pounds * Must possess basic computer skills * Must possess good communication skills and the ability to interact in a tactful and respectful manner with residents, family members and visitors * Must be able to multitask in a fast-paced work environment and prioritize duties * Must have the ability to understand and follow policies and procedures

Figure 1-3 A sample job description for a nurse assistant.

Requirements to Become a Nurse Assistant

A person who wants to become a nurse assistant must complete a state-approved training course and pass the state's certification examination. The federal government specifies that a minimum of 75 hours of training is required, and that the training must include:

- Classroom learning.
- Hands-on practice of skills in a skills lab.
- A clinical practicum (that is, the opportunity to gain supervised experience providing direct care in an actual health care setting).

Many states require more hours of training than the federally mandated 75 hours.

In addition to completing the training course, a person who wants to work as a nurse assistant must pass the state's certification evaluation. This evaluation consists of two parts: a multiple-choice written exam, and a skills test. During the skills test, the candidate is required to demonstrate randomly selected nurse assistant skills and must perform each skill satisfactorily in order to pass.

After completing the training course and passing the state's certification evaluation, a person becomes certified to work as a nurse assistant in that state. Depending on the state and the employer, a person who is certified to work as a nurse assistant may be called by many different titles, including *certified nurse assistant* or *certified nursing assistant (CNA)*, *nurse aide* or *geriatric nursing assistant (GNA)*.

WORKING AS A MEMBER OF THE HEALTH CARE TEAM

The Health Care Team

As a nurse assistant, you will be a key member of the **health care team**. The health care team consists of the person receiving care, the person's family members, and staff members and other professionals who are responsible for providing care and other services (Figure 1-4). Each member of the health care team has specialized knowledge and skills and contributes equally to achieving the health care team's goal, which is to provide personalized quality care that meets the

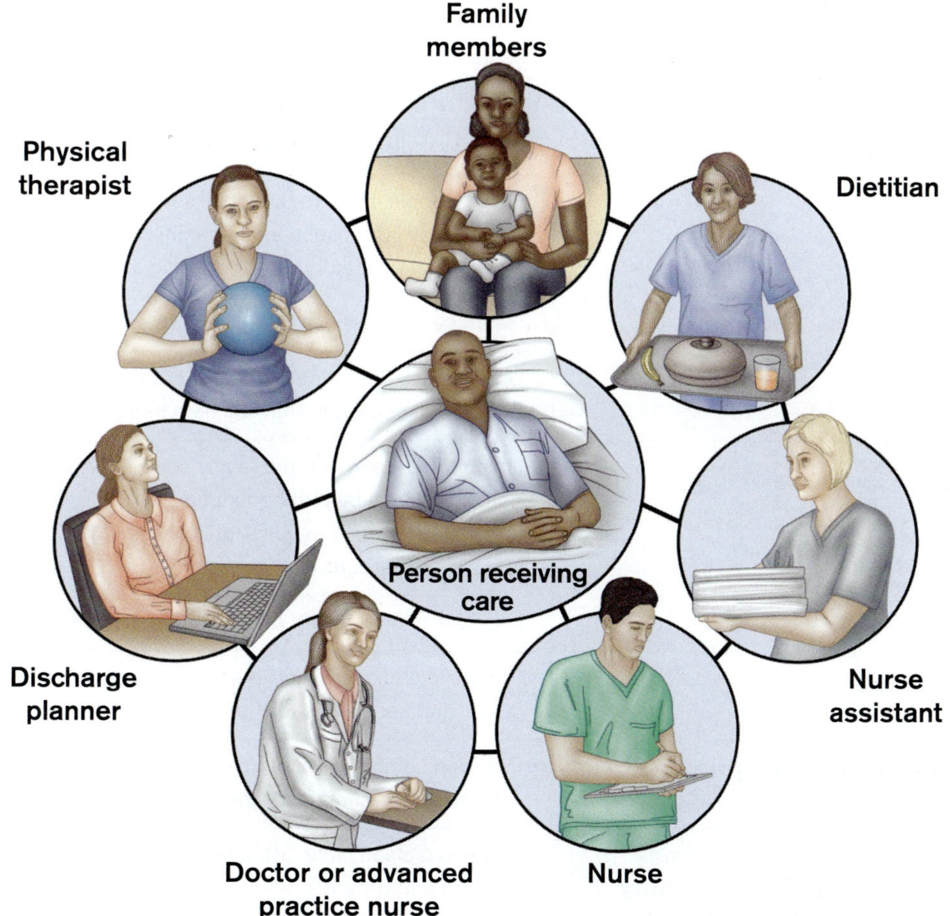

Figure 1-4 The person receiving care is always the leader of the health care team. Other team members vary depending on the individual person's needs.

person's physical, emotional, social and spiritual needs. The person receiving care is always the "captain" of the team. The other members of the health care team vary depending on the needs of the person who is receiving care. Examples of staff members who may be part of the health care team are given in Table 1-1.

Table 1-1 **Examples of Health Care Team Members***

Health Care Team Member	Responsibilities
Registered Nurse (RN)	Performs assessments, develops care plans, provides nursing care (directly and by delegating certain tasks to other nursing team members) and supervises other members of the nursing team
Licensed Practical Nurse (LPN) or Licensed Vocational Nurse (LVN)	Helps plan, deliver and supervise some types of nursing care under the direction of a registered nurse
Certified Nurse Assistant (CNA) or Home Health Aide (HHA)	Provides basic nursing care under the supervision of a RN or LPN/LVN
Doctor	Determines the person's illness or condition and supervises medical care; writes medical orders and prescribes medication and other treatments
Advanced Practice Nurse (Nurse Practitioner, Clinical Nurse Specialist)	Practices independently or along with the doctor to diagnose, treat and manage medical conditions; is qualified to do so by completing graduate-level education and training
Discharge Planner (Continuing Care Nurse, Case Manager or Utilization Manager)	Works with other members of the health care team to develop a plan for meeting the person's care needs after the person leaves the health care setting, and assists with making the necessary arrangements
Activities Director or Recreational Therapist	Plans and coordinates activities that provide opportunities for socializing, spiritual support, creativity, entertainment, exercise and community and civic involvement (for example, voting)
Physical Therapist	Helps people improve their ability to move their bodies
Occupational Therapist	Helps people improve their independence in performing actions related to everyday living, such as managing a home (for example, preparing a meal or doing laundry) or functioning in a job
Speech Therapist	Helps people improve their ability to speak, chew and swallow
Dietitian	Uses knowledge of nutrition and of the person to plan a diet that the person will enjoy and that will help him maintain or regain health
Social Worker	Helps the person and the family solve everyday problems related to the person's illness by putting him and his family in touch with resources that can help, such as meal-delivery services, adult day care services, and support groups
Psychologist	Provides mental health assessment services
Pharmacist	Provides medications ordered by the doctor or advanced practice nurse, and keeps a record of all medications
Religious Leader (for example, priest, minister, rabbi)	Provides spiritual support, as needed and requested, for the person receiving care, the family and staff members
Environmental Services Employee (may work in laundry, housekeeping or facility maintenance departments)	Ensures a clean, safe, attractive environment by maintaining the building and grounds, and by maintaining the equipment used in the facility (such as linens or wheelchairs)

* This list of team members represents only some of the many people who could be members of the health care team. The specific members of the health care team will vary depending on the person's needs.

The Nursing Team

The **nursing team** is a subset of the health care team (Table 1-2). The nursing team consists of, at minimum, a licensed nurse and a nurse assistant. Licensed nurses may be registered nurses (RNs) or licensed practical/vocational nurses (LPN/LVNs). An advanced practice nurse (APRN), who may also be called a nurse practitioner (NP) or clinical nurse specialist (CNS), may also be part of the nursing team.

Usually, nurse assistants are supervised by an RN or LPN/LVN. The nurse who supervises you may be called the *charge nurse*, *head nurse*, *primary nurse*, *supervisor* or *team leader*. The nurse will give you the authority and responsibility for completing certain tasks on his or her behalf. This is called **delegation**. After completing a task that has been delegated to you, it is important to report back to update the nurse on the person's condition, and to let the nurse know that you have completed the task.

To protect yourself, the person receiving care, and your employer, you must always work within your **scope of practice** (that is, the tasks that you are legally permitted to do). Your scope of practice is defined by the state and by your employer. Be very familiar with the tasks that you are allowed to do, as detailed in the job description given to you by your employer. Job descriptions vary from employer to employer, so you must always read each new job description carefully to make sure you know your responsibilities. Perform only the tasks listed in your job description. If the nurse delegates a task to you that is outside of your scope of practice, or that you do not feel qualified to perform safely, you must speak up and ask the nurse to reassign the task. Tasks that are usually outside of the scope of practice for a nurse assistant are described in Box 1-1.

THE ART OF CAREGIVING

Many people learn the skills of caregiving, but not everyone can perform those skills with kindness, empathy and compassion. **Empathy** is the quality of seeking to understand another person's situation, point of view or feelings. **Compassion** is the quality of recognizing another person's hardship, accompanied by a desire to help relieve that hardship. Providing skillful care in a thoughtful way is an art. As you prepare for your job, you will learn the difference between just getting your job done and providing quality care that goes above and beyond

Table 1-2 Nursing Team Members

Title	Requirements to Practice	Responsibilities
Certified Nurse Assistant (CNA) or Home Health Aide (HHA)	Certificate obtained by completing a minimum of 75 hours of training and passing a state-administered certification examination	Assists with the delivery of nursing care by performing basic nursing tasks under the supervision of a registered nurse (RN) or licensed practical/vocational nurse (LPN/LVN)
Licensed Practical/Vocational Nurse (LPN/LVN)	Certificate obtained by completing a 12- to 18-month training program AND a license obtained by passing a state-administered board examination	Helps plan and deliver certain types of nursing care under the direction of a registered nurse (RN); may also be responsible for supervising nurse assistants
Registered Nurse (RN)	Bachelor of science in nursing (BSN) degree obtained from a 4-year college OR an associate degree (ADN) obtained from a 2-year college AND a license obtained by passing a state-administered board examination	Performs assessments, develops care plans, provides nursing care (directly and by delegating certain tasks to other nursing team members) and supervises other members of the nursing team
Advanced Practice Nurse (APRN) **Clinical Nurse Specialist (CNS)** **Nurse Practitioner (NP)**	Bachelor of science in nursing (BSN) degree AND a doctorate or master's degree obtained from an accredited college or university AND a license obtained by passing a national specialty-based board examination	Independently or in conjunction with a doctor, performs medical assessments, diagnoses disease and prescribes treatments

Box 1-1 Tasks That Are Usually Outside of the Nurse Assistant's Scope of Practice*

- **Supervising or delegating nursing responsibilities to other nurse assistants.** Only a licensed nurse (an RN or an LPN) can supervise nurse assistants and delegate nursing responsibilities to them.
- **Analyzing or interpreting data.** A nurse assistant may gather data, but it is outside of the nurse assistant's scope of practice to determine the meaning of the data. For example, a nurse assistant may obtain a blood pressure measurement and note that it is higher than normal. However, determining *why* the blood pressure reading is higher than normal is the responsibility of the doctor and nurse.
- **Receiving verbal orders for the person's medical care.** The person's primary care provider (a doctor or an advanced practice nurse) may give verbal orders for the person's care over the telephone or in person. Only licensed nurses can receive these verbal orders and act on them.
- **Diagnosing illness and injury and prescribing treatments.** Only doctors and advanced practice nurses (nurses who have obtained additional training at the post-graduate level) can diagnose and order treatments (such as medications) for illnesses and injuries.
- **Administering medications and oxygen.** Medications must be administered by a licensed nurse or a doctor. In some settings, such as assisted living facilities, nurse assistants may be permitted to help the person as he takes his own medication (but they cannot actually give the medication to the person). Nurse assistants who have received advanced training in medication administration may be allowed to administer some types of medications in some states in certain settings, but this is not normally within the scope of practice for a nurse assistant.
- **Inserting or removing medical equipment.** Nurse assistants are usually not allowed to insert medical equipment (such as feeding tubes, urinary catheters or IV lines) into a person's body, or to remove these items from the person's body once they are in place.

* The nurse assistant's scope of practice may be expanded in some settings and when the nurse assistant has received additional training to perform more advanced skills.

basic expectations. Getting to know each person as an individual and seeking to meet her emotional, social and spiritual needs, in addition to her physical needs, is the key to providing the highest quality care possible (Figure 1-5).

Throughout this book, you will see references to "the five principles of care" (Figure 1-6). These principles provide a framework for providing quality care by helping you to remember to put the person in your care first. The five principles of care are:

- **Keep the person safe.** As a nurse assistant, you are responsible for protecting the people in your care from harm. You will do this by taking steps to prevent the person from physical injuries (such as skin tears, bruises or burns) and from situations that can put the person at risk for

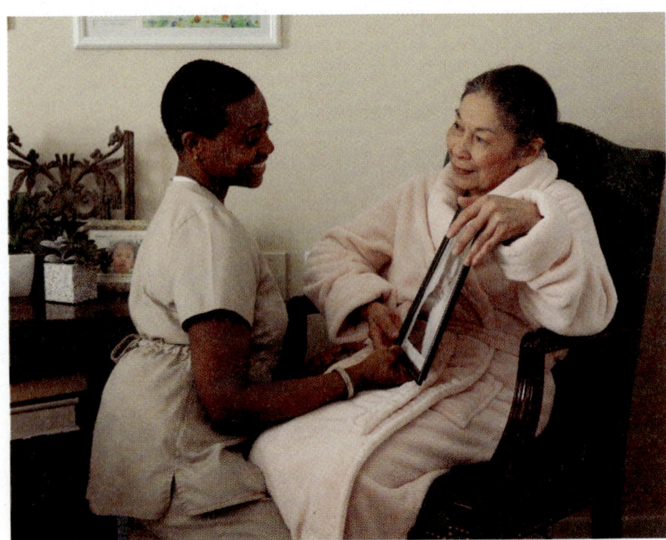

Figure 1-5 Getting to know and appreciate each person in your care as an individual is one of the keys to providing quality care.

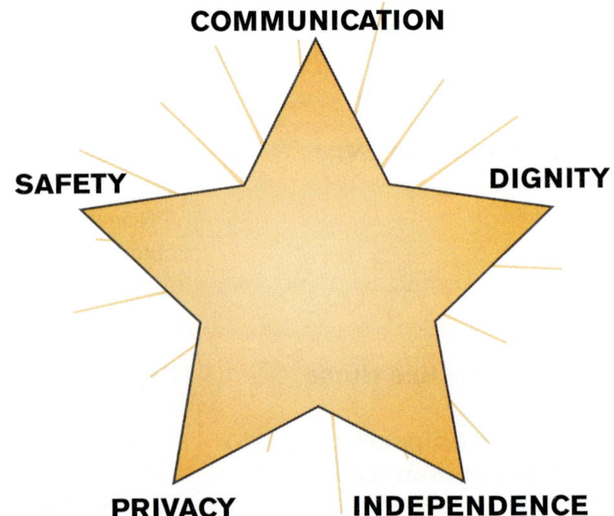

Figure 1-6 Applying the five principles of care can help you to provide "star-quality" care.

injury (such as wandering away from the facility). You will also help to keep the people in your care safe by practicing infection-control methods, such as washing your hands, consistently and correctly.

- **Protect the person's dignity.** Dignity is the quality of being worthy of respect. In addition to treating the people in your care with respect, you will help them to maintain their sense of dignity by fostering their sense of self-esteem, or self-respect. Actions you can take to help protect the person's dignity include taking care not to expose the person's body unnecessarily, avoiding talking down to the person or using baby talk, involving the person in decision making about her care, encouraging the person to do as much for herself as possible, and helping the person to have a clean and neat appearance.
- **Foster the person's independence.** Being able to make decisions and do things for oneself is important for maintaining a sense of dignity and self-esteem. In addition, it is important to encourage the people in your care to do as much for themselves as possible to maintain the abilities that they have, and to prevent future loss of function.
- **Protect the person's privacy.** Keep a person's private business private, and do not allow private things to be seen or overheard by other people.
- **Practice good communication skills.** Be available to talk, listen and respond to a person's thoughts and feelings. Tell the person about the care you plan to provide, and involve the person in making decisions about her care.

After the game show is over, Mr. McCarthy smiles and says to you, "OK, I promised I would let you do your job after my program was over, so let's get to it. Can you just give me a hand getting to the bathroom?" As you help Mr. McCarthy walk to the bathroom, you notice that he begins to tire quickly and appears to get short of breath. He says, "I never realized how much work it is sometimes just to walk." You get to the bathroom and say, "Why don't you just sit down here on the commode and rest a bit while I get your supplies together?"

How can actions like watching the game show with Mr. McCarthy and listening to him when he explains why he likes it so much help you provide better care?

While you are assisting Mr. McCarthy with bathing and dressing, what actions can you take to protect his dignity and promote his independence? How will you help to keep him safe?

After you are finished caring for Mr. McCarthy, is there any information you would share with the nurse? If so, what and why?

PROFESSIONALISM

As a nurse assistant, you will be a professional caregiver. You will have the training and knowledge to perform a certain role, that of the nurse assistant. But being a professional is about more than having certain training, credentials or qualifications. It is about having a positive attitude toward your job, and doing your job to the best of your ability at all times. Help others see you as the professional that you are through your actions and appearance.

Acting in a Professional Manner

Let's look at some of the actions that will help you excel as a nurse assistant:

- **Dependability.** Being dependable means that others can count on you. For the people in your care, this means they can trust you to come to work on time and to help them in a timely fashion. For your co-workers, this means that if they ask you to do something, they can trust you to follow through on the request.
- **Accountability.** Being accountable means taking responsibility for your actions and the results of those actions. Sometimes, you may make a mistake while delivering care. An accountable person takes responsibility for the mistake, and looks to prevent similar mistakes from occurring in the future.
- **Integrity.** Having integrity means that you behave according to an understanding of the right way to behave. One way to think about integrity is that it means doing the right thing even when no one is watching. Acting in an honest manner is one way that you show integrity. Keeping private information about the people in your care to yourself is another.
- **Conscientiousness.** Being conscientious means paying attention to the details of your work. The people in your care, and your co-workers, count on you to do your job the right way and to the best of your ability, every day.
- **Courtesy.** A person who behaves professionally is courteous to everyone. Simple courtesies can make the workplace a more pleasant environment, and increase the likelihood that others will also treat you courteously. Remember to say *please* and *thank you.* Address others as they prefer to be addressed. If you do not know how a person prefers to be addressed, err on the side of formality (for example, "Mr. Johnson" instead of "Bill"). Offer to hold the door or elevator for others, and clean up after yourself in shared areas (such as the kitchenette or the nurses' station).
- **Stewardship.** A *steward* safeguards something from harm. As a nurse assistant, you will be entrusted with the care of items belonging to others. You have an obligation to treat these items with the

same care and respect you would treat your own valued possessions. Stewardship also means using your employer's resources wisely and avoiding waste (for example, by only taking the supplies you will use for a procedure into a person's room).

- **A willingness to help.** A willingness to pitch in and work as part of a team makes many tasks much easier and safer, and contributes to a healthy work environment by helping to reduce stress.
- **The ability to communicate.** Being able to communicate effectively with the people in your care, their family members and your co-workers is a critical skill in health care. An effective communicator is a good listener, is able to express her own needs clearly and is able to advocate (speak up for) others when necessary.
- **The ability to problem solve.** This book provides guidelines to help you make the best decisions to provide the best care to each person. Each person receiving care is different, as is each situation. Using critical thinking skills allows you to look at a problem, identify possible solutions, name the pros and cons of each solution, decide which solution is best and then act on it.

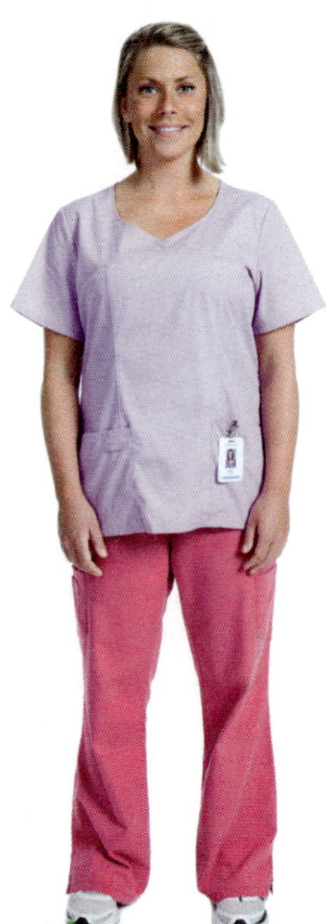

Figure 1-7 Help others see you as the professional that you are by maintaining a professional appearance.

Maintaining a Professional Appearance

As a health care professional, you are expected to look a certain way (Figure 1-7). Many of the standards that relate to a health care worker's appearance are based on principles of safety and infection control. However, maintaining a clean, neat appearance serves another purpose as well. As a nurse assistant, you represent your employer and your facility or agency. You will spend a great deal of time interacting with the people in your care, and with their family members. When you make an effort to present a neat, clean appearance, the people in your care feel more assured that you will do the same for them. Guidelines for maintaining a professional appearance are given in Box 1-2.

Box 1-2 Nurse Assistant DO's and DON'Ts

Maintaining a Professional Appearance

DO wear a clean, pressed uniform; clean shoes; and your name badge in accordance with your employer's policies.

DO bathe or shower, shampoo your hair and brush your teeth regularly.

DO keep your nails short, filed smooth, free of polish, and clean. This helps to prevent accidental scratches when you are providing care, and is also important for infection control.

DO keep your hair neatly styled and pulled back from your face. If not secured, long hair can get tangled in equipment, or a confused person or a young child may pull it. Keeping hair off your face is also important for infection control; you do not want to be reaching up to move your hair out of the way with dirty hands or gloves.

DON'T wear dangly or excessive jewelry. A confused person or a child may pull necklaces, bracelets or dangly earrings. Wearing rings and bracelets makes it difficult to wash your hands properly. Although some employers permit employees to wear a plain wedding band, it is safest to avoid wearing rings while you are at work.

DON'T wear excessive make-up.

DON'T wear fragrance (for example, perfume or cologne).

DO keep facial hair trimmed and neat.

DO try to select a uniform style that will cover tattoos.

DO remove visible body piercings.

DON'T wear undergarments that show through your clothing (for example, avoid wearing dark-colored undergarments under a light-colored uniform).

CHECK YOUR UNDERSTANDING

Questions for Review

1. **The "captain" of the health care team is the:**
   a. Doctor.
   b. Registered nurse (RN).
   c. Advanced practice nurse.
   d. Person receiving care.

2. **Which one of the following is a nurse assistant's responsibility?**
   a. Administering medications
   b. Communicating verbal orders related to the person's medical care to the nurse
   c. Assisting people with activities of daily living (ADLs)
   d. Analyzing and interpreting data

3. **At minimum, how many hours of training are required to become a nurse assistant?**
   a. 65
   b. 75
   c. 40
   d. 50

4. **A nurse assistant finds a 10-dollar bill in the linens while changing a person's bed, and places the money on the person's bedside table. This nurse assistant acted with:**
   a. Integrity.
   b. Courtesy.
   c. Dependability.
   d. Stupidity.

5. **Empathy is the quality of:**
   a. Acting in a way to gain the trust of others.
   b. Pitching in to work as part of a team.
   c. Recognizing another person's hardship, accompanied by a desire to help relieve that hardship.
   d. Seeking to understand another person's situation, point of view or feelings.

6. **To maintain a professional appearance, you should do all of the following EXCEPT:**
   a. Avoid smiling too much while at work.
   b. Keep your hair pulled back from your face.
   c. Wear a clean, pressed uniform; clean shoes; and a name badge.
   d. Keep your nails clean, trimmed, filed smooth, and free of nail polish.

7. **The goal of the health care team is to:**
   a. Minimize health care costs by spreading the workload over many people.
   b. Make sure the person is sent home from the facility as soon as possible.
   c. Provide personalized quality care that meets the person's physical, emotional, social and spiritual needs.
   d. Make decisions on behalf of the person receiving care.

8. **Which of the following statements about delegation is true?**
   a. It is outside the nurse assistant's scope of practice to decline to do a delegated task.
   b. When one person delegates a task to another, that person gives the other person the authority and the responsibility to complete the task on his or her behalf.
   c. Nurse assistants may delegate tasks to other members of the health care team.
   d. All of the above

Questions to Ask Yourself

1. *What are some of the most important qualities a nurse assistant should have?*
2. *What special qualities would you bring to your work as a nurse assistant?*
3. *What do you think the most rewarding part of being a nurse assistant will be? The most challenging part?*
4. *Think of someone you know who is currently receiving health care, or who has received health care in the past. What does the person think of the care he or she received, or is receiving?*
5. *At Morningside Nursing Facility, Mr. Flanagan spends a lot of time holding a picture of his wife. Sometimes he talks to the picture. Every day he tells you that he wants to go home. How would you respond?*
6. *Mrs. Landers clearly loves the fresh flowers her daughter brought her and wants to keep them on her bedside table, but her roommate is allergic to flowers. What would you do?*

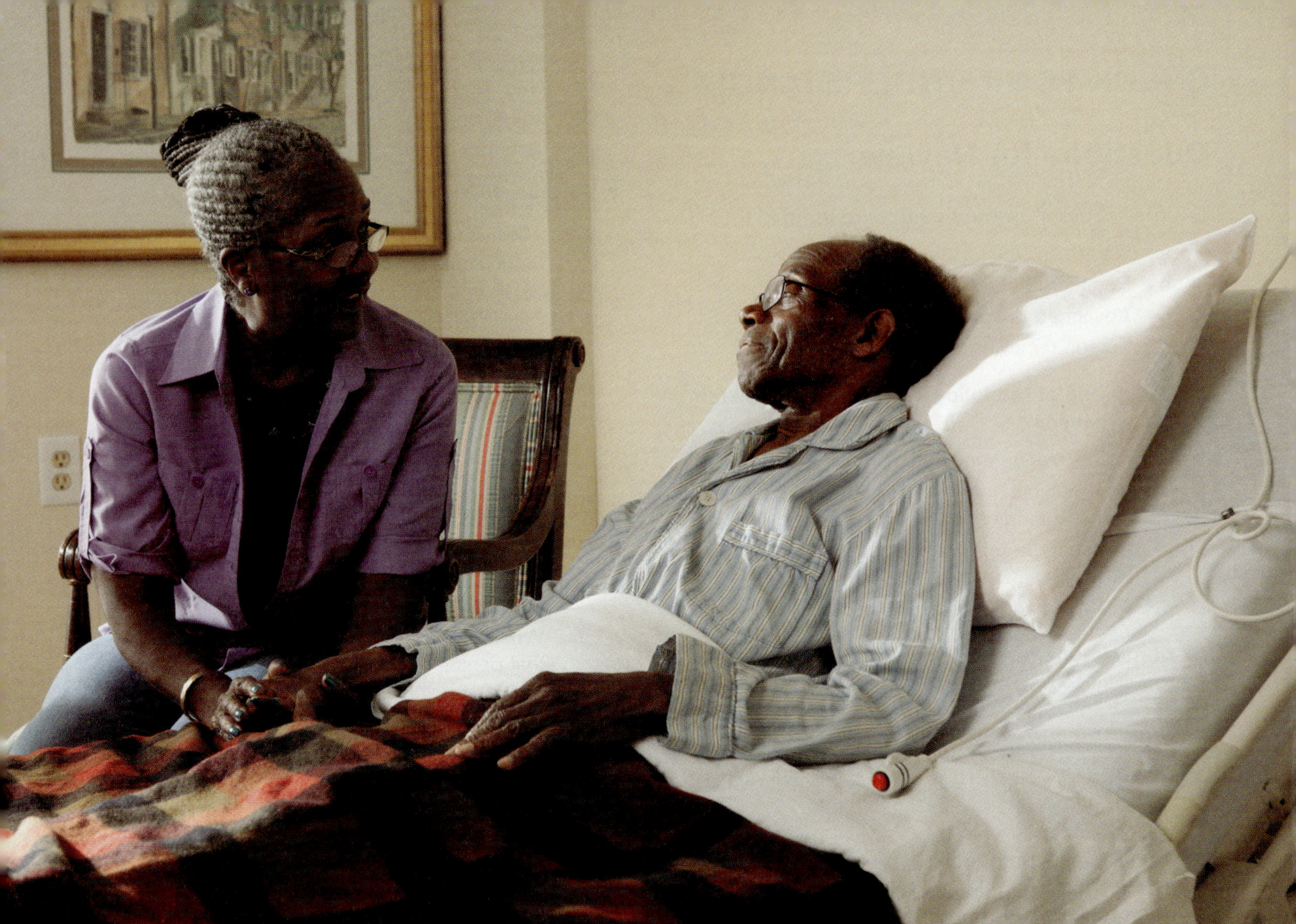

CHAPTER

2 Working in the Health Care System

Goals

After reading this chapter, you will have the information needed to:

- Identify different types of health care settings, and describe the types of services each provides.
- Discuss some differences between working as a nurse assistant in an acute care setting, a sub-acute care setting, a long-term care setting and a home setting.
- Describe government insurance programs that help to offset the costs of health care.
- Describe legislation, programs and organizations that are in place to help protect the recipients of health care, and ensure that quality standards for care are met.
- Give examples of rights that people who are receiving health care are entitled to.

Goals

- Explain how legislation brought about by the Omnibus Budget Reconciliation Act (OBRA) seeks to ensure quality care for nursing home residents.
- Discuss how the Occupational Safety and Health Administration (OSHA) seeks to protect workers from on-the-job injuries.

Key Terms:

acute care setting
patient
inpatient care
outpatient care
sub-acute care setting
long-term care setting
resident
nursing home
assisted-living facility
cognitive impairment
client
Medicare
Medicaid
Omnibus Budget Reconciliation Act of 1987 (OBRA)
ombudsman
accreditation
Occupational Safety and Health Administration (OSHA)

It was a rainy morning in April when 72-year-old Alma Renaldo was rushed by ambulance to the local hospital's emergency room. She had been talking with her husband, Luis, while she prepared breakfast. All of a sudden, while Alma was serving the plates, she suddenly collapsed and the plate she was holding clattered to the floor. She was unconscious and unresponsive. Luis called 9-1-1 and waited anxiously for the ambulance to arrive. In the emergency room, the doctors determined that Alma had experienced a massive stroke.

After spending nearly 2 weeks on life support in the intensive care unit of the hospital, Alma's condition was stable enough for her to be moved to a rehabilitation facility. The stroke had paralyzed the right side of Alma's body, left her unable to speak, and made it difficult for her to swallow without choking. In the rehabilitation facility, Alma worked with physical therapists and speech therapists to try to regain as much function and independence as possible.

Despite several weeks of therapy, Alma was not able to regain enough function to care for herself anymore. Now Alma and her family had to make a difficult decision. Would it be possible for Luis to provide the care Alma would need at home, or would other arrangements for Alma's care need to be made? Alma's and Luis' two daughters, Isabela and Maria, were both married and busy with families and careers of their own, and neither lived close by. They would only be able to provide limited support to their parents. After thinking through all of the options as a family, the Renaldos made the difficult decision for Alma to move into Morningside Nursing Home.

HEALTH CARE SETTINGS

The health care system has many parts, each with a special function. In some instances, a person may use several parts of the system to meet his or her health care needs.

Acute Care Settings

Services provided in acute care settings

Acute care settings specialize in providing care to people who become sick or injured suddenly, or who have other conditions (such as delivering a baby) that require short-term health care (Figure 2-1). Care is provided in the acute care setting until the person is medically stable. Usually, the length of stay in an acute care setting is short.

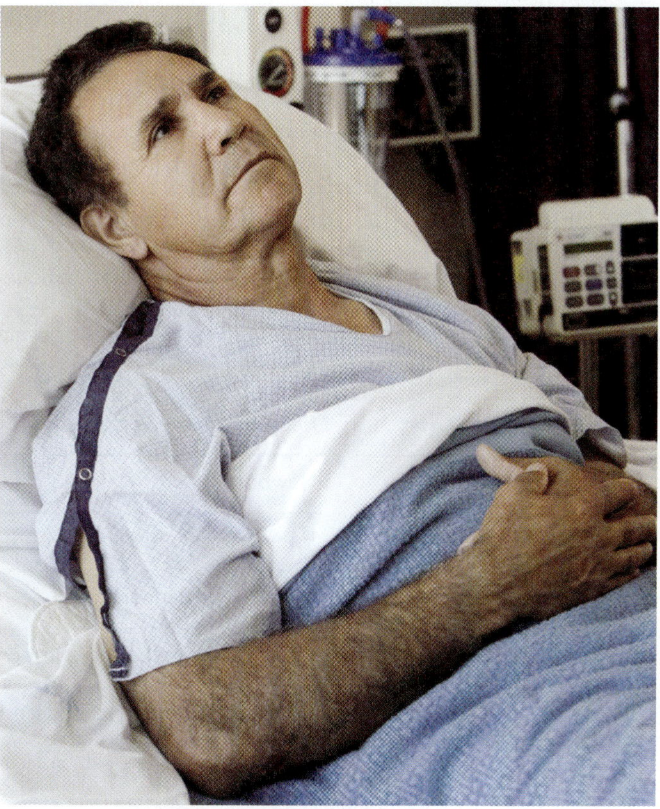

Figure 2-1 People with illnesses or injuries who are medically unstable are cared for in acute care facilities. *Image © Monkey Business Images, 2012. Used under license from Shutterstock.com.*

The most common type of acute care setting is a hospital. A person who receives care in a hospital or other acute care setting is called a **patient**. Patients who stay overnight in the hospital receive **inpatient care**. Not all hospital patients stay overnight, however. Some patients may come to the hospital to receive a specific therapy (for example, a chemotherapy treatment for cancer, or surgery to repair a broken bone) and go home the same day. This is called **outpatient care**. Outpatient care may also be delivered by other acute care settings, such as a clinic (a health care facility that is devoted to providing services such as treatments or diagnostic tests on an outpatient basis) or a surgical center (a health care facility that performs outpatient surgeries, where the person is admitted for the surgery and sent home the same day).

Many hospitals provide a wide variety of services for patients of all ages and with many different types of illnesses or injuries. Within the hospital, patients are grouped according to age or the type of care they require (Table 2-1). Other hospitals specialize in providing care for only one age group or for people with a certain type of disorder (for example, a children's hospital or a hospital that cares only for people with cancer).

What is it like to work in an acute care setting?

Many nurse assistants work in hospitals. When you work as a nurse assistant in a hospital, the people in your care will change fairly often because most patients do not stay in the facility for a very long time. A nurse assistant working in a hospital must have a special ability to form effective relationships quickly with people who are under stress. For the patient and family, receiving acute care can be very upsetting. Injuries and illnesses that require treatment in a hospital are usually quite serious, and patients (and their family members) are often very worried about the potential for recovery, the long-term effects of the illness or injury, the results of diagnostic tests and the risks associated with undergoing certain procedures and treatments. Things happen quickly in a hospital, and patients and family members may not remember or may not understand information they were given by other members of the health care team. You will become an important link between the patient and family and the other members of the health care team by telling the nurse about any questions and concerns the patient or family discuss with you.

You will also play an important role in promoting comfort and providing emotional support. The hospital environment

Table 2-1 **Examples of Clinical Services Provided Within a Hospital**

Service	Care Recipients
Medical	People who have conditions that are treated medically (for example, with drugs or other non-surgical therapies)
Surgical	People who are recovering from conditions that are treated surgically
Cardiology	People who have heart conditions
Emergency	People who have signs or symptoms of illness that require immediate evaluation and treatment by a health care professional
Intensive Care	People who are very medically unstable and who have life-threatening illnesses or conditions
Neonatal	Newborns
Obstetric	Pregnant women and newborns
Oncology	People with cancer
Operating Room	People who are having surgery
Orthopedic	People with bone and joint problems
Pediatric	Children up to 18 years of age
Psychiatric/Mental Health	People with mental illness

can be uncomfortable, with unfamiliar sounds and smells, and few comforts of home. Most patients share a room with one or more others. Depending on the person's illness or injury and hospital policy, visiting hours may be limited, so patients may not always have the comfort of having friends and family near. The compassionate care you provide can make a big difference in how the patient and family feel about their experience in the hospital.

> **Think back to Alma Renaldo's family.**
>
> ***How might they have been feeling while Alma was hospitalized and in intensive care? What factors might have contributed to these feelings?***
>
> ***What actions could staff members at the hospital take to try and help the Renaldos through this difficult time?***

Sub-Acute Care Settings

Services provided in sub-acute care settings

Being cared for in a hospital is very expensive, so patients are usually discharged from the hospital as soon as they are medically stable. However, some patients will still require treatments such as intravenous (IV) drug therapy, physical rehabilitation or wound care for complex wounds that can only be provided by health care professionals (Figure 2-2). This type of care is provided in a **sub-acute care setting**, which may be a special unit of a hospital or nursing home, or a separate facility, such as a long-term acute care hospital (LTACH). The typical length of stay for a person receiving care in a sub-acute care setting is less than 30 days.

What is it like to work in a sub-acute care setting?

The people receiving care in sub-acute care settings are often still quite ill and require a great deal of medical and nursing care. In addition to helping people receiving sub-acute care to meet their physical needs, a nurse assistant who works in a sub-acute care setting must be able to provide a great deal of emotional support. Many people who are admitted to sub-acute care settings are recovering from illnesses or injuries that significantly impact their ability to function independently. As a result, they and their family members are often very worried about what the future holds. Will the illness or injury have a permanent impact on the person's ability to function, and if so, how severe will that impact be? Will the person be able to return home, or is this the injury or illness that will make moving to a nursing home necessary? In addition, undergoing rehabilitation is very difficult, both physically and emotionally. As with all people you care for, your ability to show empathy for the person and her situation will be extremely important. You will play a very important role in reinforcing the techniques that the person learns in therapy, encouraging the person, and recognizing the person's progress toward her goal.

Long-Term Care Settings

Services provided in long-term care settings

In a **long-term care setting**, people receive assistance meeting their medical, personal and social needs over an extended period of time (Figure 2-3). The term **resident** is used to refer to a person who receives care in a long-term care setting, because

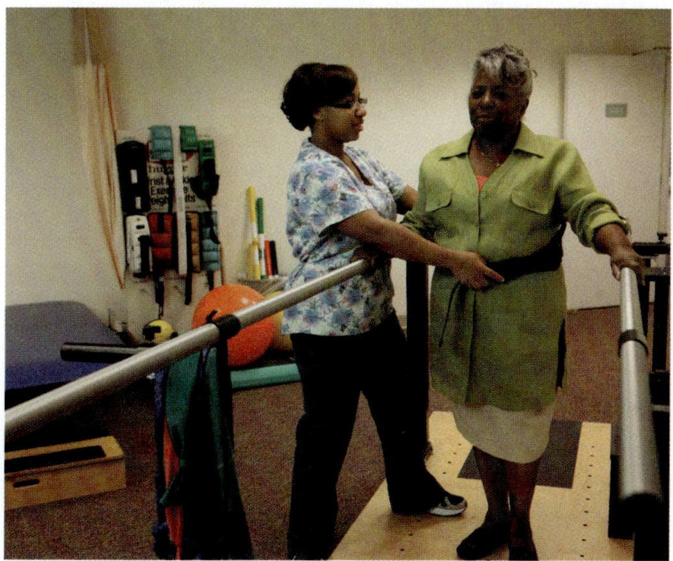

Figure 2-2 People who are well enough to leave the acute care setting but who still require treatments that are too complex to be delivered by family members at home may be admitted to a sub-acute care setting.

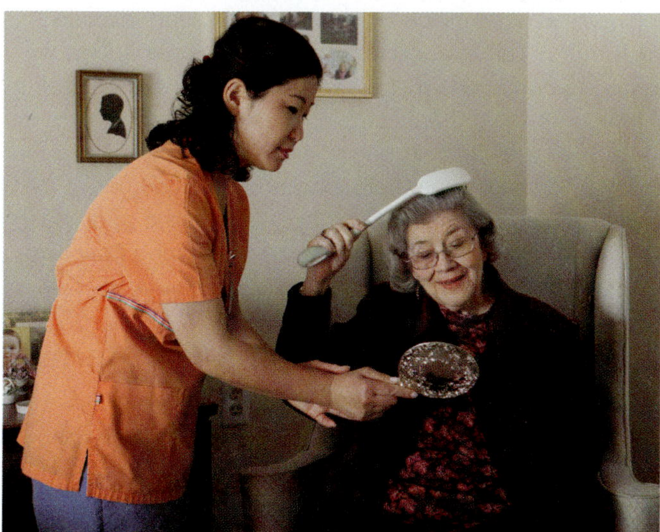

Figure 2-3 Long-term care facilities provide nursing care and supervision for people who can no longer live independently because of illness or disability. Care focuses on helping residents achieve or maintain their highest level of function.

the facility becomes the person's home, either temporarily or permanently. Short-term residents are those who leave the facility in 3 to 6 months. They tend to be younger, and may be admitted from a hospital to receive sub-acute care until they are well enough to return home. Long-term residents stay in the facility for 6 months or more. The average stay for a person in a long-term care facility is 7 months to 2 years.

There are two major types of long-term care settings, **nursing homes** and **assisted-living facilities**. People who are cared for in assisted-living facilities require some assistance with tasks such as activities of daily living (ADLs) or reminders to take medications, but are otherwise fairly independent. Most residents of assisted-living facilities live in their own apartments, but have access to shared services in the building or on the campus, such as a restaurant or dining room and areas for recreation. People who are cared for in nursing homes require a much higher level of nursing care and supervision as compared with those who live in assisted-living facilities.

Although most people who receive care in a nursing home are elderly with one or more chronic conditions (long-lasting conditions that require regular treatment), younger people with debilitating conditions (such as multiple sclerosis), mental disabilities or serious disabling injuries (such as traumatic brain injury or a spinal cord injury) may also receive care in a nursing home. The most common reason for admission to a nursing home is the loss of the ability to perform one or more ADLs independently. Many residents of nursing homes have some degree of **cognitive impairment**. Cognitive impairment is difficulty with thinking processes involving memory, reasoning, judgment and language, such as that caused by disorders like Alzheimer's disease (a form of dementia). Most residents of nursing homes also have one or more chronic conditions that can affect their physical abilities, such as heart disease, lung disease or arthritis. The effects of the medical conditions, rather than the conditions themselves, often lead to the nursing home admission. For example, someone who has arthritis may no longer be able to get in and out of bed, go to the toilet or dress without help. Someone with dementia may be physically able to function but may need a great deal of help because she has trouble remembering how to care for herself.

What is it like to work in a long-term care setting?

Nurse assistants are the key staff in providing for the needs of long-term care residents, especially those in nursing homes. Providing restorative care (care that helps people maintain abilities that they still have, and regain, to the greatest extent possible, abilities that they have lost) is a major focus for nurse assistants working in nursing homes. In addition to helping residents meet their physical needs, nurse assistants are an important source of emotional support for residents and their families. Coming to live in a long-term care facility can be a big adjustment for the person and his or her family members. Many times, a sudden event (such as a stroke or the loss of a spouse) makes admission to a long-term care facility necessary. Most people do not choose to come to live at a long-term care facility, and have little time to prepare for this change in their lives. The emotions that accompany admission to a nursing home can be complex for both the person and the family members and may include loneliness, grief, guilt and anger.

Working in a long-term care setting can be both very challenging and very rewarding. Many of the people you will care for will be nearing the end of their lives, which means you will often have to face losing people you have come to care about. Caring for people with cognitive impairments (such as dementia) can be very stressful for the person providing care. In addition to being emotionally demanding, the job is physically demanding, because nursing home residents need so much assistance with their ADLs. Despite these challenges, the ability to form long-term relationships with the people in your care, being able to help them maintain or achieve their highest level of functioning, and helping them to enjoy the best quality of life possible can be very satisfying, and are the reasons why many nurse assistants choose to work in long-term care.

You are the nurse assistant assigned to care for Mrs. Renaldo on her first day at Morningside. As you greet Mrs. Renaldo and her family members when they arrive at the facility, you can tell that everyone is very upset. Mr. Renaldo smiles sadly at you as he shakes your hand, and his voice cracks when he introduces himself, his wife and his daughters. Later, Isabela Renaldo takes you aside and says, "I'm so worried about my parents. Mama and Papa have been married for 53 years, and hardly ever spent a night apart before Mama's stroke. These last few weeks, Papa has just been rattling around the house. He doesn't know what to do with himself, and he's terribly lonely. And Mama—she can't stop crying. I think this is going to kill them both."

Think about each member of the Renaldo family. What losses do you think each of them has experienced as a result of Mrs. Renaldo's stroke?

As a nurse assistant, what things can you do to help make this time of change less difficult for Mrs. Renaldo and her family?

What will be a primary focus of care for Mrs. Renaldo going forward?

Home Settings

Services provided in home settings

Today, many people receive health care in their homes (Figure 2-4). A person who receives home health care is called a **client**. Home health care agencies provide services for clients of all ages with many different types of health care needs. For example, a home health care agency may provide sub-acute care services in a person's home, following hospitalization for the treatment of an acute injury or illness. A home health care agency may also provide services for a person who cannot manage some tasks independently, but is not quite ready or willing to move to a long-term care facility.

What is it like to work in a home setting?

Nurse assistants who work for home health care agencies are usually called home health aides. Home health aides work under the supervision of a licensed nurse, but usually visit the person's home alone to provide assistance with personal care, meal preparation and light housekeeping tasks, such as laundry. Home health aides must be confident in their own abilities and comfortable working on their own because co-workers and supervisors will not be readily available to provide hands-on assistance. Flexibility and adaptability are also important characteristics for a home health aide to have. Furniture and equipment that is available in a facility is not always available in a person's home. Finally, home health aides, like all nurse assistants, must also have excellent communication skills because often the home health aide is the only link between the client and the other members of the health care team. You will learn more about working in a home setting in Chapter 22.

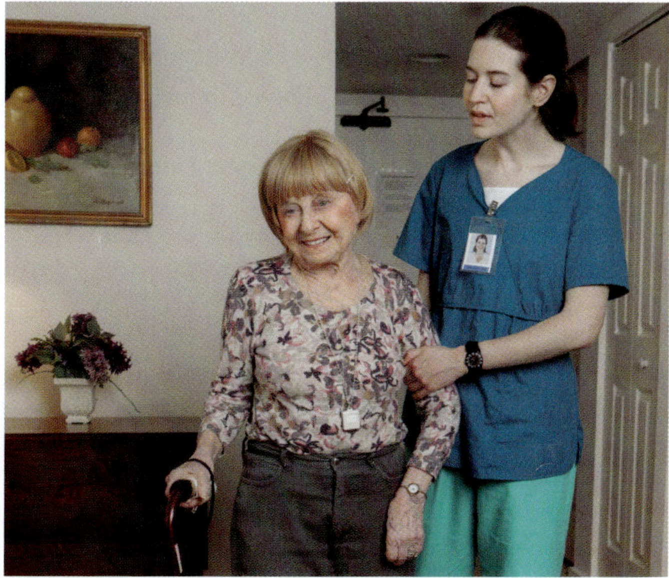

Figure 2-4 Home health agencies provide health care for people in their own homes.

PAYING FOR HEALTH CARE

Because you will be working within the health care system, it is important for you to have a basic understanding of how people pay for the services you provide. In the United States, people pay for health care in a variety of ways. Some people may pay the entire cost for health care out of their own personal earnings or savings. However, because health care can be very expensive, most people rely on insurance to pay all or part of the costs of the services they receive. Many employers offer health care insurance as part of their benefits program for employees. Usually, the employer and the employee share the cost of the insurance, which makes the insurance more affordable for the employee. People who are self-employed or unemployed may purchase health care insurance independently.

Many people receive health insurance through government programs like **Medicare** (a federally funded insurance program for people who are 65 years and older) and **Medicaid** (an insurance program for people with low incomes, jointly funded by federal and state governments). If you work for a facility or agency that receives funding from the Medicare or Medicaid programs, accurate documentation of the care you provide is essential to ensure that the people in your care continue to be eligible to receive the services they need. Proper documentation is also necessary to ensure that the facility receives the proper payment for services that have been provided.

PROTECTING THE RECIPIENTS OF HEALTH CARE

People who require health care want to know that they will receive good quality care. Many regulations and agencies exist to define standards of quality and to ensure that the care provided meets those standards.

Patient, Resident and Client Rights

People who receive health care have certain basic rights and privileges, such as:

- The right to competent care that is delivered with respect.
- The right to know the kind of care they will receive and the cost of that care.
- The right to participate in decisions made about the care they receive and who will provide it.
- The right to confidentiality and privacy.
- The right to be free from restraints and abuse.

These basic rights are similar across all health care settings. In nursing homes, these rights are called *resident rights* (Box 2-1). People receiving care in hospitals have *patient rights*, and people receiving care at home have *client rights*. When a person becomes a patient, resident or client, she is informed of her rights. Discussing these rights helps the person and the family understand what they are entitled to and

▼ Box 2-1 **Resident Rights**

DIGNITY

You have the right:

- **To be valued as an individual, to maintain and enhance your self-worth.**
- **To be treated with courtesy, respect and dignity, free from humiliation, harassment or threats.**
- **To be free from physical, sexual, mental, verbal and financial abuse.**
- **To be free from chemical and physical restraints and involuntary seclusion.**

PRIVACY

You have the right:

- **To personal privacy during care and treatment.**
- **To confidentiality concerning your personal and medical information.**
- **To private and unrestricted visits with any person of your choice, in person and by telephone.**
- **To send and receive mail without interference.**

GRIEVANCES

You have the right:

- **To voice grievances about care or services without discrimination or reprisal.**
- **To expect the facility to promptly investigate and try to resolve your concerns.**
- **To contact the ombudsman to advocate on your behalf, free from discrimination or reprisal, if you feel any of your rights have been violated.**

ACCESS

You have the right:

- **To be fully informed, both orally and in writing, of your rights and the facility's rules before admission and during your stay in the facility.**
- **To be fully informed of the services available and related costs.**
- **To not provide a third-party guarantee of payment.**
- **To be informed and to receive assistance in accessing all of your benefits through Medicare or Medicaid.**
- **To equal access to quality care for all residents.**
- **To be told in advance about care and treatment, including all risks and benefits.**
- **To look at your records and receive copies at a reasonable cost.**
- **To have reasonable access to any personal funds held for you by the facility.**
- **To retain and use personal possessions.**
- **To receive notice in advance of any plans to change your room or roommate.**
- **To organize and participate in a resident council and for your family to organize and participate in a family council.**
- **To participate in social, religious and community activities, including the right to vote.**
- **To read the results of the most recent state or federal inspection survey and the facility's plan to correct any violations.**
- **To contact your ombudsman, or the state survey agency, or any advocate or agency of your choosing.**

TRANSFER OR DISCHARGE

You have the right:

- **To remain in the facility unless there is a valid, legal reason for your transfer or discharge.**
- **To receive a 30-day written notice with the reason for the transfer or discharge, including appeal rights and information.**
- **To have a planning conference at least 14 days prior to the transfer or discharge.**
- **To receive assistance to assure a safe transfer.**
- **To be offered to hold your bed if your transfer is temporary, such as for hospitalization or therapeutic leave.**

SELF-DETERMINATION

You have the right:

- **To be offered choices and allowed to make decisions important to you.**
- **To expect the facility to accommodate individual needs and preferences.**
- **To participate in the planning of your care and services.**
- **To self-administer medications.**
- **To accept or refuse care and treatment.**
- **To choose your health care providers, including your doctor and pharmacy.**
- **To manage your own personal finances, or to be kept informed of your finances if you choose to let someone else manage them for you.**
- **To refuse to perform work or services for the facility.**

how they can expect to be treated while receiving health care.

As a nurse assistant, you will play an important role in making sure that the rights of the people in your care are upheld. Practicing the five principles of care (see Chapter 1, Figure 1-6) consistently with every person in your care is one way you can help to make sure that the person's rights are respected. As you continue through your training course, you will learn about actions you can take in specific situations to protect the rights of the people in your care.

As a resident of a nursing home, what rights will Mrs. Renaldo be entitled to?

What actions can you take as a nurse assistant to support Mrs. Renaldo's rights?

Omnibus Budget Reconciliation Act (OBRA) Regulations

The **Omnibus Budget Reconciliation Act of 1987 (OBRA)** led to legislation that was put into effect by the federal government in 1990. To guarantee that people being cared for in nursing homes received a certain level of care, this legislation established standards for staffing and operation that all nursing homes accepting federal funding must meet. OBRA legislation emphasizes the responsibility of nursing homes to provide residents with a comfortable and fulfilling lifestyle and to promote their physical, mental, emotional and spiritual well-being to the highest degree possible (Figure 2-5). OBRA legislation addresses areas such as training requirements for nurse assistants, the physical environment of the facility and the basic rights of nursing home residents (see Box 2-1). In addition, OBRA legislation establishes a mechanism for ensuring that facilities are providing care up to OBRA standards. Per OBRA, nursing homes that receive

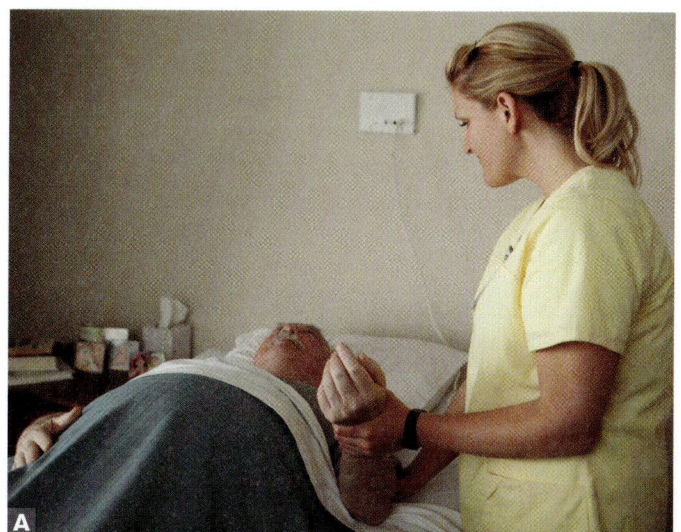

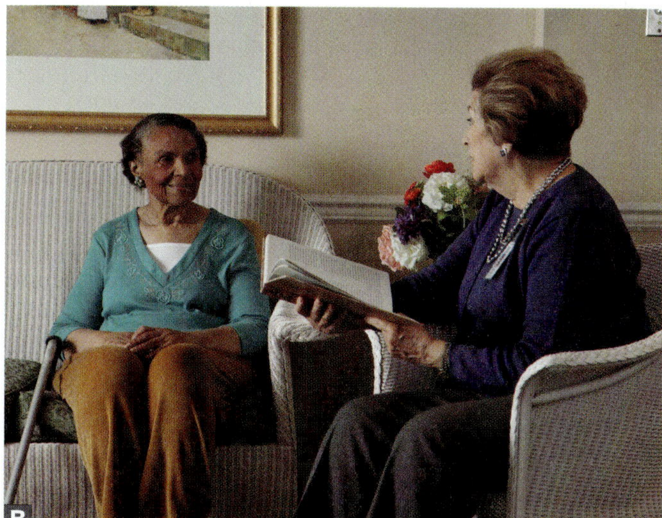

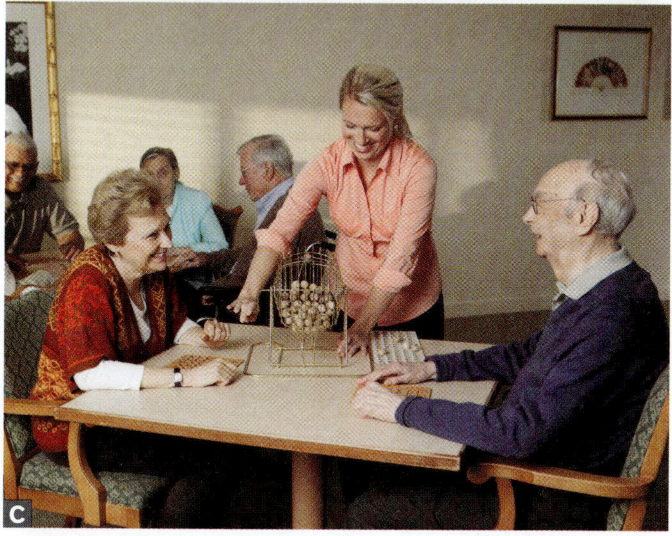

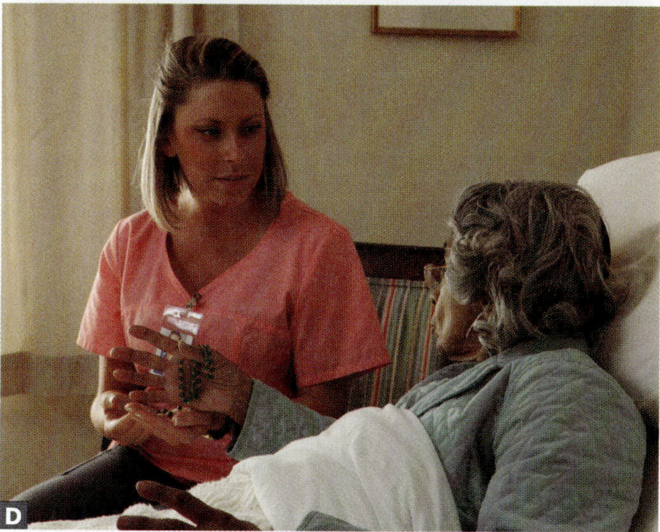

Figure 2-5 Quality care seeks to meet the person's (A) physical, (B) mental, (C) emotional and (D) spiritual needs.

federal funding must undergo routine inspections by the government, called surveys, to make sure that the facility is providing care in accordance with government standards.

Ombudsman Programs

The federal government requires each state to have an ombudsman program that serves nursing homes. **Ombudsmen** are volunteers who advocate for (act on the behalf of) nursing home residents and their family members to resolve problems related to quality of care. The ombudsman has the same goal that you have: to make sure the needs of the people in your care are met, and that their rights are respected. The ombudsman visits the nursing home regularly to talk with residents and family members (Figure 2-6). Residents, family members or even staff members may also contact the ombudsman directly if they have concerns about the quality of care that is being provided. Information given to the ombudsman is treated confidentially. After receiving permission from the person who voiced the concern to investigate further, the ombudsman talks with those involved to find out what happened and asks questions to find out what actions the facility has already taken to address the problem. After investigating the problem, the ombudsman works with the appropriate people or agencies to find a solution to the problem and make sure the resident's, family member's or staff member's concerns are addressed. The most frequent concerns reported to ombudsmen have to do with accidents, neglect of personal cleanliness, lack of respect for residents, poor staff attitudes and resident requests that go unanswered.

Government Oversight

Federal, state and local governments are all involved in establishing regulations and monitoring the quality of care provided by health care facilities and agencies in the United States. You have already learned about one important piece of federal legislation, OBRA, which applies to nursing homes that receive federal funding. However, government at all levels is involved in setting standards, and making sure these standards are met, for other types of health care facilities and agencies as well.

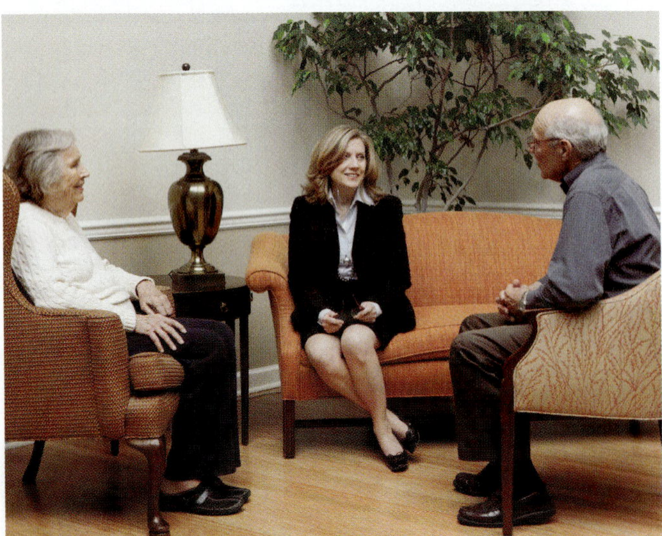

Figure 2-6 Ombudsmen advocate on behalf of nursing home residents and their families to ensure quality care.

Accrediting Organizations

Professional associations and organizations that are not associated with the government also exist to ensure that people receive quality health care. Health care facilities that meet the standards established by these organizations receive **accreditation** (official recognition that the facility provides care to a certain standard). Accreditation is another way for recipients of health care to have confidence that they are receiving quality care.

The most well-known of these organizations is The Joint Commission. You may hear The Joint Commission referred to as "JAYCO" because in the past, the name of this organization was The Joint Commission on Accreditation of Healthcare Organizations (JCAHO). The Joint Commission works to establish national standards of care, especially with regard to safety, for all types of health care facilities. Facilities that meet these standards receive accreditation and are permitted to display The Joint Commission's Gold Seal of Approval.

PROTECTING HEALTH CARE WORKERS

The **Occupational Safety and Health Administration (OSHA)** is a government agency that was established in 1970 to help protect workers in all industries (not just health care) from on-the-job injuries. OSHA establishes standards that employers must follow to protect employees from hazards. For example, OSHA has established standards relating to:

- The prevention of employee exposure to harmful substances and chemicals.
- Equipment employers must provide, and environmental standards they must maintain, to keep workers safe on the job.
- Training employers must provide to help keep employees safe on the job.
- The need for employers to monitor hazards and keep records of workplace injuries and illnesses.

As you continue reading this text, you will see references to OSHA standards that apply to health care workers.

CHECK YOUR UNDERSTANDING

Questions for Review

1. **Where is care provided for a person who requires treatment for a sudden injury or illness?**
   a. Sub-acute care setting
   b. Home setting
   c. Acute care setting
   d. Long-term care setting

2. **Mr. Bowler is 85 years old. He has dementia and requires close supervision to make sure that he does not hurt himself. He also requires a great deal of help with his activities of daily living (ADLs). What health care setting would provide the most appropriate care for Mr. Bowler?**
   a. Acute care setting
   b. Nursing home setting
   c. Hospital setting
   d. Sub-acute care setting

3. **Which legislation establishes quality standards for the care of residents of nursing homes?**
   a. Ombudsman Act (OA)
   b. Occupational Safety and Health Administration (OSHA)
   c. Omnibus Budget Reconciliation Act (OBRA)
   d. Resident Rights Act (RRA)

4. **Which of the following is a basic right of people who are receiving health care?**
   a. The right not to pay
   b. The right to competent care that is delivered with respect
   c. The right to abuse health care workers
   d. All of the above

5. **Which of the following is a government-funded insurance program for people older than 65 years?**
   a. Medicare
   b. Medicaid
   c. OBRA
   d. Social Security

6. **Mr. Johnson was admitted to the hospital for pneumonia and was hospitalized for 4 days. What word best describes Mr. Johnson?**
   a. Outpatient
   b. Resident
   c. Inpatient
   d. Client

Questions to Ask Yourself

1. *As a nurse assistant, in which type of health care setting would you most like to work? Why?*
2. *In this chapter, you read about legislation, government agencies and programs, and accrediting organizations that are in place to ensure that people who use the services provided by the health care system receive quality care. Think about words or phrases you would use to describe quality care. What are some of these words or phrases?*
3. *Mrs. O'Brien's husband is receiving care in a nursing home. Lately, when Mrs. O'Brien has come to see her husband, she has noticed that he smells of urine. Mrs. O'Brien spoke to the nurse about her concerns, but the problem has continued. What resources are available to help Mrs. O'Brien resolve this problem?*
4. *Mary is a nurse assistant at a nursing home. For each of the following actions, what resident right is Mary supporting?*
   - *Mary asks Mr. Cleary's permission before opening the dresser drawer where he keeps personal items.*
   - *Mary asks visitors to leave, shuts the door, and pulls the privacy curtain before assisting Mr. Howe to dress.*
   - *When assisting Mrs. Lyons with a bed bath, Mary makes sure to keep Mrs. Lyons covered with a bath blanket, rearranging the bath blanket as necessary so that only the body part she is washing is exposed.*
   - *Mary asks Mr. Upchurch whether he would prefer to bathe in the morning or the evening.*

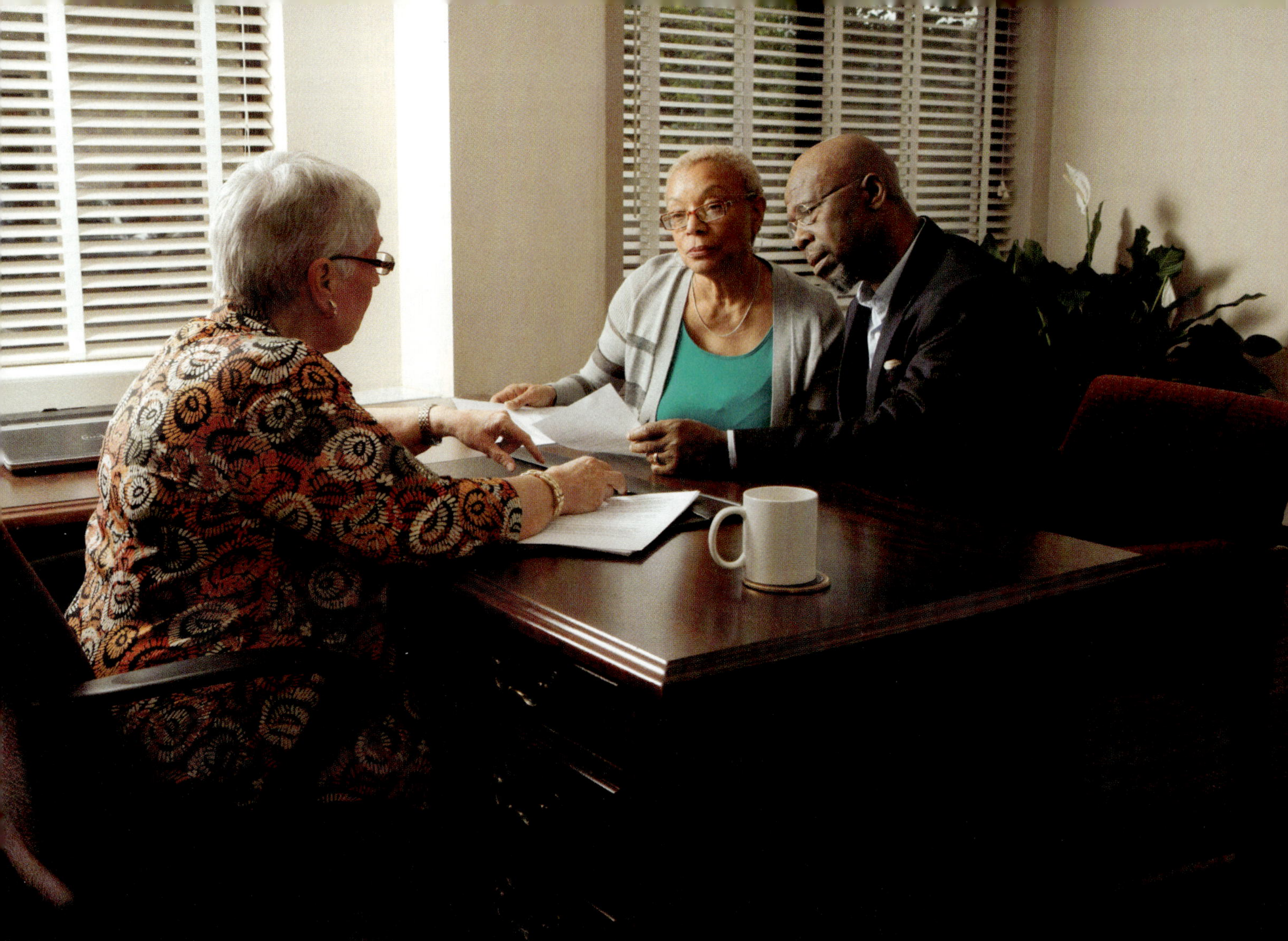

CHAPTER

3

Understanding Legal and Ethical Aspects of Health Care

Goals

After reading this chapter, you will have the information needed to:

- Explain important legal obligations health care providers have as specified by the Patient Self-Determination Act, and identify actions a nurse assistant can take to make sure Patient Self-Determination Act requirements are met.
- Explain important legal obligations health care providers have as specified by the Health Insurance Portability and Accountability Act (HIPAA), and identify actions a nurse assistant can take to make sure HIPAA requirements are met.
- Describe behaviors that can result in legal or disciplinary action, and understand how to avoid these behaviors.
- Describe types of abuse, and recognize possible signs of abuse.
- Describe the nurse assistant's responsibilities related to reporting suspected abuse.

Goals

- Describe ethical principles that health care workers can use to guide their decision making and behavior.
- List actions a nurse assistant can take to protect himself or herself from legal and ethical difficulties on the job.

Key Terms:

laws
ethics
informed consent
advance directive
durable power of attorney for health care
living will
abuse
assault
battery
negligence
fraud
larceny
ethical dilemma
ethics committee

Mrs. Geneva Millen is a 58-year-old woman who was transferred yesterday afternoon to the Golden Shepherd Rehabilitation Facility after undergoing back surgery. You are assigned to care for Mrs. Millen today. While you are passing through the common area on the unit, you overhear two other nurse assistants talking about Mrs. Millen. One of them says, "The evening and night shifts said she was really demanding after she got here. She kept putting on her call light every five minutes. I'm really glad she wasn't assigned to me today!" You notice that Mrs. Millen's call light has just come on.

Every day, you make decisions about how to behave. Some of these decisions are guided by your knowledge of our society's **laws** (rules established by a governing authority to protect citizens from harm and provide a framework for resolving conflicts). Other decisions are guided by **ethics** (moral principles or standards that we use to decide the correct action to take). In this chapter, we will take a closer look at issues relating to the law that nurse assistants should be aware of. We will also discuss how ethics can guide behavior in the workplace.

LEGISLATION THAT INFLUENCES THE DELIVERY OF HEALTH CARE

In Chapter 2, you learned about the Omnibus Budget Reconciliation Act (OBRA), legislation that was put into place to ensure standards of care for residents of nursing homes. Let's look at two other important pieces of legislation that affect the delivery of health care in all settings.

Patient Self-Determination Act

In 1991, the federal government passed the Patient Self-Determination Act. This law gives a person the right to make decisions about his or her care. These rights include the right to accept or refuse care and to develop advance directives.

Informed consent

The Patient Self-Determination Act obligates health care providers to obtain the patient's, resident's or client's permission, or **informed consent**, before going ahead with a treatment or procedure. To make sure that the person's decision is informed (that is, based on a thorough understanding of the benefits and risks associated with the proposed treatment or procedure), the health care team must give the person the information he needs in order to make the decision he feels is best. This includes explaining why the procedure or treatment is being recommended, reviewing the risks associated with the procedure or treatment, and explaining what the risks are if the person chooses not to have the procedure or treatment. If the person agrees to go ahead with the procedure or treatment, he then signs a document giving his consent. Even if a person initially consents to a procedure or treatment, he has the right to withdraw that consent and refuse the treatment or procedure at any time.

Although as a nurse assistant you will not be responsible for getting a person's written consent to perform a procedure or treatment, you still must obtain the person's verbal consent before providing care. Tell the person what you are there to do, and ask him if it is okay to continue (Figure 3-1). Make sure to explain things in a way that the person can understand. A person who is confused (for example, someone with dementia) may resist standard care, such as a bath. Although every person in your care has the right to refuse a bath (or any other care procedure), you may be able to gain the person's cooperation and consent by taking a different approach, or by coming back later and asking again. For example, a person with dementia might not agree to a bath, but maybe she will agree to freshening up at the sink. Remember that even if a person gives you consent to do something, she can withdraw that consent at any time.

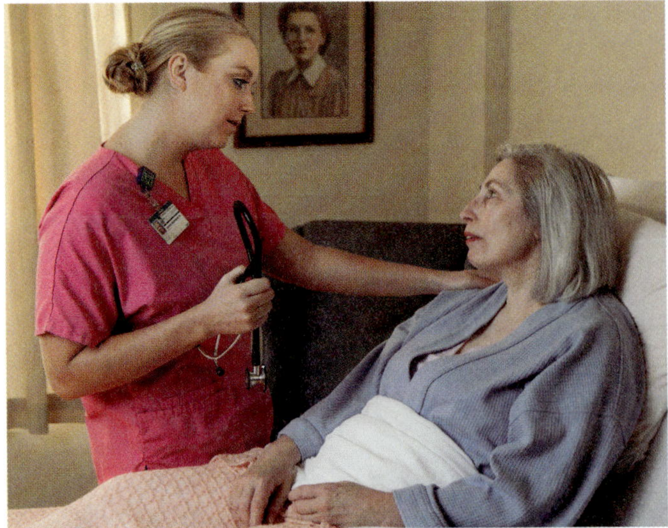

Figure 3-1 Before providing care, always explain to the person what you are there to do, and ask the person's permission to continue.

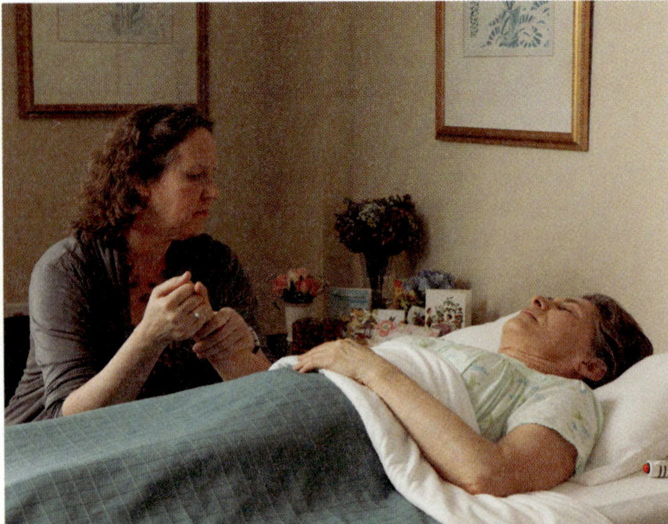

Figure 3-2 A living will is a document that allows a person to specify her wishes for care in the event that she is no longer able to express those wishes herself.

Advance directives

Under the Patient Self-Determination Act, people have the right to be informed about how they can communicate their preferences regarding health care decisions in the event that they are no longer able to make or communicate these decisions themselves. An **advance directive** is a legal document stating how the person wants health decisions made if he or she is unable to make or communicate these decisions independently in the future. There are different types of advance directives:

- A **durable power of attorney for health care** is a legal document that gives the responsibility for making decisions on the person's behalf to someone else, such as a family member, in case the person becomes unable to make these decisions on her own behalf.
- A **living will** is a legal document that gives specific directions about what steps the health care team should or should not take to prolong the person's life when death seems near. When a person's wishes are not known, health care providers must assume that the person would want life-sustaining treatments initiated. However, in some situations, a person may wish to avoid life-sustaining treatments if they would potentially cause more suffering. A living will allows the person to specify these desires so that others are aware of them and can provide care accordingly (Figure 3-2).

The Patient Self-Determination Act requires health care facilities and agencies to teach patients, residents, and clients and their family members about the purpose of advance directives, and to assist them with putting a durable power of attorney for health care, a living will or both in place, if they so desire. If a person in your care expresses concern about his or her ability to make decisions independently in the future, or a desire to put an advance directive in place, you should communicate this to the nurse immediately so that proper follow-up can take place.

Health Insurance Portability and Accountability Act (HIPAA)

In 1996, the federal government passed the Health Insurance Portability and Accountability Act (HIPAA). People who are receiving health care have the legal right to have their medical information kept secure and private. This law defines who can look at and receive information about a person's health status and care, and sets rules related to how information that is communicated in writing, verbally or electronically should be handled to protect the person's privacy.

As a nurse assistant, you play an important role in helping to ensure that a person's rights under HIPAA are protected (Figure 3-3). You will have access to

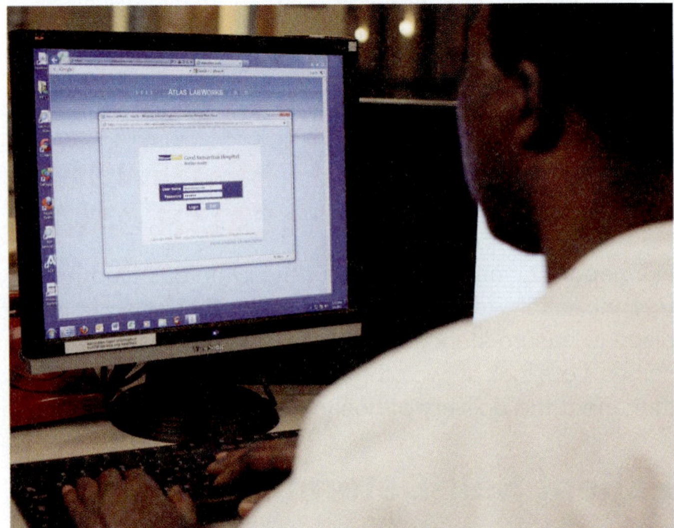

Figure 3-3 The people in your care have a legal right to have information about their health status and care kept private and secure.

information about the person's health status and treatments. This is protected information. Steps you can take to help keep this information secure include the following:

- Share information about the person's condition or the care you have provided only with those who need to know and who are also directly involved in providing care for the person (for example, the nurse).
- Avoid having conversations about the person's health status or care in places where you may be overheard by others.
- Never discuss a person's condition or care as part of casual conversations with friends or neighbors, or on social media posts (for example, Facebook or Twitter).
- Take care to secure tools used for documentation (such as the person's chart or electronic medical record) per your employer's policy. For example, return the chart to the designated area when you are finished charting, or close the computer screen. Never share the user name and password that you use to log into the computer system at work with anyone.
- If someone asks you for information about a person in your care and you are not sure whether that person has a right to this information, refer the person to the nurse. This includes the person's family members, if you are not sure the person would want them to have this information.
- Always follow your employer's policies and procedures relating to how private information about patients, residents, or clients is to be handled and secured.

You enter Mrs. Millen's room and find her crying. She tells you that she is in pain and can't get comfortable. You offer to help her change her position. While you are there, she says, "I'm just not used to this place. It's all so new and I don't know the staff. At least when I was in the hospital, I knew what to expect. I heard the staff talking about me last night."

Imagine that you were Mrs. Millen. How would you feel if you overheard staff members talking about you?

Would you say anything to the nurse assistants you overheard talking about Mrs. Millen in the common area? Why or why not?

What measures can you take to help protect Mrs. Millen's privacy going forward?

BEHAVIORS THAT CAN RESULT IN LEGAL OR DISCIPLINARY ACTION

As a nurse assistant, it is important for you to understand behaviors that could result in legal or disciplinary action being taken against you. There can be significant consequences if you commit one of these acts, ranging from disciplinary action being taken by your employer, to losing your job, to being arrested and tried in a court of law. In many cases, behaviors that result in legal or disciplinary action being taken against a nurse assistant are recorded on the nurse assistant's record in the state registry. A record of having committed one of these acts can have a very negative impact on the nurse assistant's ability to get another job in health care.

Abuse

Abuse is the willful infliction of injury or harm on another. A person can commit abuse by actively doing something to another person (for example, by hitting the person or verbally tormenting or threatening the person). Failing to provide necessary care for someone who is dependent on others for that care is also a form of abuse. Abuse can take many forms (Table 3-1).

ELDER CARE NOTE. Older people, especially those who have multiple health conditions and rely on others for care, are particularly vulnerable to being abused. This is called elder abuse, and it can take any of the forms described in Table 3-1. An older person who is being abused is often reluctant to report abuse, especially when he or she depends on the abuser for care. When caring for older people, be alert to changes in the person's behavior or appearance that might indicate that abuse is occurring (see Table 3-1).

Abuse can happen to anyone, and anyone can be an abuser. People who depend on others for care, such as children and the elderly, are at the highest risk for being abused. Caregivers can be at high risk for committing abuse when the stress of providing care becomes overwhelming. For example, many families struggle when one family member (such as a spouse or an adult child) must take on most of the responsibility for providing care to a loved one. Sometimes the stress becomes too much, which can lead to abuse. Even professional caregivers, like nurse assistants, are subject to on-the-job stress that can lead to abuse.

Abuse is never an acceptable form of behavior, and acting in an abusive manner can lead to the end of your career in health care. Many employers offer counseling to help employees manage

Table 3-1 **Forms of Abuse**

Form of Abuse	Examples	Possible Signs
Physical Abuse: Deliberately hurting another person's body	■ Hitting ■ Pushing or shoving ■ Pulling the hair ■ Biting ■ Burning ■ Choking ■ Shaking ■ Endangering the person (putting him in a life-threatening situation he cannot respond to) ■ Using restraints inappropriately	■ Cuts, bruises or other signs of injury, especially when the person seems to experience a lot of these types of injuries ■ Burns, especially when they occur in unusual places or have unusual patterns ■ Person may be withdrawn or fearful, especially in the presence of the person who is causing the abuse
Emotional Abuse: Degrading, belittling or threatening another person	■ Threatening a person with physical harm or the withdrawal of support ■ Humiliating a person ■ Teasing a person in a cruel way ■ Refusing to speak to the person or ignoring the person ■ Preventing a person from interacting with others (involuntary seclusion) ■ Using restraints inappropriately	■ Person may be withdrawn or fearful, especially in the presence of the person who is causing the abuse
Sexual Abuse: Forcing the person to take part in sexual activity of any kind	■ Inappropriately touching a person's breasts, buttocks or genitals, or forcing the person to touch someone else in an inappropriate way ■ Forcing another person to participate in sexual activities ■ Making inappropriate, sexually suggestive comments ■ Sexually exploiting the person (for example, by photographing the person's nude body)	■ Bruises, scratches or cuts around the breasts, buttocks or genitals ■ Unexplained vaginal or rectal bleeding ■ Person may refuse personal care ■ Person may be withdrawn or fearful, especially in the presence of the person who is causing the abuse
Neglect: Failing to provide for a dependent person's basic needs	■ Failing to provide food, water, clothing, shelter or necessary treatments (such as medications) ■ Failing to assist the person with personal hygiene and toileting	■ Signs of poor personal hygiene (for example, dirty hair, body odor, dirty fingernails, crusty eyes, bleeding gums or lips) ■ Dehydration ■ Weight loss ■ Pressure ulcers
Financial Exploitation: Taking or misusing another person's money or assets	■ Stealing a person's money, Social Security checks or belongings ■ Using a person's funds for a purpose other than what they were intended for ■ Using a person's checks or credit card, or withdrawing money from a person's bank account, without the person's knowledge or permission ■ Forging the person's signature on checks or legal documents	■ Person reports that money or assets are missing ■ Correspondence from banks or other financial institutions that the person did not expect or does not understand ■ Unpaid bills, even though the person has enough money to pay them

job-related stress. Take advantage of the opportunity to attend counseling sessions if they are offered. Other methods for managing stress include participating in activities that you enjoy outside of work, taking time for yourself on a regular basis to relax and recharge, and creating an environment where co-workers pitch in to help one another. Sometimes, despite all of your stress management techniques, you may find yourself becoming overwhelmed at work. Ask a co-worker to cover for you and remove yourself from the situation. Take a few minutes to get your feelings under control. If you find a situation to be too difficult to manage appropriately, you may need to ask your supervisor to reassign you.

If you have concerns that someone is abusing a person in your care, you have a legal responsibility to report your concerns to your supervisor (or to another person in the organization, per your employer's policy) (Figure 3-4). There may be times when you are unsure whether abuse has actually occurred; in these circumstances it is best to err on the side of reporting. The name of the person making the report is kept confidential unless the person permits his or her name to be used, or a court of law requires the person to testify. You are not responsible for investigating abuse, just reporting your concerns. The state agency that investigates cases of suspected abuse will follow up and investigate accordingly.

Assault and Battery

Assault is an action that causes a person to fear being touched in a harmful or unwelcome way. For example, raising your hand as if to strike a person in your care, or making a statement that suggests you will physically harm the person (such as, "If you don't stop trying to pull that IV line out I'm going to tie your hands behind your back!") could be considered assault. **Battery** is actually touching another person in a harmful or unwelcome way. Hitting, pinching or slapping a person in your care would be considered forms of battery. The inappropriate use of physical restraints (devices used to restrict a person's ability to move freely) is also considered a form of battery. Even beginning a procedure without obtaining the person's verbal consent to do so could be considered a form of battery, because you would be touching the person in an unwelcome way.

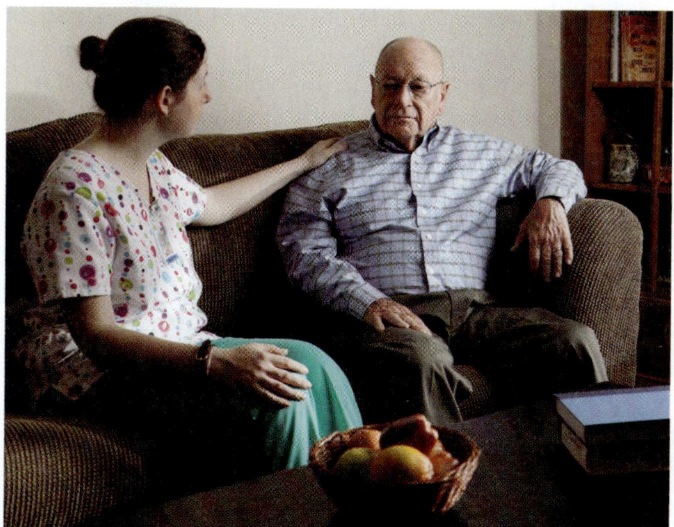

Figure 3-4 If you suspect that a person in your care is being abused, you have a legal obligation to report your concerns to your supervisor. Make careful note of the person's behavior, injuries or both so that you can give your supervisor accurate information.

Negligence

Negligence is failure to do what a reasonable and careful person would be expected to do in a given situation. Examples of negligence include the following:

- A nurse assistant has been trained in how to use the mechanical lift (a device used to assist people with moving from one place to another). While using the lift to move a person from the bed to a chair, the nurse assistant fails to lock the brakes on the lift, resulting in injury to the person.
- A nurse assistant is helping a person to get out of bed. The person repeatedly tells the nurse assistant that he is feeling dizzy, but the nurse assistant encourages him to stand up anyway, because she does not have time to wait for the person's dizziness to pass. The person stands up and then experiences a fall.
- A nurse assistant is asked to do a task that she has not been trained to do. Instead of declining to do the task, the nurse assistant attempts the task and causes injury to the person.

Fraud

Fraud is lying to gain profit or advantage. For example, a very problematic type of fraud in health care is Medicare fraud, which occurs when an individual or an organization seeks Medicare reimbursement for services that were not provided. Always document the care that you provide accurately and honestly. A health care worker can also commit fraud by misrepresenting his qualifications to others. For example, it would be fraudulent for a nurse assistant to tell a person in his care that he is a nurse, because he does not have the training or license necessary to practice as a nurse.

Larceny

Larceny is theft. As a nurse assistant, you will have access to the personal belongings of the people in your care. This is especially true if you work in a long-term care or home setting. It is never acceptable to take something that belongs to someone else, even if the person does not seem to need the item. People who are elderly or ill are particularly at risk for having money or belongings stolen from them. Family members, friends, staff members or even other people receiving care in the facility may commit larceny. If you notice that items are missing, or if you see someone taking an item that belongs to one of the people in your care, you must report this to the nurse.

A job in health care also gives employees access to things like medications. Taking medications from the people receiving care in the facility, or from the facility itself, is another form of larceny.

USING ETHICS TO GUIDE BEHAVIOR

As a nurse assistant, you have a responsibility to act within the law. However, not every decision you make with regard to how to behave or act will be guided by your knowledge of what you must do in order to avoid breaking the law. Many decisions will be guided instead by your knowledge of what is right, meaning what is good or moral. When you do what is right (that is, when you act in an ethical manner), you go beyond what is legally required.

Your own personal code of ethics is influenced by the beliefs and principles that you choose to live by. These beliefs and principles are in turn influenced by many different factors, including your upbringing, your religious or spiritual beliefs, your culture and your life experiences. Many professions also have codes of ethics that guide decision making and behavior for the people who practice that profession. For example, five ethical principles that are especially relevant to health care workers include the following:

- **Autonomy.** Every person has the right to make decisions about matters that affect him personally.
- **Justice.** All people—regardless of race, religion, culture, sexual orientation, disability or ability to pay for services—deserve fair and equal treatment.
- **Beneficence.** Health care workers are obligated to act in a way that promotes the well-being of those in their care.
- **Nonmaleficence.** Health care workers are obligated to avoid harming those in their care.
- **Fidelity.** Health care workers are obligated to act in a way that is truthful and trustworthy.

Any behavior that could cause harm to a person, either physically or emotionally, is unethical. You may have to decide the right thing to do in situations involving people in your care. For example, consider the following situation. A resident is slightly injured when another nurse assistant accidentally catches his finger in the wheelchair brake. The nurse assistant does not report the incident, so you have to decide whether to report it. If you decide not to report the incident, you may not be committing a crime. But are you acting in an ethical manner?

Later that morning, you approach the nurse to discuss the situation with Mrs. Millen. You tell the nurse that you overheard two nurse assistants talking about Mrs. Millen, and that she apparently heard them talking about her too. You ask the nurse's opinion about the best way to deal with the situation.

How is making the decision to discuss the situation involving Mrs. Millen with the nurse a reflection of your personal ethical standards? What about your ethical standards as a health care worker?

Often situations arise in health care where there may be more than one good or moral solution, depending on one's point of view. These situations are called **ethical dilemmas**. Ethical dilemmas can arise when a person receiving health care is not able to make her preferences known. When this occurs, members of the health care team have to make the decision that they feel is best for the person in their care. Different members of the team may have differing but equally valid viewpoints, depending on their own personal ethical standards and their individual knowledge of the person and the situation. In difficult situations like this, the health care team may seek the help of an **ethics committee** in resolving the ethical dilemma. Members of the ethics committee have many different areas of expertise, and an in-depth knowledge of ethical principles. After the facts of the case are presented to the ethics committee, the committee members help the health care team to find a solution that takes into account the best interests of the person receiving care.

AVOIDING LEGAL AND ETHICAL DIFFICULTIES ON THE JOB

Your work as a nurse assistant will put you in many different situations and require you to make many different decisions about how to behave or what to do. These decisions may not always be straightforward. To best serve those in your care, and to help protect yourself and your employer from legal and ethical difficulties, follow the guidelines in Box 3-1.

Box 3-1 Nurse Assistant DO's and DON'Ts

Avoiding Legal and Ethical Difficulties

DO practice the five principles of care (safety, dignity, independence, privacy, communication) with every person in your care.

DO be knowledgeable about the rights of the people in your care, as outlined in the Resident Rights portion of OBRA, the American Hospital Association's The Patient Care Partnership, or the National Association for Home Care and Hospice's Patient Rights.

DO be aware of legislation that protects the rights of the people receiving health care, such as the Patient Self-Determination Act and the Health Insurance Portability and Accountability Act (HIPAA).

DO be aware of ethical principles that guide the actions of health care workers: autonomy, justice, beneficence, nonmaleficence and fidelity.

DO be familiar with your employer's policies and procedures.

DO be familiar with your scope of practice, as defined by your job description, your employer and your state.

DON'T perform tasks or make decisions that are outside of your scope of practice.

DON'T accept gifts of personal belongings or money from those in your care or from their family members. Although the gift is often a genuine gesture of gratitude and appreciation for a job well done, accepting such a gift could set you up for accusations of illegal or unethical behavior later. Most employers have policies that prohibit employees from accepting gifts from those in their care, or from their family members.

DO seek help from your supervisor if you are not sure of the correct legal or ethical action to take in a situation.

CHECK YOUR UNDERSTANDING

Questions for Review

1. A nurse assistant is careless and fails to check the linens for personal items before stripping the bed and sending the soiled linens to the laundry. As a result, a resident's dentures are put through the washing machine and damaged. This is an example of:

a. Larceny
b. HIPAA violation
c. Negligence
d. Abuse

2. You suspect that one of your home health clients is being abused by her son. The woman becomes withdrawn and fearful whenever he is in the room, and you have noticed some strange bruises on her arm. What should you do?

a. Call the police immediately.
b. Confront the son and tell him to stop, or you will call the police.
c. Report your concerns to your supervisor at the agency.
d. Nothing; this is a private family matter.

3. Which legislation supports a patient's, resident's or client's right to make decisions on his or her own behalf?

a. Health Insurance Portability and Accountability Act (HIPAA)
b. Advance Directive Act
c. Patient Self-Determination Act
d. Patient Autonomy Act

4. Mrs. Underwood has dementia and has signed a document giving her husband the authority to make decisions about her care on her behalf. What is this document called?

a. Durable power of attorney for healthcare
b. Living will
c. Informed consent form
d. Beneficence form

5. Which of the following actions supports a person's legal rights under HIPAA?

a. A nurse assistant closes the door to a person's room before having a conversation with the person about her care.
b. A hospital stops documenting patient care on paper records and begins using a computer instead.
c. A nursing home has a policy that says all residents will receive equal treatment, regardless of their ability to pay for services.
d. A nurse obtains informed consent from a person before the person undergoes a surgical procedure.

Questions to Ask Yourself

1. *One of the friends you made during nurse assistant training is posting comments about situations and the people she cares for on a social networking site. Last night, she wrote "My thoughts and prayers are with the Miller family." Would you say anything to your friend about her posts? Why or why not?*
2. *You are providing care for Miss Eller. She is dying. She says she would like for you to have a ring that belonged to her sister, who died last year. What should you say?*
3. *You see a co-worker slapping a person in her care. What should you do?*
4. *You meet some people in the grocery store who recognize you as the nurse assistant who is providing care for their aunt, Mary. They ask you specific questions about her medical condition. How do you reply?*
5. *One of your home health clients tells you that he hides his pills and does not take them. He shows you his hiding place for the pills because he trusts you. What should you do?*
6. *You see a nurse assistant removing a watch belonging to one of the residents in her care from the resident's bedside table drawer while the resident is attending an activity session. What are possible reasons the nurse assistant could be removing the watch? Are all of them necessarily unethical or illegal?*

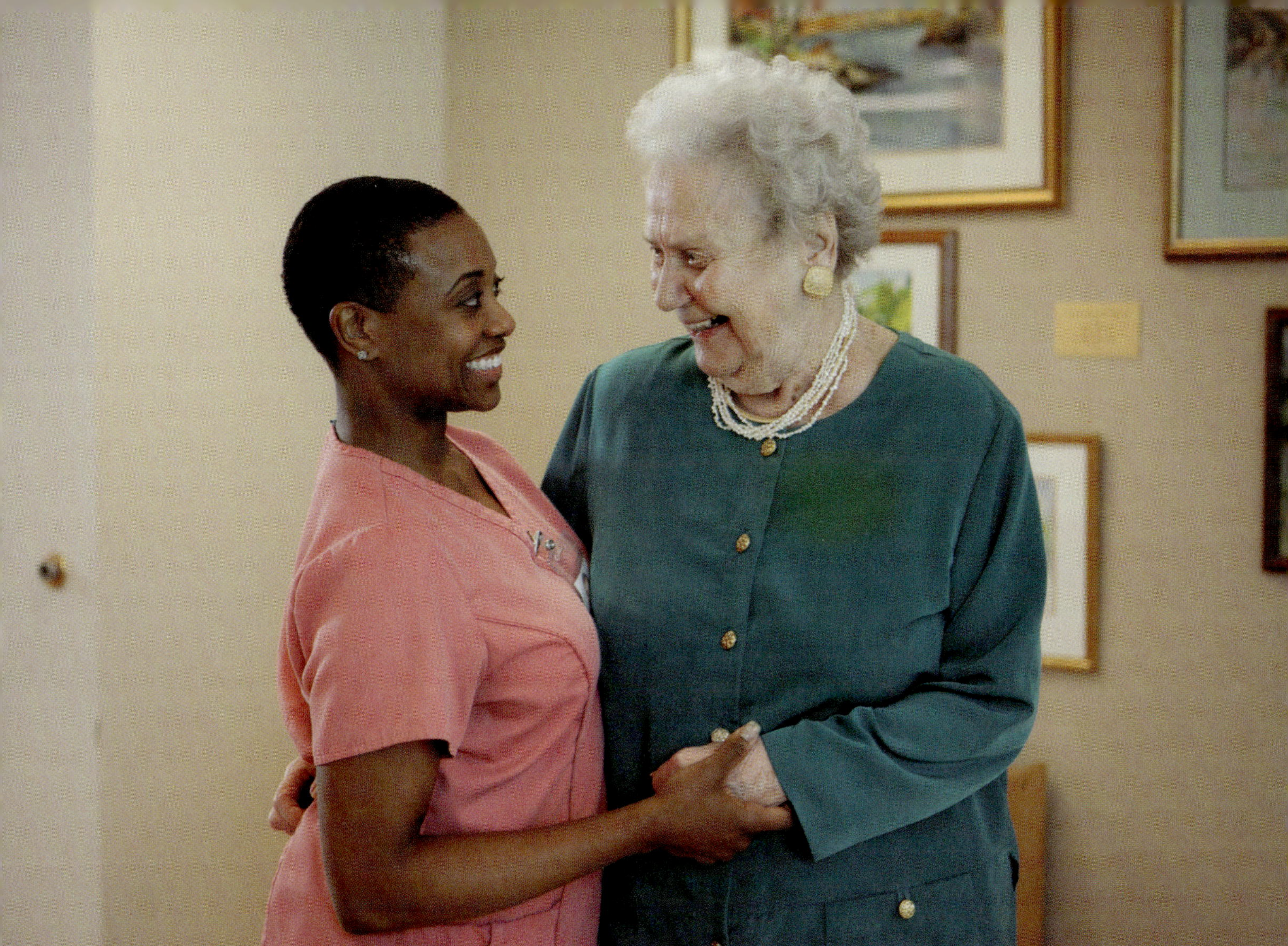

Understanding the People in Our Care

CHAPTER 4

Goals

After reading this chapter, you will have the information needed to:

- List the stages of human growth and development, and describe some of the physical changes and developmental tasks a person who is in each stage may face.
- Explain the five levels of human needs as defined by Maslow, and describe actions a nurse assistant can take to help a person meet his or her needs at each level.
- Explain the concepts of sexuality and intimacy, and understand how a nurse assistant can respect others' sexuality and need for intimate relationships.
- Describe preferences a person may have while receiving health care that may be influenced by the person's culture.
- Describe how a nurse assistant can help to support a person's spirituality.

Key Terms:

- **human growth**
- **human development**
- **sexuality**
- **sexual behaviors**
- **gender identity**
- **sexual identity**
- **intimacy**
- **masturbation**
- **erection**
- **transgender**
- **transsexual**
- **heterosexual**
- **homosexual**
- **bisexual**
- **culture**
- **spirituality**

Mrs. Josie McMillen, age 77, came to live at Morningside Nursing Home 3 years ago after health problems made it impossible for her to remain in her own home. Mrs. McMillen has many chronic health problems, including severe rheumatoid arthritis in the joints of her hands. You have cared for Mrs. McMillen for the past 2 years, and you can always tell when she is having a flare-up of her arthritis. On those days, Mrs. McMillen has little interest in eating, socializing or doing anything else because the pain is so bad. She often just wants to stay in bed and watch her favorite religious program on the television, or listen to one of her favorite books from the Bible on CD.

Mrs. McMillen's husband died many years before Mrs. McMillen came to live at Morningside. Over the years, Mrs. McMillen developed a close friendship with Mr. Frank Knoll, a man who attended her church. Mr. Knoll's wife had also died several years previously. One day, Mr. Knoll invited Mrs. McMillen to lunch after church, and soon they were spending more and more time together. But eventually, Mr. Knoll's house became too much for him to take care of on his own, so he decided to sell his house and move in with his daughter and son-in-law. Usually, Mr. Knoll's daughter or son-in-law brings him to Morningside to visit with Mrs. McMillen at least once a week. Mrs. McMillen tells you often how much she looks forward to Mr. Knoll's visits. She says, "He always makes me laugh, and it's so good to talk to him."

Throughout the first few chapters of this book, you have learned how important it is to appreciate each person in your care as the individual that he or she is. Our upbringing, our beliefs and values, our culture, our life experiences and the qualities we are born with (for example, our personality, sense of humor, or brown eyes) all combine to make each of us a unique individual. But at the same time, there are many experiences and needs that all humans share. In this chapter, we'll take a look at some of the things that all human beings have in common.

HUMAN GROWTH AND DEVELOPMENT

All people move on the same basic track through life. They begin as infants, then grow into children, develop into teens, mature into adults and become elderly. The process of moving from one stage of life to the next is called human growth and development. Human growth and development is characterized by changes. **Human growth** refers to physical changes, such as growing bigger and cutting teeth in infancy, or developing breasts or a beard in adolescence. **Human development** refers to social changes (the way the person relates to others), emotional changes (the way the person feels and expresses those feelings) and cognitive changes (the way the person thinks and understands the world).

There are many different theories related to human growth and development. Scientists who study human growth and development typically divide the process into separate stages. Although ages are given here as a point of reference, it is important not to confuse *ages* with *stages*, because there is no definite age at which someone can or should be able to do something. One common way of defining these stages is as follows (see also Table 4-1):

- **Infancy (birth to 1 year).** When babies are born, they have been growing and developing since conception, about 9 months. At birth, babies are called neonates, and by the time they are 1 month old, they are called infants. Infancy is a time of rapid growth and development changes.
- **Toddlerhood (1 to 3 years).** During toddlerhood, the child is very busy learning about his world. Physical coordination increases, allowing the toddler to be quite active and develop the skills necessary for tasks such as dressing, eating and using the toilet.
- **Preschool age (3 to 5 years).** Preschool-age children can do many things for themselves; have friends; may go to nursery school or kindergarten; and spend a great deal of time "pretending" to be grown-ups. However, they still see the world through young children's eyes and imagine and fear things adults know cannot be possible.

Table 4-1 **Stages of Human Growth and Development**

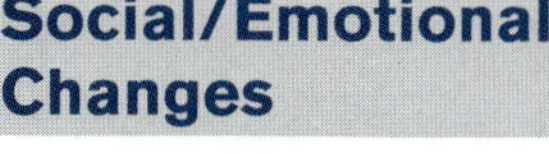

Stage	Physical Changes	Social/Emotional Changes	Cognitive Changes
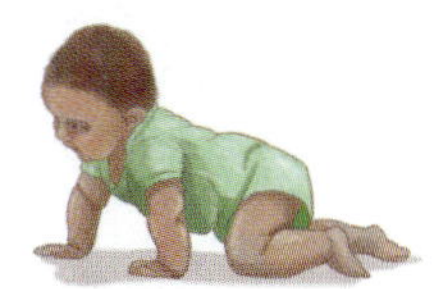 **Infancy: birth to 1 year**	■ May triple in weight and increase greatly in length by 1 year ■ Begins to control body movement: lifts head; holds and throws objects and puts them in mouth; rolls over, sits up, crawls, climbs, takes first steps with assistance; and stands ■ Begins cutting teeth and taking solid food	■ Cries to communicate ■ Begins to smile and laugh ■ Begins to trust caregivers and cry at the sight of strangers	■ Uses senses to explore the world ■ Begins to say a few short words
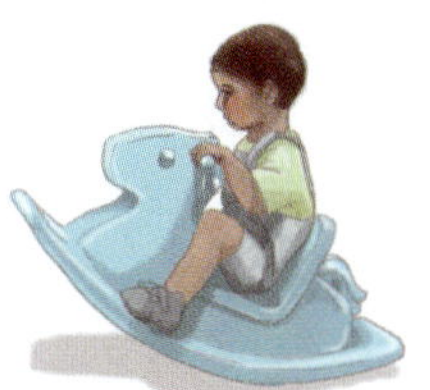 **Toddlerhood: 1 to 3 years**	■ Does many things that require coordination of large muscles in arms and legs: walks, runs, jumps and climbs ■ Plays with toys ■ Has 6 to 12 baby teeth and eats regular table food ■ Learns to use the toilet and eats, drinks and dresses with little or no help ■ Needs to rest frequently during the day	■ Likes to play alone or side by side with another child, and tends not to share toys ■ Independence increases, and the toddler does not like to be told what to do ■ Throws temper tantrums when desires are not met ■ May be afraid when separated from parents or other familiar caregivers	■ Able to follow simple instructions when given slowly and clearly ■ Responds fairly well to adult language and can point to objects named by adults ■ Has a strong, self-oriented point of view and is unable to understand others' points of view ■ Begins to put words together to make short sentences ■ Understands that objects taken out of sight still exist ■ Likes to choose own activities and toys
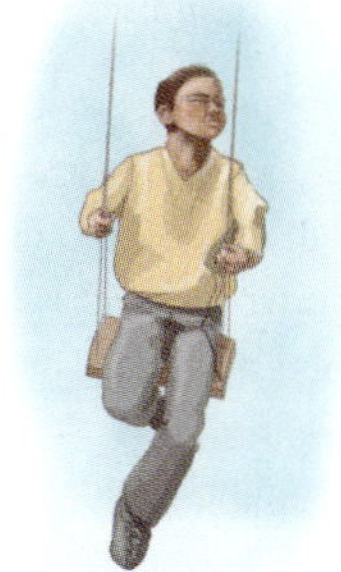 **Preschool Age: 3 to 5 years**	■ Has improved large-motor skills ■ Has more control over small-motor skills such as drawing or writing ■ Does many things to take care of self such as dressing, eating and using the toilet	■ Has a strong sense of identity ■ Makes own choices ■ Plays easily with other children and enjoys games involving sharing and taking turns ■ Looks up to and imitates adults ■ Likes routine and may feel insecure if schedule is changed too often	■ Learns new words quickly and may start to read some words; counts and enjoys learning things with numbers ■ Groups objects that are alike and is able to pick out objects that do not fit with others ■ Follows directions ■ Has strong curiosity and imagination and asks many questions ■ Has a strong, self-oriented point of view and sometimes is unable to understand others' points of view

Continued on next page

Table 4-1 **Stages of Human Growth and Development** *continued*

Stage	Physical Changes	Social/Emotional Changes	Cognitive Changes
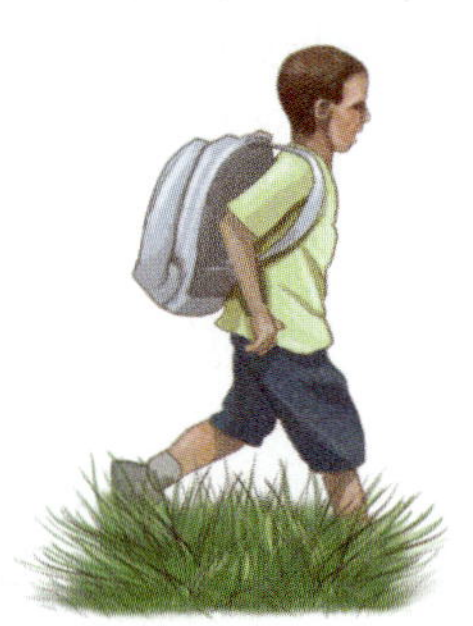 **School Age: 5 to 12 years**	■ Grows steadily ■ Develops muscle tone, balance, strength and endurance and is physically well coordinated ■ Uses large muscles for games and sports, cycling and dance ■ Uses small muscles to write, draw and do crafts ■ Enters puberty at about age 10 to 12 for girls and age 12 for boys	■ Begins to form lasting relationships with friends ■ Forms small, close-knit groups that exclude other children, especially those of the opposite sex ■ Spends more time away from parents or other caregivers ■ Begins to understand that other people also have feelings ■ Has many emotions and sometimes has difficulty expressing them; may have dramatic mood swings that accompany hormonal changes when going through puberty	■ Pays attention longer, remembers longer and follows more complex directions ■ Ability to think logically and make decisions increases ■ Starts to organize new information in meaningful ways ■ Behaves more responsibly ■ May question and resist adult decisions
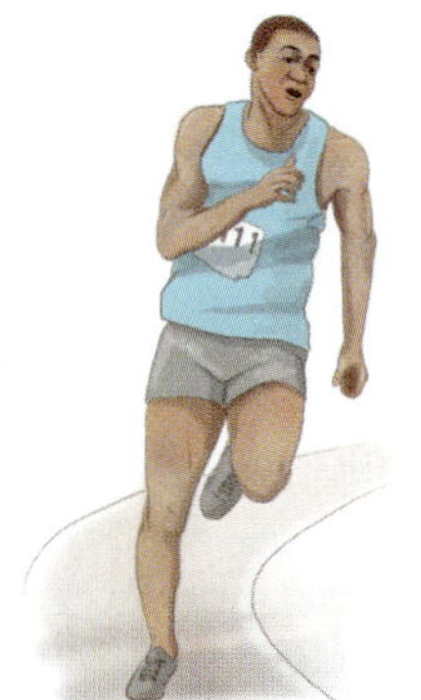 **Adolescence: 12 to 20 years**	■ Reaches reproductive maturity: in girls, breasts develop, hips widen, pubic and underarm hair appears and menstruation begins; in boys, penis and testes grow to adult size, ejaculations begin, pubic and facial hair develops, voice deepens and neck and shoulders grow ■ Girls tend to be taller than boys of the same age at the beginning of this age range and tend to be shorter at the end	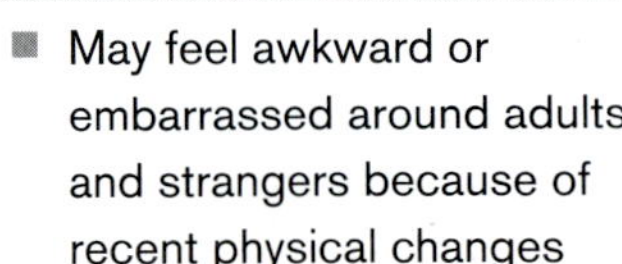 ■ May feel awkward or embarrassed around adults and strangers because of recent physical changes ■ Assumes more responsibility for own behavior ■ Often rebels against adult authority	■ Able to think logically and understand abstract concepts ■ Imagines alternatives when making a decision, which makes decision making more difficult ■ Plans for the future ■ Becomes more self-conscious and concerned with physical appearance ■ Is easily disappointed and discouraged ■ May set unreasonable goals
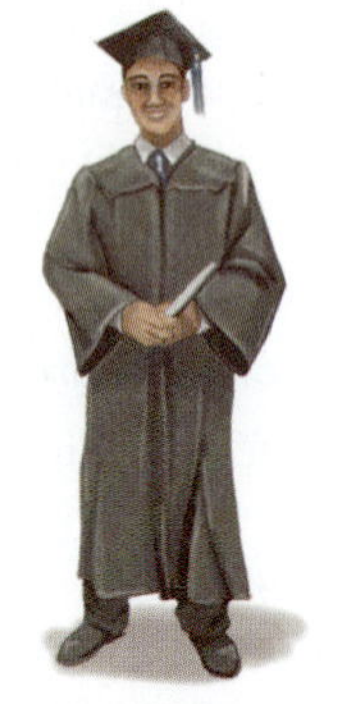 **Young Adult Years: 20 to 45 years**	■ Muscle strength, bone density and senses are at their peak ■ Gets sick infrequently, and recovers quickly from illnesses and injuries ■ Women may experience physical changes of pregnancy	■ Establishes lasting and intimate relationships with friends and partners ■ Makes commitments ■ May begin a family	■ Functions at higher level than children and adolescents, although some young adults continue to think and reason much like adolescents and children ■ Is able to imagine being in another person's situation and recognize how another feels ■ Has better-developed moral reasoning

Table 4-1 **Stages of Human Growth and Development** *continued*

Stage	Physical Changes	Social/Emotional Changes	Cognitive Changes
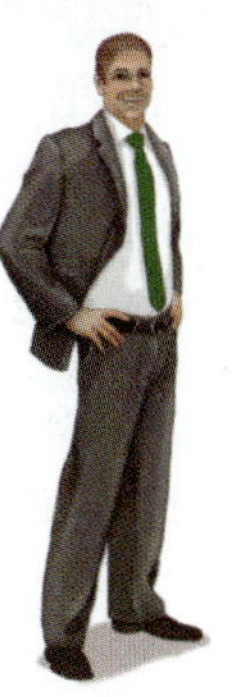 **Middle Adult Years: 45 to 64 years**	■ May develop chronic illnesses, although some find that existing health conditions disappear or become less problematic ■ May have slight decreases in senses, physical strength and coordination ■ Women experience menopause 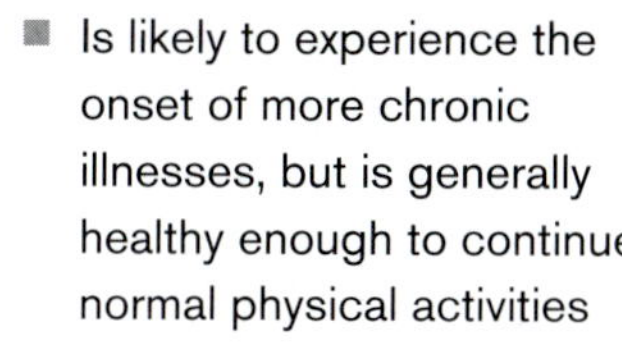	■ Begins to feel anxious about aging ■ Feels more satisfied by work ■ May become depressed as children grow up and leave, or may delight in the new freedom ■ Often takes on more responsibility for caring for aging parents ■ May have to cope with the loss of one or both parents ■ May become a grandparent	■ Increases in mental growth and has high levels of intellectual performance ■ Finds this is often the most creative time of life
Young-Old Years: 65 to 75 years	■ Is likely to experience the onset of more chronic illnesses, but is generally healthy enough to continue normal physical activities	■ May retire from a job, which can lead to increased energy, productivity and creativity; feelings of loss; or both ■ May have to cope with death of a spouse, friends or other family members (such as siblings) ■ May have to cope with losses of independence, such as those caused by giving up a driver's license, moving out of one's own home or accepting the need for someone else to enter the home to provide care	■ Generally maintains intellectual abilities and may pursue new interests and hobbies 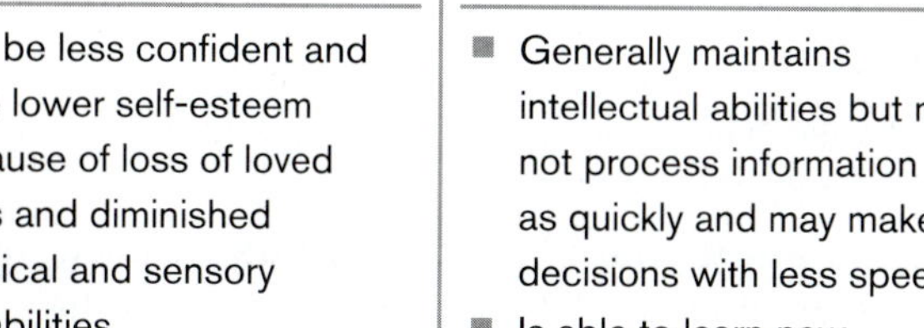
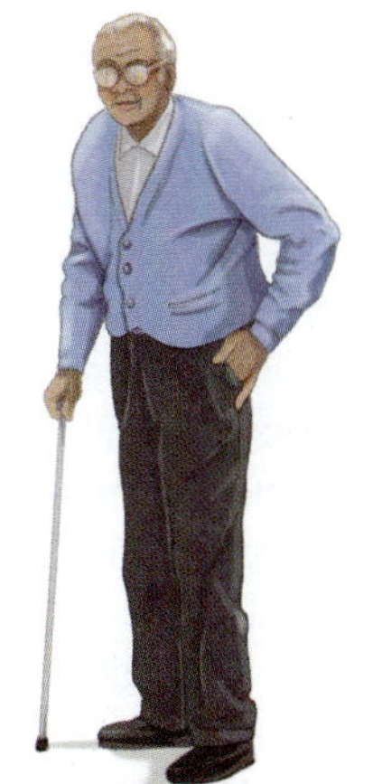 **Middle-Old Years: 75 to 85 years**	■ May have decreased vision, with loss of night vision and less depth and color perception ■ May experience some hearing loss and a decreased sense of smell and taste ■ May have less strength and balance and may be prone to accidents and falling ■ May be noticeably shorter because of spinal column shrinkage ■ May adjust less quickly to cold	■ May be less confident and have lower self-esteem because of loss of loved ones and diminished physical and sensory capabilities ■ Often has to cope with major life changes, such as the death of a spouse or the need to sell a house and move	■ Generally maintains intellectual abilities but may not process information as quickly and may make decisions with less speed ■ Is able to learn new information and skills but needs more time to learn

Continued on next page

Table 4-1 **Stages of Human Growth and Development** *continued*

Stage	Physical Changes	Social/Emotional Changes	Cognitive Changes
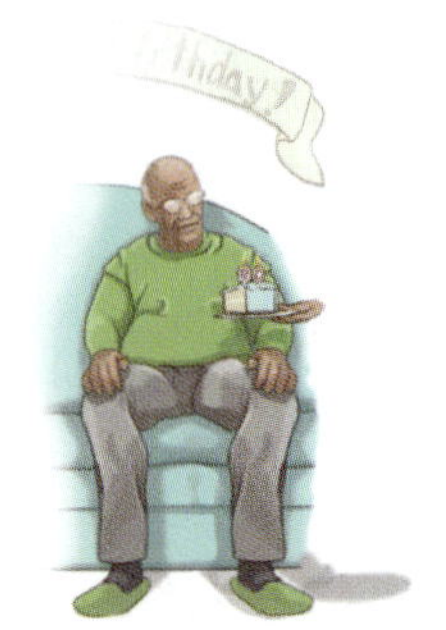 Old-Old Years: 85 years and older	■ Physical abilities may continue to decrease, both as a result of normal changes of aging and illness or injury	■ May struggle with accepting failing health or increased dependency on others for assistance and care ■ May begin to think about and plan for own death ■ May look back and reflect on own life	■ Generally maintains intellectual abilities but may not process information as quickly and may make decisions with less speed ■ Is able to learn new information and skills but needs more time to learn

- **School age (5 to 12 years).** School-age children seem like miniature adults at times. They can hold very interesting conversations and have firm opinions. Throughout the school-age years, the child goes through many growth spurts, leading to steady increases in height and weight.
- **Adolescence (12 to 20 years).** During adolescence, children leave their childhood ways behind and gradually move into adulthood. Their bodies reach full size during these years, and their minds begin to work like those of adults. Social and emotional experiences are intense as strong friendships and early love relationships develop. Some adolescents begin sexual relationships and may parent children of their own.
- **Young adult years (20 to 45 years).** For most people, the young adult years are filled with beginnings: living on one's own away from parents, starting a career, beginning a relationship with someone who may eventually be a life partner or spouse. Many young adults begin a family by conceiving or adopting children.
- **Middle adult years (45 to 65 years).** During the middle adult years, many people experience the satisfaction of enjoying what they began in their 20s and 30s. Their careers are often at their peak, children are growing or grown, and finances may be secure enough to allow for more leisure time. During this stage, many people become caregivers to aging parents, and may experience the loss of a parent. Many middle adults also become grandparents.
- **Young-old years (65 to 75 years).** During this period, the person may retire from a job. For some people, this is a welcome event, but others may struggle with the change in role or the need to adjust to living on a fixed income. The person may begin to notice changes in physical abilities related to the process of aging, or the onset of disease or disability.
- **Middle-old years (75 to 85 years).** Many people continue to enjoy good health, although others will begin to experience health problems. The person may need to come to terms with an increased need to rely on the help of others with tasks such as maintaining the house or driving. The person may begin to experience repeated losses, such as the loss of independence associated with having to give up a driver's license or home, or the deaths of a spouse or other family members and friends.
- **Old-old years (85 years and beyond).** During this stage, people look back on their lives and begin to prepare for their own deaths. Often, the person must cope with increasing losses: the deaths of friends, family members, and possibly a spouse; physical limitations caused by the process of aging; and the increasing loss of independence. Many older adults become mentors to younger people by sharing the perspectives and knowledge only a lifetime of experiences can provide.

Being able to recognize the developmental stage of a person in your care will help you to better understand the person's needs, behavior and responses to situations. This understanding will also help you to communicate more effectively with the person, in terms that are appropriate for the person's developmental level. However, always remember that the characteristics given in Table 4-1 are general guidelines, not rules. You should expect to see many individual differences among those in your care.

ELDER CARE NOTE. Many people have beliefs about aging that are not based in fact. These beliefs can lead to ageism (having preconceived negative ideas about aging or elderly people). For example, although many of the people who

become residents of nursing homes are elderly and have some form of cognitive impairment (such as dementia), dementia is not a normal or expected consequence of aging. Similarly, neither is incontinence (an inability to control the release of urine or feces). Many older adults enjoy relatively good health and are able to remain quite independent well into their later years. As a nurse assistant, it is important to understand each person in your care as the unique individual that he is, and to avoid making assumptions about what the person can do or should do based on his age.

Remember Mrs. McMillen, whom you met at the beginning of this chapter? What developmental tasks might she be facing at this point in her life?

BASIC HUMAN NEEDS

To live and to be healthy and happy, certain basic needs must be met. Many years ago, Abraham Maslow, a famous psychologist, developed a theory about people and their needs. According to Maslow's theory, people have needs on different levels. A person must meet lower level needs before she can meet higher level needs. To illustrate his theory, Maslow organized human needs into a pyramid, called a hierarchy, from lowest to highest (Figure 4-1).

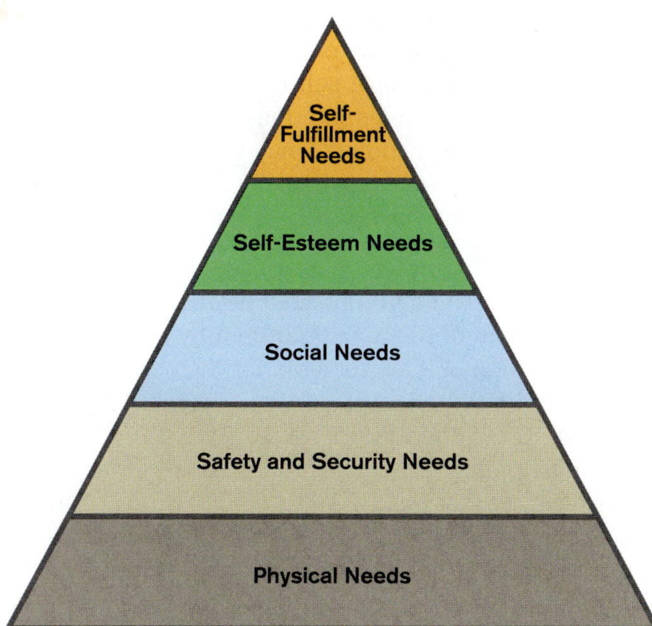

Figure 4-1 Maslow's hierarchy of needs.

Maslow defined five levels of needs: physical needs, safety and security needs, social needs, self-esteem needs, and self-fulfillment needs. As a nurse assistant, you play a large role in helping people meet their physical, safety and security, social, and self-esteem needs. As the needs at these first four levels are met, the person turns inward to meet the self-fulfillment needs at the top of the pyramid on his or her own.

Maslow's theory is just one of many theories about basic human needs, but it provides a good framework for caregiving. Understanding the idea that basic needs must be met before more advanced needs can be met will help you provide better care. For example, a person who is having difficulty breathing is not going to have the interest or energy to try to meet higher level needs, such as the need to socialize with others. By helping people to meet their most basic needs first, you can make it easier for them to meet their higher level needs.

Physical Needs

Physical needs are basic requirements for life, such as food, water, oxygen, exercise, sleep, the ability to eliminate bodily wastes and the ability to experience human touch. As a nurse assistant, many of your daily responsibilities will have to do with helping people to meet basic physical needs (Figure 4-2). For example, you will help people with eating, toileting, and walking or other forms of exercise. You will help to ensure that the people in your care are able to rest by maintaining a quiet, restful environment and providing clean linens. You will help meet the person's need for physical contact by gently squeezing her hand, patting her arm or giving her a hug.

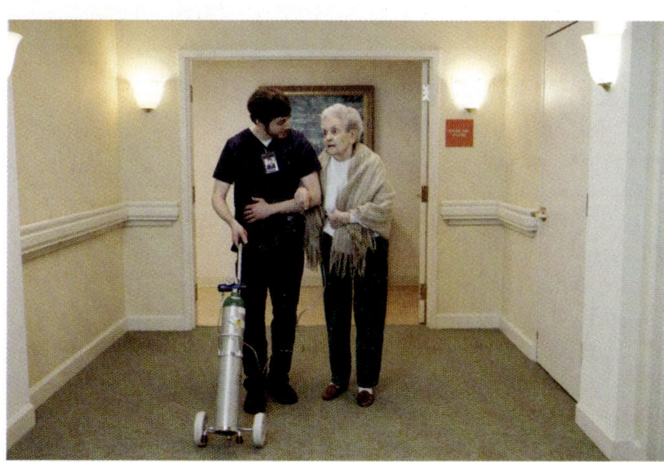

Figure 4-2 Physical needs must be met before a person can think about meeting higher level needs.

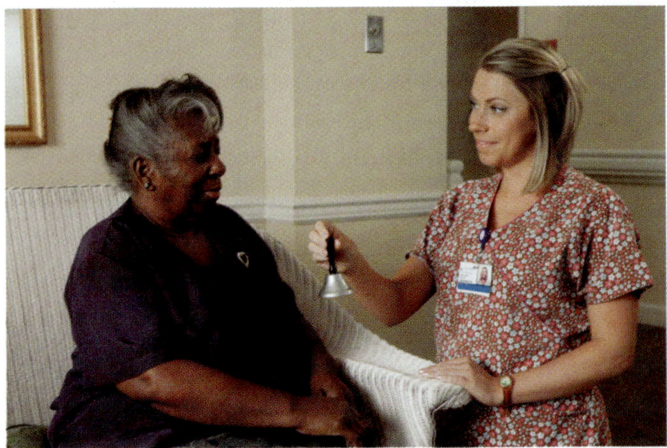

Figure 4-3 Making sure the person has a way to call for help if she needs it is one way nurse assistants help to meet the person's need to feel safe and secure.

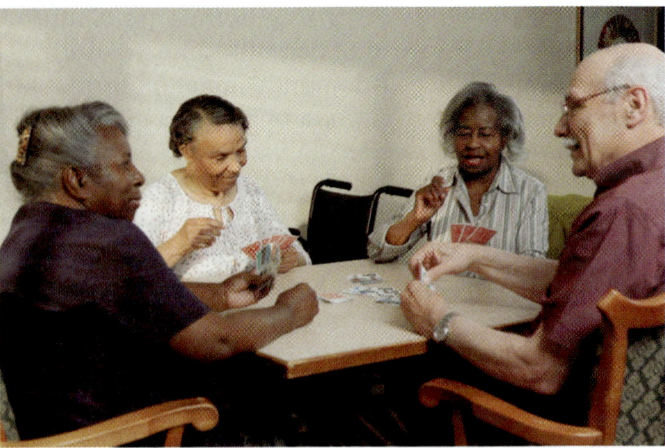

Figure 4-4 All people have the need to interact socially with others.

Safety and Security Needs

Remember that safety is one of the five principles of care. As you continue through this course, you will learn many different actions that you can take to keep the people in your care safe and secure. For example, you will take steps to prevent the spread of microbes that can cause infection, lock the brakes on equipment with wheels to prevent injuries, and keep a close eye on people who may be confused and at risk for wandering away from the facility.

In addition to helping the people in your care *be* safe, you will help them to *feel* safe (Figure 4-3). When we feel safe, we can relax and rest. Simple actions, such as checking on each person in your care frequently and answering requests for help promptly, build trust and help the people in your care to feel safe and secure. What makes someone feel safe and secure may vary from person to person, so make an effort to find out each person's preferences. For example, one person may feel more secure with the door to her room closed, while another may want to leave the door to her room open.

Social Needs

Most people need to be liked, loved and accepted by individuals and groups (Figure 4-4). These are social needs. No one wants to be ignored, to feel left out or to feel unloved or lonely. As a nurse assistant, you can help meet the social needs of the people in your care many times each day. You can be especially helpful when a person's family and friends cannot be with her. Take the time to sit with the person and look through a photo album together, help with a crossword puzzle or just talk with the person for a little while. In long-term care facilities, there are many ways you can help residents to meet their social needs. For example, planned activities (such as games, holiday celebrations and musical performances) give residents an opportunity to meet other residents and socialize. You will also help residents to meet their social needs by assisting them to the dining room for meals, so that they can enjoy the company of others while eating.

Self-Esteem Needs

People need to feel good about themselves, and that they are worthy of the respect of others. People who are in need of health care often feel that they are no longer important and that they cannot contribute in a meaningful way. The loss of ability and independence that may come with illness, injury or advanced age can affect a person's self-esteem. A loss of cognitive ability (such as that which occurs with dementia) can also affect a person's self-esteem. For a person with dementia, even a simple question like "What do you want to wear today?" may be very difficult to answer. The person's inability to answer the question easily can have a very negative impact on her self-esteem.

As a nurse assistant, you help to protect and build the self-esteem of those in your care by allowing them to do as much as possible for themselves, and recognizing their accomplishments. Take an interest in the person, and encourage him to talk about past accomplishments (such as raising a family or serving in the military) that make him feel proud. Make sure you communicate with the person at a level she understands, to make it easier for her to respond appropriately. (For example, instead of asking a person with dementia what she wants to wear, offer her two choices of outfits so that she can easily pick one.) Show the person that he is still worthy of the respect of others by treating him with respect yourself (for example, address the person in the way that he likes to be addressed). On a very basic level, helping the person with bathing and grooming also builds self-esteem by helping the person feel confident and attractive to others (Figure 4-5).

Self-Fulfillment Needs

Self-fulfillment means that a person feels satisfied with herself and her life. When a person's self-fulfillment needs are satisfied, she believes that she is doing what she is best suited to do (Figure 4-6). For example, a person may experience self-fulfillment by writing a great book, working toward finding a cure for a disease, becoming a terrific parent or working to provide good care for the elderly. Because each person excels in different areas of life, each person's self-fulfilling experience will be different.

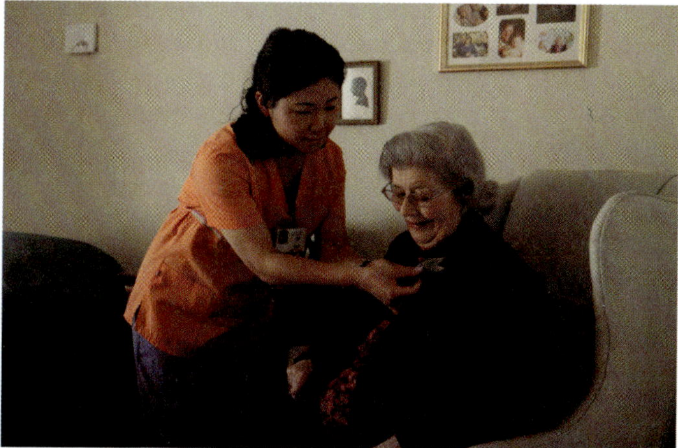

Figure 4-5 Helping a person to look and feel her best helps to build the person's self-esteem.

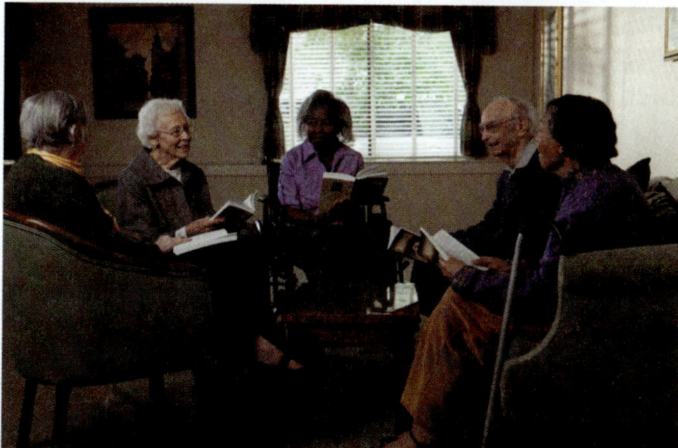

Figure 4-6 This resident of a nursing home, a retired teacher, continues to find self-fulfillment by leading a book discussion group at the facility.

This morning, when you go to Mrs. McMillen's room to help her with her morning care, you can tell that she is not having a good day. As you help her get out of bed and to the bathroom, she tells you that she did not sleep well the night before, and that the pain is really bad. She says, "Frank is supposed to come today and we were going to have lunch, but I don't know if I even have the energy. Maybe I should call him and tell him not to come."

Which needs of Mrs. McMillen's are a priority now? How are these needs affecting her ability to meet her other needs?

What can you do to help Mrs. McMillen meet her needs?

SEXUALITY AND INTIMACY

All people are sexual beings, and have a need for sexual expression and sexual pleasure. How we perceive ourselves and express ourselves sexually is called **sexuality**. Sexuality is related to many different concepts, including **sexual behaviors** (physical activities, such as sexual intercourse and masturbation, related to obtaining sexual pleasure and reproducing), **gender identity** (a person's inner sense of being male or female), and **sexual identity** (a person's sexual orientation and preferences with regard to sexual partners).

The need and ability of a person to feel emotionally close to another human being and to have that closeness returned is called **intimacy**. Intimacy includes all the good feelings that people have for one another, such as liking, loving, sharing and caring (Figure 4-7). To express

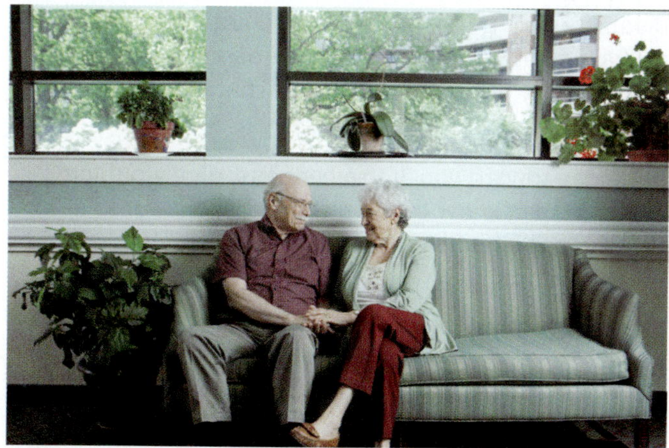

Figure 4-7 All people have the need to develop close emotional ties with others.

their feelings of intimacy, people may kiss, hug, touch or hold hands, or they may simply engage in private conversations. Intimate relationships may or may not involve sexual activity.

ELDER CARE NOTE. It is important to remember that *all* people, young and old alike, have the need to think of themselves as sexual beings and engage in intimate relationships (which may or may not involve sexual activity).

Sexual Behaviors

Sexual behaviors include activities a person engages in to derive sexual pleasure or to reproduce, such as sexual intercourse with a partner or **masturbation** (touching or rubbing one's own genitals for sexual release or pleasure).

As a nurse assistant, you must respect the right of those in your care to engage in sexual behaviors, and provide the necessary privacy. Since many people might be embarrassed to ask for privacy, you must look for cues that a person or couple may want to be alone. When a couple is together, excuse yourself and say what time you will be back. As always, knock on the person's door and wait for a reply before entering. Be aware that a person who is confused may engage in sexual behaviors, such as masturbation, outside of the privacy of his or her room. If this occurs, help the person back to his or her room and provide the necessary privacy.

You will also have the responsibility of protecting the people in your care from unwanted sexual advances. Although everyone has the right to express himself or herself sexually, he or she must only exercise that right with someone who is a willing participant. A person who is confused may not be able to consent to sexual activity, because he or she may not understand what is happening. Similarly, a person with a developmental disability may be physically old enough to engage in sexual activity, but may not be emotionally ready or intellectually able to understand what is happening.

Sometimes, a person may make unwanted sexual advances toward you. If this happens, gently but firmly let the person know that you want the behavior to stop. You can say something such as:

- "I really like you as a person, but I don't like it when you touch me that way."
- "I really enjoy providing care for you, but I feel uncomfortable when you talk to me that way."
- "I want you to stop touching me like that. Please do not do that again."

At the same time, you must be careful not to misread something that may look like sexual attraction. For example, a man may have an **erection** while you are providing care. This physical change does not necessarily mean that he is attracted to you or that he is thinking about you sexually. An erection may mean the man has a full bladder, is thinking about something else that is sexually exciting, is feeling afraid or is feeling pleasure. You and the man may feel embarrassed. To make the situation more comfortable, you may want to talk about something unrelated or simply continue the task without talking.

Gender and Sexual Identity

Gender identity refers to how a person perceives his or her "maleness" or "femaleness." Most children recognize whether they are male or female by the age of two. They know by looking at their bodies whether they are girls or boys. Some people have a personal feeling that their gender does not match the physical body they were born with. They may be males who feel themselves to be female, females who feel themselves to be male, or people who do not strongly identify themselves as either male or female. Such people are called **transgender**. Transgender individuals may or may not become **transsexuals**, people who alter their physical appearance to more closely match the gender they most strongly identify with. A person who is transsexual may take hormones, have surgical procedures or both to alter his or her body to better match his or her inner sense of gender identity.

Sexual identity refers to a person's preferences with regard to sexual partners. A person can be attracted to someone of the opposite sex, the same sex or both. A person who is attracted to people of the opposite sex is called **heterosexual** (some also use the word "straight"), and a person who is attracted to people of the same sex is called **homosexual** (some also use the word "gay" to refer to a man who is attracted to other men, or "lesbian" to refer to a woman who is attracted to other women). A person who is attracted to people of both sexes is called **bisexual**.

Respecting Others' Sexuality

As a nurse assistant, you will provide care for people whose feelings and beliefs about sexuality will differ from yours. For example, you may have been raised with the belief that people who are not married should not have sex, that masturbation is wrong or that homosexual relationships are wrong. Regardless of your own beliefs and feelings, you must avoid being judgmental of those in your care, and treat every person in your care with respect and consideration.

CULTURE

Culture is a shared set of beliefs, values, customs and practices that characterizes a group of people or a society. Our culture affects how we view the world and respond to life's experiences. It helps us to understand who we are and how we fit into our society. Culture may be based on a common ethnic heritage, on a common geographic location, on common religious beliefs or on a combination of these (Figure 4-8).

Here in the United States, you may have the opportunity to care for people from many different cultures. It is important to understand how culture influences behavior. A person's cultural beliefs, values, customs and practices can influence many preferences a person receiving health care, or her family members, may have, such as preferences regarding:

- What foods are eaten, how they are prepared, when they are served and how they are served.
- Personal care rituals, such as when and how to bathe, or clothing selections.
- Who can provide care, especially care that involves exposing the person's body.
- Which family member should be consulted about the person's care.
- What type of touch is acceptable.
- What type of eye contact is acceptable.
- Social customs, such as what actions are considered polite and impolite.
- How illnesses should be managed and treated.
- What rituals should be followed leading up to and after death.
- What rituals should be followed leading up to and after giving birth.

Although information is available about cultural preferences, it is risky to make assumptions about what a person might prefer based on the person's name, nationality or physical appearance. The best approach is to be aware of areas where a person's culture may influence preferences, ask what the person's preferences are and then respect those preferences, even if they seem strange to you. Asking about the person's preferences shows the person you are interested in him or her as an individual, and can also prevent misunderstandings due to a lack of knowledge about the person's culture.

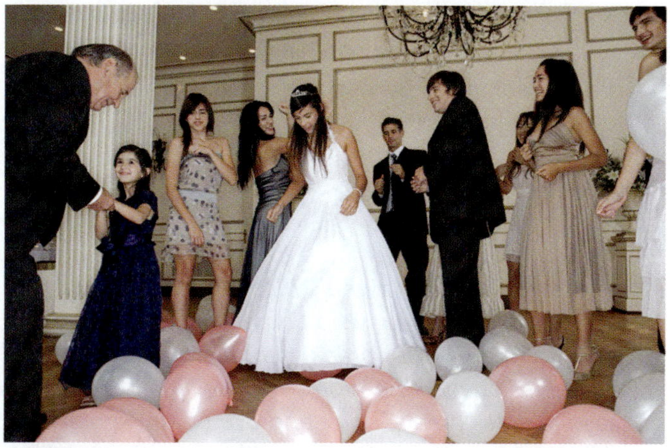

Figure 4-8 Quinceañera, a festive celebration surrounding a girl's fifteenth birthday, is a common tradition in many Hispanic cultures. *Image © AISPIX by Image Source, 2012. Used under license from Shutterstock.com.*

SPIRITUALITY

Spirituality is a belief in something greater than oneself that helps a person assign meaning and purpose to life. For many people, organized religion is closely linked to spirituality. However, many people are spiritual without participating in a formal, organized religion. Spirituality has to do with having an awareness of the purpose and meaning of life, and finding guidance and comfort in that awareness. Having a strong sense of spirituality can strengthen a person's ability to cope with difficult situations. Spiritual beliefs (such as the belief in a power greater than oneself) and practices (such as attending a religious service or engaging in quiet meditation or prayer) can provide mental relief by reducing stress and worry and increasing feelings of hope and gratitude.

As a nurse assistant, there are many things you can do to support and foster a person's sense of spirituality (Figure 4-9). A person may find it comforting to have you read from a book that is meaningful to him (such as a religious text or a book of poetry), to engage in a meaningful activity or ritual with him (such as prayer) or to help him with activities that strengthen his spirituality (such as writing in a journal, attending a religious service or visiting with a clergy member). Remember that you do not have to share the person's spiritual beliefs and practices in order to help the person benefit from those beliefs and practices.

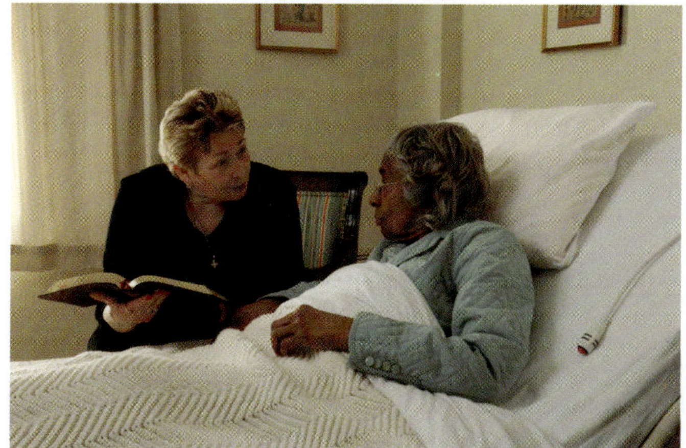

Figure 4-9 For many people that you care for, religious or spiritual beliefs will be a source of strength and comfort.

CHECK YOUR UNDERSTANDING

Questions for Review

1. **You are providing care for 13-year-old Kathy Harrison at her home while she is recovering from injuries caused by a car crash. She has stitches along her forehead and across one cheek. Her friends call, but she doesn't want to see them. She may be worrying that:**
   a. She will have to tell her friends that she cannot leave the house to go to the mall.
   b. Her friends will think she is ugly.
   c. Her mother won't let them come over.
   d. Her friends will bring her schoolwork.

2. **A nurse assistant helps Mrs. Smith, a resident of a nursing home, to meet her social needs by:**
   a. Ensuring Mrs. Smith has enough to eat.
   b. Helping Mrs. Smith get ready to attend a group activity.
   c. Encouraging Mrs. Smith to do as much for herself as possible.
   d. Making sure that Mrs. Smith feels safe and secure.

3. **Mr. Jameson always talks about his days as a leader in his union but he hardly ever talks about the present. When he starts to talk about the past, you should:**
   a. Tell him not to dwell on the past.
   b. Tell him how interesting it must have been in those days and ask him some questions about it.
   c. Change the subject by asking him what he would like to do today.
   d. Remind Mr. Jameson that he is retired now.

4. **A nurse assistant helps a person meet his self-esteem needs in all of the following ways EXCEPT:**
   a. Addressing the person in the way he prefers to be addressed.
   b. Doing everything for the person so that that he does not have to do anything.
   c. Taking care to protect the person's privacy and modesty.
   d. Taking an interest in the person as an individual.

5. **Sexuality is:**
   a. The physical act of having sexual intercourse.
   b. The ability to form intimate relationships with others.
   c. How a person perceives of herself and expresses herself sexually.
   d. Knowing whether you are a girl or a boy.

6. **A nurse assistant must care for people from many different cultures. How should the nurse assistant handle this?**
   a. The nurse assistant should advise people that when they are in the health care facility, they must follow the health care facility's policies and procedures.
   b. The nurse assistant should seek to understand each person as an individual, and accommodate the person's preferences whenever possible.
   c. The nurse assistant should use his or her own cultural beliefs to guide care.
   d. The nurse assistant should avoid caring for people who are from a different culture.

7. **Which of the following statements about older adults is true?**
   a. Older adults are not capable of learning new skills or concepts.
   b. Older adults may be sexually active and continue to need to have close, intimate relationships with others.
   c. Most people start to become confused as they age and become incapable of taking care of themselves.
   d. Older adults usually become depressed because they no longer have anything to contribute to their families, communities or society in general.

8. **Which of the following actions helps to meet a person's safety and security needs?**
   a. Encouraging the person to do as much for himself as he is able
   b. Answering the person's requests for help promptly
   c. Locking the person in his or her room
   d. Providing the person with privacy when he or she has visitors

Questions to Ask Yourself

1. *Mr. Robinson was admitted to the nursing home where you work last week. Mr. Robinson has a partner, Mr. Benning, who comes to visit him every day. You are on your break with another one of the nurse assistants who works on the floor, and he says to you, "I really don't approve of Mr. Robinson's relationship with Mr. Benning. It's just not natural." Do you think your co-worker's feelings might negatively affect his ability to care for Mr. Robinson? What would you say to your co-worker?*

2. *You are Mrs. Sokoloski's home health aide. Mrs. Sokoloski is receiving home care because she has several health issues that make it difficult for her to provide for her own personal care. Previously, Mrs. Sokoloski's husband took care of her and managed the house, but he died suddenly last month. Today, you make Mrs. Sokoloski lunch and sit with her while she eats. She just pushes the food around on the plate and she looks like she is on the verge of crying. She says to you, "Ralph and I used to always eat together. I'm so lonely and I miss him so much." What needs does Mrs. Sokoloski have? How can you help her to meet those needs?*

3. *Mrs. Kipper has dementia and is a resident in the nursing home where you work. Today, you found Mrs. Kipper half undressed and trying to get into bed with Mr. Lyons, another resident who also has dementia. When you arrived in the doorway of Mr. Lyons' room, Mr. Lyons was pushing Mrs. Kipper away and yelling, "Get out!" How should you handle this situation?*

4. *Mrs. Ali, a patient in the hospital where you work, has very different religious beliefs from your own. Today, she asks you to help her with a ritual that involves praying aloud together and reading from a religious text. How would you respond?*

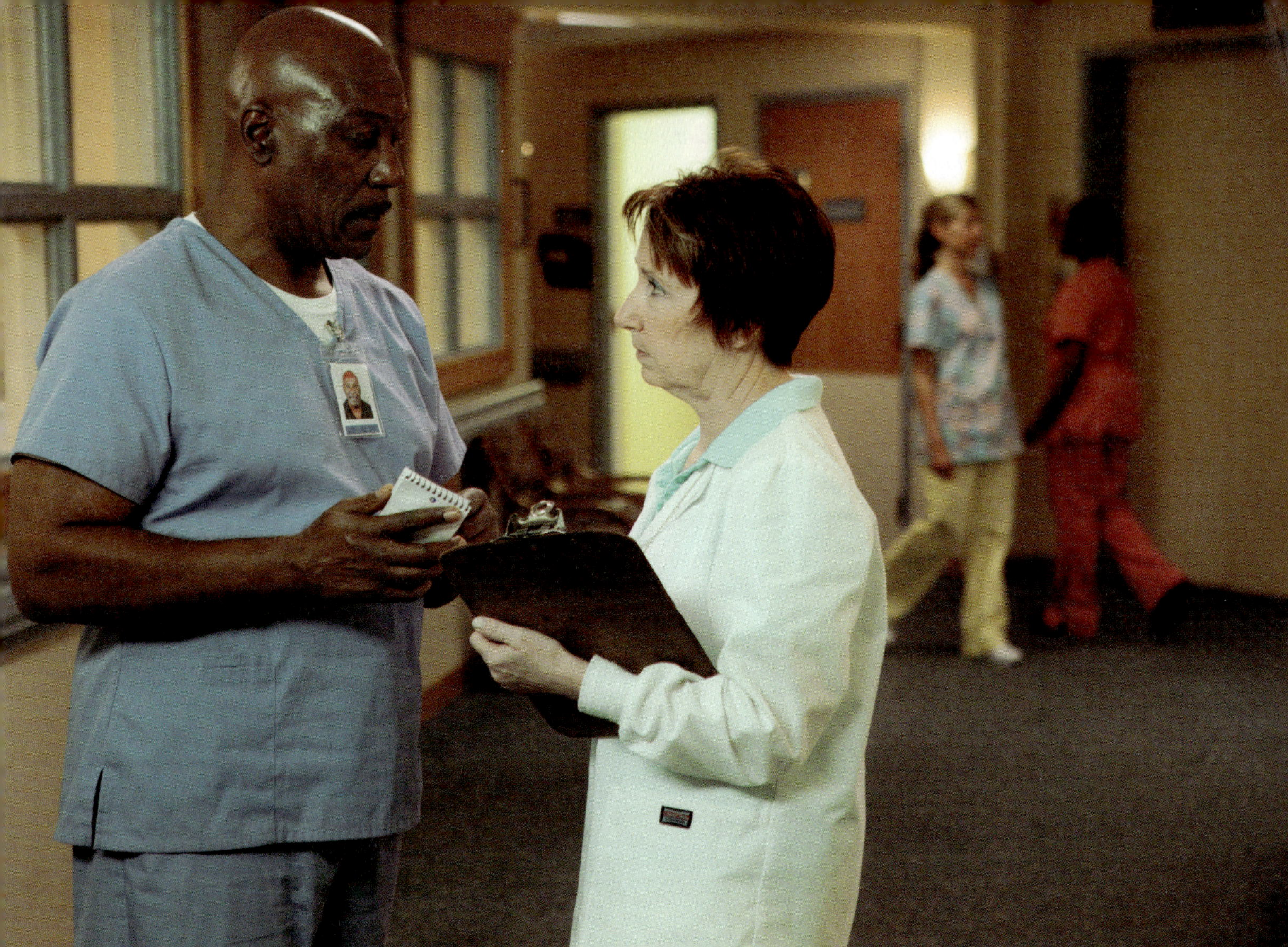

CHAPTER

5 Communicating with People

Goals

After reading this chapter, you will have the information needed to:

- Describe a model for effective communication.
- Explain the difference between verbal and nonverbal communication.
- List strategies for enhancing communication.
- List strategies for communicating with people with sensory impairments.
- Describe communication techniques that can be effective when it is necessary to discuss difficult topics.
- Describe how nurse assistants use communication skills to assist with teaching and reinforcing new information and skills.
- Describe the nurse assistant's role in communicating with family members.
- Describe a process for determining the meaning of unfamiliar medical words.

Goals

- Describe the nurse assistant's role in making and reporting observations.
- Describe guidelines for recording information.
- Describe guidelines for using the telephone.

Key Terms:

communication **nonverbal communication** **recording (documenting)** **care plan**
verbal communication **reporting** **medical record**

As you are walking down the hall, you notice that Mrs. Whitchurch's call light has come on again. You knock on her door and enter when she tells you to come in. When you ask Mrs. Whitchurch how you can help her, she says, "Oh, dear, I need to use the commode again." As you help Mrs. Whitchurch to the commode, you realize that this is the third time since you started your shift 2 hours ago. After you get Mrs. Whitchurch back in bed, you take the commode bucket to the bathroom to empty it. You notice that it does not contain much urine, and the urine is cloudy and strong-smelling. When you come back out of the bathroom, Mrs. Whitchurch says to you, "I just can't get comfortable. I feel like I need to go again, but I know I don't have any urine to pass." You decide you had better share your observations with the nurse right away.

Communication is the process of giving and receiving information. Good communication skills are essential to providing quality care. As a nurse assistant, you must be able to communicate effectively with those in your care, as well as other members of the health care team.

COMMUNICATION BASICS

Most people think that communication is something we all do naturally every day. However, you probably realize from personal experience how common it is for people to misunderstand one another. Good communication skills need to be learned.

Communication Model

Figure 5-1 shows a model for effective communication. You can see that effective communication involves a *sender*, the person who is providing information, and a *receiver*, the person to whom the information is being sent. The people who are communicating with each other repeatedly switch roles, sending and receiving messages back and forth. The information that the sender provides is called the *message*. After receiving the sender's message, the receiver becomes the sender and delivers his own message, called *confirmation*. This back-and-forth flow of information is very important, because this is how the sender knows that his message has been received and understood.

Communication Methods

People express themselves both verbally and nonverbally. **Verbal communication** involves the use of spoken language and written language, as well as American Sign Language, the system of hand movements used by many people with hearing impairments. **Nonverbal communication** is the sharing of information and feelings through body language, including gestures, body position, movement, facial expressions and tone of voice.

As a nurse assistant, you will use both verbal and nonverbal methods to communicate with others. For example, when you are caring for a person with dementia, it is often most effective to show, as well as tell, the person what you need him to do. If you want the person to sit down, you could say, "Mr. Greene, please sit here" (verbal communication) while patting the seat of the chair (nonverbal communication). To reassure a person, you might say, "I'm here for you" (verbal communication) while gently resting your hand on the person's hand (nonverbal communication). You must also be aware of the methods others are using to communicate with you. Paying attention to a person's nonverbal body language can give you important information, in addition to what the person may tell you. For example, a person may not complain of pain, but the way she carries her body or the expression on her face when she moves a certain body part may tell you that something is wrong.

Strategies for Effective Communication

To be a skilled communicator, you must be able to express yourself clearly in a way the other person can easily understand. You must also be able to receive information from the other person, which requires good

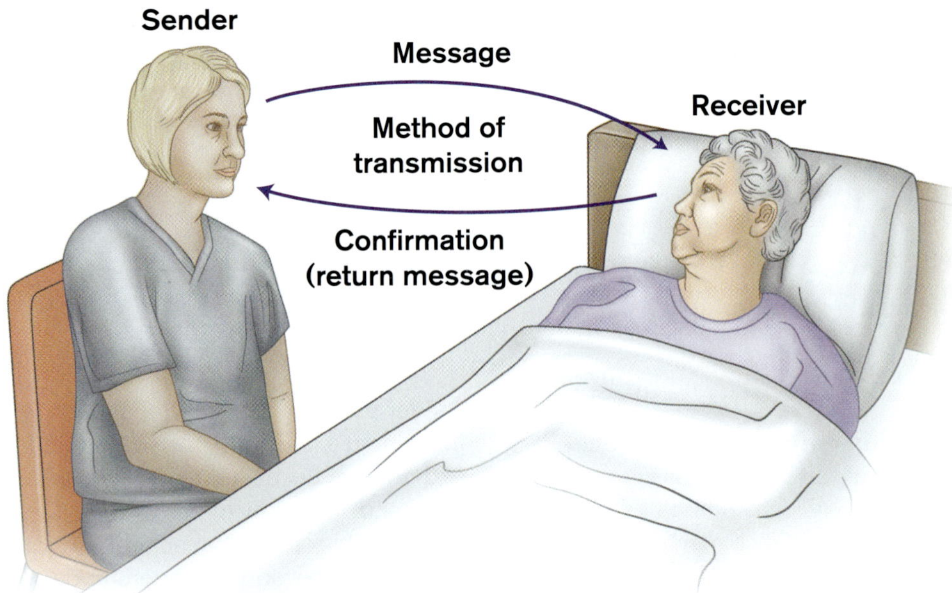

Figure 5-1 Communication involves a sender and a receiver. The sender sends a message. The receiver then provides confirmation that she received the message. Communication continues in this way, with the sender and receiver switching roles.

listening and observing skills. Strategies for effective communication include the following:

- **Make sure your message is clear.** Communication can fail when the other person does not fully understand your message. Tips for ensuring that your message is clear are given in Box 5-1.
- **Provide and seek confirmation.** When you are the receiver, confirm that you have received the sender's message by repeating, in your own words, what the sender said. If you have misunderstood the sender's message, this will be clear to the sender and she can correct any misunderstandings immediately. Sometimes, when you are the sender, it may be necessary to prompt the receiver to provide confirmation. One effective way to do this is to ask an open-ended question. An open-ended question is one that requires more than a simple "yes" or "no" answer, such as "Could you repeat back the plan for tomorrow?" This type of question requires the person to repeat, in his own words, what he understands your message to be, which will allow you to correct any misunderstandings as needed. If you ask a close-ended question (one that can be answered with a simple "yes" or "no"), such as "Do you understand what is happening tomorrow?" the person might say "yes" even if he did not fully understand your message.

Box 5-1 **Ensuring a Clear Message**

When speaking:

- Use words that the person understands. Avoid using terms or abbreviations that are unfamiliar to the person you are communicating with. Use the simplest words you can to get the message across.
- Talk slowly enough to express your thoughts clearly and to give the person time to think about what you are saying. Pause periodically to give the person the opportunity to respond or ask questions.
- Speak loudly enough to be heard, but not too loudly. If the person is having trouble hearing you, move closer to her.
- If the person speaks a different language than you do, hand gestures, drawings and picture boards can be effective for communicating simple messages. More complex messages may require the aid of a translator to ensure that your meaning is clear.

When writing:

- Write neatly. If your handwriting is hard to read, print instead.
- If you are writing something for a person with limited eyesight, use large letters. Write with a thick black or dark blue pen on white paper.
- Be specific. For example, if you are noting the time, be sure to write a.m. or p.m.
- Spell correctly. If you are not sure of the spelling, look the word up in a dictionary or ask.

- **Be an active participant in the conversation.** When you are the receiver, give the sender your full attention. Be an active listener. Avoid interrupting the person, or thinking about what you are going to say next. Instead, really focus on what the person is trying to tell you, both verbally and nonverbally. Ask questions as necessary to make sure you understand the person correctly. As appropriate, prompt the person to give you more information or to continue talking by repeating the person's own statement back to him. For example, if Mr. Jones says to you, "I just don't feel like myself today," you could respond by saying, "You don't feel like yourself today, Mr. Jones?" This type of response indicates to Mr. Jones that you were listening to what he said, and that you would like him to tell you more about how he is feeling.
- **Be mindful of the nonverbal messages you are sending.** Remember that your body language sends a message too (Table 5-1). Pay attention to things like your tone of voice, your facial expressions, your gestures and how you hold your body, and make sure that your nonverbal messages match your verbal ones.
- **Remember the importance of touch.** A caring touch, such as a hand on a shoulder, a pat on the back or a hug, is often a good way to make someone feel special or emphasize what you are saying. However, as you know, touching is not considered appropriate in all cultures, and some people simply do not like to be touched. Be sure you are aware of the person's comfort level with this form of communication before using it!

You find the nurse down the hall, at the medication cart. She is busy trying to make sure that all of the residents receive their medications on time. You say, "Mary, I need you to check on Mrs. Whitchurch. I've helped her to the commode three times in the last 2 hours, and each time, she passes only a small amount of cloudy, strong-smelling urine. She also told me that she can't get comfortable and she feels like she needs to urinate, even right after using the commode." Mary tells you that she will check on Mrs. Whitchurch as soon as she is finished giving Mr. Ivers his medication.

What strategies for effective communication were used here?

COMMUNICATING WITH THOSE IN YOUR CARE

In your work as a nurse assistant, your ability to communicate can have a positive impact on the health and well-being of the people in your care.

Table 5-1 Body Language

	Sends a Positive Message	Sends a Negative Message
Tone of Voice	■ Moderate volume ■ Calm, relaxed pace ■ Clear	■ Too loud or too soft ■ Sharp, rushed pace ■ Mumbling ■ Sighing loudly
Facial Expressions	■ Smiling ■ Concerned (depending on the situation)	■ Frowning ■ Grimacing ■ Eye rolling ■ Yawning
Gestures	■ Sitting down ■ Patting a person's arm or holding a person's hand ■ Nodding as the person speaks ■ Making good eye contact (unless this is considered disrespectful in the person's culture)	■ Checking watch or looking toward door ■ Glancing away from the person as he or she talks
Body Position and Movement	■ Positioning yourself to be at eye level with the person ■ Leaning toward the person as he or she talks	■ Standing over the person ■ Crossing your arms ■ Tapping your feet ■ Slouching

Communicating with People with Sensory Impairments

We rely very much on our senses of hearing and sight for effective communication. Many of the people in your care will have difficulty seeing or hearing. When you are caring for a person with impaired sight or hearing, there are strategies you can use to enhance communication.

Visual impairment

Visual impairment may have many causes, such as cataracts (a clouding of the lens of the eye that is caused by aging, injury or other diseases) or diabetes. When caring for a person with impaired sight, use your communication skills to help orient the person to surroundings and events.

- Knock on the person's door or tell him right away that you are there so that you don't startle him. Stand where he can see you, and call him by name: "Good morning, Mr. Wilson." Then tell him who you are.
- Describe the person's surroundings and tell him what is going on. Describe the people or events in a way that helps to create a mental picture: "Mr. Wilson, your daughter Susan is here, and she's wearing a beautiful red dress." Or "It's sunny today, and the patio door is open if you would like to go outside."
- As you move through a skill, describe each step as you are doing it. When using a piece of equipment, describe it to the person. If it doesn't cause an infection control risk and if he is interested, let him touch what you are holding.
- When helping the person move around, encourage him to hold your arm just above your elbow for support, describe where you are going and mention things that are in your path: "We're going up three steps now."

Hearing impairment

Some people who are hearing-impaired may be deaf, whereas others may have problems hearing only certain sounds. Learn what the people in your care can and cannot hear. Hearing aids improve some hearing problems but are not always completely effective. If the person uses a hearing aid, encourage her to wear it whenever she is awake, and ask her from time to time whether it is working well. Help her use and care for the hearing aid properly (see Chapter 13). Other ways you can help improve communication with a person with impaired hearing include the following:

- Always approach the person from the front, and gently touch the person on the hand or arm to gain the person's attention before speaking.
- If someone hears more clearly in one ear than the other, find out which ear is better, and position yourself near that ear when you talk.

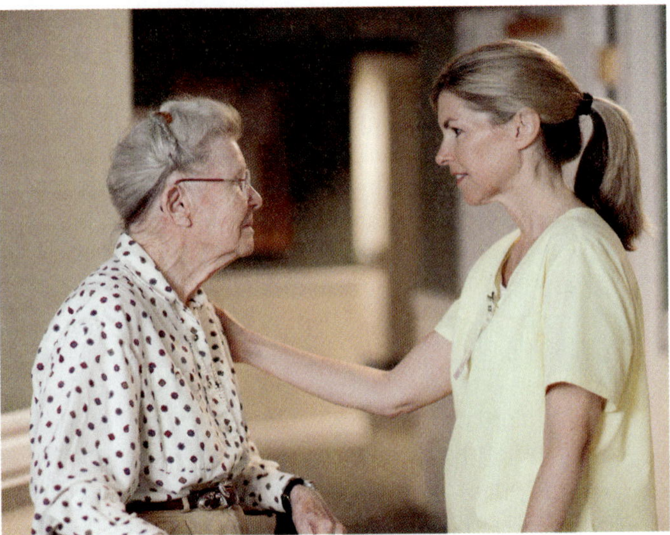

Figure 5-2 When speaking with a person who is hearing impaired, face the person so that she has a good view of your face and mouth.

- Be aware that hearing-impaired people often learn to read lips and rely on watching your mouth move. When speaking with the person, position yourself so that she can see your mouth and facial expressions (Figure 5-2). Pronounce your words slowly and clearly, and speak in short sentences.
- If the person does not seem to understand what you say, change your words, not the volume of your voice, unless you spoke too softly. Shouting sometimes creates more distress for the person, and she still may not understand what you are saying.
- Reduce background noise as much as possible, because television or radio sounds can be very distracting to the person with a hearing impairment during conversation.
- Use gestures to help explain what you are saying. Or, if the person can read, write messages on paper. When you have important information to get across, make sure that the person understands you by asking her for confirmation.

Communicating About Difficult Topics

People receiving health care and their family members may face difficult situations, which are often accompanied by complex emotions. The people in your care, or their family members, may express these emotions and thoughts to you. For example, a person who has just been admitted to a nursing home might say, "My family doesn't care about me anymore." Or a family member whose mother is in the last stage of a terminal illness might say, "I wish she would just die." Comments like this may make you feel uncomfortable, afraid, nervous or unsure about how to respond.

Your first response might be to try and end the conversation quickly by leaving the room or changing the subject. Or, you might say something like "You don't really mean that" or "Don't be silly." However, these sorts of responses cut off communication with the person. Because part of your job is to listen and talk with those in your care, it is important to keep lines of communication open. The following suggestions may help you when it is necessary to communicate about difficult topics:

- Show the person that you care about her feelings by stopping what you are doing, paying full attention and making eye contact. If it is appropriate, hold or gently squeeze her hand or touch her on the shoulder. Sometimes all the person needs is for someone to listen. If the person feels your interest and concern, your silent support can sometimes help more than words (Figure 5-3).
- Encourage the person to talk by asking a question that focuses on what she is telling you (for example, "Are you saying that you miss being close to another person?") Or confirm the person's message by repeating it in your own words: "It sounds like you are saying that you miss seeing and hearing from your family."
- If the person needs answers or help that you are unable to provide, involve other members of the health care team. Tell the person in your care that you will talk with someone who may be able to help. Then be sure to follow through.

Teaching and Reinforcing New Information and Skills

As a nurse assistant, you play an important role in helping the people in your care achieve or maintain their best level of health and functioning. One way you will do this is by using your communication skills to provide people with information and skills that can help them to remain independent and regain their health to the greatest extent possible (Figure 5-4). You will also use your communication skills to provide ongoing support and encouragement as the person learns new skills and behaviors.

Because you will spend the most time with the person every day, you will often be in a good position to help reinforce (strengthen) the teaching that another member of the health care team has started. For example, the physical therapist has been working with Mr. Wilson to teach him how to walk with a cane. You can reinforce these lessons by observing Mr. Wilson's use of the cane when you help him to get from one place to another, and reporting your observations about Mr. Wilson's ability to use the cane to the nurse or physical therapist. You may also be responsible for teaching a person how to do certain things that are within your scope of practice. For example, Mrs. Simmons has weakness on her left side because of a stroke. You can show Mrs. Simmons techniques that will make it easier for her to dress herself.

As you provide care, you may recognize that a person does not fully understand information he has been given or skills he has been taught. For example, the person may make a comment or ask a question that alerts you to the need for more teaching. Reinforce the information the person has already been given, and then make sure to report the person's need for more information to the nurse. For example, Mr. Rivera, a 78-year-old man in your care who had a stroke, takes medication that increases the amount of time it takes for blood to clot. Even a small cut may cause serious bleeding. The nurse has instructed you to have Mr. Rivera switch from shaving with a safety razor to shaving with an electric razor to help prevent nicking his skin. One morning, while helping Mr. Rivera shave, you have the following conversation with him.

Mr. Rivera: "I don't see why I have to use this electric razor. I've been shaving with my safety razor for years, and I never had a problem."

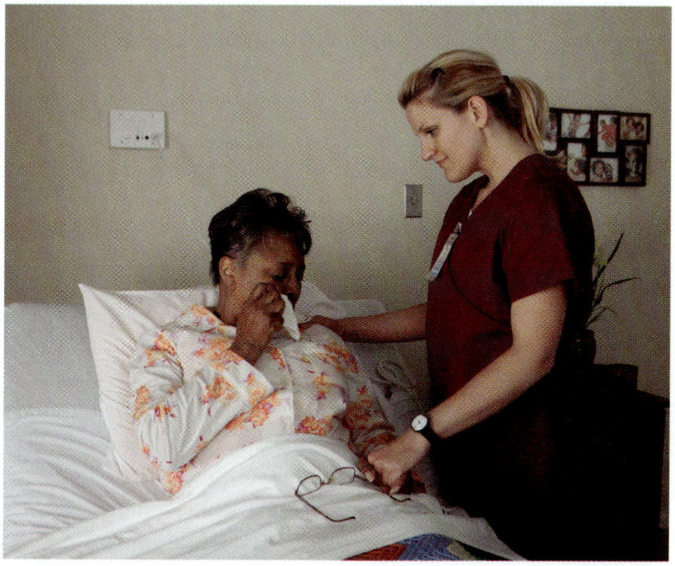

Figure 5-3 Sometimes a willingness to listen and a gentle touch are more powerful than words for communicating your care and concern.

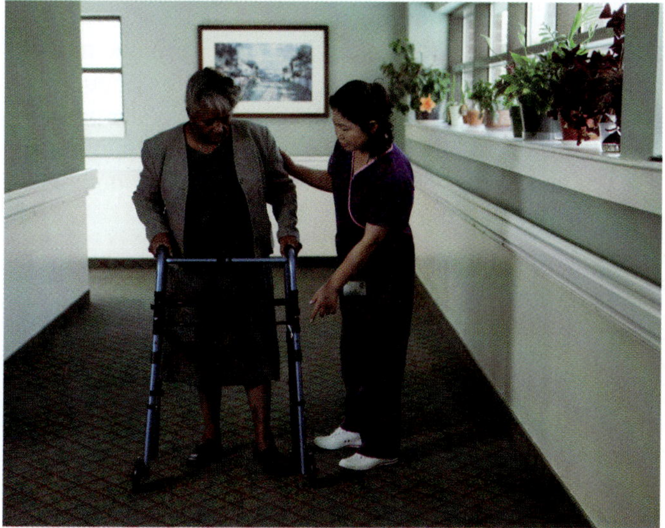

Figure 5-4 Nurse assistants use their communication skills to help the people in their care achieve or maintain their best level of health and function.

You could say: "I know you like the safety razor better, Mr. Rivera, but because of the kind of medication you are taking, it is important that you don't cut yourself. The electric razor doesn't nick your skin, so it is safer for you to use."

Mr. Rivera: "I don't like electric razors, but I don't like bleeding either, so I guess I'd better try it."

By providing Mr. Rivera with an explanation for the change, you have helped him become more accepting of it. You should also report this conversation to the nurse, because it is possible that Mr. Rivera needs more information about the medication he is taking (for example, why he is taking it and how it works).

In about half an hour, Mary finds you and says, "Mrs. Whitchurch's primary care provider has requested that we obtain a 'clean catch' urine sample because she suspects a urinary tract infection. Can you make sure to obtain this sample the next time Mrs. Whitchurch uses the commode? I explained to Mrs. Whitchurch that she will need to start the flow of urine, then stop it, and then collect the urine sample from the restarted flow, but she might forget, so be sure to remind her."

How will you use your communication skills to reinforce the information Mary has given Mrs. Whitchurch?

COMMUNICATING WITH FAMILY MEMBERS

As a nurse assistant, you must be able to communicate effectively with the family members of the people in your care. Because you will spend a great deal of time with the person and provide the most assistance with routine activities, you will often be the first member of the health care team family members ask for information about the person's physical health and abilities, emotional status and overall well-being. If a family member asks a question that you are not qualified to answer, make arrangements for the family member to speak with the nurse.

Be aware that the way you communicate with family members contributes to the overall impression they have of the care their loved one is receiving. You can help family members feel more comfortable by explaining your role in providing care, and explaining why you do things in a certain way. Build a relationship with the family by getting to know the family members, learning about their family history, talking with them and listening to them (Figure 5-5). Family members often can provide valuable information, for example, about what techniques they have found to be most effective in caring for their loved one. Welcome their input and feedback. The information provided by family members can make your job easier and increase the quality of the care you provide.

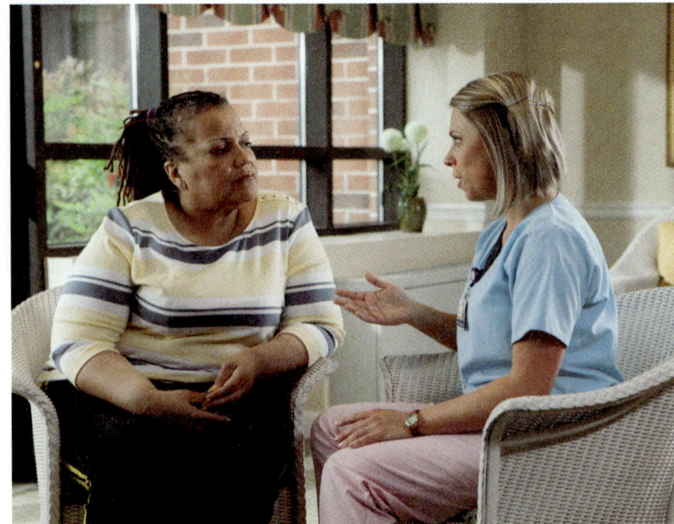

Figure 5-5 Communicating with family members is an important part of the nurse assistant's job, too.

Sometimes, family members may voice a complaint or a concern about their family member's care. When this happens, it is important to respond in a professional manner, and to seek a solution to the problem. Avoid becoming defensive or angry. Instead, use your communication skills to gain a full understanding of the family member's concerns and to reassure the family member that you understand her concerns and will take the appropriate measures to resolve them.

COMMUNICATING WITH OTHER MEMBERS OF THE HEALTH CARE TEAM

The members of the health care team must communicate effectively with each other in order to ensure coordinated, high-quality care. As a nurse assistant, you are in a position to gather important information about those in your care on a daily basis, and you must know how to report and record this information so that it is available to other members of the health care team who need it.

Understanding Medical Words and Abbreviations

To communicate effectively with other members of the health care team, you must be able to understand and use medical words and abbreviations. For students who have never worked in a health care setting, learning medical words may seem to be an overwhelming task. Some of the words are long, some are difficult to pronounce and spell and many of them are not used in everyday conversation. However, it is often possible to break long, complex words into smaller parts, making it easier to determine the meaning of the word.

A word can contain the following parts:

- **Root.** The root is the foundation of the word. All medical words have at least one root, and some may have two.
- **Prefix.** A prefix may be added before the root to make the root more specific.
- **Suffix.** A suffix may be added after the root to make the root more specific.
- **A combining vowel.** A combining vowel, which may be an "o," an "a" or an "i," is added between the root and the suffix to join them together and make the word easier to say.

To determine the meaning of an unfamiliar word, first identify each of its parts, and determine what they mean. For example, let's look at the word *cholecystectomy*. In this word, the root is *cholecyst*, which means "gallbladder." The suffix is *–ectomy*, which means "removal of." So the word *cholecystectomy* means "removal of the gallbladder." Now, let's look at the word *hypoglycemia*. The root is *glyc*, and means "sugar." The prefix is *hypo-*, which means "under." The suffix is *–emia*, which means "blood disorder." So the word *hypoglycemia* means "low blood sugar." Appendix A contains a list of commonly used roots, prefixes and suffixes. Familiarizing yourself with these will help you to determine the meaning of unfamiliar words.

You will also notice that the members of the health care team often use abbreviations, or shortened forms of words and phrases, when communicating with each other. Using abbreviations can make communication more efficient by saving time and space. Sometimes abbreviations are formed from the initial letters of each word in a phrase, such as "DON" for "director of nursing." Others are just shortened versions of a word, such as "cath" for "catheter." Some abbreviations used in health care do not seem to relate to the words they stand for at all, such as "NPO." This is because "NPO," which means "nothing by mouth," comes from the Latin phrase "*nils per os*." When using abbreviations, it is very important to only use those that have been approved by your employer. This helps to ensure that the meaning of the abbreviation is clear to everyone. Common abbreviations that are often used in health care are also listed in Appendix A.

Reporting

Reporting is the verbal exchange of information between members of the health care team. Reporting happens routinely at the change of shift, when the staff members who are finishing their shift update the staff members who are coming on duty. Reporting also happens throughout the shift, when it is necessary to communicate a change in a person's condition to other members of the health care team. Typically, you will report to the nurse before and after you finish providing care for a person, and whenever else you think it is necessary.

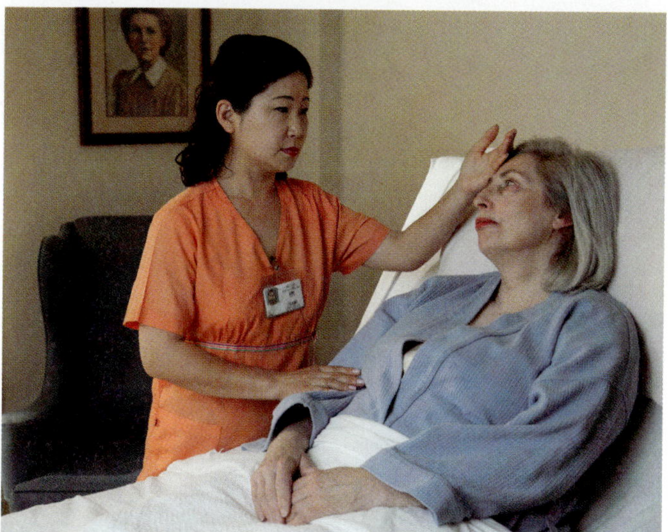

Figure 5-6 Objective observations are observations you make based on one of your five senses. Here, this nurse assistant is using her sense of touch to determine that the person's skin is hot and dry.

You spend a great deal of time with the people in your care. As a result, you will often be the first to notice a change in the person's condition, abilities or emotional status that should be reported to the nurse. Observations you make about the person's condition can take two main forms:

- **Objective observations** relate to information that you obtain directly, using one of your five senses. For example, you may feel that a person's skin is hot and dry (Figure 5-6), or you may measure a person's blood pressure using a blood pressure cuff.
- **Subjective observations** relate to information that you cannot detect with one of your five senses or cannot measure using equipment (Figure 5-7). For example, a person may tell you that she has a headache or that she did not sleep well the night before. These observations are subjective because you cannot detect the person's pain or tiredness with your own senses. Instead, you must rely on what the person is telling you.

As you make observations, you must decide what information to pass on to other members of the health care team. When deciding what to report, focus on the word *change*. Report observations that indicate changes in the person's:

- Mood.
- Mental awareness.
- Level of independence.
- Behavior.

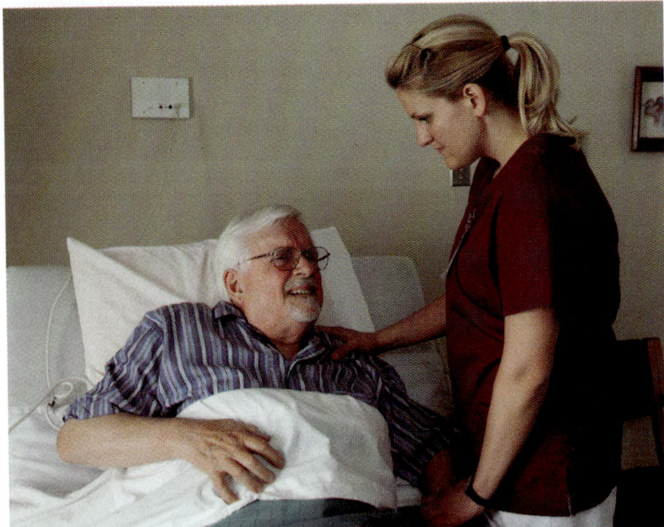

Figure 5-7 Subjective observations are observations that you make based on what the person tells you. Here, this person is describing pain that he is having to the nurse assistant. The nurse assistant cannot feel his pain herself, but she knows it exists because the person is telling her about it.

- Vital signs.
- Urine or bowel movements.
- Skin condition or color.
- Appetite.
- Sleep habits.
- Comfort level.

If you are ever in doubt about whether you should report an observation to the nurse, remember the following guideline: "When in doubt, report." It is best to share your observations with the nurse and let the nurse determine whether additional follow-up is needed.

Remember that the members of the health care team who do not have the opportunity to spend as much time with the person as you do rely heavily on your observations. When reporting, include as many accurate details as possible, and focus on facts rather than your personal opinions. Look at the following examples:

Example 1. Mrs. Damon is recovering from a broken hip. You are to help her stand three times a day. Usually she is able to stand for 2 or 3 minutes each afternoon. Today, using your arm for support, Mrs. Damon stood for 5 minutes.

Helpful: "Mrs. Damon stood for 5 minutes this afternoon. She leaned on my arm. In the past, she has only been able to stand for 2 or 3 minutes at a time."

Less helpful: "Mrs. Damon stood for longer than usual."

Example 2. Since his stroke, Mr. Rivera has been working with an occupational therapist to relearn how to shave using an electric razor. When he started therapy last week, he had a hard time holding the razor and making his hand move the right way. He got frustrated and asked you to finish the job. Today you notice that he shaved his whole face.

Helpful: "Mr. Rivera has made progress with his shaving skills. He is able to shave his whole face."

Less helpful: "Mr. Rivera is doing better holding the razor."

Example 3. Mrs. Kline has dementia. This morning while you were trying to help her with her morning care, she picked up a brush, threw it at you, and yelled "Get out!" Usually, Mrs. Kline is cooperative when you provide care.

Helpful: "This morning while I was trying to help Mrs. Kline get dressed, she picked up her hairbrush and threw it at me, telling me to get out. She does not usually behave like this."

Less helpful: "Mrs. Kline tried to hit me with a hairbrush this morning."

Think back to the observations you made when you were helping Mrs. Whitchurch to use the commode. Which of these observations were objective? Which were subjective?

How did promptly reporting your observations and providing factual details lead to better care for Mrs. Whitchurch?

Recording

Recording, also called documenting, is the written exchange of information between members of the health care team. Recording takes place on various forms, which are contained in the person's **medical record** (a legal document that details the person's condition, the measures taken by the health care team to diagnose and manage the condition, and the person's response to the care provided). Traditionally, medical records have been kept on paper, but electronic medical records (kept on a computer) are becoming increasingly more common (Figure 5-8).

When working with a person's medical record, it is very important to remember what you learned in Chapter 3 about maintaining the person's confidentiality. Always return paper records to their proper location in the nurse's station when you are finished using them. If electronic medical records are in use, always log off the computer when you are finished using it. Remember that only the members of the health care team who are directly involved in providing care to the person need to have access to the person's medical record.

Key forms

The medical record contains many different forms. There are three forms that are of particular interest to

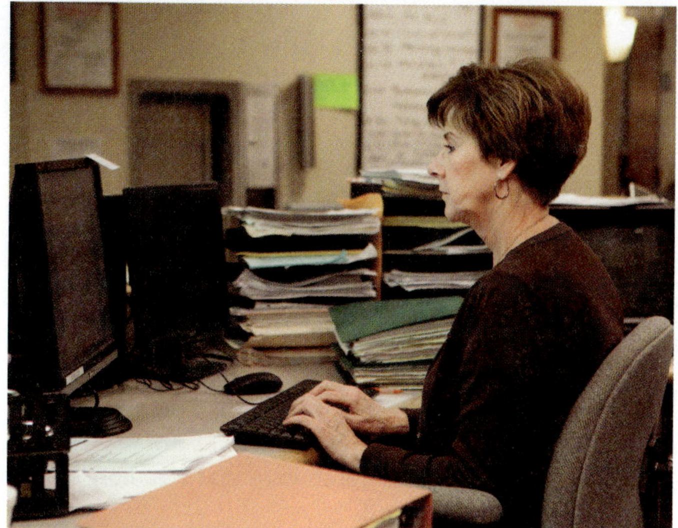

Figure 5-8 Electronic medical records are becoming more common.

the nurse assistant: the care plan, the flow sheet and nursing notes.

- **Care plan.** Each day, the first form you will refer to is the person's **care plan**. The care plan details the care the person requires, and the methods, equipment and frequency for providing that care. Because the person's condition may change, the care plan is updated frequently, so you must check it every day. The care plan may take the form of a computer print-out, or it may be kept on a card in a file.
- **Flow sheet.** A flow sheet is used to track changes in measurements (such as vital signs, intake and output, and weight) over a period of time.
- **Nursing notes.** This form is used by the nursing staff to document the person's condition, the nursing care provided to the person, and any significant events that took place during the shift or visit. Some employers allow nurse assistants to record certain types of information in the nursing notes. Others will require you to report your observations to the nurse so that he or she can update the nursing notes.

Guidelines for recording

Depending on your employer's policy, you may be responsible for recording. For example, some employers allow nurse assistants to record information on the flow sheet, but not the nursing notes. Others allow nurse assistants to document the care they provide and the observations they make in the nursing notes as well.

If you are expected to record, it is important to do it correctly and accurately. The medical record is a legal document. As such, it is a formal accounting of the care a person receives while in the facility, and can be used as evidence should a legal problem or dispute arise. In addition, other members of the health care team rely on what is documented to evaluate the person's condition (for example, how well the person is responding to treatment) and to make decisions about future care measures. Also, it is important to understand that in facilities and agencies that receive federal funding (for example, Medicare or Medicaid payments), accurate documentation is essential to ensure that the facility receives the proper payment for services that were provided, and that the person continues to receive services he is eligible for.

Whenever you record information in the person's medical record, include the date, the time and your initials or signature. When documenting, usually a 24-hour clock (also called military time) is used to express the time (Figure 5-9). Other guidelines for proper documentation are given in Box 5-2.

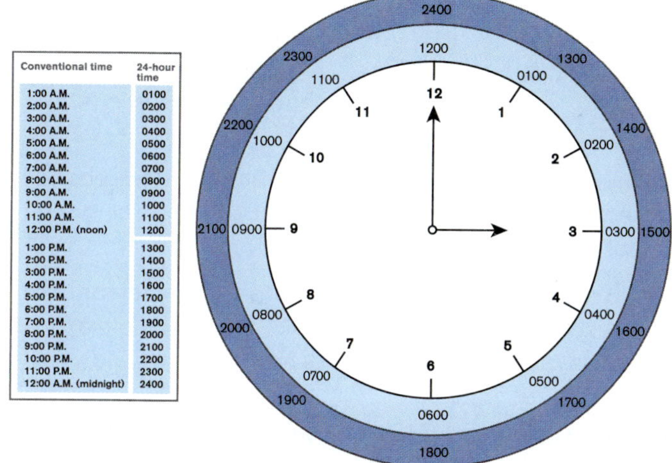

Conventional time	24-hour time
1:00 A.M.	0100
2:00 A.M.	0200
3:00 A.M.	0300
4:00 A.M.	0400
5:00 A.M.	0500
6:00 A.M.	0600
7:00 A.M.	0700
8:00 A.M.	0800
9:00 A.M.	0900
10:00 A.M.	1000
11:00 A.M.	1100
12:00 P.M. (noon)	1200
1:00 P.M.	1300
2:00 P.M.	1400
3:00 P.M.	1500
4:00 P.M.	1600
5:00 P.M.	1700
6:00 P.M.	1800
7:00 P.M.	1900
8:00 P.M.	2000
9:00 P.M.	2100
10:00 P.M.	2200
11:00 P.M.	2300
12:00 A.M. (midnight)	2400

Figure 5-9 A 24-hour clock is usually used for documenting time in medical records. On a 24-hour clock, the hours between 1:00 a.m. and 12:00 p.m. (noon) are the same as they are on a 12-hour clock. To indicate a time in the afternoon, add "12" to the time on the 12-hour clock. For example, 3:00 in the afternoon would be expressed as "1500." When using a 24-hour clock, the first two numbers indicate the hour and the last two numbers indicate the minutes (for example, 3:19 a.m. = 0319).

While waiting for Mrs. Whitchurch's test results to come back, the primary care provider started her on an antibiotic and asked the nursing staff to measure Mrs. Whitchurch's temperature at regular intervals throughout the day and night.

What form will you use to record Mrs. Whitchurch's temperature measurements?

Why is it important to record Mrs. Whitchurch's temperature measurements correctly and accurately?

At the nursing home where you work, nurse assistants are allowed to document in the nursing notes. How would you document the observations that you made when you first suspected that Mrs. Whitchurch might have a problem? What details would you include?

Box 5-2 Nurse Assistant DO's and DON'Ts

Recording

DO make sure that you are recording the information on the correct person's medical record.

DO include the date, the time and your initials or signature for every entry you make.

DO use proper medical terminology and abbreviations, per your employer's policy.

DO record facts, not opinions.

DO use black ink.

DON'T erase mistakes. Instead, follow your employer's policy for correcting mistakes. For example, your employer may require you to draw a line through the mistake and initial it.

DO record promptly after providing care or making observations.

DON'T record care before you have actually provided it.

DO record only care that you have personally provided and observations that you have personally made.

DO remember that, in a legal situation, care that was not recorded is considered care that was not provided.

Using the Telephone

In your work, you may be required to use the telephone to receive or make calls (Figure 5-10). When using the telephone:

- **Be professional.** Know how to use the telephone system to make outgoing calls, answer incoming calls, put someone on hold, transfer a call and use any other features.
- **Identify yourself.** When you answer the telephone, greet the caller and state your name, your title and the unit where you work, and ask how you can be of assistance (for example, "Hello, this is Melissa Schmidt, CNA, 3 West speaking. How can I help you?"). When you are placing a call, identify yourself as soon as the other person picks up.
- **Be courteous.** Answer the telephone as soon as you hear it ring. Speak slowly and clearly, in a pleasant tone of voice. If you have to put a caller on hold, do it for only a short time. If the wait is going to be longer than a minute, get back on the line to let the caller know, and offer to take a message.
- **Take accurate messages.** If you are asked to take a message, write it down carefully and repeat it to the caller to make sure the information is correct. Include the date and time of the call on the message, and sign your name. Make sure that your message is complete. To make sure that you have not made any mistakes, check over what you have written before you deliver the message. Put the message where the person is most likely to find it.
- **Respect privacy.** Callers may ask questions about someone's health or may request other personal information. Be aware that even confirming that a person is receiving care in the facility could be considered a breach of privacy. Do not provide any information unless you are sure that your employer permits it, and be sure that any information you provide is correct. If you are unsure about what information to provide to the caller, ask your supervisor.

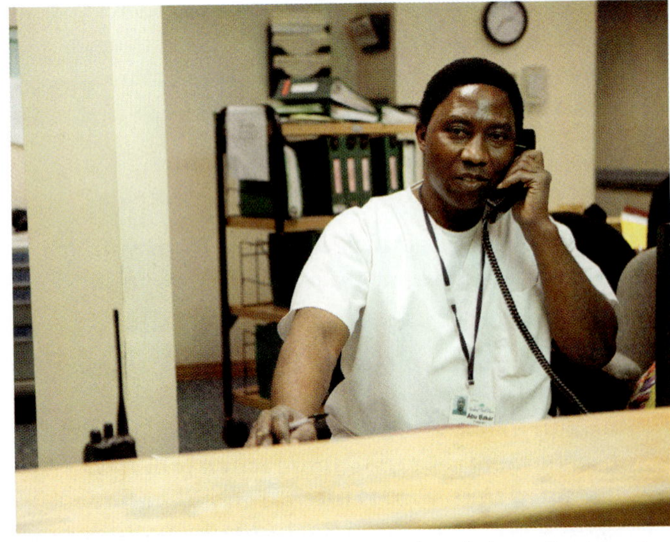

Figure 5-10 Answer the telephone promptly and pleasantly, state who you are and ask what you can do to help the caller.

CHECK YOUR UNDERSTANDING

Questions for Review

1. **When you are the sender, what should you do after you deliver your message?**
   a. Expect the person to do what you told him.
   b. Ask for confirmation that the message was understood.
   c. Communicate the next message.
   d. Look for written communication.

2. **When entering the room of a person who is blind, you should:**
   a. Walk up quietly and touch the person on the back.
   b. Knock on the door, wait for a response and introduce yourself.
   c. Knock on the door and go in.
   d. Talk in a low voice.

3. **Mrs. James is deaf. What can you do to make sure she understands the information you have just given her?**
   a. Get help from a translator.
   b. Write the information down for her.
   c. Speak in the loudest voice possible.
   d. All of the above

4. **Mrs. Morgan's daughter always watches closely how you provide care to her mother, and seems critical of some of the things you do. What would be the best way for you to handle this situation?**
   a. Ask Mrs. Morgan to tell her daughter that she likes the care you provide.
   b. Tell Mrs. Morgan's daughter that her mother likes the care she is receiving.
   c. Tell Mrs. Morgan's daughter that what you are doing is the right and only way to provide care.
   d. Explain to Mrs. Morgan's daughter what you are doing and why you are doing it, and ask her what care measures she found to be effective when she was caring for Mrs. Morgan at home.

5. **Mrs. Goldstein has recently been diagnosed with diabetes and must eat meals at regular times. Today is a fasting day in her religion. She knows that she needs to eat because of her disease, and she knows that her religion says that sick people don't have to fast. Yet when you serve her food, she tells you that she feels funny about eating. You could:**
   a. Tell her that she shouldn't feel bad.
   b. Avoid talking about religion and serve her food without saying anything.
   c. Tell her that she doesn't really have to eat if she doesn't want to.
   d. Tell her that you can understand that it must feel strange to eat on a fasting day and encourage her to talk about it.

6. **Which of the following is a subjective observation?**
   a. Mrs. Lyons tells you she feels sick to her stomach.
   b. Mr. Upton has a red sore forming on his big toe.
   c. Mr. Halladay's blood pressure measurement is 130/90 mm Hg.
   d. Mrs. Harper ate only 50% of her meal.

7. **Which of the following observations should you report to the nurse?**
   a. Mrs. Zimmer is having difficulty having a bowel movement.
   b. Mr. Thomas does not seem like himself today.
   c. Mrs. Nolan told you that she does not want to attend the group activity today.
   d. All of the above

8. **Which document details the care the person requires, and the methods, equipment and frequency for providing that care?**
   a. The electronic medical record
   b. The nursing notes
   c. The flow sheet
   d. The care plan

9. **It is 2:00 in the afternoon. How would you express this using the 24-hour clock?**
   a. 2 p.m.
   b. 0200
   c. 1400
   d. 2 a.m.

10. **Why is it important to record care and observations accurately and correctly?**
   a. The medical record is a legal record of the care provided.
   b. Other members of the health care team rely on the medical record to evaluate the person's condition and make decisions about future care.
   c. Federal reimbursement (payment) depends on accurate documentation of the services that were provided.
   d. All of the above

Questions to Ask Yourself

1. *Mrs. Alvarez has just been admitted to the nursing home where you work. You can tell that she is upset, and her family is worried. What communication strategies will you use to help Mrs. Alvarez and her family members feel better about this situation?*

2. *You are a home health aide. Today, while you were changing Mr. Linkins' bed linens, he tells you that he has decided to stop taking his blood pressure medicine because it makes him have to use the bathroom too frequently. He asks you not to tell the nurse, because she will get angry with him. How*

would you respond to Mr. Linkins? Would you report Mr. Linkins' comment to the nurse, despite the fact that he asked you not to? Why or why not?

3. *Mr. Diaz is recovering from a stroke. Per his care plan, you are to encourage him at each meal to walk from the entrance to the dining room to his place at the table, a distance of about 15 feet. Today, Mr. Diaz was able to walk to his place at the table for lunch, but he was too tired to try to walk the distance at dinner. How would you phrase your report to the nurse?*

UNIT 2

PROMOTING SAFETY

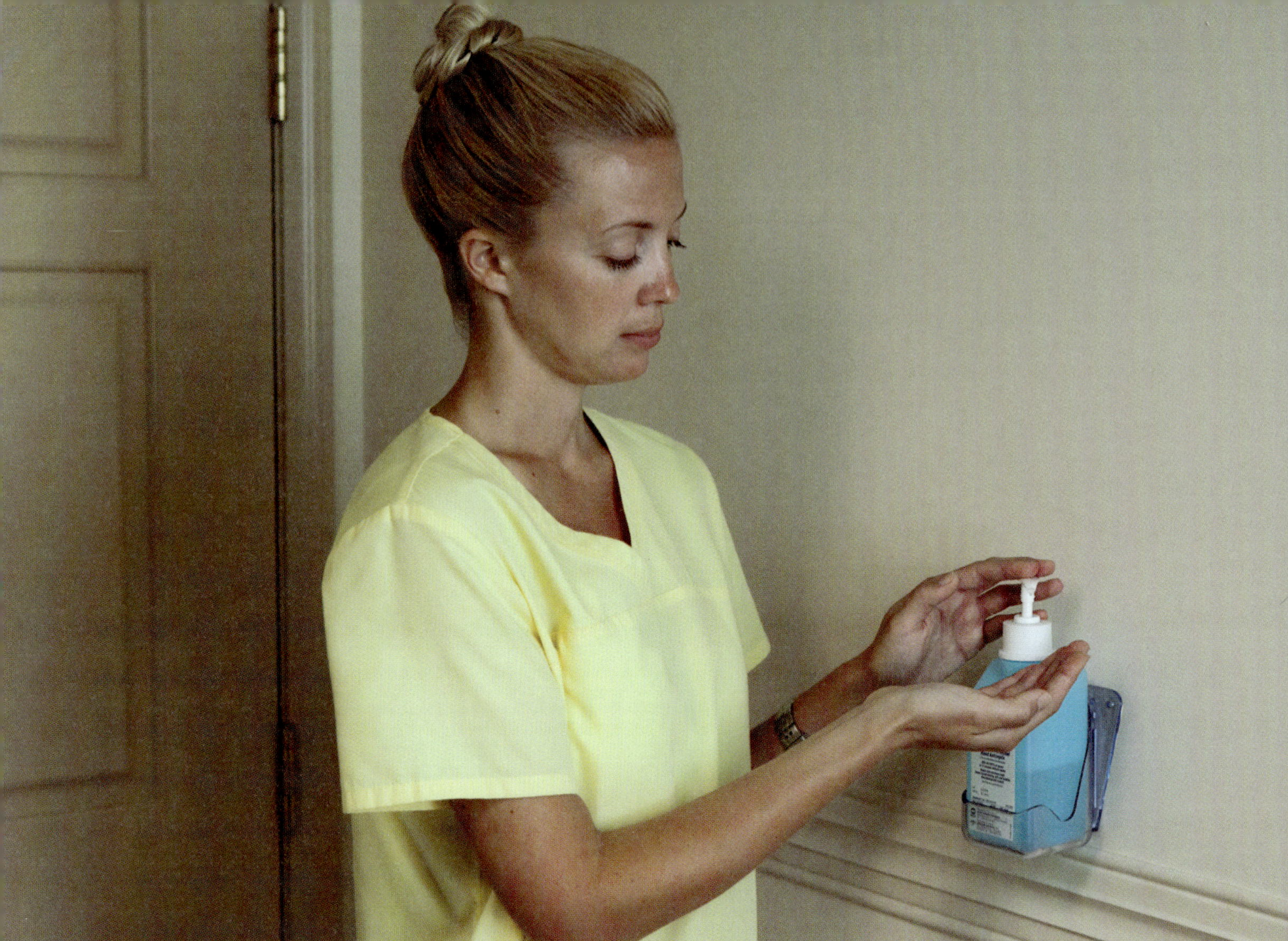

CHAPTER 6 Controlling the Spread of Infection

Goals

After reading this chapter, you will have the information needed to:

- Understand how infections can be spread from one person to another.
- Recognize the signs and symptoms of an infection.
- Take measures to control the spread of microbes that can cause infection.
- Apply standard precautions and transmission-based precautions.
- Understand your role and your employer's role in protecting you from exposure to bloodborne pathogens on the job.

After practicing the corresponding skills, you will have the information needed to:

- Wash your hands in a way that controls the spread of microbes that can cause infection.
- Put on and take off personal protective equipment (PPE) correctly.
- Open and close a trash bag correctly and double-bag contaminated trash and laundry.

Key Terms:

microbes (microorganisms)

pathogens

infection

mucous membranes

chain of infection

contaminated

health care–associated infection

infection control

body fluids

disinfectant

sterilization

personal protective equipment (PPE)

high-efficiency particulate air filter (HEPA) mask

standard precautions

transmission-based precautions

sharps container

tuberculosis

bloodborne pathogens

human immunodeficiency virus (HIV)

acquired immunodeficiency syndrome (AIDS)

hepatitis

occupational exposure

During morning report at Metropolitan Hospital Center, your supervising nurse tells you about your new patient, Louise Wang, a 53-year-old woman who was admitted through the emergency room from Morningside Nursing Home last night. Because she was diagnosed with highly contagious staph pneumonia, she is in isolation in Room 117. Last year, she had part of her bowel removed because of colon cancer, and she uses an ostomy appliance (a bag worn on the outside of the body) for the elimination of feces. The feces pass through a surgically made opening in her abdomen and into the ostomy appliance. In addition to assisting Mrs. Wang with changing her ostomy appliance, you will need to help her with a complete bed bath and with transferring from the bed to the chair, because she is very weak. The nurse also tells you that Mrs. Wang is originally from China but speaks and understands English very well.

You decide to visit Mrs. Wang immediately because you think she might be afraid. Before going into her room, you wash your hands and put on a gown, mask and gloves. Outside her room, you notice the sign posted on her closed door. The sign requests visitors to report to the nurses' station.

You knock gently, then a little louder when you hear no response. When you finally hear a faint "Come in," you open the door to see the back of a small woman lying in bed. You walk toward the bed, gently calling Mrs. Wang's name and telling her who you are. When she turns toward you and sees your masked face, her eyes open wide before she turns back to face the wall.

WHAT CAUSES INFECTION?

Louise Wang is in a room by herself because she has *Staphylococcus pneumonia* (staph pneumonia), a disease that other people could catch from her. Colds and flus also are diseases that people can get from one another. Have you ever caught a cold or flu from someone? You can lessen your chances of getting sick and avoid passing on an illness to someone else by learning about what causes infections and how infections can spread.

Microbes (microorganisms) are tiny living things that are too small to see but are all around us. Microbes can only be seen using a microscope. Examples of microbes include bacteria, viruses, fungi, yeasts and molds. Most microbes grow rapidly wherever they have warm temperatures, moisture, darkness and food. These characteristics make the human body an ideal place for microbial growth! Some microbes are harmful to humans and some are not. Harmful microbes that cause disease are called **pathogens**. A disease caused by a pathogen is called an **infection**.

Microbes are everywhere, even in and on our bodies. Many of the microbes that live in and on our bodies are harmless, and some even perform useful functions. However, even microbes that are useful and necessary in certain areas of the body can cause disease if they spread to another part of the body where they are not normally found. For example, certain bacteria in the stomach and bowel help to digest food. But if these same bacteria are present in the kidney or bladder, they can cause an infection.

The body has many natural defenses against infection. Healthy, intact skin and **mucous membranes** help to prevent microbes from entering the body. Reflexes, such as coughing and sneezing, help to expel microbes from the body. Finally, white blood cells carried in the blood are able to destroy pathogens that enter the body. These natural defense mechanisms help to keep us healthy. In addition, modern medicine has made other tools available to help us fight and prevent infections, such as antibiotic medications and vaccinations. Even though our bodies have ways of protecting us from infection and there are medications available to treat some infections, *prevention* is still the optimal goal. Some infections can be fatal, especially in people who are not otherwise healthy, and some infections cannot be treated with medication.

THE CHAIN OF INFECTION

Many infections can be passed from one person to another. However, for this to occur, six requirements must be met. These six requirements are called the **chain of infection** (Figure 6-1). Eliminating just one link in the chain can prevent an infection from spreading. Let's take a closer look at the six links in the chain of infection:

1. **Pathogen.** For an infection to occur, a microbe capable of causing disease must be present.
2. **Reservoir.** *Reservoir* is a French word that means "storehouse." Here, we are using it to mean a place where microbes can grow and multiply. Possible reservoirs for microbes include the bodies of people and animals, bodies of water, and food.
3. **Portal of exit.** *Portal* comes from the Latin word for "gate." For an infection to occur, the microbe must have a way of leaving the reservoir, or a *portal of exit*. The portal of exit varies depending on the pathogen and the reservoir. When the reservoir is a human or animal body, the portal of exit may be the respiratory tract, the digestive tract, the genitourinary tract or breaks in the skin.
4. **Method of transmission.** The way a pathogen gets from one person to another is called the pathogen's method of transmission. The method of transmission may be direct or indirect. In *direct transmission*, the pathogen is passed from one person to another through close physical contact, such as touching, kissing, having sex or breathing infected air. *Indirect transmission* means that pathogens are spread by way of a **contaminated** surface or object. Usually this situation occurs when an infected person touches something and then someone else touches that same object. For example, if you have a cold and blow your nose into a tissue, and someone else picks up the tissue to throw it away without wearing gloves, that person can get your cold by indirect contact. The germs will spread from your nose secretions to the tissue to the other person's hand.
5. **Portal of entry.** Just as the pathogen must have a way of leaving the reservoir, it must also have a way of gaining entry to a new reservoir. This is called a *portal of entry*. In the case of person-to-person (or animal-to-person) transmission, potential portals of entry include the respiratory tract, the digestive tract, the genitourinary tract, the eye and breaks in the skin.
6. **Susceptible host.** Finally, the pathogen must enter a susceptible host, or a person who is capable of becoming infected with that particular pathogen. Some factors increase a person's susceptibility to infection, including very young or very old age, poor general health, and the presence of medical devices that are placed in the body (such as urinary catheters). Many of the people you will care for will have risk factors that increase their susceptibility to infection.

HEALTH CARE–ASSOCIATED INFECTIONS

A **health care–associated infection** is an infection that a person gets while receiving care in a health care facility. You may also hear health care–associated infections referred to as *nosocomial infections*. Health care organizations that seek to provide quality care

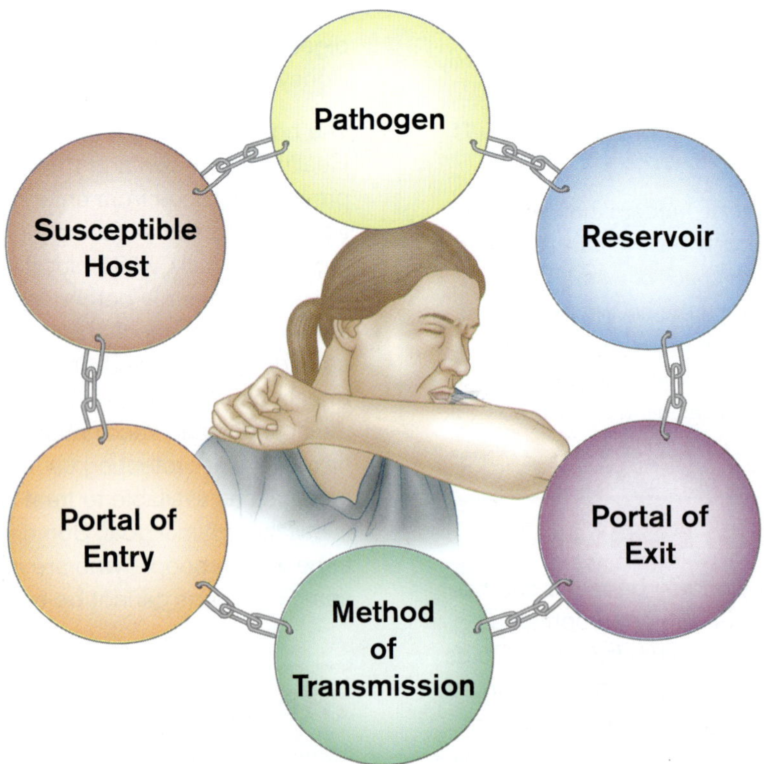

Figure 6-1 The chain of infection. Breaking just one link in this chain can stop an infection from occurring.

make it a priority to prevent health care–associated infections from occurring. If a person develops an infection while in a health care facility, he may need to stay in the facility longer so that the infection can be treated, delaying the person's recovery and driving up health care costs. In addition, developing a health care–associated infection can put the person at risk for serious complications and even death. As noted earlier, many people who are receiving care in health care facilities are more susceptible to developing infections, and if they do develop an infection, it is harder for their bodies to overcome it. In addition, some of the microbes that commonly cause health care–associated infections are very difficult to treat. Over time, these microbes have become resistant to the antibiotics (such as methicillin and vancomycin) used to treat the infections they cause, which means that these medications are no longer effective for eliminating the infection. Examples of these hard-to-treat super bugs include the following:

- **Methicillin-resistant *Staphylococcus aureus* (MRSA).** Staph infections are spread by direct contact, and can cause serious skin infections. If the bacterium enters the body (for example, through a cut on the skin), the person can develop serious infections of the blood, lungs, heart or bone.
- ***Clostridium difficile*, or C-diff.** *C. difficile* is a microbe that is passed from the body in feces. Contact with surfaces or hands contaminated by the microbe spreads the infection to others. The bacteria invade the bowel, causing diarrhea and abdominal pain. *C. difficile* produces spores that can live on hands and surfaces for a long time. When a person is known to have *C. difficile* infection, you must always wash your hands with soap and water, because alcohol-based hand rubs are not effective for removing *C. difficile* from the hands. In addition, a disinfectant containing bleach must be used to clean hard surfaces.
- **Vancomycin-resistant enterococcus (VRE).** This microbe can infect wounds, the intestinal tract and the urinary tract.

The basic infection control measures that you will learn about in this chapter are extremely effective for preventing the spread of these very dangerous microbes, as well as other microbes that can cause health care–associated infections. The key is to use these infection control methods properly and consistently.

HOW TO RECOGNIZE AN INFECTION

An infection occurs when pathogens grow inside the body. Almost any part of the body can become infected. You can recognize a possible infection in a person's body by certain signs and symptoms (Box 6-1). The signs and symptoms of infection vary according to the pathogen and the place in the body where the infection is occurring. If you notice that someone in your care has one or more of the signs and symptoms in Box 6-1, report your observations to the nurse. By recognizing infections early, you help to ensure that the person receives prompt treatment, which in turn helps to prevent the spread of infection to other people. Remember that not all people with infections will show common signs and symptoms of infection. This is why it is important to practice infection control with *every* person in your care, even when you do not observe any signs or symptoms of infection.

Box 6-1 **Common Signs and Symptoms of Infection**

- High body temperature
- Red or draining eyes
- Stuffy nose
- Coughing
- Headache
- Sore throat
- Flushed face
- Loss of appetite
- Nausea
- Stomach pain
- Diarrhea
- Vomiting
- Cloudy or smelly urine
- Joint pain
- Muscle ache
- Skin rash
- Sores
- Redness around a wound or incision
- Drainage from a wound or incision
- Swelling

ELDER CARE NOTE. In older adults, fever may not be present even if an infection is present. That's because many older adults have other chronic conditions, are taking medications, or have changes in their immune system that can interfere with the body's ability to produce a fever. So be alert for other possible signs and symptoms in older adults, such as:

- **A new onset of confusion or increased confusion (if the person is already confused).**
- **Changes in eating or appetite.**
- **New onset of the loss of bladder or bowel control or more frequent episodes of incontinence.**
- **Loss of the ability to complete tasks the person is usually able to do.**
- **Fatigue or lethargy.**
- **Flu-like symptoms.**

Box 6-2 General Actions That Help to Control the Spread of Microbes

- **Cleanse your hands frequently, using soap and water or an alcohol-based hand rub.**
- **Take care of your body.** Eat well, exercise and get enough rest to keep your immune system healthy.
- **Get vaccinated.** Vaccines are available to prevent many infectious diseases, including influenza and hepatitis B. Receiving appropriate vaccinations and keeping them up to date helps to protect you from getting these infectious diseases.
- **Stay home if you are sick.** If you must report to work when you are not feeling well, be sure to discuss your illness with your supervising nurse so that he or she can make decisions about what tasks you can do and what care you can safely provide to others.
- **Recognize and report signs and symptoms of infection.** Be on the lookout for any signs of infection and report any findings immediately to the nurse.
- **Maintain cleanliness.** Keep yourself, those in your care, and the environment clean.
- **Ensure single use of personal equipment.** Make sure each person in your care has his or her own personal items such as bedpans, urinals, washbasins, emesis basins, toothbrushes, toothpaste, lotion and soap. These items should never be shared.
- **Handle linens properly.** When handling bed linens, be sure to keep dirty linens away from your uniform. Avoid shaking dirty linens, because this can spread microbes into the environment. Place dirty linens in the laundry bag in the person's room before you carry the bag to the laundry hamper outside the room. Place wet and soiled linens in a plastic or leakproof laundry bag.
- **Cover bedpans and urinals.** To contain fluids when carrying them from one place to another, always cover bedpans and urinals.
- **Prepare food carefully.** When preparing food for yourself or for those in your care:
  - Wash your hands first.
  - Rinse off the tops of cans before opening them.
  - Wash fruits and vegetables before using them.
  - Ensure that cooked foods (especially meat) reach the proper temperature.
  - Wash, dry and store dishes and utensils after each use.
  - Wash cutting boards used to prepare meat and poultry with hot soapy water immediately after use. Use separate cutting boards for cutting meat or poultry and for cutting vegetables that are not going to be cooked.
- **Serve meals immediately.** After food arrives from the dietary department of a hospital or nursing home, or as soon as you prepare food in a person's home, serve it immediately.
- **Store foods carefully.** Make sure people do not store food in their rooms, unless the food is nonperishable and is stored in a tightly sealed container. If a person wants to save part of a meal for later, explain to her that unrefrigerated food can grow bacteria that can make her ill, and tell her that you will bring her a fresh serving of the food later, if she wants it.

HOW TO CONTROL THE SPREAD OF MICROBES

Health care workers take certain actions to control the spread of microbes that can cause disease. This practice is called **infection control**. Protecting those in your care from infections is an important part of ensuring their safety, one of the five principles of care. You probably already practice some types of infection control in your daily life without thinking much about it. If you cough or sneeze, for example, do you cover your mouth with a tissue or cough or sneeze into your elbow to control the spread of germs? If someone you know has a cold or flu, do you try to keep your distance from that person so that you will not catch the cold or flu yourself? Do you always wash your hands after using the bathroom? If you do these things, you already are using infection control methods. Box 6-2 summarizes general actions that can be taken to help control the spread of microbes. Four common methods of infection control used in health care settings include hand washing (also called hand hygiene), decontaminating objects and surfaces, using personal protective equipment (PPE) and taking isolation precautions.

Hand Washing

Washing your hands is ***the most important thing*** you can do to control the spread of microbes (Figure 6-2). As a nurse assistant, you wash your

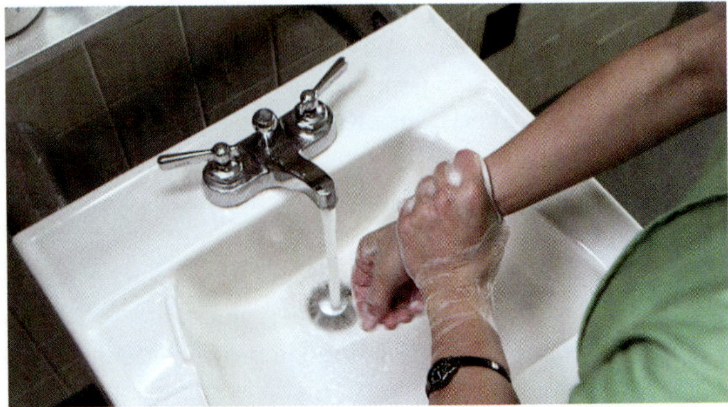

Figure 6-2 Washing your hands is the single most important thing you can do to protect yourself and others from infection.

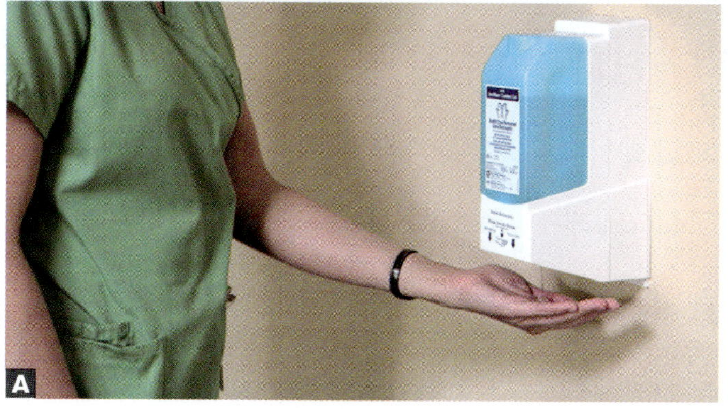

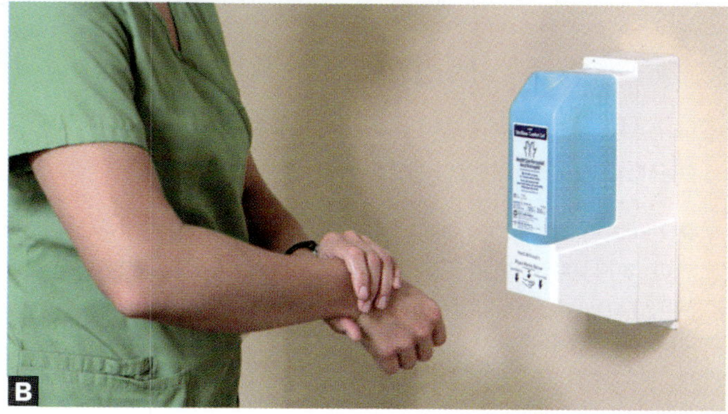

Figure 6-3 An alcohol-based hand rub may be used as an alternative to washing with soap and water if your hands are not visibly soiled with blood or other body fluids. To use an alcohol-based hand rub, (A) dispense the recommended amount of product into the palm of one hand, and (B) rub your hands together, covering all surfaces, until the product dries.

hands in a special way to ensure that all surfaces are clean. You should wash your hands whenever they are visibly soiled with dirt or **body fluids**, and at specific times throughout the day (Box 6-3). Guidelines for proper hand washing are given in Box 6-4. The specific procedure for hand washing is explained step by step in Skill 6-1.

When your hands are visibly soiled, you must wash them with soap and water. However, if your hands are not visibly soiled with dirt or body fluids, you may use an alcohol-based hand rub to decontaminate your hands instead of washing with soap and water. When using an alcohol-based hand rub, use the amount of product recommended by manufacturer. Rub it thoroughly over all surfaces of the hands, including the nails and between the fingers, until the product dries (Figure 6-3).

Sometimes you may think that hand washing is an inconvenience when you have so much else to do. But the one time you decide to skip hand washing may be the time you infect yourself or someone else with microbes from another person.

Box 6-3 When to Wash Your Hands

- As you are coming on duty
- Before and after contact with a person in your care
- Before and after putting on gloves
- After using the bathroom
- After coughing, sneezing or blowing your nose
- After smoking
- After handling dirty supplies or equipment
- Before handling food
- Before handling clean supplies or equipment
- Before going home
- Any other time you think it may be important

Keeping Objects and Surfaces Clean

When you work in any health care setting, you can help control the spread of infection if you understand exactly what is meant by *clean* and what is meant by *dirty*. Clean items or surfaces are considered to be free of dirt and pathogens. Dirty items or surfaces are considered contaminated because they contain dirt or pathogens. An unused item is considered to be clean until it comes in contact with a person or his environment. It is then considered dirty and cannot be reused for another person. In a hospital or nursing home, clean, unused supplies (such as linens and dressings) are stored in the clean utility room. Used supplies that must be cleaned or laundered are returned to the dirty utility room. The dirty utility room also has trash containers for disposing of disposable supplies.

As a nurse assistant, one of your responsibilities is to help keep the person's environment clean. You may also be responsible for cleaning some types of equipment after you use it. Health care workers use many strategies to remove microbes from objects and surfaces. Simply washing the object or surface with soap and water will remove dirt and some microbes. Or you can use **disinfectant** to kill microbes on the object or surface (Figure 6-4). The facility will specify which disinfectant solution to use, or you may make a disinfectant solution by mixing a solution of 1½ cups bleach to 1 gallon of water. When using a bleach solution, always ensure good ventilation and wear gloves and eye protection. Let the disinfectant or bleach solution stand on the surface for the recommended amount of time (for example, 1 to 3 minutes for a

Box 6-4 Nurse Assistant DO's and DON'Ts

Hand Washing

DO keep your fingernails trimmed short and use a nailbrush or orange stick to remove dirt and microbes from underneath them.

DON'T wear artificial nails or nail polish. Microbes can be very difficult to remove from the spaces created when artificial nails lift or nail polish peels and cracks.

DON'T wear rings to work. The tiny spaces in jewelry are difficult to clean and can harbor microbes. In addition, it is difficult to remove microbes from underneath the jewelry.

DO push your watch above your wrist, put it in your pocket or pin it to your uniform. This enables you to wash your wrists along with your hands.

DO apply hand lotion to help prevent the chapping and dryness that can occur with frequent hand washing.

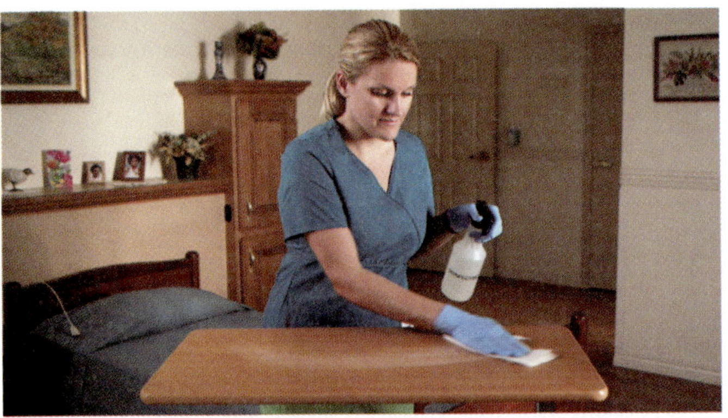

Figure 6-4 One of your responsibilities as a nurse assistant is to keep the person's environment clean. Here, a nurse assistant is using a disinfectant solution to clean an over-bed table.

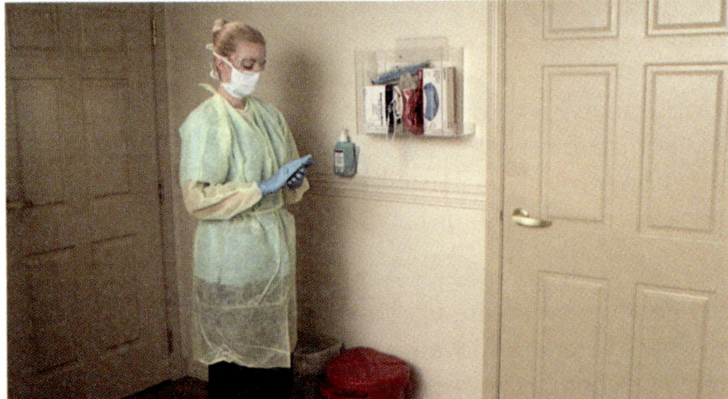

Figure 6-5 Personal protective equipment (PPE) helps to protect your skin, mucous membranes and uniform from becoming contaminated with microbes.

disinfectant solution, 10 to 15 minutes for a bleach solution). When it is necessary to destroy all of the microbes on an object or surface, **sterilization** is used. Objects that are going to be placed inside a person's body (for example, indwelling urinary catheters) must be sterile. Sterilization is achieved using gas, chemicals, dry heat or pressurized steam. In facilities, a special department (often called Central Supply) is usually responsible for sterilizing objects. In the home setting, boiling an object in water for 20 minutes is an effective means of sterilization.

Using Personal Protective Equipment

Personal protective equipment (PPE) is used to prevent microbes from contaminating your uniform, skin or mucous membranes. Properly using PPE eliminates a portal of entry for potential pathogens, and helps to keep you safe from infection. PPE includes gloves, gowns, masks and eyewear (Figure 6-5).

PPE is usually put on outside of the person's room, and removed and discarded inside the person's room. When it is necessary to put on multiple types of PPE, items are put on in the following order: gown, mask, protective eyewear, gloves. When it is necessary to remove the PPE, the order is as follows: gloves, protective eyewear, gown, mask. Removing PPE in the proper order helps to protect you from contaminating yourself or your uniform. Guidelines for the proper use of PPE are given in Box 6-5. Skill 6-2 describes step by step how to put on and remove each article of PPE.

Gloves

Disposable gloves are typically made of vinyl, nitrile or latex. These gloves are meant to be worn once and then discarded. Gloves should fit properly, and be free of rips or tears. Gloves are worn whenever there is a possibility that you will come in contact with a person's blood or body fluids (Box 6-6). For example, you wear gloves when you provide mouth care, perineal care or care for someone who has a draining wound or open sores on the skin. You also wear gloves when there is a break in the skin on your own hands.

You may need to change gloves several times during one procedure to avoid contaminating clean surfaces

Box 6-5 Nurse Assistant DO's and DON'Ts

Using Personal Protective Equipment (PPE) Properly

DO choose gloves that fit your hands properly.

DON'T wear gloves as a "second skin" throughout the day. Replace your gloves as often as necessary throughout a procedure to avoid contaminating clean surfaces with dirty gloves, and always discard your gloves and wash your hands when you have finished the procedure.

DON'T wash or disinfect disposable gloves for re-use. They are meant to be worn once and discarded.

DON'T use gloves that have rips, tears or punctures, or that appear discolored.

DO change masks and gowns if they become moist.

DO put on and take off PPE in the proper order.

by touching them with dirty gloves. Always wash your hands after removing your gloves and before putting on a new pair. When you are finished caring for one person, always remove and discard your gloves and wash your hands before leaving the room or assisting another person.

Some people are allergic to latex, a material commonly used to make disposable gloves. If you or the person you are caring for develops skin redness, a rash, hives, itching, a runny nose, sneezing, itchy eyes, a scratchy throat or difficulty breathing while you are providing care using latex gloves, wash the area in contact with the gloves immediately, and notify the nurse. In the future, you will need to use disposable gloves made of vinyl or nitrile when providing care.

Recall that you will be responsible for helping Mrs. Wang with changing her ostomy appliance and with bathing.

Should you wear gloves when assisting Mrs. Wang with these activities? Why or why not?

Box 6-6 When to Wear Gloves

- When there is a possibility that you will touch blood or other body fluids
- When you are providing care that requires you to touch mucous membranes
- When the person in your care has broken skin, or you have broken skin on your hands
- When you must handle items or surfaces soiled with blood or other body fluids

Gowns

A gown is worn to protect your clothes and body from splashes and sprays of blood and body fluids. The gown must completely cover you from your neck to your knees. A gown is worn only once and then is placed in a laundry hamper (if it is made of fabric) or thrown away (if it is made of paper). Because a damp or wet gown will not protect you, you must change your gown if it becomes wet.

Masks

A mask covers your nose and mouth to protect you from inhaling pathogens into your lungs. You may also wear a mask when it is important to protect the person from pathogens you may exhale. The mask should fit snugly over your nose and mouth. Use a mask only once. Change your mask if it becomes moist, because moisture reduces the effectiveness of the mask.

There are two types of masks you may use. A surgical (face) mask is most commonly used. These masks are effective for providing a barrier that large droplets cannot pass through. When a person is known to have a disease that is caused by very small droplets suspended in the air (called aerosols) a **high-efficiency particulate air filter (HEPA) mask** must be worn. HEPA masks must be specifically fitted to the person who will be wearing them. These masks actively filter the air to prevent aerosols from passing through.

Protective eyewear

Wear protective eyewear, such as goggles or a face shield, to keep body fluids from splashing into your eyes when cleaning items or disposing of fluids. Protective eyewear may be reusable or disposable.

Taking Isolation Precautions

Isolation precautions are actions taken to isolate pathogens to prevent them from spreading throughout the facility. Isolation precautions are based on the pathogen's method of transmission. The goal of these precautions is to contain the pathogen and limit others' exposure to it as much as possible. There are two major types of isolation precautions: **standard precautions** and **transmission-based precautions**.

Standard precautions

Standard precautions (sometimes called universal precautions) are precautions that health care workers take with *every* person to protect themselves and others from pathogens that are transmitted in body fluids. You must practice standard precautions whenever you come into contact with body fluids, such as when assisting with a medical procedure or when providing personal care—even if you think the person in your care is not infected. Box 6-7 lists standard precautions. Memorize these precautions and make them a way of life as you work as a nurse assistant.

Transmission-based precautions

When a person's primary care provider suspects or confirms that the person has an infection that can be spread to others, you must take additional precautions to prevent the spread of the infection to other people. These precautions are referred to as transmission-based precautions. The primary care provider decides which transmission-based precautions must be followed. This decision is based on two things: *the pathogen* and *how that pathogen spreads*. When transmission-based precautions are in effect, you will usually put on the appropriate PPE before entering the person's room, and remove it at the doorway right before leaving the person's room. The three types of transmission-based precautions are airborne precautions, droplet precautions and contact precautions.

- **Airborne precautions** are used when caring for a person who is known or thought to have an illness that is transmitted through the air. For example, **tuberculosis** (Box 6-8) and measles are spread in this manner. Airborne pathogens (pathogens expelled into the air when an infected person breathes, coughs or sneezes) can travel a long distance on air currents and through ventilation systems. Therefore, airborne precautions include placing the person in a private room and keeping the door closed, wearing a HEPA mask when providing care, and having the person wear a mask when he or she must leave the room.
- **Droplet precautions** are used when caring for a person who is known or thought to have an illness that is transmitted by large droplets in the air, such

Box 6-7 **Standard Precautions**

1. **Wear disposable gloves** whenever the possibility exists that you could come into contact with blood or body fluids. This includes when you are providing care and situations where you must handle items soiled with blood or other body fluids. Also wear gloves whenever you have broken skin on your hands.
2. **Wash your hands** and skin surfaces thoroughly and immediately if your skin becomes soiled with blood or other body fluids, or if you have handled potentially soiled items. Also wash your hands after removing gloves, and before putting on gloves. If your hands are not visibly soiled with blood or other body fluids, you may use an alcohol-based hand rub to decontaminate your hands after removing gloves and before putting on a clean pair.
3. **Wear personal protective equipment (PPE)** as indicated by the situation. A gown must be worn whenever the possibility exists that your uniform could be soiled by the splashing of blood or other body fluids. Protective eyewear, a mask, or both must be worn whenever the possibility exists that blood or other body fluids could splash into your eyes, nose or mouth.
4. **Handle sharp objects carefully.** Protect yourself and others from injury caused by sharp objects that may be soiled by blood or other body fluids (such as razors and needles) by disposing of them in a **sharps container**. Never recap a sharp object before disposing of it, because you could cut yourself while trying to replace the cap.
5. **Clean up blood or body fluid spills promptly,** using an approved disinfectant or a freshly mixed solution made by adding 1½ cups of bleach to 1 gallon of water. Be sure to wear appropriate PPE when cleaning up the spill.
6. **Handle contaminated articles carefully.** Put articles that have been contaminated with blood or body fluids into a puncture-proof, labeled biohazard bag. Place a second bag over the first if the outside of the first bag may have become contaminated. Skill 6-3 describes step by step how to handle a plastic trash bag and how to double-bag contaminated waste.
7. **Practice respiratory hygiene and cough etiquette.** Take measures to contain respiratory secretions that can spread infections such as influenza. Encourage people who enter the facility with visible signs of a respiratory illness to cough or sneeze into a tissue to contain respiratory secretions, dispose of tissues properly and clean their hands with soap and water or an alcohol-based hand rub after sneezing, coughing or handling dirty tissues. People with signs of respiratory illness may also be provided with masks or physically separated from other people (for example, in common waiting areas) to further limit the spread of infections carried by respiratory secretions.

▼ Box 6-8 Tuberculosis and the Health Care Worker

As a nurse assistant, you may care for people with tuberculosis, a bacterial infection of the lungs that is spread through the air from one person to another. People with tuberculosis are most likely to spread the disease to people they spend time with every day. The bacteria are put into the air when the person with tuberculosis coughs, sneezes or talks.

In most people who become infected with the pathogen that causes tuberculosis, the body is able to fight the pathogen and keep it from growing and multiplying in the body. The pathogen becomes inactive, but remains alive in the body and can become active later. Many people with tuberculosis infection never develop active tuberculosis disease. However, in others, the pathogen that causes tuberculosis becomes active later in life, and the person develops tuberculosis. Although tuberculosis primarily affects the lungs, it can affect the bones, brain, kidneys and other organs as well. If not treated, tuberculosis can be fatal. Treatment is complex and involves taking many different medications over an extended period of time.

Because health care workers are at risk for exposure to the pathogen that causes tuberculosis, health care facilities routinely screen employees for infection. Many states also require health care workers to be screened for tuberculosis infection as a requirement for employment. Screening can be done using a skin test called the Mantoux test, which involves placing a small amount of tuberculin (a protein made from the bacteria that causes tuberculosis) under the skin using a needle or tines. After a few days, the area will become red and swollen if the person is infected with the pathogen that causes tuberculosis. A blood test may also be used to screen for tuberculosis. Remember that a positive result on a screening test does not mean that you have active tuberculosis. The pathogen that causes tuberculosis may be alive in your body, but inactive. If a screening test indicates exposure to tuberculosis, other follow-up tests, such as sputum testing or chest x-rays, are ordered to rule out active tuberculosis.

as a respiratory virus or meningitis. These droplets are spread by sneezing, coughing, laughing, singing and talking. The droplets do not travel far. Droplet precautions are similar to airborne precautions, except a surgical (face) mask can be worn instead of a HEPA mask.

- **Contact precautions** are used when caring for a person who is known or thought to have an illness that can be spread by direct or indirect contact. Some types of wound infections and skin infections can be spread in this way. Contact precautions include wearing a gown and gloves when providing care, and containing and disposing of contaminated items properly.

When transmission-based precautions are in effect, a sign may be posted outside the person's room so that all health care workers and visitors (if permitted) are aware of the precautions that must be taken. Make sure visitors and other health care workers follow these precautions.

Having transmission-based precautions in effect can be very difficult for the person. How would you feel if the door to your room had to be closed all the time for isolation? Perhaps you would feel as if no one wanted to be near you or that no one liked you. You might feel lonely, angry, depressed, embarrassed, afraid or all of these things! What if the people caring for you could not come near you without wearing gowns, masks and gloves? Even though you must follow transmission-based precautions as ordered, you can also be sensitive to the person's feelings. Make sure the person knows why the transmission-based precautions are being taken, and stress that these precautions will help to speed her recovery and prevent others from getting sick. Explain the purpose of the PPE you are wearing. This can help the person get used to seeing you in protective clothing. Make a special effort to check in on the person often, and take time to talk with her. Spending time with the person and offering reassurance can help the person feel better about the time spent in isolation, and the need for the transmission-based precautions.

You know from the nurse's report that droplet precautions are in effect for Mrs. Wang because staph pneumonia is contagious. As you enter Mrs. Wang's room, she turns her face away and covers her eyes so that you can't see her tears.

"Good morning, Mrs. Wang," you say and then introduce yourself. You explain that you will be taking care of her today. Mrs. Wang looks at you and smiles sadly.

What might be bothering Mrs. Wang?

How could you provide emotional support to Mrs. Wang, in addition to providing physical care?

What information would you give Mrs. Wang about the transmission-based precautions that are being used?

BLOODBORNE PATHOGENS AND WORKPLACE SAFETY

As a nurse assistant, you are responsible for keeping yourself and others safe from *all* infections. However, some infections pose particular risk to you as a health care worker, because of their long-term effects on your health if you become infected. Many of the most serious infections that health care workers may be exposed to are caused by **bloodborne pathogens**. Infection occurs when blood from an infected person enters the bloodstream of a person who is not infected. In the workplace, this could happen if you stick yourself with a contaminated needle (a "needlestick injury") or cut yourself with broken glass that has been soiled with blood. You could also become infected through direct contact with another person's blood if it comes in contact with your eyes, mucous membranes or an area of broken skin on your body.

Bloodborne diseases that pose particular risk to health care workers are **human immunodeficiency virus (HIV)** infection and hepatitis B, C and D.

- **HIV** is a virus that that invades and destroys the cells that help us to fight off infections. A person who is infected with HIV may look and feel healthy for many years. However, during this time, the virus is breaking down the person's immune system. Eventually, most people who are infected with HIV develop **acquired immunodeficiency syndrome (AIDS)**. A person with AIDS is unable to fight off infections that a healthy person would be able to resist or control. The person dies from one of these infections, or another complication of HIV infection. Although medications have been developed to help slow the progression of HIV infection, currently there is no cure.
- **Hepatitis** is inflammation of the liver, an organ that performs many vital functions for the body. There are many different types and causes of hepatitis. Hepatitis B, hepatitis C and hepatitis D are caused by infection with bloodborne viruses. Chronic infection with the viruses that cause hepatitis B, C or D can lead to liver failure, liver cancer and other serious conditions. A vaccine is available to protect against hepatitis B virus (HBV). Vaccination for HBV also offers protection from hepatitis D virus (HDV). However, there is no vaccine to protect against hepatitis C virus (HCV).

You and your employer share the responsibility for protecting you from **occupational exposure** to bloodborne pathogens. Remember that the standard precautions we take with every person (see Box 6-7) are designed to prevent accidental exposure to blood and other body fluids. This is because you may not know whether a person is infected with a bloodborne pathogen or not, and it is important to protect yourself and others from accidental exposure. To effectively limit your risk for exposure to bloodborne pathogens while you are on the job, you must practice standard precautions consistently and correctly. Your employer also has responsibility for keeping you safe from bloodborne pathogens on the job by making sure you have the equipment and training you need to lower your risk. Standards that employers must follow to keep their employees safe from occupational exposures to bloodborne pathogens are outlined in the Bloodborne Pathogens Standard issued by the Occupational Safety and Health Administration (OSHA) in 2001 (Box 6-9).

Box 6-9 Bloodborne Pathogens Standard

To protect health care workers from exposure on the job to bloodborne pathogens, employers are required to adhere to the following standards:

- **Exposure control plan.** The facility must have a plan that outlines actions that will be taken if an employee is exposed to blood or other body fluids on the job. The plan must be reviewed annually and made available to all employees in written form. Employees are responsible for reporting exposure incidents so that proper follow-up (for example, medical testing) can be provided.
- **Proper training.** Employers must provide training about risks associated with bloodborne pathogens and how to minimize these risks to all employees who may be exposed to bloodborne pathogens on the job. Training usually occurs during employee orientation and then at regular intervals thereafter.
- **Proper equipment.** Employers are responsible for providing personal protective equipment (PPE) for employee use.
- **HBV vaccination.** Employers must offer employees who have a risk of exposure to blood an opportunity to receive at no cost a vaccination that protects against hepatitis B. An employee may refuse the vaccination, but if at any time the employee later decides to accept the vaccination, the employer must provide it.
- **Work practice controls.** The employer is responsible for establishing and enforcing procedures for handling contaminated waste, laundry and so on, and supplying the equipment needed to follow these procedures. The employer must also ensure that necessary systems are installed and running to maintain a safe environment (for example, ventilation systems).
- **Engineering controls.** The employer is responsible for making equipment available that limits the employee's risk for needle-stick injuries, such as sharps containers.

CHECK YOUR UNDERSTANDING

Questions for Review

1. **When you take dirty linens to the laundry hamper you should:**
   a. Shake them first.
   b. Hold them away from your uniform.
   c. Take only one sheet at a time to prevent contamination.
   d. Save steps by tossing them into the laundry hamper from a short distance.

2. **What is the most important thing you can do to control the spread of microbes?**
   a. Bag all contaminated linens.
   b. Wash your hands.
   c. Always cover bedpans and urinals when carrying them from place to place.
   d. Eat a well-balanced diet and stay healthy.

3. **You should practice standard precautions:**
   a. When you provide care for any person.
   b. Only when you provide care for people infected with HIV or HBV.
   c. Only when a person is in isolation.
   d. Only when you need to wash your hands.

4. **What is one time when you must wear gloves?**
   a. When you give someone a back rub
   b. When you cough or sneeze
   c. When you serve meal trays
   d. When you touch blood or other body fluids

5. **If you have a cut or open sore on your hand, what must you do to protect yourself from infection?**
   a. Avoid providing care for people with infections.
   b. Stay away from work until the wound heals.
   c. Wear gloves while providing care.
   d. Handle only clean items.

6. **Which of the following is a reason to place someone in isolation?**
   a. The person has a contagious disease.
   b. The person had surgery.
   c. The person is demanding and cannot get along with others.
   d. The person wants the privacy of a single room.

Questions to Ask Yourself

1. *How can you control the spread of infection when you provide care for a person with an open wound?*
2. *How can you spread infection if you have a cold?*
3. *In the past, how have you possibly spread pathogens through direct and indirect contact? Think of three ways.*
4. *What will you do in the future to avoid spreading pathogens by direct and indirect contact? Think of three ways.*
5. *Airborne precautions are in effect for Mr. Thompson. You are changing Mr. Thompson's linens when you realize that you brought only one sheet instead of two. How would you handle this problem? What would you do first?*
6. *When you put on gloves to help Mr. Wilson with mouth care, he eyes the gloves and says, "I don't have AIDS, you know. Why are you wearing those things?" How should you respond?*
7. *Emma Jones, who works as a nurse assistant, became engaged over the weekend. She wants to wear her new engagement ring to work on Monday so that she can show it off. What does she need to consider when deciding whether to wear the ring?*
8. *The nurse asks for your help to position a person on his side. The person has a large, open, draining wound that needs cleaning. The nurse explains to you that a great deal of solution will be used to clean the wound and that it is likely to splash. What personal protective equipment (PPE) should you put on and why?*

Skill 6-1
Hand Washing

PREPARATION

1. Gather your supplies:
   - Soap
   - Paper towels
   - Orange stick or nail brush (optional)
   - Lotion (optional)
2. Remove your watch or push it up on your forearm. If you are wearing long sleeves, push them up.

PROCEDURE

3. Turn on the water and adjust the temperature until it is comfortably warm.
4. Put your hands under the running water to wet your hands and wrists, keeping your hands and wrists below the level of your elbows.
5. Apply soap from the dispenser.
6. Rub your hands together vigorously to work up a lather.
7. Wash vigorously for at least 20 seconds (Figure 1, A–D), paying particular attention to:
   - The wrists (grasp and circle with your other hand).
   - The palms and backs of your hands.
   - The areas between the fingers.
   - The nails (rub against the palms of your hands, or use an orange stick or nail brush to clean underneath them).

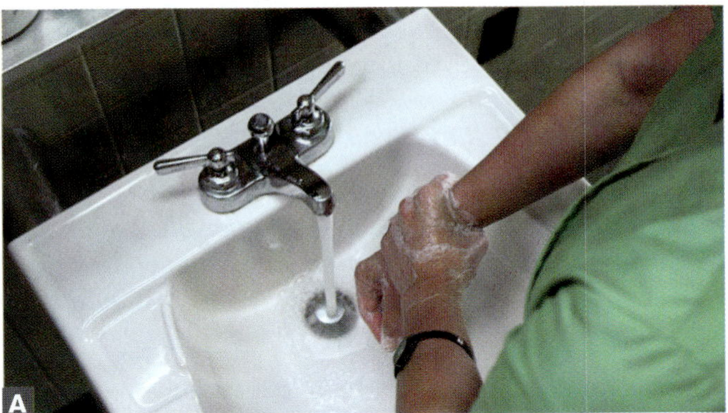

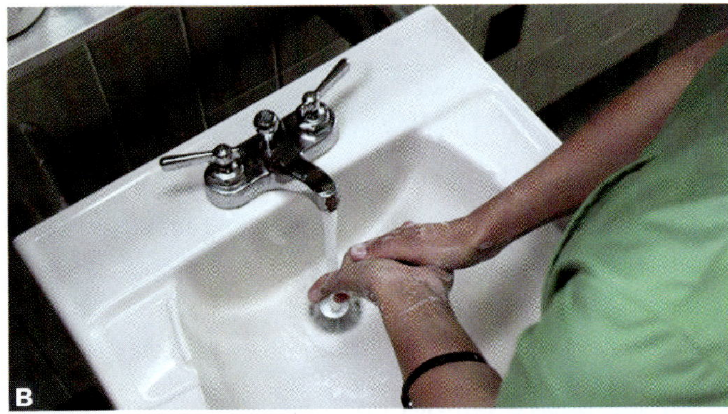

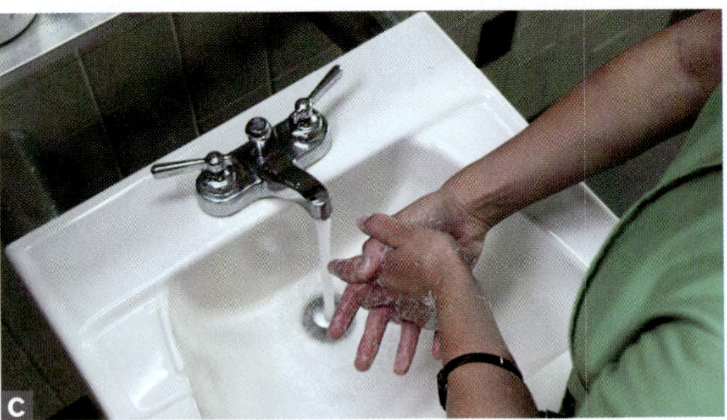

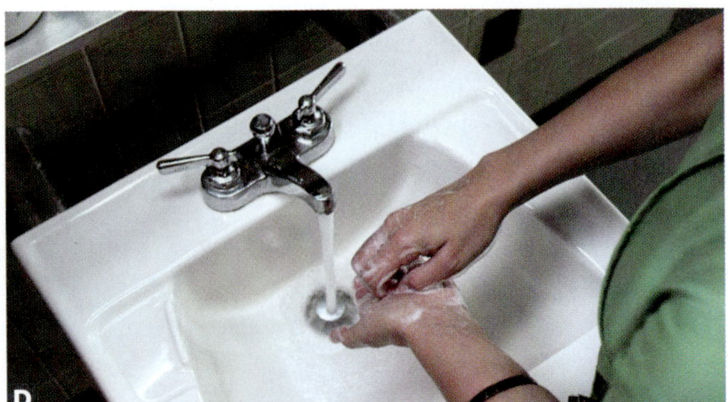

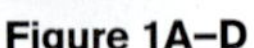
Figure 1A–D

8. Rinse your hands and wrists under the running water, keeping your hands lower than your elbows and the fingertips down (Figure 2).

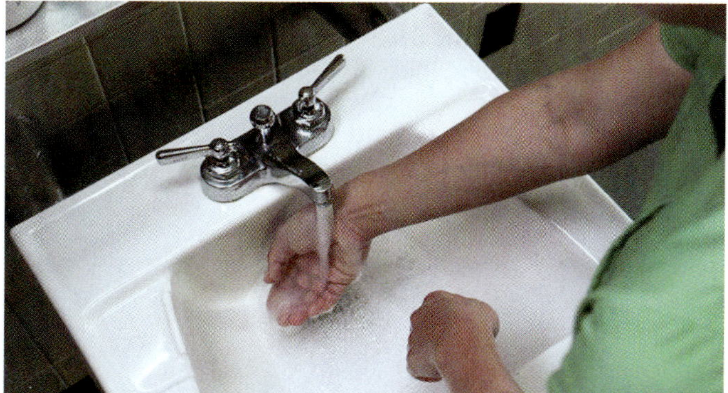

Figure 2

9. Using a clean, dry paper towel, dry your hands thoroughly, beginning at the fingertips and moving back toward the elbow (Figure 3). Drying your hands thoroughly keeps them from becoming chapped. Discard the paper towel in a facility-approved waste container.

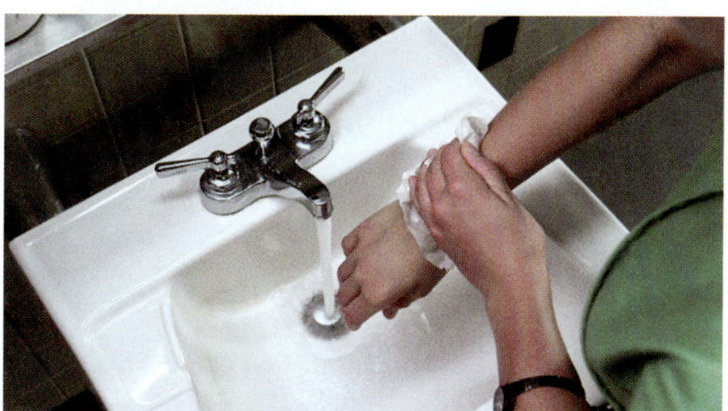

Figure 3

10. Use another clean, dry paper towel to turn off the faucets (Figure 4). Discard the paper towel in a facility-approved waste container.

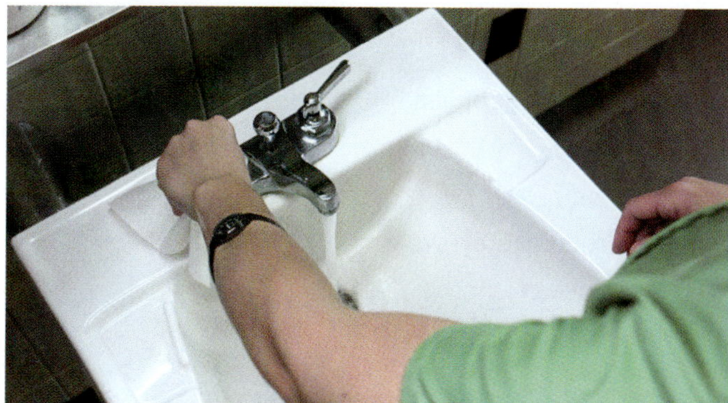

Figure 4

11. Exit the hand-washing area by pushing the door open with your shoulder and hip. If the door has a handle, turn the handle using a paper towel to avoid contaminating your clean hands.

12. If desired, apply a small amount of hand lotion to prevent chapping and dryness.

Skill 6-2

Using Personal Protective Equipment (PPE)

PREPARATION

1. Gather your supplies:
   - Gown
   - Mask
   - Protective eyewear
   - Gloves
2. Wash your hands.

PROCEDURE

Putting on a Gown

3. Slide your arms through the armholes, keeping the opening of the gown in the back.
4. Fasten the ties at the back of your neck and at your waist, making sure the edges of the gown overlap so that your back is completely covered (Figure 1).

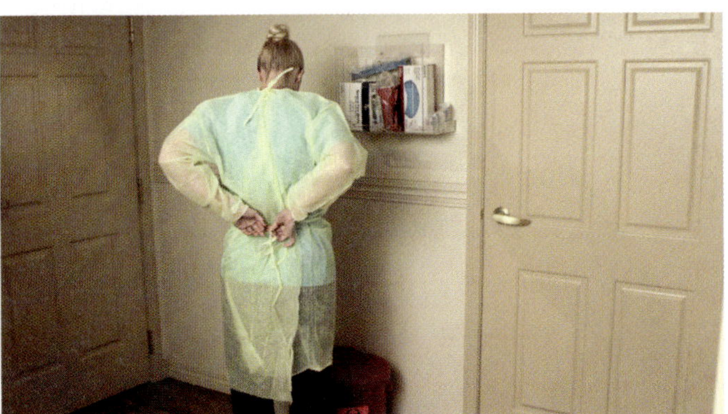

Figure 1

Putting on a Mask

5. Put the mask over your mouth and nose.
6. Tie the top strings behind your head, then tie the bottom strings or place the elastic loops around your ears (Figure 2).

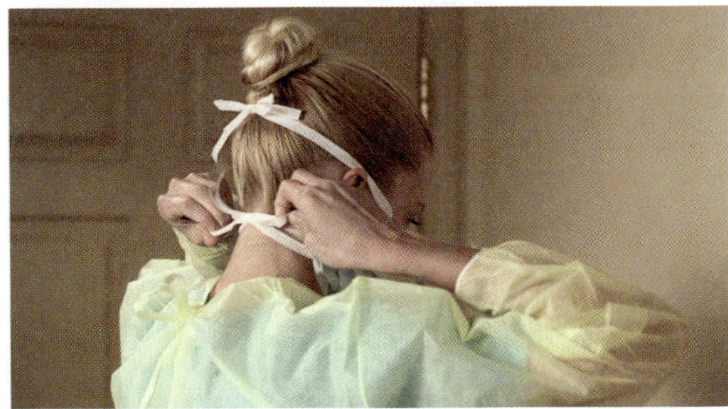

Figure 2

7. Adjust the mask for comfort. If necessary, bend the nose wire to fit.

Putting on Protective Eyewear

8. Place the earpieces over your ears or the headband around your head and adjust the fit.

Putting on Gloves

9. Inspect both gloves carefully for tears.
10. Put the gloves on carefully so that they do not tear. Pull the gloves up over the gown cuffs (Figure 3).

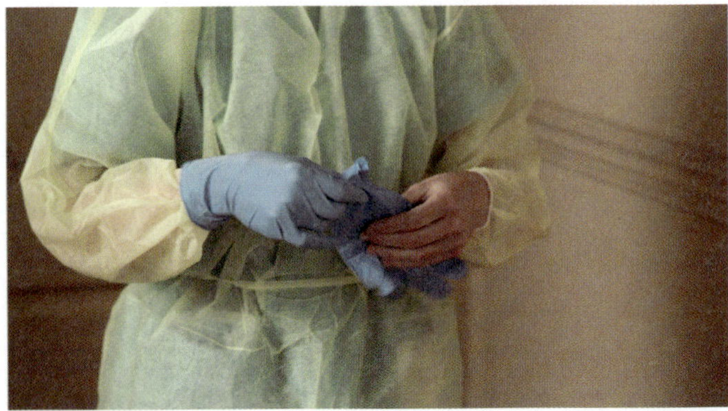

Figure 3

Taking off Gloves

11. Make a cuff on your dominant hand by grasping the glove and pulling it partway down toward your fingers (Figure 4). Do not touch the clean inside of the glove.

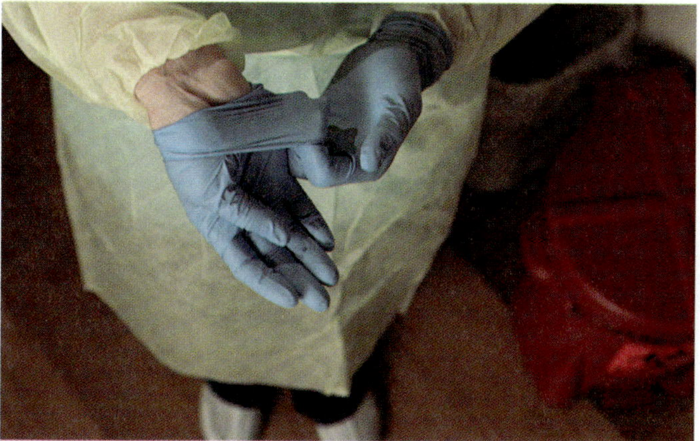

Figure 4

12. Using the fingers of your dominant hand, pull the glove on your non-dominant hand off by pulling it inside out and rolling it into a ball. Be careful not to let the outside (contaminated side) of the glove touch your bare hand as you pull the glove off. (Figure 5).

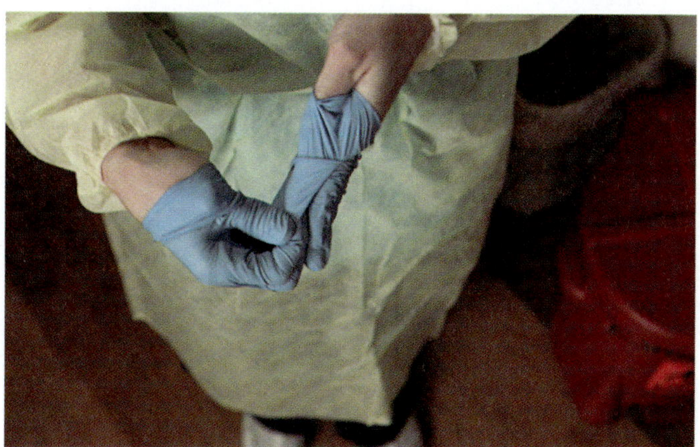

Figure 5

13. Continue to hold the glove that you have removed in your dominant (still-gloved) hand. With your bare non-dominant hand, place your fingers under the cuff of the glove on your dominant hand, touching only the clean inside of the glove (Figure 6).

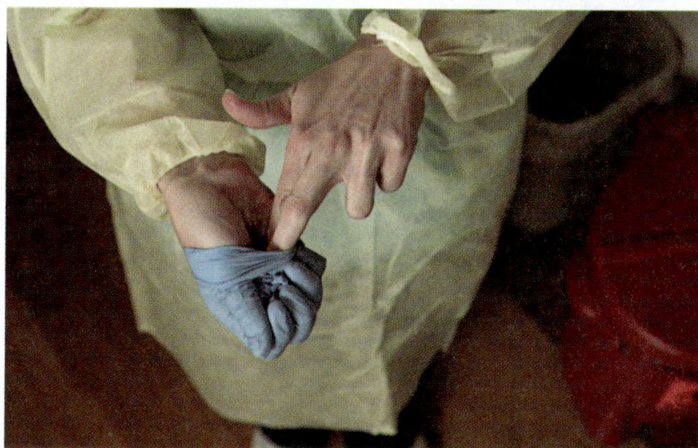

Figure 6

14. Remove the glove by pulling it down so that the other glove is contained inside (Figure 7).

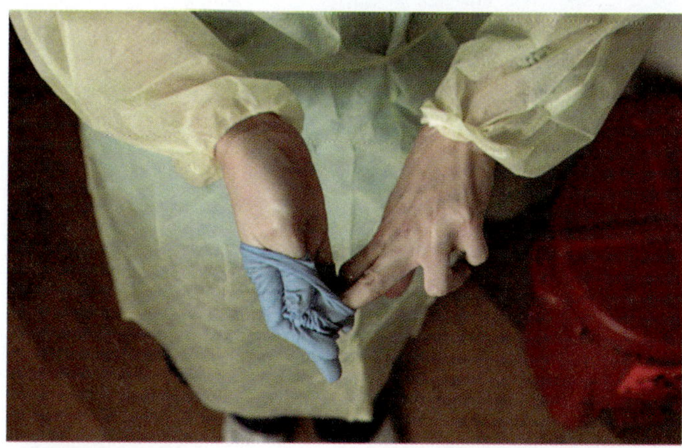

Figure 7

15. Discard the gloves in a facility-approved waste container.

Taking off Protective Eyewear

16. Touch only the earpieces or the head band.
17. Place the eyewear in the appropriate container for reprocessing, or discard in a facility-approved waste container.

Continued on next page

Skill 6-2
Using Personal Protective Equipment (PPE) *Continued*

Taking off a Gown

18. Untie the neck and waist strings.
19. Pull off one gown sleeve by slipping your fingers under the cuff and pulling the sleeve just over your fingertips (Figure 8).

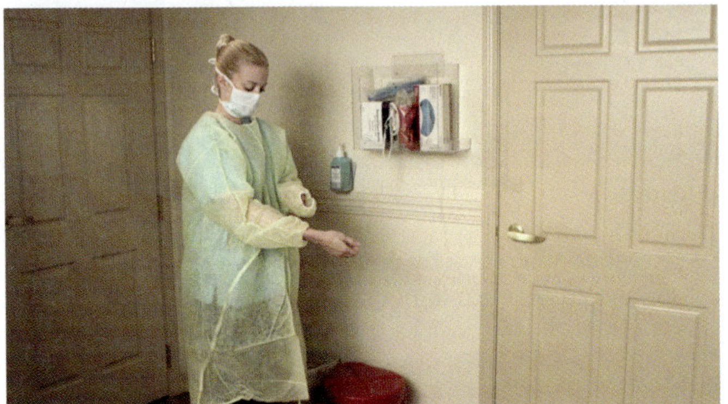

Figure 8

20. Grasp the other sleeve with the covered hand and pull it off.
21. Continue holding that sleeve in your covered hand. Grasp the inside of the first shoulder of the gown with your uncovered hand and pull the gown off the shoulder (Figure 9). Continue to bring the gown forward and turn it inside out as you pull it over your covered hand.

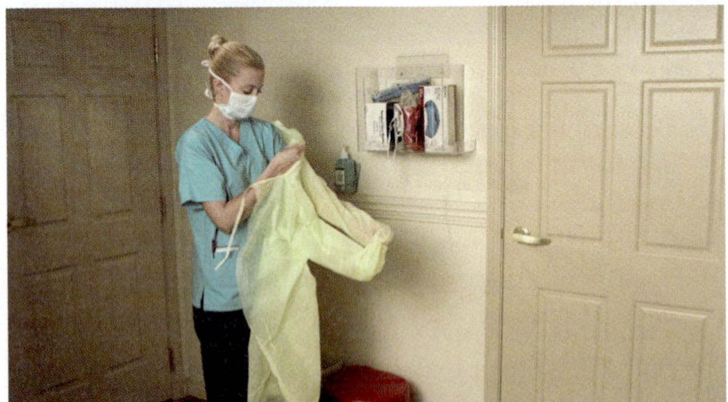

Figure 9

22. Fold the outer, contaminated surface inward and roll up the gown (Figure 10).

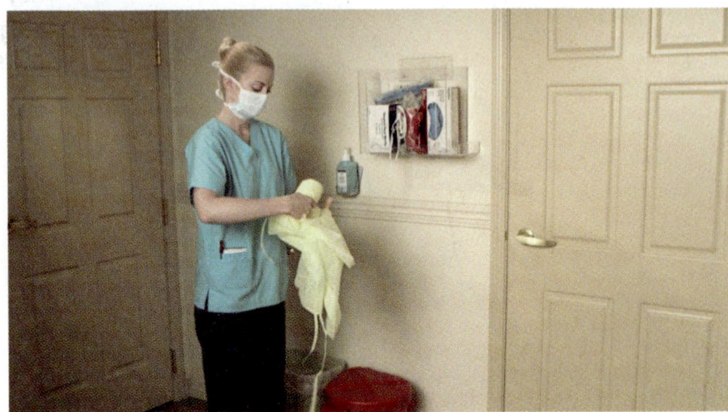

Figure 10

23. Discard the gown in a facility-approved waste container, or place the gown in the laundry hamper, if it is not disposable.

Taking off a Mask

24. Untie the bottom strings and then the top strings, or pull the elastic loop from around one ear and then the other.
25. Hold the mask by the strings (Figure 11) and discard it in a facility-approved waste container.

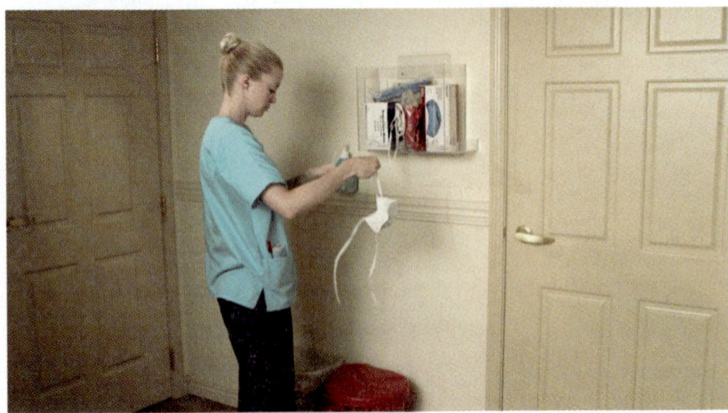

Figure 11

COMPLETION

26. Wash your hands.

Skill 6-3
Handling a Plastic Trash Bag

PREPARATION

Gather supplies:

- Plastic trash bag(s)

PROCEDURE

Opening a Plastic Trash Bag

1. Open the plastic trash bag and make a cuff around the opened edge (Figure1).

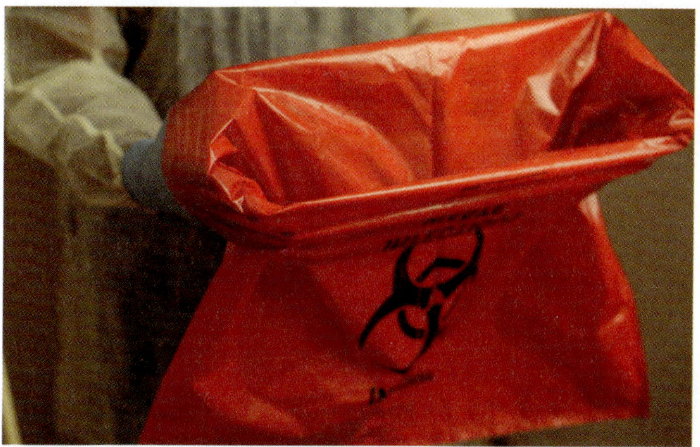

Figure 1

2. Put the opened bag on a clean surface within easy reach of your work area.

Closing a Used Plastic Trash Bag

3. Put your fingers under the cuffed edge of the used plastic trash bag.
4. Pull the cuffed edges together and close the bag by tying a knot. Touch only the outside of the bag because the inside of the bag is contaminated.

Double-Bagging a Bag That Is Contaminated with Body Fluids

5. Arrange for a co-worker to assist you at a certain time.
6. Remove the bag from the trash or laundry container inside the person's room, close it and carry it to the door of the person's room.
7. Have your co-worker prepare a clean bag by folding down a cuff at the top of the clean bag and labeling the bag "contaminated." Have your co-worker hold the clean bag under the cuff and stand by the doorway.
8. Put the bag with contaminated items into the clean bag that your co-worker is holding under the cuff (Figure 2).

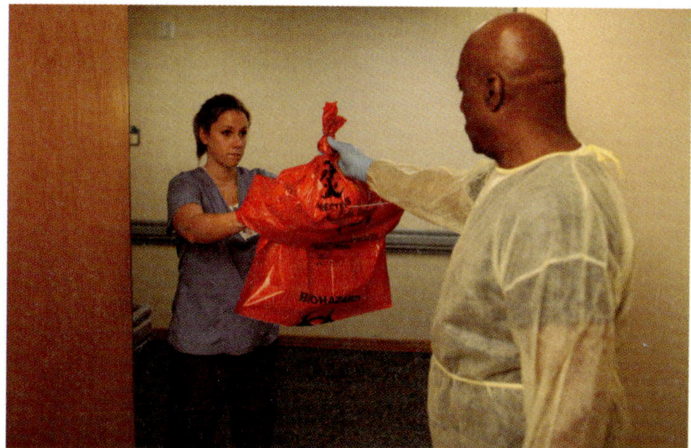

Figure 2

9. Have your co-worker close the outside bag by raising the cuffed area and tying a knot.
10. Have your co-worker take the bag to the area designated for disposal or laundering of contaminated items.
11. Wash your hands.

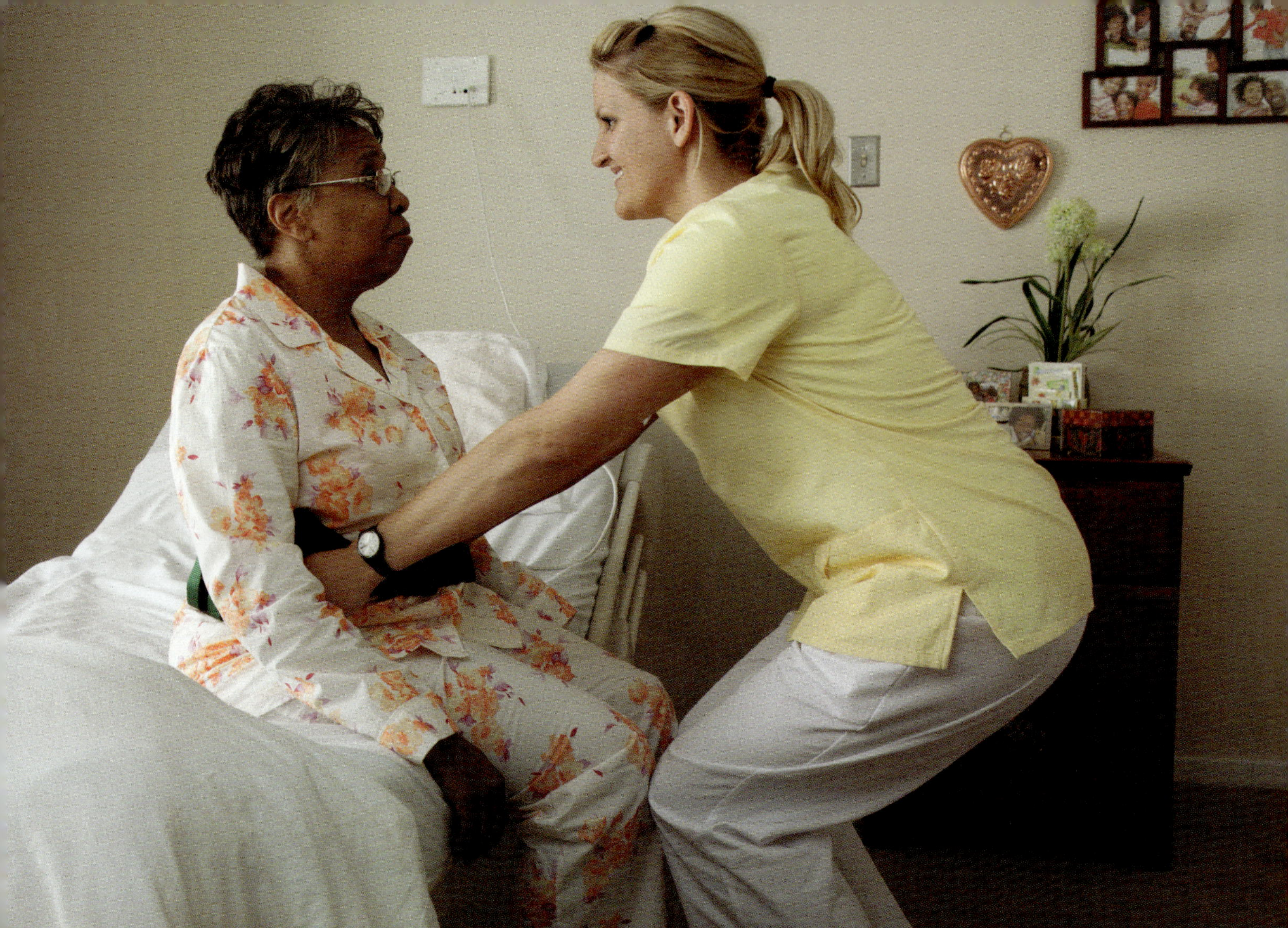

CHAPTER

7 Preventing Injuries

Goals

After reading this chapter, you will have the information needed to:

- Use proper body mechanics and lifting technique to protect your body from injury on the job.
- Describe the safe use of equipment with moving parts.
- Be aware of factors that place those in your care at risk for injury.
- Take measures to prevent common accidents (such as falls, electrical shocks, burns and poisoning) from occurring.
- Ensure that proper follow-up takes place if an incident does occur.
- Understand the hazards associated with restraint use, and describe alternatives to restraint use.

Foods and beverages that are too hot can also cause burns. If food is steaming or a plate is too hot to touch, wait until the food stops steaming or the plate has cooled a little before serving the meal. Also make sure hot beverages have cooled a bit before serving them. If a person has trouble keeping a firm grip on the cup, spills can occur, leading to burns. Serving the beverage in a cup with handles and a lid can help the person hold the cup more securely (Figure 7-7).

Some people may use heating pads to promote comfort. Place the heating pad in its cloth cover or wrap a towel around it before placing it against the person's skin. Set the temperature according to the person's care plan, and avoid leaving the heating pad in place for longer than 20 minutes. Check the skin underneath the pad every 5 minutes for excessive redness or blisters. Do not allow the person to lie on top of the heating pad, because this increases the likelihood of burns.

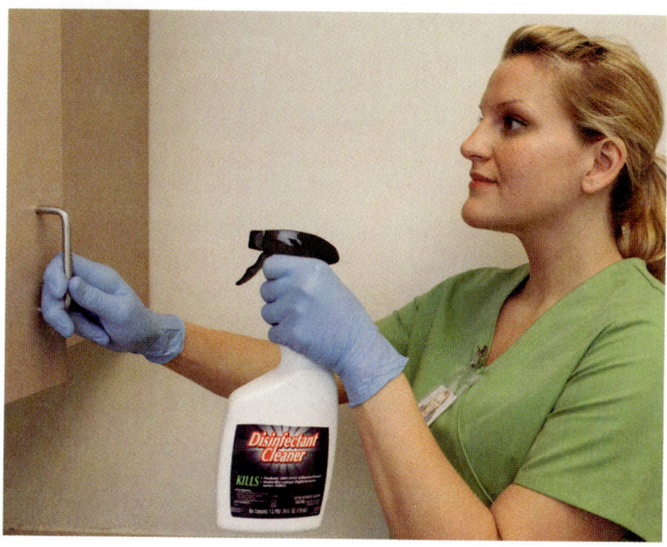

Figure 7-8 All containers should have a clear label stating what is inside. Keep cleaning supplies, medications and other potentially poisonous substances in a locked cabinet or closet.

Poisoning

A poison is any substance that causes injury, illness or death if it enters the body. Cleaning supplies, fluids used for car and home maintenance, and certain plants can all cause poisoning if a person swallows them. Poisoning can also occur if a person takes the wrong medication, or too much of it. To reduce the risk for accidental poisoning, make sure all containers are clearly and accurately labeled. Store all medicines, cleaning materials and other potentially poisonous substances in locked cabinets and closets (Figure 7-8).

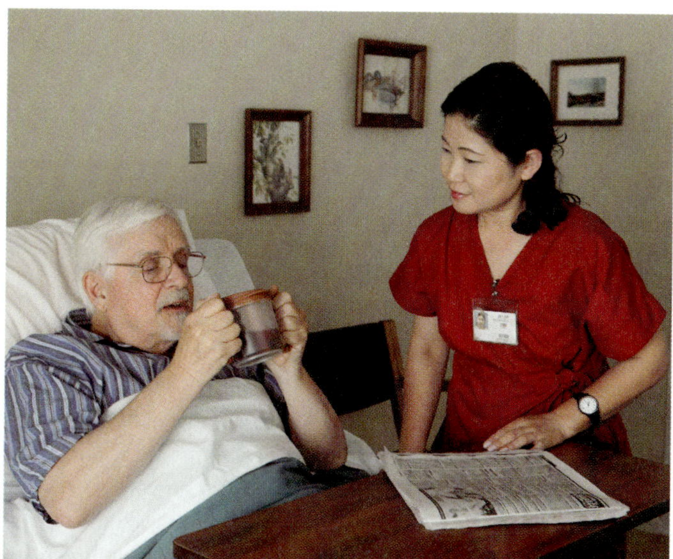

Figure 7-7 Take special precautions to prevent burns caused by spilling hot liquids or foods when a person has weak or unsteady hands.

It is 11:00 and your new resident, Mr. Rivera, has arrived with his wife. The admissions paperwork has been completed and you've helped to get Mr. Rivera settled in his room and his belongings put away. You show Mr. Rivera how to use the call signal and ask him to please call you before he gets out of bed or the chair, so you can help him.

Knowing what you know about Mr. Rivera, what risk factors does he have for injury?

In addition to showing Mr. Rivera how to use the call signal and reminding him to use it whenever he wants to get up, what other measures will you take to help keep Mr. Rivera safe?

Reporting Incidents

An **incident** is something unusual that happens to a person receiving care, a staff member or a visitor to the facility and has the potential to cause harm. You must verbally report all incidents, even those that do not result in injury, to the nurse. In addition, you must complete a written incident report, per your employer's policy.

When reporting an incident and completing an incident report, it is important to provide facts, not opinions. The goal is not to assign blame. It is to provide a factual account of what happened so that appropriate steps can be taken to prevent a similar incident from happening in the future. Report the incident and complete the incident

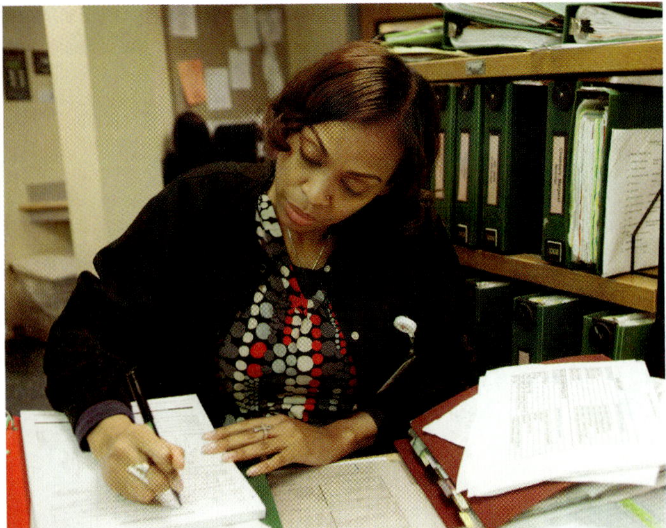

Figure 7-9 Following an incident, an incident report must be completed. The incident report helps management identify trends and prevent similar incidents from occurring in the future.

report promptly, while the details of what happened are still fresh in your mind (Figure 7-9).

A complete incident report contains answers to the following questions:

- Who was the person involved in the incident?
- Was the person confused before or after the incident?
- Was the person alone?
- What happened to the person? Was the person injured? If so, describe the injury.
- What caused the incident? (For example, was water on the floor?) Remember to state only facts, not opinions.
- Where did the incident happen?
- When did the incident happen (time, date)?
- Who gave assistance or first aid?
- What kind of assistance or first aid was given?
- Were there witnesses to the incident? If so, who?
- Did the person receive medical treatment?

Also include other information that would be a useful part of the record or that is required by your employer.

A WORD ABOUT RESTRAINTS

A **restraint** is any device that inhibits a person's freedom of movement. Restraints can be physical or chemical. A physical restraint is attached on or near a person's body to limit the person's freedom of movement or ability to reach part of her body. Examples of physical restraints include wrist restraints, mitt restraints, jacket restraints and vest restraints. Devices such as side rails and lap trays can also be considered physical restraints, if the person is not able to move them out of the way independently. Chemical restraints are medications used to subdue a person, so that the person is unable to function normally.

In the past, it was thought that restraints helped to keep people safe by preventing them from getting up without assistance and falling or wandering away from the facility. However, now we know that restraints can cause very serious complications, and even death (Box 7-3). In addition, the use of restraints can rob a person of his or her dignity. As a result, restraint use is decreasing in all health care settings. Today, many health care facilities, especially nursing homes, strive to be restraint free. The Omnibus Budget Reconciliation Act (OBRA) states that people receiving care in nursing homes and in their own homes have the right to be free of restraints, and establishes strict guidelines for their use.

Restraints must *never* be used as a convenience for the nursing staff, or to punish or discipline a person.

Box 7-3 Complications Associated with Restraints

- **Strangulation** (cutting off the air supply) can occur with some types of restraints (such as vest restraints or seat belts) if they are not applied properly, or if the restraint moves and gets tangled around the person's neck.
- **Entrapment and other serious injuries.** A person who struggles to get free from the restraint is at risk for serious injuries, such as suffocation and broken bones. For example, a person who tries to climb over side rails may become caught in the side rails (entrapment). Attempting to get up while restrained can cause the chair or wheelchair to tip over on the person, or the person may trip and fall.
- **Mental effects.** A person who is restrained may become more agitated and confused. Other adverse mental effects include depression and loss of self-esteem.
- **Complications of immobility.** Not being able to move freely puts the person at risk for pressure ulcers, contractures, blood clots, pneumonia, incontinence, constipation and loss of muscle tone and balance.
- **Tissue and nerve damage.** A restraint that is applied too tightly can cut off the blood supply to the body part beyond the restraint, leading to tissue and nerve damage.
- **Bladder and bowel elimination problems.** If the person is not offered the opportunity to use the bathroom frequently enough, the person may become incontinent of urine, feces or both.

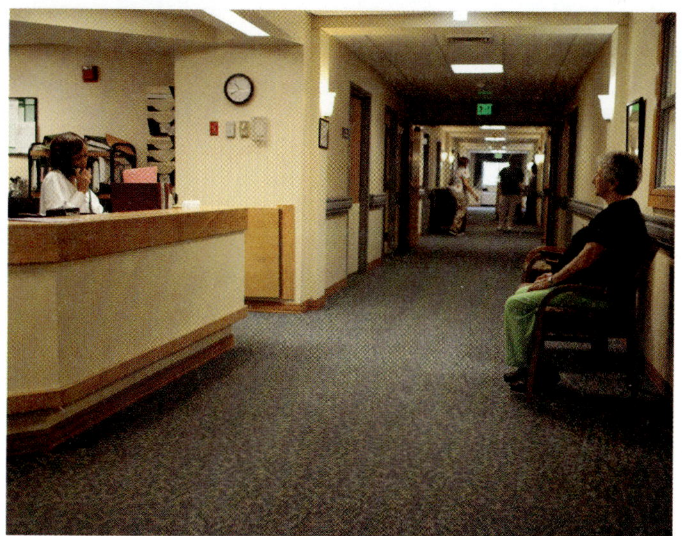

Figure 7-10 Alternatives to physical or chemical restraints must always be tried first. The better you know the person, the more able you will be to predict the person's behavior and take measures to keep the person safe. This nurse assistant knows that this resident tends to try to get out of her chair or bed when she is feeling lonely, so the nurse assistant decided to bring the resident to the nurse's station where she will feel less lonely and the staff will be able to see her if she tries to get up unassisted.

As a nurse assistant, you must seek ways to keep the people in your care safe without using restraints. Providing company and distraction is one way to do this (Figure 7-10). Involve the person in meaningful activities, such as exercise, games, hobbies or musical entertainment. Activities provide gentle physical and mental stimulation, help the person feel useful and improve the person's self-esteem. Ask family members or volunteers to sit with the person, or bring the person to the nurse's station with you while you complete paperwork. Check in on the person very frequently, and offer a snack or beverage, or assistance using the bathroom. Getting to know the person as an individual will help you think of creative ways to keep the person safe without using restraints.

In some very specific situations and health care settings, it may be necessary to apply a restraint. For example, it may be necessary to apply a wrist restraint to a hospitalized person who is confused and keeps removing a medical device that is essential to his care, such as an intravenous (IV) line. If restraints are in use in the facility where you work and applying them is part of your job description, your employer will teach you how to properly apply the types of restraints that are in use in the facility. If you are asked to apply a restraint, make sure that the conditions listed in Box 7-4 have been met first. Make sure you understand exactly how to use the restraint, and use the right size for the person's height and weight. Follow your employer's procedure and the manufacturer's instructions for securing the restraint. After the restraint is applied, you must help keep the person safe (Box 7-5).

PERFORMING SKILLS SAFELY

In Unit 3, you will begin to learn the skills you will need to provide hands-on care. Completing all of the steps of a skill, correctly and in the correct order, is important to protect those in your care, and yourself, from injury. Although you may learn how to do these skills one way during your training, your employer may have specific ways of doing certain skills, which will be detailed in a procedures manual. Always follow your employer's procedure manual.

There are certain steps that you should always take before starting a skill and after completing the skill. In this book, we call these steps "Preparation Steps" and "Completion Steps." Performing these steps routinely promotes safety and efficiency, and helps to protect the person's rights. These steps are summarized in Box 7-6. In addition, your instructor will give you a handout listing these steps, and you can keep this handout with you when performing skills in this course. It is important to memorize and perform these steps every time you provide hands-on care. Let's take a closer look at why each of the preparation and completion steps is important.

Box 7-4 **OBRA Conditions That Must Be Met Before a Restraint Can Be Applied**

- A primary care provider (doctor or advance practice nurse) must write the order for the restraint. The order must specify the type of restraint, the purpose of the restraint and how long the restraint is to be used.
- All alternatives to physical or chemical restraint must be tried and the person's response to these alternatives must be documented before resorting to the use of a physical or chemical restraint.
- There must be a clear medical reason for the restraint. A restraint is never to be used for staff convenience or to discipline a person.
- The person must be given an explanation of how the restraint works, why it is needed and how long it will be used. Family members must also be given this information if the person wants them to have it, or if the person is not able to make decisions about care independently.

Box 7-5 **Care for a Person Who is Restrained**

- Check on the person very frequently. She may need to be reassured that she hasn't been abandoned. Many people injure themselves by trying to get out of restraints without assistance.
- Release the restraints every 2 hours and help the person go to the bathroom, stretch, change positions and do range-of-motion exercises. Inspect the person's skin for reddened areas and report any concerns to the nurse. Offer the person a snack or a drink. Release the restraints more often if the person seems to be anxious, needs to go the bathroom or is in distress.
- Observe the person carefully and report any changes in behavior (such as increased agitation, drowsiness or decreased appetite) immediately to the nurse.
- Report and record the care you provide and the observations you make.

Preparation Steps

Before beginning any skill, always complete the following steps:

- **Wash your hands.** This is essential to prevent the spread of infection.
- **Gather your supplies.** Having everything you need before you start promotes efficiency.
- **Knock, greet the person and ensure privacy.** Before entering a person's room, you must always knock and ask permission to enter. Greet the person by name, and if you do not know him well, check his identification photo or wristband to make sure that the person you are speaking to is the person who is supposed to receive the care that you are about to provide! Also tell the person who you are. It is especially important to introduce yourself if the person does not know you well, is confused or has impaired vision. Shut the door to the room behind you and pull the privacy curtain to protect the person's privacy during the procedure.
- **Explain the procedure.** Tell the person what you are there to do and how he can help you. Then, as you work through the skill, tell the person what you are doing and remind him of how he can help. Remember to explain the skill in a way that the person can understand. Also, be aware that a person who is unconscious may still be able to hear you and may still be aware that someone is doing something to him, so it is important to perform this step with every person in your care.
- **Adjust equipment for body mechanics and safety.** Many of the skills you will do while the person is in bed. If the person is in an adjustable bed and will be staying in bed throughout the skill, raise the bed to a comfortable working height to protect your back. If the person will be getting out of the bed, lower the bed to the height specified in the person's care plan. This height will allow the person to place both feet flat on the floor with the hips, knees and ankles at right angles, which will make it easier and safer for him to get out of bed. Make sure the wheels on any equipment with wheels are locked.

Completion Steps

When you are finished with a skill, always perform the following steps:

- **Ensure the person's comfort and good body alignment.** Before leaving the person, smooth the sheets on the bed, make sure he is warm enough, and make sure he can easily reach items such as drinking water, the television remote or reading material. Make sure the person is in good body alignment to promote comfort and prevent complications such as pressure ulcers.
- **Adjust equipment for safety.** If you raised the bed during the skill, return it to the level specified in the person's care plan to make it safer for him to get out of bed independently. Check the wheels on any equipment again to make sure they are locked. Place the person's method of calling for help within reach. In many facilities, this will be the call light control, but it may also be a small hand bell or other way of making noise. If side rails are in place on the bed, lower or raise the side rails according to the person's care plan.
- **Clean up your work area.** Show respect for the person's living space and prevent the spread of infection by cleaning up after every skill. Dispose of disposable items. Place linens in the linen hamper for laundering. Clean and put away reusable equipment according to your employer's policy. Disinfect surfaces as required.
- **Wash your hands.** This is essential to prevent the spread of infection.
- **Report and record.** Reporting to the nurse lets the nurse know that you have completed the assigned task and gives you the chance to update the nurse on any changes in the person's condition. Record your observations and the care you provided according to your employer's policy.

▼ Box 7-6 **Preparation and Completion Steps**

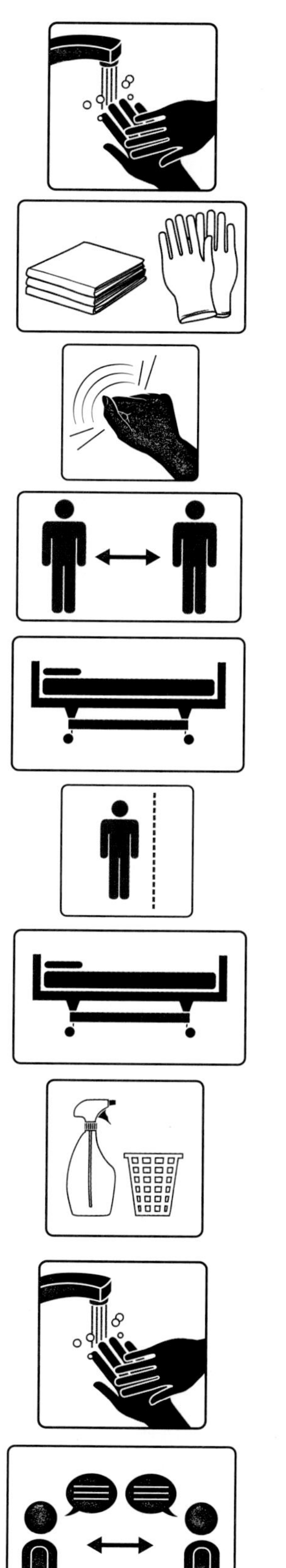

PREPARATION STEPS

Wash your hands.

Gather your supplies.

Knock, greet the person and ensure privacy.

Explain the procedure.

Adjust equipment for body mechanics and safety.

COMPLETION STEPS

Ensure the person's comfort and good body alignment.

Adjust equipment for safety.

Clean up your work area.

Wash your hands.

Report and record.

The steps listed here represent general principles of good care and should be followed throughout your training. However, your employer may have specific preparation and completion steps that you should follow; always check your employer's procedure manual.

CHECK YOUR UNDERSTANDING

Questions for Review

1. **Which of the following is part of good body mechanics?**
   a. Independence
   b. Communication
   c. Entrapment
   d. Alignment

2. **Which of the following moves increases your stability?**
   a. Moving your feet close together
   b. Bending at the waist
   c. Spreading your feet apart
   d. Relaxing your stomach muscles

3. **Before using any equipment, you should:**
   a. Check to make sure it is working properly.
   b. Unplug it.
   c. File an incident report.
   d. Stand up straight.

4. **Mrs. Singer is a home health client. Complications of diabetes have caused her to lose feeling in her legs. Because of her condition, what type of injury is Mrs. Singer at high risk for?**
   a. Poisoning
   b. Burns
   c. Entrapment
   d. Electrical shock

5. **All of the following are risk factors for falling EXCEPT:**
   a. Poor eyesight.
   b. Being overweight.
   c. Poor mobility.
   d. Medication effects.

6. **You are a new employee and the nurse has asked you to assist Mr. Thompson out of bed using a mechanical lift device. Although you have used mechanical lifts before, you are not familiar with the kind of mechanical lift used in this facility. What should you do?**
   a. Go to help Mr. Thompson. The lift probably works the same way the lifts you used at your previous place of employment did.
   b. Ask the nurse or another nurse assistant to show you how to use the lift.
   c. Help Mr. Thompson to get out of bed without using the lift.
   d. Practice using the lift with another resident before going to assist Mr. Thompson.

7. **All of the following are potential complications of restraints EXCEPT:**
   a. Death.
   b. Low self-esteem and depression.
   c. Nerve and tissue damage.
   d. Drowning.

8. **You work in a hospital and the nurse has asked you to apply a wrist restraint to Mrs. Schneider because she has repeatedly pulled her intravenous (IV) line out. Before applying the restraint, you must make sure of all of the following EXCEPT:**
   a. Mrs. Schneider is able to remove the device independently.
   b. The doctor or advance practice nurse has written an order for the restraint.
   c. Mrs. Schneider understands the reason for the restraint.
   d. You have been properly trained in how to apply the restraint, and applying restraints is part of your job description.

9. **Restraints must be released at least:**
   a. Every shift.
   b. Every hour.
   c. Every 2 hours, and more often if necessary.
   d. Whenever a relative visits.

Questions to Ask Yourself

1. *Mrs. Kennedy has poor vision and uses a walker. What special measures would you take to make sure her room is safe?*
2. *Mr. Lightfoot's legs are unsteady when he gets up quickly from his chair. Today, he is anxiously waiting for a phone call from his daughter. What risk factors does Mr. Lightfoot have for falling, and what can you do to help keep him safe?*
3. *Mrs. Simpson, a resident at the nursing home where you work, has been wandering into other residents' rooms. The nurse tells you to strap her into a wheelchair so that she can't wander. What should you do?*

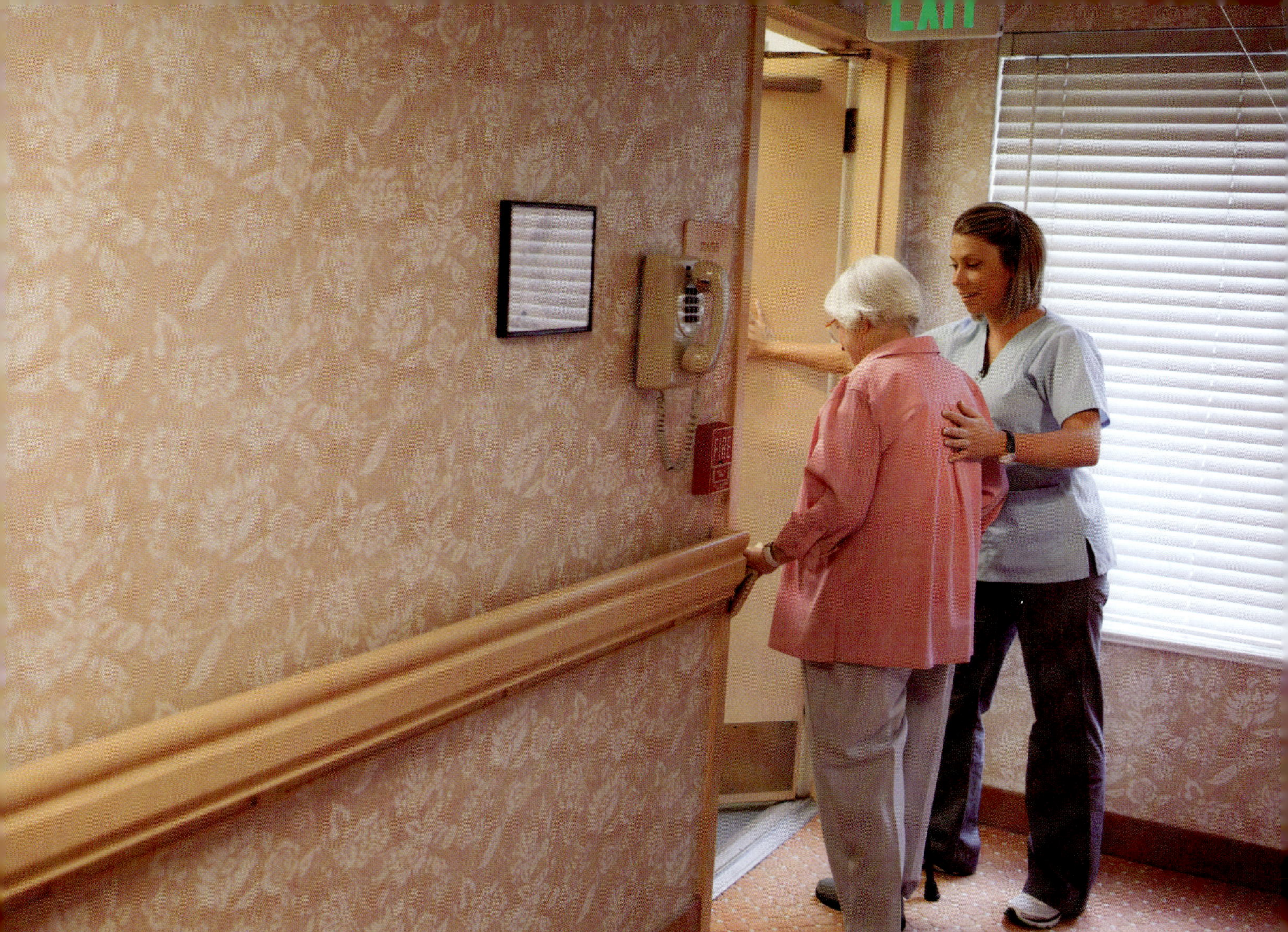

CHAPTER 8

Responding to Emergencies

Goals

After reading this chapter, you will have the information needed to:

- Recognize and respond to common medical emergencies, including stroke, myocardial infarction, choking, bleeding, shock, seizure, fainting and burns.
- Prevent a fire emergency from occurring.
- Keep people safe in the event of a fire emergency.
- Keep people safe during weather emergencies and other events that disrupt the facility's ability to function normally.

After practicing the corresponding skills, you will have the information needed to:

- Clear the airway of a conscious choking adult.

Key Terms:

emergency

disaster

first aid

cerebrovascular accident

myocardial infarction

cardiopulmonary resuscitation (CPR)

automated external defibrillator (AED)

shock

seizure

epilepsy

You have been caring for Mrs. Schulman, one of your home health clients, for 3 years. For as long as you have known Mrs. Schulman, part of your duties have been to help her get ready to go to the synagogue with her daughter on Friday evenings. But this Friday afternoon, when you arrive at Mrs. Schulman's house, she tells you she doesn't feel like attending the service. The only other time you can remember Mrs. Schulman missing Friday evening prayers was last winter, when she was hospitalized for pneumonia. Mrs. Schulman asks you to please call her daughter and tell her not to come pick her up. She says, "I just feel really strange, not like myself at all. My left leg feels numb ... like I might fall if I try to put weight on it. And my left arm feels weak and strange too. If you could just make me a cup of tea and help me get ready for bed, I think that might be best. I'm sure I'll feel better in the morning." You tell Mrs. Schulman that you are worried about her, and that you'd like to talk to someone else about her symptoms and find out what you should do.

An **emergency** is a situation that arises suddenly and requires immediate action to keep a person safe. Emergencies can be medical in nature, involving an acute illness or injury that requires immediate attention to prevent the person from dying or experiencing permanent long-term effects. Emergencies can also be environmental, involving changes to a person's environment that affect the person's health and safety. Examples of environmental emergencies include fires, weather emergencies (such as snow storms, tornadoes and hurricanes) and **disasters** (severe events that cause widespread damage and destruction, affecting many people and disrupting normal functioning of the community). As a nurse assistant, you must know how to respond in the event of an emergency to keep the people in your care safe.

MEDICAL EMERGENCIES

Recognizing and Responding to Medical Emergencies

The following steps guide your actions in an emergency and ensure your safety and the safety of others.

1. **Recognize the emergency.** Sometimes it will be obvious that a person is in distress. Other times, however, a medical emergency may only be signaled by a slight change in the person's behavior or appearance. As a nurse assistant, you will have in-depth knowledge of what is normal for each person in your care. A change from normal could signal an emergency and should be reported immediately (Figure 8-1).
2. **Check.** Stay calm, and check the scene and the person. First, make sure there is nothing that could hurt you or cause further injury to the person, such as a downed wire in the area. Next, look for clues that may help you understand what happened. Finally, check the person: tap her shoulder or hand and shout to see if he or she is conscious.
3. **Call.** Next, call for help. In a hospital, there is usually a code you can dial to call for help from within the facility. In other health care settings, you may be required to dial 9-1-1 or another emergency number. Know your employer's policies and procedures related to calling for help in an emergency.
4. **Care.** Provide appropriate care (according to the situation and your level of training) until help arrives. Help the person rest comfortably, and provide reassurance because the person is likely to be frightened and upset. In the sections that follow, we will review basic **first aid** for some common medical emergencies. To expand your knowledge of how to respond to emergencies, it is strongly recommended that you take American Red Cross First Aid/CPR/AED training in addition to the nurse assistant training course.

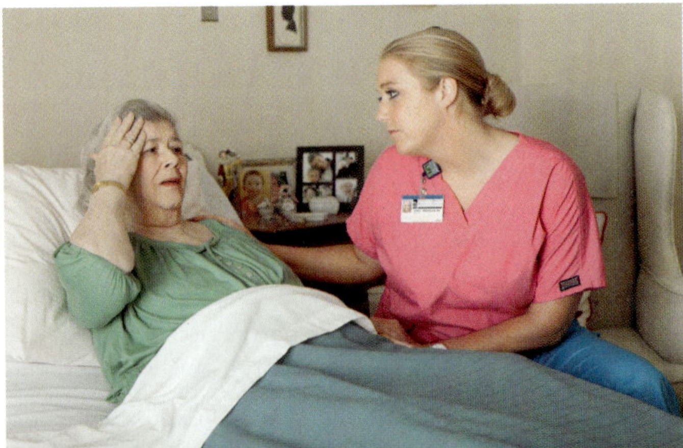

Figure 8-1 Your knowledge of what is normal for each person in your care can help you detect when something is wrong. Sometimes the only sign of a medical emergency is a slight change in the person's appearance or behavior.

5. **Report and record.** Your observations about what happened before, during and after the emergency are important to share with other members of the health care team. These observations should be reported to the nurse and documented on the appropriate forms, per your employer's policy. Note whether the person complained of any symptoms before the event, the time the symptoms started and how long the symptoms lasted. Be specific. For example, "She was breathing at a rate of 25 breaths per minute" is more specific than "She was having trouble breathing." If you arrived on the scene to find the person in distress and unconscious or otherwise unable to tell you what happened, note anything unusual that you observed while you were checking the scene and the person. Also report and record exactly what you did to help the person (for example, "I helped her to sit up and held her there.")

Observations Into Action!

In older people, the signs and symptoms of an emergency may be very general and non-specific, and they may be barely noticeable to someone who does not know the person well. Because you will spend a lot of time with the people in your care and you will get to know what is normal for each of them, you will be in a good position to notice subtle changes that could be a sign of a medical emergency. General signs and symptoms that could signal a medical emergency in an older person include the following and should be reported to the supervising nurse right away!

- **Headache**
- **A change in the person's usual level of activity**
- **A change in mental status (such as agitation, the new onset of confusion, or increased confusion in a person who is already confused)**
- **Lethargy (extreme drowsiness or sleepiness)**
- **Difficulty sleeping**

Common Medical Emergencies

Stroke

A stroke, or **cerebrovascular accident**, occurs when blood flow to a part of the brain is interrupted, resulting in the death of brain cells. A stroke can also be caused by bleeding into the brain tissue. Strokes can cause permanent brain damage, but with quick action, sometimes the damage can be stopped or reversed.

The signs and symptoms of a stroke can vary from person to person. A person who is having a stroke may show any of the following signs and symptoms:

- Slurring of words
- Drooping of the features on one side of the face (for example, the eyelid and the corner of the mouth)
- Trouble seeing in one or both eyes
- Weakness or numbness in an arm or leg
- A sudden, severe headache
- Dizziness or loss of balance
- Confusion, or a loss of consciousness
- A generally ill appearance, or abnormal behavior

The "FAST" check (Figure 8-2) is a quick way of checking for signs of a stroke:

Face. Ask the person to smile. Is there weakness or drooping on one side of the face?
Arm. Ask the person to raise both arms. Is there weakness or drooping of one of the arms?
Speech. Ask the person to say a simple sentence or phrase. Does the person have trouble speaking, or is her speech slurred?
Time. If the person has difficulty performing any of these actions or shows other signs of stroke, call for help immediately. Prompt medical attention may reduce the amount of disability the person experiences as a result of the stroke.

If you think that a person is having a stroke, follow your employer's procedure for calling for help. Stay with the person and provide reassurance until help arrives. Monitor the person's breathing and check for any changes in his condition. If the person is drooling or has trouble swallowing, place him on one side to keep the airway clear. Note when the person's symptoms started. This is important information to report because some of the medications used to treat stroke are only effective within a certain time frame after the onset of symptoms.

You are concerned about the numbness and weakness Mrs. Schulman is reporting on her left side. You do the "FAST" test with Mrs. Schulman and see that she is not able to raise her left arm. You suspect that Mrs. Schulman has had a stroke, and decide to call 9-1-1, per your employer's policy. Then you call Mrs. Schulman's daughter.

What information should you be ready to give the emergency services dispatcher?

What care will you provide to Mrs. Schulman while you are waiting for the ambulance to arrive?

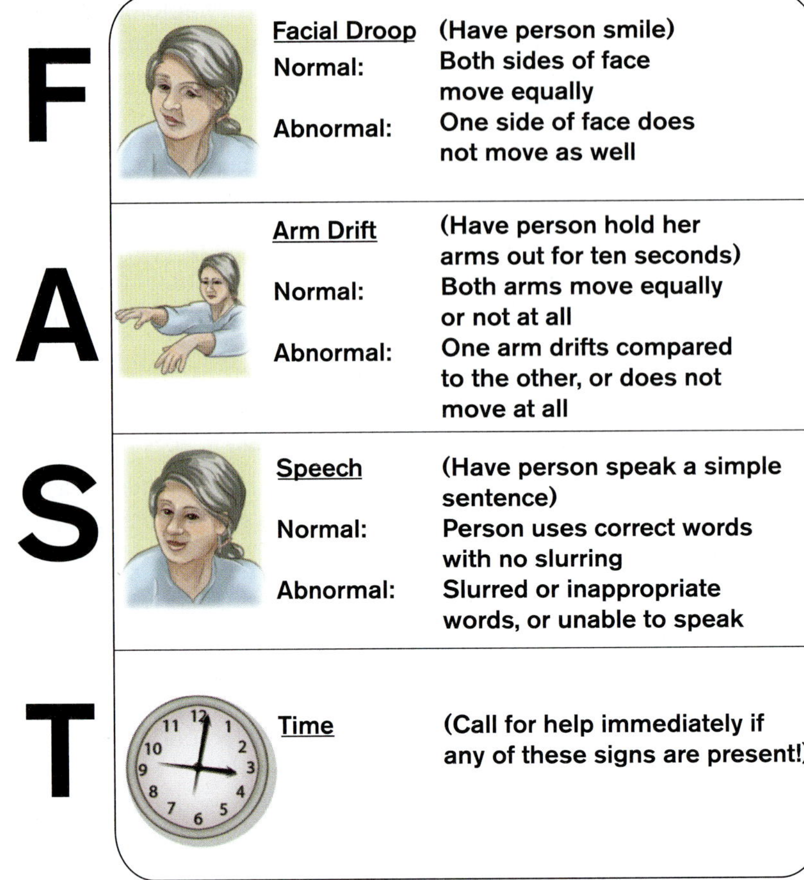

Figure 8-2 "FAST" recognition and reporting of stroke symptoms can help to minimize the lasting effects of stroke.

Myocardial infarction

A **myocardial infarction**, or heart attack, occurs when blood flow to part of the heart muscle (the myocardium) is blocked, causing the cells in that area to die. As a result, the heart's ability to pump blood throughout the body can be affected. If a large area of the heart is damaged, the heart may stop beating (cardiac arrest). Signs and symptoms of a heart attack vary from person to person, and can be different in women than they are in men. A person who is having a heart attack may show any of the following signs and symptoms:

- Chest pain, discomfort, pressure, or squeezing that lasts longer than 3 to 5 minutes and is not relieved by resting, changing position, or taking nitroglycerin, or that goes away and then comes back
- Discomfort or pain that spreads to one or both arms, the back, the shoulder, the neck, the jaw or the upper part of the stomach
- Dizziness, lightheadedness or loss of consciousness
- Trouble breathing, including noisy breathing, shortness of breath and breathing that is faster than normal
- A heartbeat that is faster or slower than normal, or irregular
- Nausea
- Pale, ashen or slightly bluish skin
- A cold sweat
- A feeling of anxiety or doom
- Extreme fatigue (tiredness)

Although men most often have the classic signs of a heart attack (for example, chest pain), women often have more subtle signs, such as a squeezing sensation in the chest, extreme fatigue, nausea, breaking out in a cold sweat, dizziness or lightheadedness, and shortness of breath.

If you think a person in your care is having a heart attack, stay with her and follow your employer's procedure for calling for help. Encourage the person to remain calm and quiet while you are waiting for help to arrive.

If the person loses consciousness, stops breathing, or has no pulse, the person is in cardiac arrest and will require **cardiopulmonary resuscitation (CPR)** and possibly defibrillation (delivery of an electric shock to the heart muscle to restore a normal rhythm). An **automated external defibrillator (AED)** is a portable electronic device that delivers a defibrillation shock automatically or with a push of a button to help the heart restore an effective pumping rhythm (Figure 8-3). The proper use of an AED along with CPR has been shown to improve survival rates among people experiencing cardiac arrest. You should know the location of AEDs in your facility, because you may be asked to retrieve the AED in an

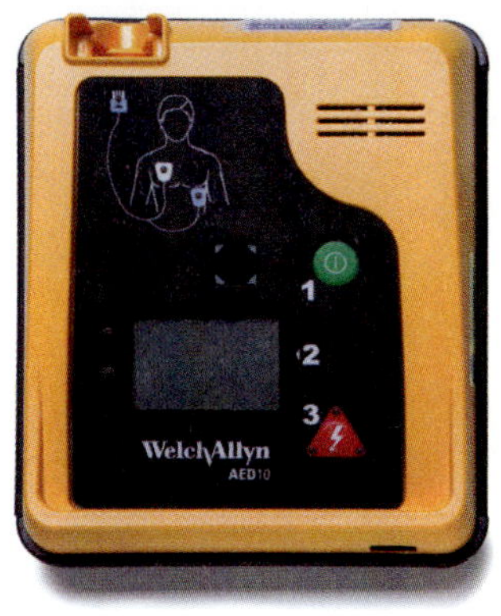

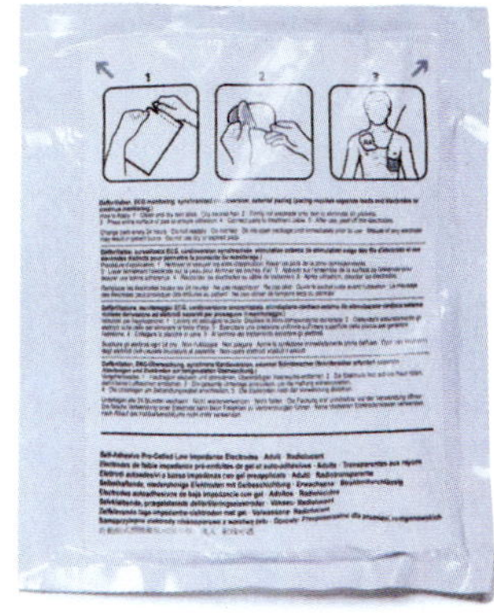

(AED) is often used along
en a person is in cardiac
acility in case you need to

sters CPR. You
ning barrier devices
ng resuscitated and
bes in saliva, blood
ou can access them
CPR and using an
ourse, but you are
erican Red Cross
these skills.

omes either partially or
ct. Many of the people
choking. For example,
oke or multiple
to swallow or clear
problems or poorly
ability to chew food
ng. Eating while talking
so lead to choking.

o choke, you will need
erson to speak to you.
coughing forcefully,
sit up if she is lying
eep coughing. If the
object and clear the

l is coughing weakly
d while breathing,
and the person
must call for help
e procedure for giving
g adult (Skill 8-1).
, cough or breathe,
she will lose consciousness quickly unless the airway is cleared. Call for help immediately, and then, if the person is conscious, follow the procedure for giving first aid to a conscious choking adult (see Skill 8-1). If the person becomes unconscious, you must follow a different procedure. The procedure for helping an unconscious person who is choking is not taught as part of this course. This skill is taught as part of the American Red Cross First Aid/CPR/AED course, which you are strongly encouraged to take in addition to your nurse assistant training course.

Bleeding

Bleeding can be internal or external. Internal bleeding is not immediately obvious, but external bleeding is. Severe bleeding, whether it is internal or external, is life-threatening. To provide care for a person who is bleeding externally, first take standard precautions by putting on gloves. If you think the blood might spray or splatter, you may need eye and face protection as well. Control the bleeding by covering the wound with a sterile dressing and firmly pressing against the wound with your gloved hand until the bleeding stops (Figure 8-4, A). Apply a pressure bandage over the dressing to maintain pressure on the wound and to hold the dressing in place (see Figure 8-4, B). If blood soaks through the first dressing and bandage, continue to apply pressure and add a second dressing and bandage. If the

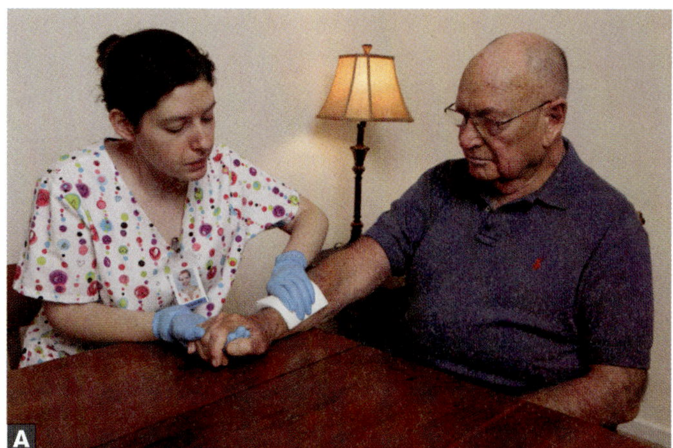

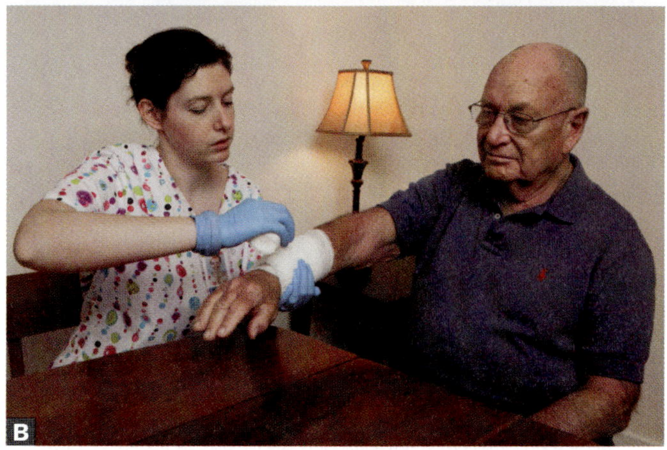

Figure 8-4 First aid for external bleeding. (A) Cover the wound with a sterile dressing and apply pressure. (B) Apply a pressure bandage to secure the dressing.

bleeding does not stop, you must call for help. Stay with person, and observe the person closely for signs that may indicate that the person's condition is worsening, such as breathing that is faster or slower than normal, changes in skin color and restlessness. Provide reassurance, and keep the person calm. Remember to wash your hands immediately after removing your gloves.

Shock

Shock is a condition in which the circulatory system fails to deliver enough oxygen-rich blood to the body's tissues and vital organs. There are many causes of shock, including massive blood loss, heart failure, severe allergic reactions and severe infections that overwhelm the body.

A person who is in shock may show any of the following signs or symptoms:

- Excessive thirst
- Restlessness or irritability
- Nausea or vomiting
- Altered level of consciousness
- Pale or ashen, gray, cool, moist skin
- A blue tinge to lips and nail beds (cyanosis)
- Rapid breathing and rapid pulse

The treatment for shock depends on the underlying cause. For example, if the shock is caused by severe blood loss, the bleeding must be stopped. Shock that is caused by a severe allergic reaction is treated by administering epinephrine. People who know they are severely allergic to something may carry epinephrine with them in the form of an auto-injector (Figure 8-5). You can learn how to assist someone with using an auto-injector in the American Red Cross First Aid/CPR/AED course.

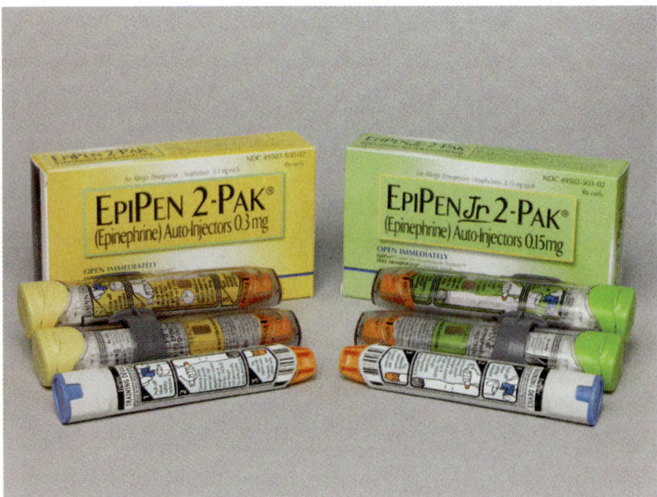

Figure 8-5 A person who is at risk for anaphylactic shock as a result of a severe allergy may carry an auto-injector like this one with her. The auto-injector contains epinephrine, a medication used to treat life-threatening allergic reactions. *Photo courtesy of Dey Pharma, L.P.*

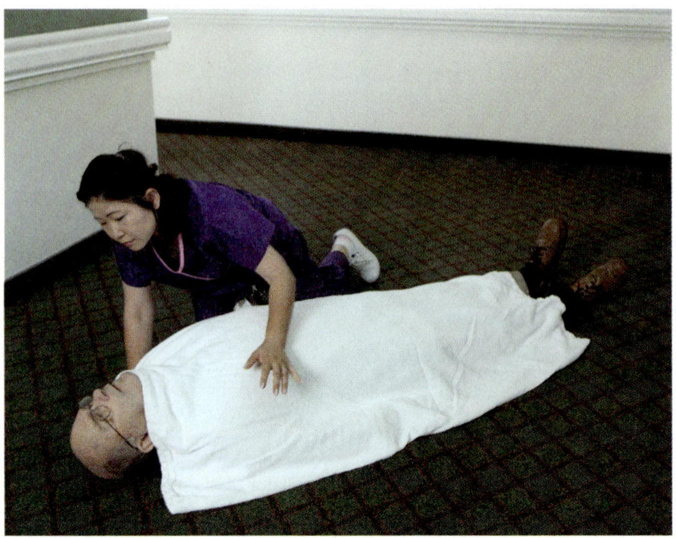

Figure 8-6 Help a person who is in shock to lie down on his back, and keep him from becoming too chilled or too hot.

To provide first aid for a person who is in shock, first call for help immediately. Take any measures that you can to address the cause of the shock (for example, control external bleeding or assist the person with using an auto-injector, if you have been trained to do so). Keep the person from becoming chilled or overheated, and help the person to rest comfortably (Figure 8-6). Even though the person is likely to be thirsty, do not give the person anything to drink or eat. The person may need surgery, which is safest when the stomach is empty. Comfort and reassure the person until medical help arrives.

Seizure

A **seizure** is the result of abnormal electrical activity in the brain, which leads to temporary and involuntary changes in body movement, function, sensation, awareness or behavior. Seizures can have many different causes. Some people may have **epilepsy**, a chronic seizure condition that can often be controlled with medication. Other causes of seizures include fever, infection and injuries to the brain tissue.

Although usually we think of a seizure as involving convulsions (uncontrolled body movements caused by contraction of the muscles) and loss of consciousness, sometimes a person having a seizure will just become very quiet and have a blank stare. A person with epilepsy may experience something called an *aura* (an unusual sensation or feeling) before the onset of a seizure.

Most seizures last only a few minutes. Your main goal is to protect the person from injury during the seizure. Remove nearby furniture or other objects that the person could accidentally hit during the seizure. Do not try to hold or restrain the person, or put anything in the person's mouth or between the teeth to prevent the person from biting his tongue. When the seizure is over, place the person on one side (Figure 8-7) to prevent him from choking on

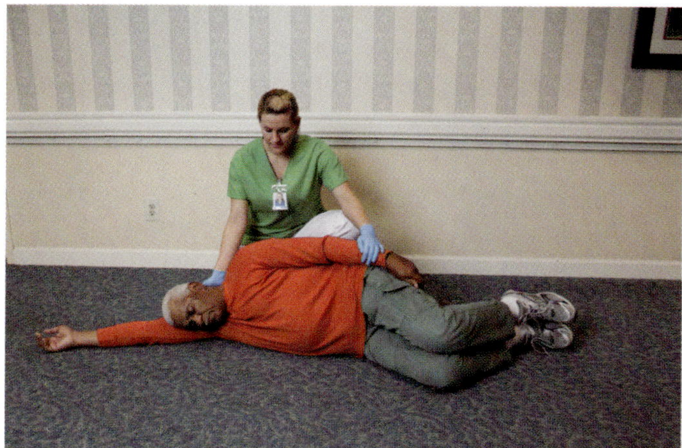

Figure 8-7 When the seizure is over, place the person in the recovery position. Turning the person onto his side helps to prevent him from choking on fluids (such as saliva or vomit) that may pool in the mouth.

secretions that may have pooled in the mouth. The person may be drowsy and disoriented or unresponsive for a period of time. He may be very tired and want to rest. Stay with the person until he is fully recovered from the seizure and aware of his surroundings.

Fainting

Fainting is a temporary loss of consciousness caused by a sudden decrease in the blood supply to the brain. Fainting may be a sign of a serious medical issue, such as a heart condition, but it can also be caused by factors such as hunger, being too hot, standing for long periods of time, medication side effects, fatigue or strong emotions. A person who is about to faint often becomes pale, begins to sweat, and then loses consciousness and collapses. The person may feel weak or dizzy. A fainting spell might be prevented by having the person lie down or sit with her head level with her knees (Figure 8-8). If the person does begin to faint, lower the person to the floor using good body mechanics, and position her flat on her back. Loosen tight clothing, such as a tie, collar or scarf. Make sure the person is breathing. Do not give the person anything to eat or drink. If the person vomits, turn her onto one side to prevent her from choking. The person will usually recover quickly with no lasting effects; however, she should receive a medical evaluation after the fainting episode.

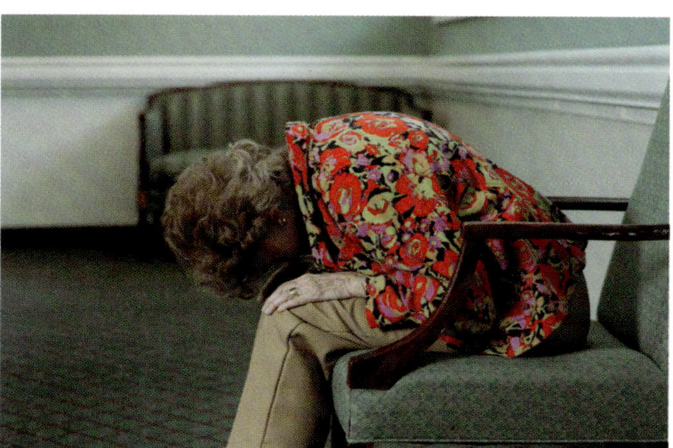

Figure 8-8 A person who feels faint may be able to prevent the fainting episode by sitting down and placing her head near her knees.

Burns

Burns are injuries to the skin and possibly the underlying structures (for example, bone and muscle) as a result of exposure to heat, radiation, an electric shock or chemicals. Burns can range in severity from minor (for example, a sunburn) to life-threatening. If a person is burned, you should *always* call 9-1-1 when:

- The burn is causing the person to have trouble breathing, or there are signs of burns around the mouth and nose.
- The burn covers more than one body part or a large area of the body.
- The person's head, neck, hands, feet or genitals are burned.
- The burn involves underlying structures (for example, muscles or bone) and the person is younger than 5 years or older than 60 years.
- The burn was caused by exposure to chemicals, an explosion or electricity.

While waiting for help to arrive, first try to remove the source of the burning. For a burn caused by heat, cool the burn with large amounts of cold running water. For a chemical burn, remove the chemical from the skin by flushing the area with large amounts of running water (if the chemical is liquid) or brushing the chemical off using gloved hands and then flushing the area with water. Be careful not to get the chemical on yourself, or on another area of the person's body. If the burn was caused by an electrical shock, turn off the power at its source before attempting to assist the person. If you cannot turn the power off at the source, do not touch the electrical wire or the person.

Cover the burned area loosely using a sterile, dry dressing. Provide reassurance, and monitor the person for the development of shock.

FIRE EMERGENCIES

A fire in a health care facility can be devastating. Many people who are receiving health care have limitations in mobility, hearing, vision or understanding—all of which interfere with their ability to successfully react to a fire. As a nurse assistant, you must know how to prevent a fire from occurring, and what to do if a fire does occur.

Preventing Fire Emergencies

For a fire to occur, the following must be present: fuel (something that burns), heat (something to ignite the fuel) and oxygen (Figure 8-9). Removing any one of these elements will stop a fire from increasing.

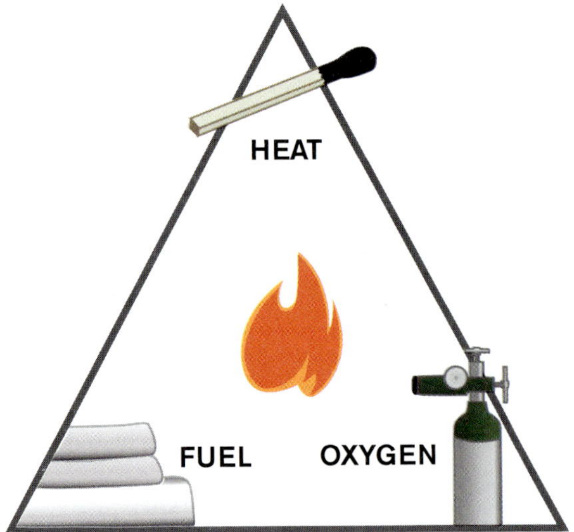

Figure 8-9 Three elements must be present for a fire to start: fuel (something to burn), heat (something to ignite the fuel) and oxygen.

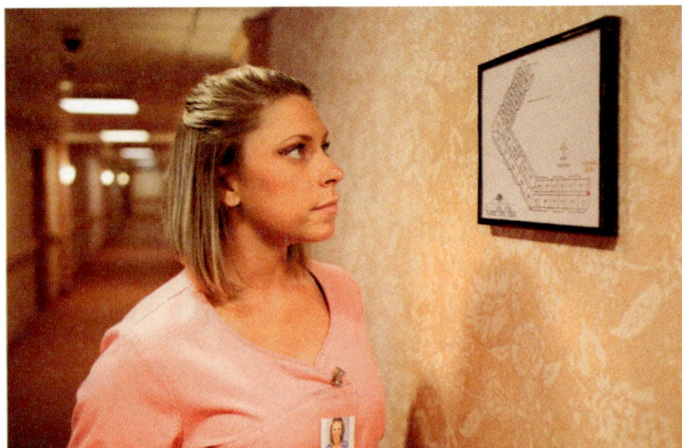
Figure 8-10 Knowing what to do in the event of a fire can save your life and the lives of others.

Remember that many people who receive health care require oxygen therapy, which increases the risk for fire. Take the following precautions to help prevent fires:

- Supervise the people in your care whenever they smoke.
- Follow your employer's rules about smoking. If you provide care for people who smoke, make sure they smoke only in appropriate places and safely extinguish their smoking materials. Make sure the person uses any protective equipment (such as a smoking apron) per your employer's policy.
- Keep materials such as matches and lighters in a secure place, out of reach from children and confused people.
- Never permit smoking around a person who is using oxygen.
- Report any electrical equipment that is not working properly or is not well-maintained to your supervisor.

Responding to Fire Emergencies

If a fire does break out, you must know how to respond. Your facility will have a fire emergency plan, which will specify the method used to alert others to fire (for example, a phone number to call or the location of fire alarm pull boxes). The fire emergency plan will also specify when and how to evacuate the people in the building, as well as any special measures to take to prevent a fire from spreading. Be familiar with your facility's fire emergency plan and participate in the periodic drills that are held to practice putting the plan into action (Figure 8-10).

The word "RACE" can help you to remember how to react to a fire emergency:

- **R**escue. Stop what you are doing and remove anyone in immediate danger from the fire to a safe area. Get out as safely and quickly as possible. The less time you and others are exposed to poisonous gases, heat or flames, the safer everyone will be. Box 8-1 describes how to move people to safety in the event of a fire emergency.
- **A**larm. Activate the nearest fire alarm pull station (if applicable). Call 9-1-1 (or another number, per your employer's policy) to report the location and current extent of the fire.
- **C**ontain. Close all doors and windows that you can safely reach to contain the fire. As you leave an area, close the door behind you.
- **E**xtinguish. Only attempt to extinguish the fire if it is safe for you to do so. If the fire is relatively small and contained, you may be able to put it out using a fire extinguisher.

Generally, to use a fire extinguisher, pull the safety pin out, aim the hose at the base of the fire, squeeze the handle, and spray using a side-to-side sweeping motion (Figure 8-11). There are three major types of fires, classified as type A, B or C (Table 8-1). Most fire extinguishers are ABC fire extinguishers, which means

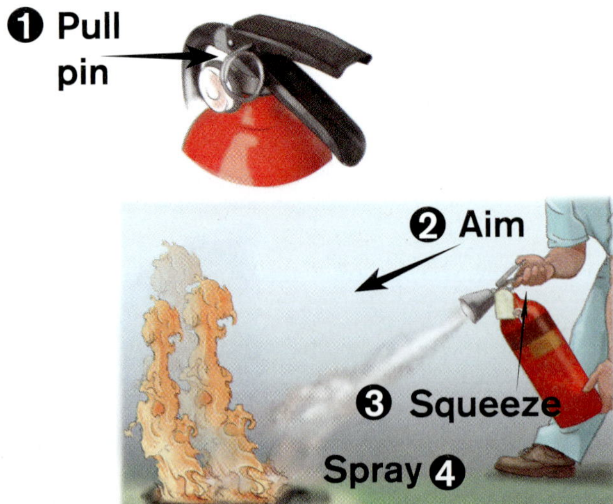

Figure 8-11 If you need to use a fire extinguisher, remember the word "PASS": **P**ull the pin out, **A**im the hose at the base of the fire, **S**queeze the handle, **S**pray in a side-to-side motion.

Box 8-1 Removing People to Safety in a Fire Emergency

- Touch doors with the back of your hand before you open them. If the door is hot, do not open it. Leave the area another way. If the door is cool, stand to one side and open it slowly. If you see heavy smoke on the other side, close the door.
- Stay low. Smoke rises, and it is easier to breathe when you are closer to the floor.
- Use stairs, not an elevator.
- If your clothing or that of another person catches fire, stop, drop (to the ground), and roll over and over (to extinguish the flames).
- Move people who cannot walk in their beds or in wheelchairs.
- People may be frightened and confused. Help to reassure them by remaining calm and explaining what is happening. Reassure people that you will help move them to a safe area. After people are moved to a safe place, make sure a staff member remains with them to keep them from wandering into dangerous areas. The presence of a staff member is especially important for people who have impaired vision or hearing or who are confused.

Table 8-1 Types of Fires and Fire Extinguishers

Type	Description	How to Put the Fire Out
A	A fire that uses ordinary dry materials as fuel, such as wood, paper or leaves	Type ABC fire extinguisher, or Type A fire extinguisher, or water.
B	A grease fire (kitchen fires are often grease fires)	Type ABC fire extinguisher, or Type B fire extinguisher, or smother the fire by sprinkling baking soda over it or putting the lid on the pan and removing the pan from the heat source. **NEVER USE WATER!**
C	An electrical fire, such as one caused by frayed wiring	Type ABC fire extinguisher, or Type C fire extinguisher. **NEVER USE WATER!**

they are effective against all types of fires. In the event that an ABC fire extinguisher is not available, you must use an extinguisher specific to the type of fire, or take other measures as summarized in Table 8-1.

WEATHER EMERGENCIES, DISASTERS AND OTHER EVENTS WITH WIDESPREAD IMPACT

Environmental events can occur that put people in immediate danger and affect the ability of the facility to function normally, resulting in an emergency situation. For example, weather emergencies such as ice or snow storms can result in power outages, an inability to receive supplies for an extended period of time, and staffing shortages. When this occurs, the facility's ability to follow normal routines to provide care may be disrupted, and an emergency exists. When an event affects many people and causes widespread damage and destruction in the community, it is called a disaster. Disasters can be caused by natural events (such as tornadoes, hurricanes or floods), or they may be caused by man (such as bombings, chemical leaks and nuclear accidents).

As a nurse assistant, you must be prepared in the event of a weather emergency or disaster. Know what types of weather emergencies are common in the area where you live, and familiarize yourself with actions you should take to keep yourself and others safe should such an emergency arise. Box 8-2 summarizes actions you take in the event of some common weather emergencies. You can learn more about other weather emergencies that may be more common in your area by visiting the American Red Cross website or your local American Red Cross chapter.

Your employer will have a disaster preparedness plan that specifies the actions the staff should take in the event of a disaster. Make sure you know your role and responsibilities. Often, when a major event such as a hurricane is predicted and there is time to prepare, the disaster preparedness plan will specify that patients or residents are to be evacuated to another facility. The disaster preparedness plan will also specify measures that should be taken to cope with the event if it occurs suddenly, there is no time to evacuate, and the normal functioning of the facility will be affected for an extended period of time.

▼ Box 8-2 Weather Emergencies

General Precautions

- Listen for weather reports on the radio or television. In a hospital or nursing home, know which staff members are assigned to listen to the reports.
- Have a flashlight, a battery-operated radio and fresh batteries available.
- Make sure you have access to a supply of fresh water.

Hurricanes. A hurricane occurs when the winds of a large tropical storm (that is, a storm that begins over warm ocean water) increase to 74 miles per hour or more.

A hurricane *watch* means a hurricane is possible in your area within the next 48 hours. If a hurricane watch is issued in your area:

- Prepare for a possible evacuation, per your employer's disaster preparedness plan.
- Check outdoor areas: remove or secure loose objects and prepare to board up windows.

A hurricane *warning* means hurricane conditions are expected within 36 hours. If a hurricane warning is issued in your area:

- Follow your employer's disaster preparedness plan for evacuating patients or residents to another facility (if an evacuation order is issued).
- If you are not told to evacuate, move people into interior rooms or hallways. Keep people away from windows. If a person cannot easily get of bed, move the person in his bed into a hallway, or push the bed against the wall. Assign a staff member to stay with people who have been moved to safety.
- Cover people with blankets or bedspreads to protect them from flying glass in case windows break.
- Close the doors to rooms and close fire doors.
- Make sure doorways to halls, fire doors and exits are not blocked.
- Monitor weather conditions carefully.

Tornadoes. A tornado is a spinning, funnel-shaped windstorm that moves along the ground. Tornadoes can arise very suddenly.

A tornado *watch* means that weather conditions are favorable for a tornado in your area. If a tornado watch is issued in your area:

- Be alert to weather conditions (for example, dark or greenish clouds, funnel clouds), blowing debris and the sound of an approaching tornado. A tornado often sounds like a freight train. Inform other staff members if you see or hear anything.
- Move people to the basement of the building. If the building has no basement, a windowless room on the lowest level of the building is the next best option.
- Close the doors to rooms and close fire doors.
- Make sure doorways to halls, fire doors and exits are not blocked.
- Follow evacuation procedures if necessary.

A tornado *warning* means a tornado has been sighted or indicated on weather radar in the area. If a tornado warning is issued in your area:

- *Immediately* move yourself and others to the basement of the building or a windowless room on the lowest level of the building.

Earthquakes. An earthquake occurs when the plates that make up the Earth's surface move against each other, causing the Earth to shake. This activity in the Earth may cause buildings to shake, windows to shatter and objects to shift or fall. It also can cause fires to start and can generate large ocean waves. Earthquakes can occur in most states, and they may occur at any time without warning. If you are inside when an earthquake occurs, stay inside and protect yourself and others from falling or shifting objects by taking cover under a large, heavy object (such as a desk or table) and holding on. If you are outside when an earthquake occurs, stay outside but move away from buildings, trees and overhead wires.

After the earthquake:

- Be prepared for aftershocks (smaller quakes that occur after the first tremor).
- Check yourself and others for injuries. Never try to move seriously injured people unless they are in danger of further injury.
- Do not use equipment or services requiring electricity, gas, water or sewage disposal because these systems may be damaged. If you smell gas or see a broken line, shut off the main valve or inform the person responsible. Do not try to turn utilities back on.
- Never smoke or light candles. Earthquakes can create gas leaks, and an open flame from a match or cigarette lighter can cause an explosion.
- Use the telephone only in a life-threatening emergency.
- Watch for fallen power lines.
- Listen to a battery-operated radio for updated information about the emergency.
- Clean up spilled medicines, drugs, flammable liquids and other materials.
- Open cabinets and closet doors cautiously. The items inside may have shifted and could fall on you when you open the door.

In the event of a disaster, you will play a very important role in helping to reassure and calm the people in your care. Many of the people in your care will have characteristics that make them more vulnerable during times of crisis. For example, a person who has recently experienced an upsetting event (such as separation from or loss of a loved one) might be less able to cope with the emotional impact of the disaster. A person who is dependent on others for care will understandably be very frightened during an event that disrupts the normal routine of the facility. A person with dementia will not be able to understand what is happening, and will become very upset by the change in the normal routine. People who speak a language other than English may fear that they will not be able to communicate their needs. By staying calm, knowing what to do and offering reassurance, you can help the people in your care to feel safe.

In a disaster situation, staff members who are on duty may be required to stay at the facility for longer than one shift because conditions outside may make it unsafe or impossible for people to travel to and from the facility. If you are on duty and a disaster occurs, your primary responsibility is assisting the people in your care. However, naturally, you will be concerned about the health and safety of your own family while you cannot be with them. Developing a home disaster preparedness plan that describes what family members should do if they are away from home or apart from each other when a disaster occurs can give you peace of mind. Review the plan frequently with family members so that you are confident everyone knows what to do. Also, make sure you are prepared in the event that you must remain in the facility for longer than one shift. For example, if you require medication to manage a chronic condition, make sure you have enough on hand to see you through the emergency.

CHECK YOUR UNDERSTANDING

Questions for Review

1. **What should you do if a fire alarm sounds while you are at work?**
   a. Leave the building and go home.
   b. Ask another nurse assistant what to do.
   c. Follow your employer's policies for responding to a fire alarm.
   d. Ignore the fire alarm, because it is probably only a fire drill.

2. **If your clothing catches fire, you should:**
   a. Run, cover and cool.
   b. Stop, drop and roll.
   c. Call the fire department.
   d. Blanket, bathe and bandage.

3. **Which of the following could be a sign of a stroke?**
   a. Profuse sweating
   b. Convulsions
   c. Fainting
   d. Drooping on one side of the face

4. **You are helping a person to eat when he begins to choke. He is making a high-pitched wheezing sound, and it is difficult for him to answer you when you ask if he needs help. What should you do?**
   a. Perform cardiopulmonary resuscitation (CPR).
   b. Call for help immediately, and then begin administering back blows and abdominal thrusts.
   c. Watch him carefully for a minute to see if he is able to cough up the object on his own.
   d. Call for help immediately, and then provide reassurance until help arrives.

5. **You are with a group of residents in the day room when suddenly one of the residents loses consciousness and slumps over in her chair. What should you do?**
   a. Call for help immediately.
   b. Splash water on the resident's face to revive her.
   c. Move furniture out of the way to protect her from further injury.
   d. Administer cardiopulmonary resuscitation (CPR).

6. **How should you position a person who has had a seizure after the seizure is over?**
   a. Flat on his back
   b. On his side
   c. Seated, with his head between his knees
   d. On his stomach

7. **One of your co-workers has cut herself with a knife while cutting up fruit for a smoothie-making activity with the residents, and she is bleeding quite heavily. What is the first thing you should do?**
   a. Call 9-1-1 and monitor her for shock.
   b. Put on a pair of gloves and then go to her aid.
   c. Put a dressing over the cut and apply pressure to stop the bleeding.
   d. Rinse the cut with water.

8. You are a home health nurse on duty and a tornado watch has been issued for your area. Which area in the client's home would be the best place to move the client to safety?

a. The dining room, which has large windows
b. A windowless bathroom on the ground floor
c. The client's room
d. The front hall

9. Which of the following could by a sign of a myocardial infarction?

a. Blurred vision
b. Nausea
c. Aura
d. Shock

Questions to Ask Yourself

1. *You enter Mr. Lee's room and see flames shooting out of the trash can. What should you do?*
2. *You are alone at Mrs. Jones's house and she begins to choke on a piece of hot dog. What should you do?*
3. *You are with Mr. Smith in the bathroom and you notice that he is sweating profusely, clutching his chest and gasping for air. What do you do?*
4. *You are caring for Mr. White in his home and he begins to have a seizure. What should you do?*
5. *You wake Mrs. George and notice that the left side of her mouth is drooping. What should you do?*

Skill 8-1
First Aid for a Conscious Choking Adult

1. Check the scene and the person.
   - Ask the person if he or she is choking.
   - Identify yourself and ask the person if you can help.
   - If the person is coughing forcefully, encourage continued coughing. Otherwise:
2. Call, or have someone else call 9-1-1 (or follow your employer's procedure).
3. **Give five back blows.** Position yourself behind the person, lean him forward and strike him firmly between the shoulder blades using the heel of your hand (Figure 1).

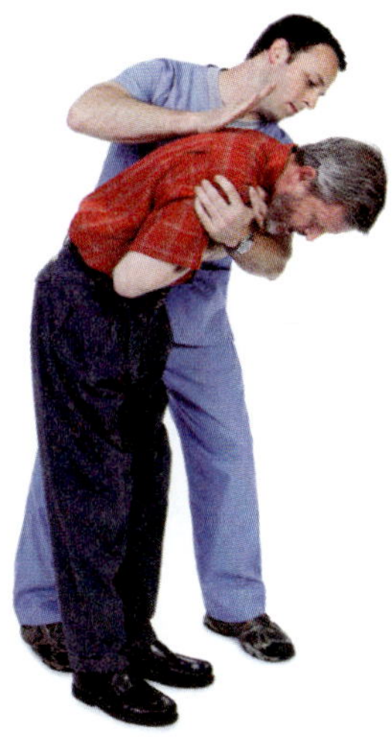

Figure 1

4. **Give five abdominal thrusts.** Still standing behind the person, wrap your arms around his waist. Place the thumb side of your fist just above the person's belly button. Clasp your fist with your other hand and give quick, upward thrusts into the abdomen (Figure 2).

   Note: If the person is pregnant or too big for you to reach around, you will need to give chest thrusts instead of abdominal thrusts. To give chest thrusts, place the thumb side of your fist over the center of the person's breastbone instead of above the person's belly button, grab your fist with your other hand and give quick, upward thrusts (Figure 3).

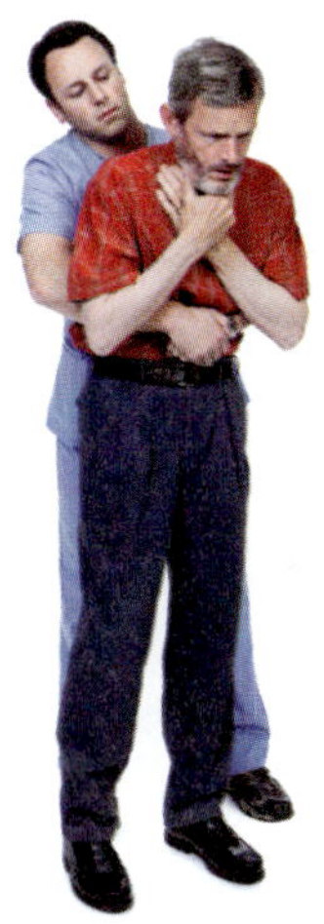

Figure 2

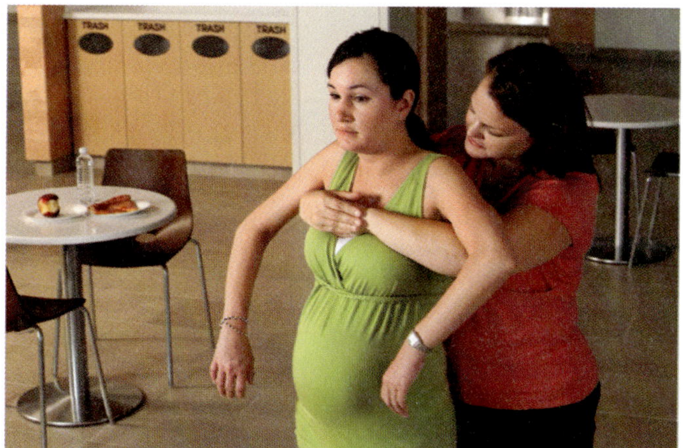

Figure 3

5. Continue giving back blows and abdominal thrusts until:
   - The object is forced out.
   - The person becomes unconscious.
   - The person can breathe or cough forcefully.
6. Document your observations and actions per your employer's policy. Be aware that the person will need to receive a medical evaluation after the emergency has passed.

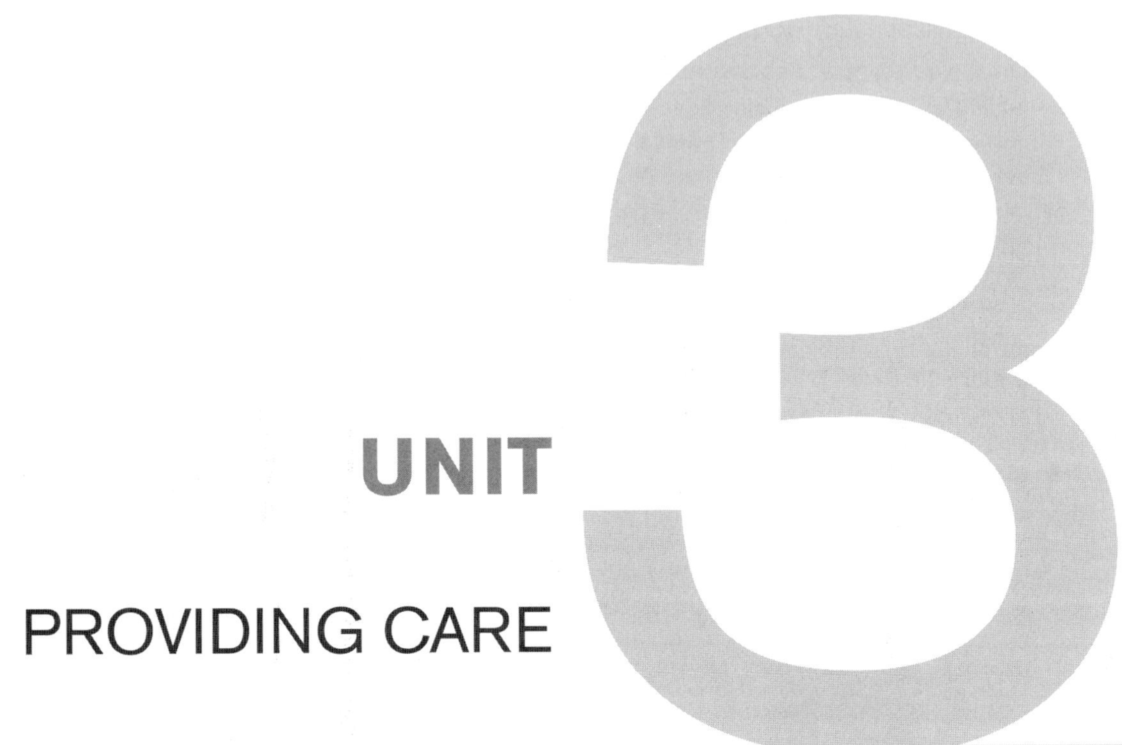

UNIT 3

PROVIDING CARE

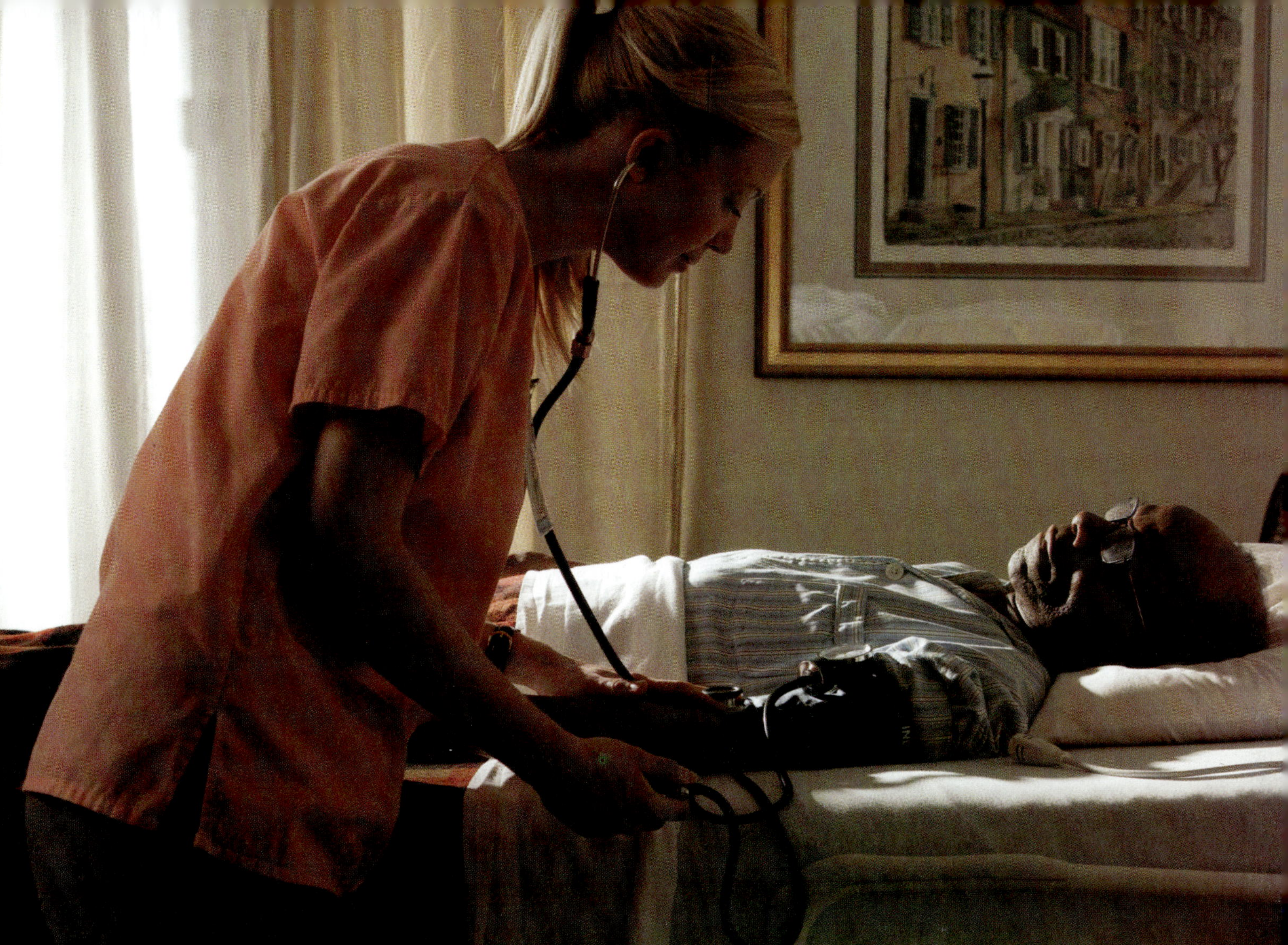

Measuring Vital Signs, Weight and Height

CHAPTER
9

Goals

After reading this chapter, you will have the information needed to:

- Discuss the importance of measuring vital signs accurately.
- Describe factors that can affect each of the four vital signs: temperature, pulse, respirations and blood pressure.
- Describe equipment used to measure each of the four vital signs.
- Discuss considerations related to measuring each of the four vital signs safely and accurately.
- Describe when weight and height measurements are obtained.
- Discuss considerations related to measuring weight and height accurately.

Continued on next page

Continued from previous page

Goals

After practicing the corresponding skills, you will have the information needed to:

- Use an electronic thermometer to measure a person's oral, rectal, axillary or tympanic temperature.
- Evaluate a person's radial and apical pulse.
- Evaluate a person's respirations.
- Measure a person's blood pressure.
- Measure a person's weight and height.

Key Terms:

vital signs	**hypothermia**	**dyspnea**	**hypertension**
fever	**stethoscope**	**hypotension**	**sphygmomanometer**

Mrs. Parker, a resident of Morningside Nursing Home, is 82 years old and came to live at Morningside after her husband died and severe arthritis and other health problems made it difficult for her to manage on her own. You always enjoy seeing Mrs. Parker. Usually you can find her in the common area, chatting to anyone who will listen. She knows all of the staff and other residents by name and always remembers something special about everyone. Whenever she sees you, she always asks about your son, and how he is doing playing basketball for the high school team.

Today, however, you discover Mrs. Parker in bed, with a dry, hacking cough. When she tries to talk to you, she coughs even more. Between coughs she manages to tell you that she aches all over. Her face looks flushed, and when you touch her, she feels warm and dry. You tell Mrs. Parker you would like to take her vital signs. Her vital signs are as follows: temperature, 99.3°F (orally); pulse, 110 beats/min and weak; respirations, 26 breaths/min and shallow; and blood pressure, 134/94 mm Hg (higher than Mrs. Parker's usual blood pressure).

VITAL SIGNS

In health care, there are four basic measurements that can tell us a great deal about how a person's body is functioning. These four measurements—temperature, pulse, respirations and blood pressure—are called **vital signs** because they represent functions that are essential for life ("vital" comes from the Latin word for "life"). Health care workers often use their own language for talking about vital signs. They talk about a person's TPR, which stands for *temperature, pulse* and *respiration*; and BP, which stands for *blood pressure*.

As a nurse assistant, you will be responsible for measuring and recording the vital signs of those in your care. These measurements are always taken when a person is first admitted to a health care facility, at regular intervals throughout the person's stay at the facility (for example, every day or every week), and before the person is discharged from the facility. When a person first starts receiving care, you may be asked to take the person's vital signs frequently because these frequent readings help the health care team determine what is normal (or baseline) for that person. After the baseline is established, the person's primary care provider (that is, the doctor or advanced practice nurse) may order the person's vital signs to be taken on a less frequent but regular basis. The frequency varies from one person to another. You may also take a person's vital signs on an "as-needed basis," such as when you notice a change in the person's usual condition, or when the nurse asks you to. For example, it may be necessary to measure a person's blood pressure before the nurse gives the person certain types of medications.

Accuracy when measuring vital signs is extremely important. Vital sign measurements often affect decisions that are made about the person's medical care. The importance of these readings to the person's care makes it essential that you measure these signs accurately, record them correctly and report any changes in them promptly to the nurse. The other members of the health care team are depending on you to give them accurate information in a timely manner.

When you are measuring a person's vital signs, remember that although obtaining these measurements may be a routine task to you, having these measurements taken may carry special significance for the person receiving care. Some people will be worried about what the measurements will reveal about their health status. Many people will be embarrassed by having a rectal temperature taken. Always observe the five principles of care when you measure a person's vital signs, and be sensitive to the person's feelings about having these measurements taken.

You find your supervising nurse on the unit and say, "Nancy, I'm worried about Mrs. Parker. She's developed a dry, hacking cough; her skin is hot and dry to the touch; she tells me that she aches all over; and she barely feels like talking! I took her vital signs, and her temperature is a little high. Her pulse rate and respiratory rate are also high, and her pulse is weak and her breaths are shallow. Her blood pressure is higher than it normally is, too. I have the measurements written down, but can you go check on Mrs. Parker?" The nurse thanks you for providing such a thorough report and says, "I'll go right away to check on her."

A short time later, while you are giving Mrs. Parker some juice, Nancy returns with a medication to lower Mrs. Parker's temperature. Shortly after Mrs. Parker takes the medicine, the doctor arrives, examines her and orders an antibiotic and a medication to help control the cough.

You could have just reported your observations about Mrs. Parker's condition, but instead you decided to obtain Mrs. Parker's vital sign measurements and include them in your report as well. How did taking Mrs. Parker's vital signs help you to communicate more effectively with the nurse?

How did Mrs. Parker benefit from your actions? What could have happened if you delayed reporting your observations, or if the vital sign measurements you took were not accurate?

Temperature

Body temperature indicates the amount of heat produced by the body. Normally the body maintains a fairly constant temperature. A special area in the brain regulates the body temperature and makes adjustments as needed to keep it within the normal range. A person's temperature usually moves up and down within the normal range, depending on factors such as the time of day, the person's level of activity, the person's emotional status and the temperature of the surrounding air. **Fever** is a temperature above the normal range and is a common response to infection. **Hypothermia** is a temperature below the normal range.

ELDER CARE NOTE. In older people, the body temperature may decrease, or only slightly increase, in response to an infection. Always report even slight variations in an older person's temperature, whether they are higher or lower than what is normal for the person.

We use a range of numbers to describe temperatures that are considered normal for most people. The normal range varies both according to where on the body the temperature is measured, and the age of the person (Figure 9-1):

- **Site.** Common places to measure a person's body temperature include the mouth (an *oral* temperature), rectum (a *rectal* temperature), ear (a *tympanic* temperature) and armpit (an *axillary* temperature). Because of the variation that occurs from site to site, it is very important to note the site where you obtained the temperature, in addition to the actual measurement! Follow your employer's policy regarding how to note the site. A common practice is to write an "O" after the measurement if the temperature was taken orally, an "R" if the temperature was taken rectally, a "TY" if the temperature was taken in the ear, and an "A" if the temperature was taken in the armpit.
- **Age.** Body temperature is usually higher in newborns and lower in older adults.

Body temperature is measured in degrees. Degrees can be measured on two different scales, Fahrenheit (°F) or Celsius (°C). In the United States, the Fahrenheit scale is used most commonly. Table 9-1 summarizes normal temperature ranges and average temperatures in degrees Fahrenheit and degrees Celsius for each of the major sites where temperature can be measured. The ranges and averages given in Table 9-1 are for adults younger than 65 years. Remember that in adults older than 65 years, the body temperature is normally 1 to 2 degrees lower than the ranges and shown in Table 9-1.

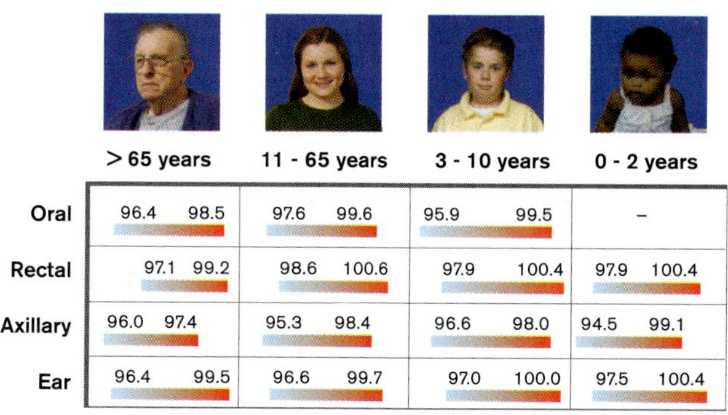

	> 65 years	11 - 65 years	3 - 10 years	0 - 2 years
Oral	96.4 98.5	97.6 99.6	95.9 99.5	–
Rectal	97.1 99.2	98.6 100.6	97.9 100.4	97.9 100.4
Axillary	96.0 97.4	95.3 98.4	96.6 98.0	94.5 99.1
Ear	96.4 99.5	96.6 99.7	97.0 100.0	97.5 100.4

Figure 9-1 Normal temperature ranges vary according to the site where the temperature was measured and the age of the person. (Data taken from the Welch Allyn website.)

Table 9-1 **Normal Range of Body Temperatures in Adults Younger Than 65 Years***

Site	(°F)		(°C)	
	Normal Range	Average	Normal Range	Average
Oral	97.6–99.6	98.6	36.4–37.5	36.9
Rectal	98.6–100.6	99	37–38.1	37.5
Axillary	95.3–98.4	96.8	35.2–36.9	36
Ear	96.6–99.7	98.1	35.9–37.6	36.7

*In adults older than 65 years, the normal temperature ranges and averages are typically 1° to 2° lower than those given here.
Data taken from the Welch Allyn website.

Observations Into Action!

The following may be signs of a medical problem and should be reported to the nurse right away.

- **A temperature that is higher than normal for the person**
- **A temperature that is lower than normal for the person**

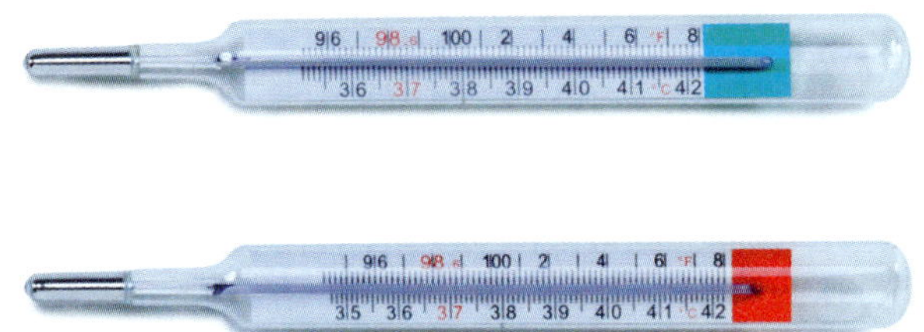

Figure 9-2 Glass thermometers vary slightly in appearance, depending on their use.

Equipment used to measure temperature

A thermometer is used to measure temperature. Several different types of thermometers are used in health care settings.

Glass thermometer

A glass thermometer contains mercury or a mercury-like substance in a thin glass tube with a bulb on the end (Figure 9-2). The glass tube is marked with a scale in degrees Fahrenheit or degrees Celsius (Figure 9-3). When the bulb is placed in the person's mouth, rectum or armpit, the person's body heat causes the substance inside the thermometer to expand and move up the tube, indicating the person's body temperature. To obtain an accurate temperature, the glass thermometer must be left in place for 3 to 10 minutes, depending on where the temperature is being measured.

Glass thermometers for oral and rectal use differ in the colors of their tips (see Figure 9-2). The oral glass thermometer, which is used for taking oral and axillary temperatures, has a blue tip. Rectal thermometers have a red tip. (Remember "Red for Rectal.") Never use a rectal thermometer to take an oral or axillary temperature.

Glass thermometers are fragile and can break easily. The mercury that many glass thermometers contain is highly toxic and must be cleaned up and disposed of properly. If you break a glass thermometer, do not touch the mercury, and prevent others from doing so as well. Notify the nurse so that the proper procedures can be followed for cleaning up the broken glass and disposing of the mercury. Even if the thermometer contains a non-toxic, mercury-like substance, broken glass still presents a hazard to you and to others. Because of the hazards associated with mercury and broken glass, many health care facilities no longer use glass thermometers. You can learn more about the proper care and use of a glass thermometer in Appendix D, Skills D-1 and D-2.

Electronic thermometer

An electronic thermometer is a battery-operated device with a heat-sensitive probe that is placed in the person's mouth, rectum or armpit to measure the temperature (Figure 9-4). The probe is covered with a disposable cover (sheath) before use. As with glass thermometers, the probe is color-coded according to

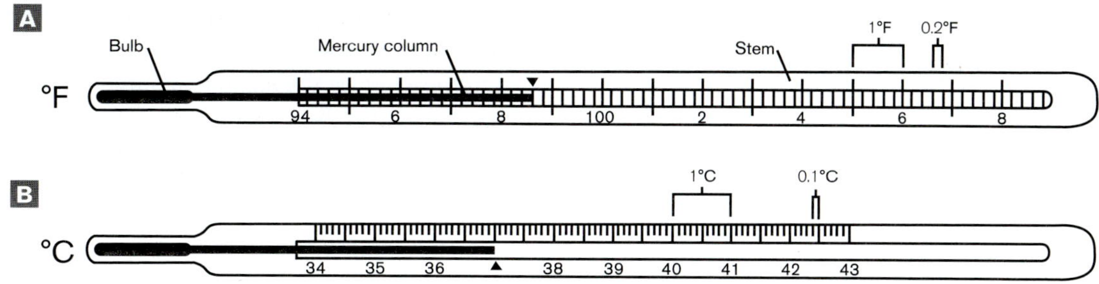

Figure 9-3 Glass thermometers are marked in either degrees Fahrenheit (F) or degrees Celsius (C). The column on a glass thermometer is marked with a series of long and short lines extending from 94° to 108° Fahrenheit, or from 34° to 43° Celsius. On a Fahrenheit thermometer (A), each long line on the thermometer represents 1 degree, and each of the four shorter lines between the long lines represents 0.2 degree. On a Celsius thermometer (B), each long line represents 1 degree, but each shorter line in between represents 0.1 degree.

its intended use (blue for oral or axillary use, and red for rectal use). Never use a rectal probe to take an oral or axillary temperature! When the device is finished measuring the person's temperature (usually in less than 1 minute), it beeps and displays the measurement on a screen. Skill 9-1 describes how to use an electronic thermometer to measure a person's oral, rectal or axillary temperature.

Tympanic thermometer

A tympanic thermometer is a special type of electronic thermometer that uses a specially designed probe to measure heat waves given off by the eardrum (Figure 9-5). (The medical term for the eardrum is *tympanic membrane.*) The probe is covered with a disposable cover and inserted into the person's ear canal. The device beeps and displays the temperature measurement on a screen within a few seconds. See Skill 9-1 to learn how to use a tympanic thermometer to measure a person's tympanic temperature.

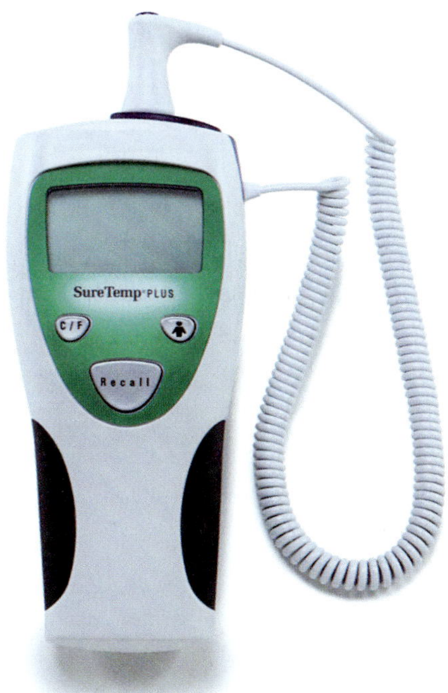

Figure 9-4 An electronic thermometer.

Ensuring safety and accuracy when obtaining a temperature

Obtaining an accurate temperature measurement safely requires you to use the right equipment in the right way. It also requires you to consider conditions the person may have that make one method of obtaining a temperature preferable over another one.

Equipment considerations

- **Glass thermometers.** Before using a glass thermometer, always inspect the thermometer to make sure that it is not chipped, cracked or broken. To prevent the spread of infection, wash the thermometer with cool water and soap before and after using it. (Never use hot water to wash a glass thermometer because this can cause the thermometer to break.) Before inserting the thermometer, move the mercury or mercury-like substance into the bulb by "shaking down" the thermometer with a quick downward flick of your wrist (Figure 9-6). The mercury or mercury-like substance must start below the 94° F mark on a Fahrenheit thermometer or the 34° C

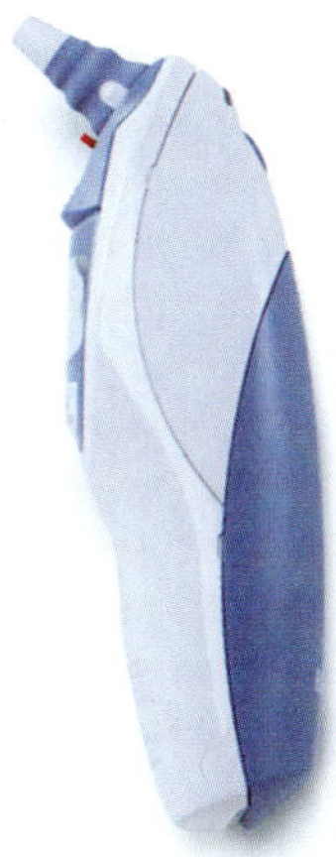

Figure 9-5 A tympanic thermometer.

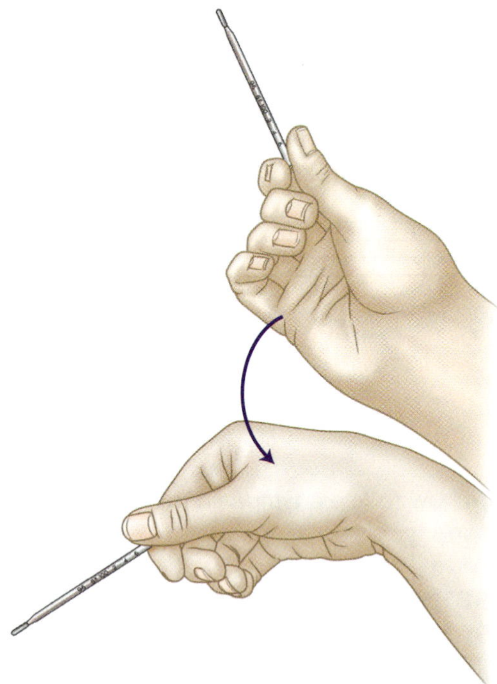

Figure 9-6 "Shake down" a glass thermometer before use by holding it firmly by the stem and snapping your wrist in a quick downward motion.

mark on a Celsius thermometer in order to give an accurate temperature reading. Be sure to place the thermometer properly, and leave it in place for the specified amount of time.

- **Electronic thermometers.** Make sure the electronic thermometer is fully charged. If you notice that the electronic thermometer is giving faulty readings (for example, a temperature that is extremely high or extremely low, or the same temperature for every person), report the problem to the nurse so that the device can be taken out of service and repaired. Electronic thermometers are used for many people, so always practice proper infection control procedures. Remember not to put the thermometer down on dirty surfaces, and if the thermometer has a cord, keep the cord in your hand and make sure that the only part of the device that contacts the person or his surroundings is the probe cover. To ensure an accurate measurement, be sure to place the thermometer probe properly, and leave it in place for the specified amount of time.

Person-specific considerations

The method used to take a person's temperature depends on several factors. Using the wrong method to take a person's temperature can affect the person's safety, the accuracy of the measurement or both.

- **Oral method.** Generally, the oral method is the preferred way to measure a person's body temperature because it is easy, causes the person minimal discomfort and embarrassment, and gives a measurement that accurately reflects the internal body temperature. Situations that may make taking an oral temperature unsafe or result in inaccurate measurements, and what to do in these situations, are summarized in Table 9-2.

Table 9-2 **Obtaining Accurate Temperature Measurements Safely**

Situation	Avoid	Do This Instead
The person has consumed food or a beverage or smoked a cigarette within the past 15 minutes.	The oral method, because the temperature of the food, fluid or cigarette smoke can influence the temperature inside the mouth, resulting in an inaccurate reading.	Wait 15 minutes before taking the oral temperature, or use another method if allowed.
The person has had recent mouth surgery or has a mouth disease.	The oral method, because the thermometer may cause injury.	Take temperature using rectal, axillary or tympanic method.
The person is confused.	The oral method with a glass thermometer, because the person may bite down on the thermometer and break it, causing injury.	Take temperature orally using an electronic thermometer, or use rectal, axillary or tympanic method.
The person is unconscious or paralyzed on one side of the body.	The oral method, because the person may not be able to keep the mouth closed around the thermometer, resulting in an inaccurate temperature reading.	Take temperature using rectal, axillary or tympanic method.
The person has trouble breathing or breathes through mouth, or the person has a tube in the nose and cannot keep the mouth closed.	The oral method, because the person will not be able to keep the mouth closed around the thermometer and still breathe.	Take temperature using rectal, axillary or tympanic method.

Continued on next page

Table 9-2 **Obtaining Accurate Temperature Measurements Safely** *continued*

Situation	Avoid	Do This Instead
The person is receiving oxygen.	The oral method, because oxygen cools the temperature inside the mouth, resulting in an inaccurate reading.	Take temperature using rectal, axillary or tympanic method.
The person has a blocked rectum or hemorrhoids, or has recently had rectal surgery.	The rectal method, because the thermometer may cause injury.	Take temperature using oral, axillary or tympanic method.
The person has diarrhea.	The rectal method, because this method can be uncomfortable for the person.	Take temperature using oral, axillary or tympanic method.
The person has certain heart conditions.	The rectal method, because placing the thermometer in the rectum may stimulate the urge to strain and may increase the workload of the heart.	Take temperature using oral, axillary or tympanic method.

- **Rectal method.** The rectal method for measuring a person's body temperature also accurately reflects internal body temperature, but it can cause the person embarrassment and discomfort. A rectal temperature is obtained when taking an oral temperature might cause injury or inaccurate results. Situations that would make taking a rectal temperature unsafe or that could result in inaccurate measurements are summarized in Table 9-2.
- **Axillary method.** The axillary method is the least accurate way to measure a person's body temperature. Take an axillary temperature only if the person cannot tolerate having an oral or a rectal temperature taken. To ensure that the results obtained are as accurate as possible, pat the armpit dry with a tissue before placing the thermometer (moisture can affect the measurement), and make sure the person stays seated or lies down while the temperature is being measured.

Pulse

Each time the heart beats, it pushes blood through the arteries, vessels that carry blood away from the heart and throughout the body. The heartbeat creates a wave of blood, which you can feel pass through the artery if you put your fingers over certain places on the body where the artery lies close to the surface of the skin (Figure 9-7). Between beats, the heart rests. Then it beats again, causing another wave that you can feel. The wave that you can feel is called the *pulse*.

Characteristics of the pulse

The pulse provides information about how a person's heart is working. When you evaluate a person's pulse, you note several things:

- **The pulse rate.** When you count the number of times you feel a person's pulse beat in a minute, you know how fast the person's heart is beating. This number is called the *heart rate* or *pulse*

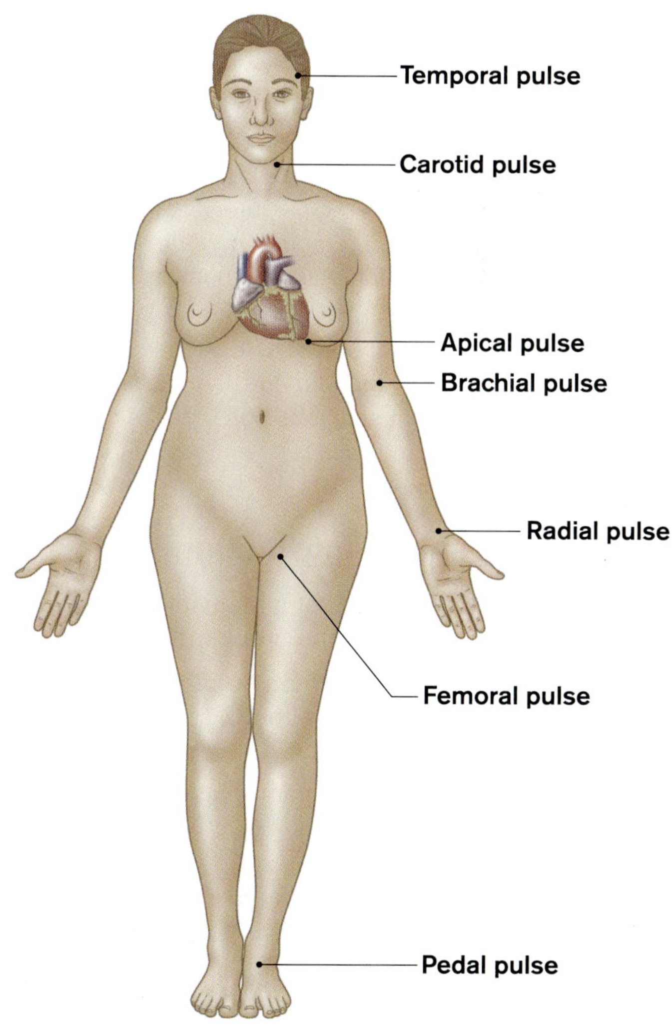

Figure 9-7 Pulse points.

Table 9-3 **Normal Resting Pulse Rates**

Age Group	Normal Resting Pulse Rate
Adults and children older than 10 years	60 to 100 beats/min*
Children between the ages of 1 and 10 years	70 to 130 beats/min
Infants between the ages of 1 and 11 months	80 to 120 beats/min
Newborns between the ages of 1 and 30 days	100 to 150 beats/min

*In well-trained athletes, the normal resting pulse rate may be between 40 and 60 beats/min.

Data from National Institutes of Health.

rate. Activity, pain, fever, significant blood loss, and emotions such as anger, fear, agitation or excitement can cause the pulse rate to increase. Sleep, some medications, and conditions such as depression can cause the pulse rate to decrease. In adults, the pulse rate is normally between 60 and 100 beats/min (Table 9-3).

- **The pulse rhythm.** When you describe the pulse rhythm, you describe how regular the pulse is. A pulse that comes at regular intervals (like the ticking of a clock) has a *regular rhythm*. If the length of time between pulses is uneven, the rhythm is *irregular*.
- **The pulse force.** If the pulse is easy to feel, it is described as a *full* or *strong pulse*. A *bounding* pulse is a pulse that seems to push up against your fingertips. A *thready* pulse is a weak pulse that is very difficult to feel.

Observations Into Action!

The following may be signs of a medical problem and should be reported to the nurse right away:

- **A pulse rate that is less than 60 beats/min or greater than 100 beats/min**
- **A pulse that is irregular**
- **A weak (thready) or bounding pulse**

Sites for evaluating the pulse

Most of the time, you will evaluate the person's pulse at her wrist. This is called a radial pulse. In some situations, you may evaluate the person's pulse over her heart. This is called an apical pulse. The technique used to evaluate an apical pulse differs from the technique used to measure the pulse at the wrist and other pulse points.

- **Radial pulse.** The radial pulse is evaluated by placing your fingers over the radial artery, on the inside of the wrist, and counting the number of pulsations that you feel in 1 minute. In addition to counting the number of pulsations, you also note the rhythm and force of the pulse. Be sure to press lightly against the wrist. If you press too hard, you can flatten the artery and you will not be able to feel anything. Skill 9-2 describes step by step how to evaluate a person's radial pulse.
- **Apical pulse.** When evaluating an apical pulse, you place a **stethoscope** over the apex of the heart and count each pulse beat by listening to it rather than feeling it. (Box 9-1 describes the parts and use of a stethoscope.) The apical pulse is evaluated when the person has a very weak or irregular pulse that is difficult to detect at the radial artery, and when the person has certain heart conditions. The apical method is also used for infants and young children. Skill 9-3 describes how to evaluate a person's apical pulse.

Ensuring accuracy when evaluating the pulse

To ensure accuracy when measuring a person's pulse, evaluate factors that could increase the person's pulse rate before beginning. For example, if the person has just come back from physical therapy or undergone a painful procedure, or if the person is emotionally upset, it might be best to give the person time to rest and relax before checking the pulse. When you are taking a radial pulse, make sure the person's arm is resting comfortably on the bed (or on her lap if she is seated). Avoid placing your thumb over the person's radial artery (when taking a radial pulse) or holding the diaphragm of the stethoscope with your thumb (when taking an apical pulse) because your thumb has its own pulse, which you might confuse for the person's pulse. Wait until the second hand gets to the "12" before you count starting, and count for 1 full minute.

Mrs. Parker's pulse rate was high (110 beats/min). What factors could be responsible for her increased pulse rate?

Respirations

Respiration is the process of breathing. When we breathe, we take oxygen into the body and expel carbon dioxide (a waste product) from the body. Both of these functions are vital to life.

▼ Box 9-1 Using a Stethoscope

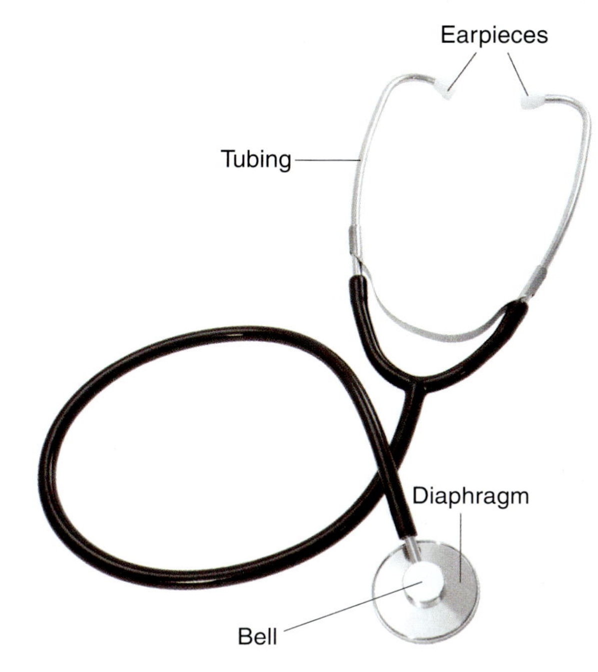

A stethoscope allows the user to listen to sounds produced inside the body. The stethoscope consists of an amplifying device (used to make sounds louder), tubing (used to conduct the sound to the user's ears), and two earpieces. The amplifying device has a large flat side, called the *diaphragm*, and a small rounded side, called the *bell*. The diaphragm is used to listen to high-pitched sounds, such as a heartbeat or blood passing through the arteries. The bell is better for listening to low-pitched sounds. Depending on your needs, you can rotate the amplifying device to use either the diaphragm or the bell side.

Before using a stethoscope, check the tubing for cracks or holes that could distort the sounds. Wipe both the earpieces and the amplifying device with an alcohol wipe before and after each use. Fit the earpieces into your ears with the tips facing forward (toward your nose). You will know they are in place correctly if you cannot hear any outside sound. Next, tap on the amplifying device to check your ability to hear through the stethoscope. If you do not hear the tap, rotate the amplifying device and tap again. When you are able to hear the tap, the stethoscope is ready to use.

Characteristics of respirations

When you are evaluating a person's respirations, as when you are evaluating the person's pulse, you note several things:

- **The respiratory rate.** This is the number of respirations that occur in 1 minute. You count respirations by observing the person's chest rise (inhalation, or taking the breath in) and fall (exhalation, or letting the breath out). One inhalation plus one exhalation equals one respiration. The same factors that can increase the pulse rate also can increase the respiratory rate (for example, exercise, fever, pain, significant blood loss, and emotions such as anger, fear, agitation or excitement). Likewise, the same factors that decrease the pulse rate can decrease the respiratory rate (for example, sleep, certain medications, and certain conditions such as depression). In adults, the normal respiratory rate is between 15 and 20 breaths/min. In infants and children, the normal respiratory rate is faster.
- **The respiratory rhythm.** This is the regularity with which the person breathes. In normal breathing, the breaths are evenly spaced.
- **The respiratory depth.** A person's respirations may be described as *deep* or *shallow*.

Normally, a person breathes quietly and easily. The breaths seem effortless and are evenly spaced. Both sides of the chest rise and fall equally. **Dyspnea** is the medical term for breathing that is difficult or seems like it takes a lot of effort.

Observations Into Action!

Difficult, irregular or noisy breathing is considered abnormal. Report the following signs of abnormal breathing to the nurse right away:

- **A respiratory rate that is greater than 20 breaths/min or less than 15 breaths/min**
- **A respiratory rhythm that is irregular**
- **Respirations that are shallow or deep**
- **Respirations that are strained or difficult (dyspnea)**
- **Respirations that do not cause both sides of the chest to rise and fall together**

Ensuring accuracy when evaluating respirations

Respiration is the one vital function that we can control to a certain extent. Although we breathe without having to think about it, we do have some control over whether our breaths are deep or shallow, and whether they are fast or slow. We also have the ability to interrupt the normal pattern of breathing, by holding our breath. Because just knowing that you are evaluating her breathing can cause a person's breathing to change, it is best to evaluate respirations without the person being aware that you are doing it. Usually, you evaluate a person's respirations after evaluating her pulse. If you keep your fingers on the person's wrist (as if you are still checking the pulse), the person may not be aware that you are evaluating her respirations, which can lead to a more accurate evaluation. Count the person's respirations for 1 full minute, counting one rise and one fall of the chest for each respiration. Skill 9-4 describes step by step how to evaluate a person's respirations.

Mrs. Parker's respiratory rate was 26 breaths/min. What factors could have contributed to her increased respiratory rate?

Blood Pressure

Blood pressure measures the pressure of the circulating blood on the walls of the arteries. Each time the heart beats, it pumps blood into the arteries. The pressure of the blood against the walls of the arteries when the heart pumps is called the *systolic pressure*. The pressure of the blood against the walls when the heart relaxes is called the *diastolic pressure*. The systolic pressure is always higher than the diastolic pressure. A blood pressure reading consists of these two numbers, which are written like a fraction. The larger systolic reading goes on the top, and the smaller diastolic reading goes on the bottom. For example, in the reading 118/78 mm Hg, 118 is the systolic pressure, and 78 is the diastolic pressure. Blood pressure is measured in "millimeters of mercury," or mm Hg.

In adults, the healthy range for blood pressure is less than 120/80 mm Hg. **Hypotension** is the word used to describe low blood pressure, and **hypertension** is the word used to describe high blood pressure. A blood pressure that remains high over time can damage the arteries and place strain on the heart.

It is important for you to know what blood pressure is considered normal for each of the people in your care. Men frequently have higher blood pressures than women, and some ethnic groups tend to have higher blood pressures than others. In addition, blood pressure tends to increase with age. When you are measuring a person's blood pressure, be aware that it is normal for the blood pressure to vary throughout the day, within a relatively narrow range. For example, blood pressure is usually higher late in the day, as compared with the morning. It is higher when a person is sitting or standing, as compared with when the person is lying down. Emotional stress can also cause blood pressure to increase.

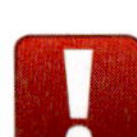

Observations Into Action!

The following may be signs of a medical problem and should be reported to the nurse right away:

- **A blood pressure that is significantly higher than the person's normal blood pressure**
- **A blood pressure that is significantly lower than the person's normal blood pressure**

At times, you may be asked to measure the person's blood pressure first in one arm and then the other, or to obtain a series of blood pressure measurements (for example, with the person lying flat, then sitting up and then standing). Follow the nurse's instructions or the person's care plan.

Equipment used to measure blood pressure

The traditional way of measuring a person's blood pressure is with a stethoscope and a **sphygmomanometer**. The sphygmomanometer has three parts: a *cuff* that is placed around the person's arm, a *bulb* that is squeezed to fill the cuff with air, and a *manometer*, a gauge for measuring the blood pressure (Figure 9-8). There are two styles of manometers. A mercury manometer is an upright gauge that contains a column of mercury. The level of the mercury shows the pressure readings. An aneroid manometer shows the pressure readings on a round dial with an arrow that points to the numbers. Although there is no mercury in an aneroid manometer, the unit of measure is still mm Hg (millimeters of mercury).

The fabric cuff contains a rubber bladder, which is connected by tubing to the bulb. A valve at the base of the bulb opens and closes to control the flow of air into the bladder. The valve is controlled by a screw. If you turn the screw to the left or down, it opens the valve and lets the air escape from the bladder, deflating the cuff. If you turn the screw to the right or up, it closes the valve so that when you pump air into the bladder with the bulb, the valve keeps the air inside the bladder, making the cuff tight.

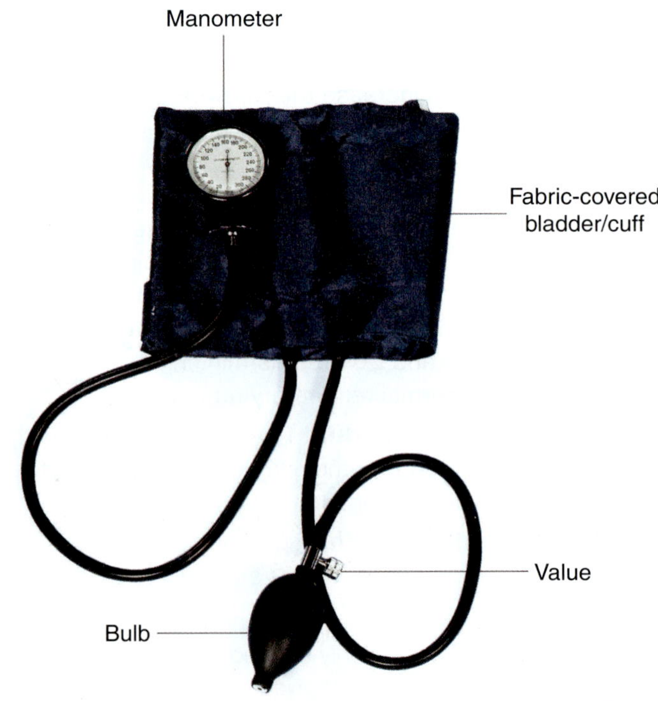

Figure 9-8 A sphygmomanometer is used to measure blood pressure.

When you take a person's blood pressure, you use the stethoscope to listen for changes in blood flow through the brachial artery of the arm. Inflating and then deflating the cuff that is wrapped around the person's arm allows you to cause these changes in blood flow, which are used to identify the systolic and diastolic pressures. As you pump air into the cuff, the cuff pressure increases until it is high enough to stop the blood flow through the brachial artery. At this point, you do not hear anything through the stethoscope. As you turn the valve to deflate the cuff and release the pressure on the brachial artery, the cuff pressure eventually matches the systolic blood pressure. At that point, you will begin to hear pulse sounds through the stethoscope. The reading on the manometer at the time that you hear the first pulse sound is the systolic pressure. As the cuff pressure drops to equal the diastolic pressure in the artery, the sounds that you hear change. The last sound that you hear before the pulse sounds fade away is the diastolic pressure. Skill 9-5 describes how to measure a person's blood pressure using a sphygmomanometer and a stethoscope.

An electronic sphygmomanometer measures and displays the person's blood pressure automatically after you place the cuff on the person's arm. Some electronic models are completely automatic, while others require you to inflate the cuff. It is not necessary to use a stethoscope with an electronic sphygomomanometer.

Ensuring safety and accuracy when measuring blood pressure

Guidelines for ensuring safety and accuracy when measuring a person's blood pressure are given in Box 9-2.

Throughout the rest of your shift, you measure and record Mrs. Parker's vital signs every 4 hours. After you leave for the day, the nurse assistant caring for Mrs. Parker continues to measure and record her vital signs every 4 hours. The next morning, the doctor calls and asks the nurse for an update on Mrs. Parker's condition. The nurse looks at Mrs. Parker's chart and reports that Mrs. Parker's temperature has decreased overnight.

Why is it significant that Mrs. Parker's temperature has decreased overnight?

How did regularly obtaining and recording Mrs. Parker's vital sign measurements help to promote efficient communication among members of the health care team? How does efficient communication benefit Mrs. Parker?

Box 9-2 Nurse Assistant DO's and DON'Ts

Measuring Blood Pressure

DO position the person comfortably in the bed or chair with the arm supported at heart level. If the person is seated in a chair, make sure his feet are flat on the floor.

DO allow the person to sit quietly for at least 5 minutes before measuring the blood pressure.

DO select the correct cuff size. Different cuff sizes include "average adult," "small adult," "large adult," "adult thigh" (used when blood pressures cannot be taken in the arms), and "bariatric" (for obese adults). Cuffs also come in a range of sizes for children. You can determine the correct cuff size by using a tape measure to measure around the person's upper arm, halfway between the elbow and shoulder. Using a cuff that is too big or too small can result in an inaccurate reading.

DON'T place the cuff over the person's clothing. This can result in an inaccurate reading and make it difficult to hear the pulse sounds.

DO wrap the cuff smoothly and snugly. This helps to ensure an accurate reading.

DO position the cuff correctly, with the arrow over the brachial artery. This is necessary to ensure an accurate reading.

DON'T place the cuff on an arm with a cast or an intravenous (IV) line, on an arm that is on the same side as a mastectomy (surgical removal of the breast), on a paralyzed or weak arm, or an arm with a dialysis shunt. These conditions can affect circulation in the arm, which can cause an inaccurate reading. In addition, you could injure the person when you decrease circulation by inflating the cuff.

DO give the vessels in the arm time to relax between blood pressure measurements. If you make a mistake or cannot hear the pulse sounds clearly and need to try again, deflate the cuff completely and wait 1 minute before attempting to measure the blood pressure again. Trying to take the pressure too soon can result in inaccurate measurements, in addition to causing the person discomfort.

WEIGHT AND HEIGHT

Although they are not vital signs, weight and height measurements also provide important information about a person's health status. A person's height is usually only measured on admission to the health care facility, but weights are obtained periodically. As with a person's vital signs, the frequency with which a person's weight is measured varies from person to person. Also as with vital signs, accuracy is extremely important. For people with certain medical conditions, such as heart failure, changes in weight are used to help monitor the person's condition, and even small changes can be significant. Also, medication dosages are sometimes based on weight.

Equipment Used to Measure Weight and Height

Depending on the situation, a person's height and weight can be measured in different ways:

- When a person can stand independently long enough to be weighed, an upright scale (Figure 9-9, A) is used. The upright scale is also used to measure the person's height. Skill 9-6 describes step by step how to measure a person's weight and height using an upright scale.
- When a person is able to get out of bed but is not able to stand long enough to be weighed using an upright scale, a chair scale (see Figure 9-9, B) may be used to weigh the person. Some chair scales have a seat mounted on the scale and you simply help the person to sit in the seat. Other chair scales are designed to be used with a wheelchair. When using this type of chair scale, you first weigh the empty wheelchair, and then you weigh the wheelchair with the person in it. The person's weight is the difference between the two measurements.
- If the person is unable to get out of bed at all, a sling scale is used to weigh the person. The person's height can be measured while the person lies in bed, using a tape measure.

Ensuring Accuracy When Measuring Weight

Weight measurements can be used to evaluate a person's medical condition or nutritional status over time. For example, you may be asked to obtain a person's weight every day, or every week. Since weight varies throughout the day, a consistent process and technique can help to ensure that the weights you obtain are accurate, and make weight comparisons more reliable. For example, always use the same scale in the same place. Weigh the person at approximately the same time of day each time, and have the person wear the same type and amount of clothing. Consistently give the person an opportunity to use the bathroom before obtaining the weight measurement. Finally, make sure the scale is balanced (it should read "0" without any weight on it.)

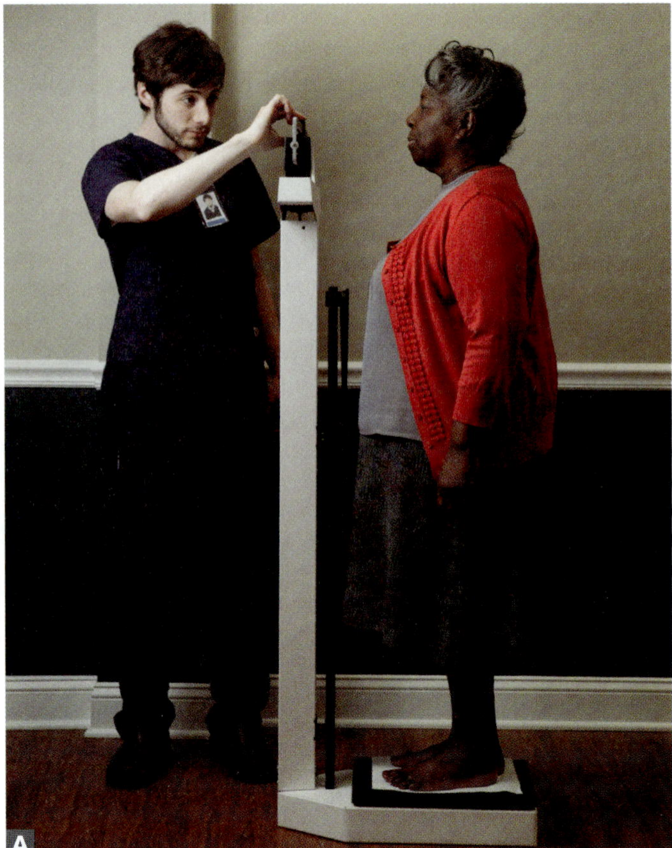

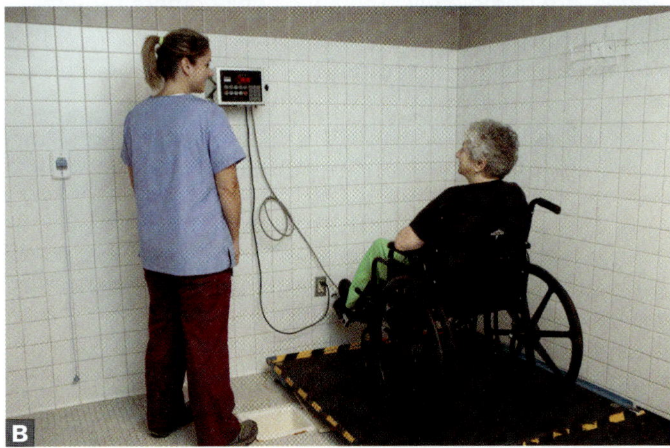

Figure 9-9 Depending on the situation, different types of scales may be used to weigh a person. (A) An upright scale. (B) A chair scale.

CHECK YOUR UNDERSTANDING

Questions for Review

1. **Temperature, pulse, respirations and blood pressure usually are taken together and are referred to as:**
   a. Life measurements.
   b. Vital signs.
   c. Routine measurements.
   d. Monitoring.

2. **Mrs. Tyler has just been admitted to the nursing home. What measurements will you obtain?**
   a. Blood pressure, temperature, respiratory rate, pulse rate
   b. Height
   c. Weight
   d. All of the above

3. **What instrument is used to listen to sounds when obtaining a blood pressure or an apical pulse measurement?**
   a. Stethoscope
   b. Diaphragm
   c. Sphygmomanometer
   d. Thermometer

4. **Mr. Rollins is receiving oxygen therapy. You could use any of the following methods to take his temperature EXCEPT the:**
   a. Oral method
   b. Axillary method
   c. Rectal method
   d. Tympanic method

5. **Which of the following measurements is outside of the normal range for an adult?**
   a. Temperature, 99° F
   b. Respirations, 13 breaths/min
   c. Pulse, 63 beats/min
   d. Blood pressure, 107/70 mm Hg

6. **Where is the brachial pulse located?**
   a. The inside of the elbow
   b. At the top of the heart, just under the left nipple
   c. On the inside of the wrist at the base of the thumb
   d. On the inside of the groin where the thigh meets the hip

7. **What equipment is nee ... e a radial pulse?**
   a. Sphygmomanometer
   b. Stethoscope
   c. Watch with a second hand
   d. All of the above

8. **Mrs. Wilson's pulse is very weak. How would y describe her pulse?**
   a. Shallow
   b. Thready
   c. Bounding
   d. Irregular

9. **Which of the following factors can affect a person's vital sign measurements?**
   a. Illness
   b. Emotions
   c. The time of day
   d. All of the above

10. **The nurse has asked you to measure Mr. Simon's temperature rectally. What equipment will you use?**
    a. A tympanic thermometer
    b. An axillary thermometer
    c. An electronic thermometer with a blue probe
    d. An electronic thermometer with a red probe

Questions to Ask Yourself

1. *You are getting ready to assist Mrs. Perkins to the bathroom when she tells you that she feels very dizzy. You decide to take her vital sign measurements, which are as follows: temperature, 97° F (oral); pulse, 80 beats/min; respirations, 15 breaths/min; and blood pressure, 90/52 mm Hg. Which of these measurements is significant and why?*
2. *When you go into Mrs. Clement's room to take her oral temperature, you notice a cup of coffee on her over-bed table. What should you consider, and what should you do?*
3. *When you take Mr. Wilson's pulse at 8:00 a.m., the rate is 72 beats/min and the rhythm is regular. When you take it again at 9:00 a.m., the rate is 56 beats/min and irregular. What should you do?*
4. *Mrs. O'Neill wants to talk with you while you are trying to measure and record vital signs. How should you handle this situation? What should you say to her?*

SK
.ı 9-1

ʋsing an Electronic Thermometer to Measure a Person's Temperature

PREPARATION

1. Wash your hands.
2. Gather your supplies:
   - **Oral or axillary temperature:**
     - Electronic thermometer with blue probe
     - Probe cover
     - Tissues
     - Pen and paper
   - **Rectal temperature:**
     - Electronic thermometer with red probe
     - Probe cover
     - Lubricating jelly
     - Gloves
     - Tissues
     - Pen and paper
   - **Tympanic temperature:**
     - Tympanic thermometer
     - Probe cover
     - Pen and paper
3. Knock, greet the person and ensure privacy.
4. Explain the procedure.
5. Adjust equipment for body mechanics and safety: Raise the bed to a comfortable working height. Make sure the wheels are locked.

PROCEDURE

6. Turn the thermometer on by removing the probe from the location in the machine where it is stored (electronic thermometer) or by pushing the button (tympanic thermometer).
7. Place the probe cover on the probe. For an electronic thermometer, insert the probe into the probe cover by pushing firmly until you feel the cover snap into place (Figure 1). For a tympanic thermometer, place the probe cover over the cone-shaped probe.
8. Position the person appropriately.
   - **Oral or axillary temperature:** Position the person in Fowler's position (sitting up with the head of the bed elevated) or the supine position (lying on the back).

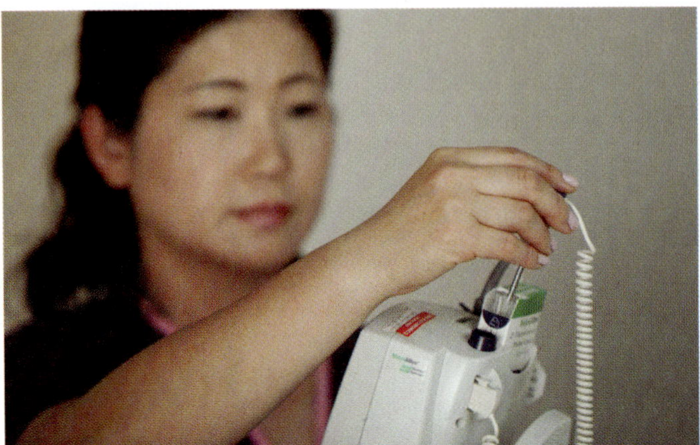

Figure 1

   - **Rectal temperature:** Help the person lie on one side with his back toward you and the top knee flexed.
   - **Tympanic temperature:** Position the person in Fowler's position.
9. If taking a rectal temperature, lubricate the tip of the probe by placing a small amount of lubricating jelly on a tissue and dipping the tip of the probe in it. Put on the gloves.
10. Place the thermometer.
    - **Oral temperature:** Put the probe under the person's tongue and slightly to one side (Figure 2A). Ask the person to close his lips around the thermometer.

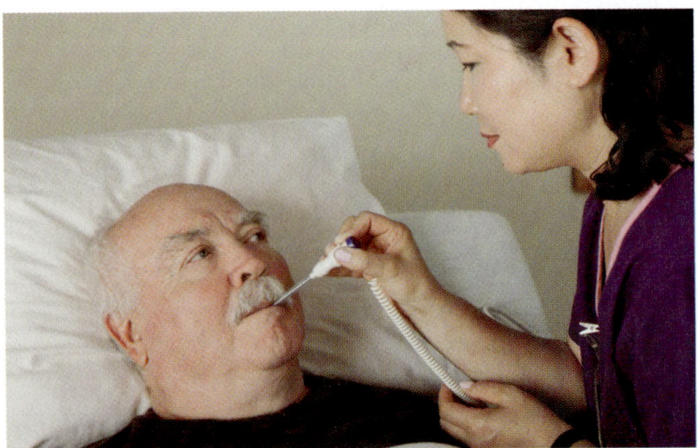

Figure 2A

- **Rectal temperature:** Adjust the top covers and the person's clothing as necessary to expose the buttocks. Lift the person's upper buttock and insert the probe into the anus no more than 1 inch in an adult or 1/2 inch in a child (Figure 2B). Stay with the person and hold the probe in place.

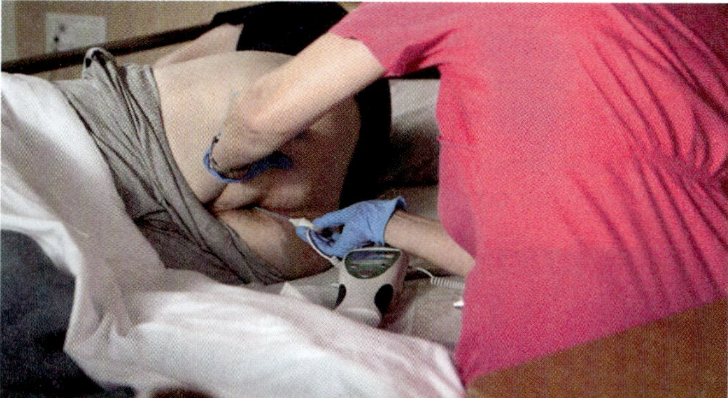

Figure 2B

- **Axillary temperature:** Expose the person's underarm and pat the skin dry with a tissue, if necessary. Put the probe in the middle of the person's underarm and then bring the person's arm across his chest to hold the probe in place (Figure 2C).

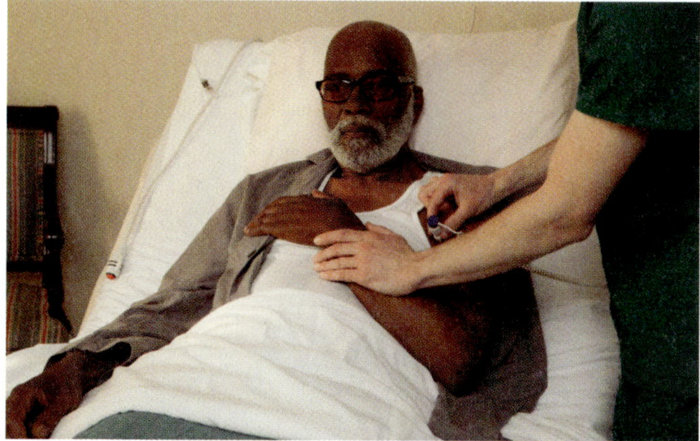

Figure 2C

- **Tympanic temperature:** Grasp the top of the person's ear and pull *up and back* (in an adult) or *down and back* (in a child younger than 3 years) to straighten the ear canal. Insert the probe into the ear canal, pointing it down and forward, toward the person's nose (Figure 2D).

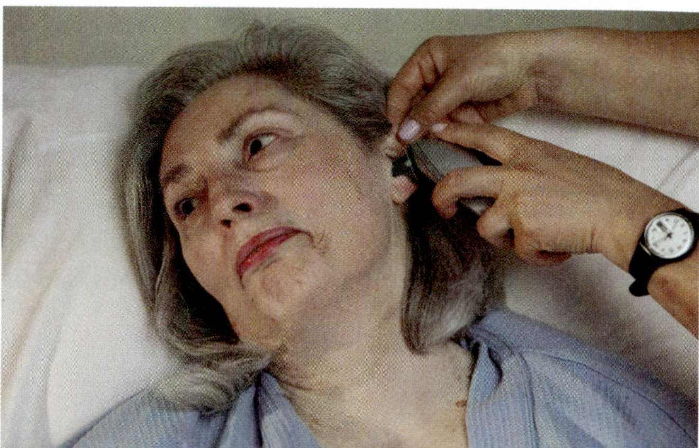

Figure 2D

11. When the thermometer beeps, remove the probe and read the temperature measurement on the screen.
12. Eject the probe cover into a facility-approved waste container and return the probe to its home. (Be aware that returning the probe to its home clears the display screen, so be sure to make note of the temperature measurement first.)
13. Help make the person comfortable.
    - **Rectal temperature:** Wipe the lubricating jelly from the person's buttocks with a tissue and discard the tissue in a facility-approved waste container. Adjust the person's clothing to cover the buttocks.
    - **Axillary temperature:** Adjust the person's clothing to cover the underarm area.
14. Remove and dispose of your gloves. Wash your hands.
15. Write down the person's name, the time, the temperature measurement, and the method used to obtain the temperature (***O*** for oral, ***R*** for rectal, ***A*** for axillary or ***TY*** for tympanic).
16. Continue obtaining other vital sign measurements, or follow the completion steps.

COMPLETION

17. Ensure the person's comfort and good body alignment.
18. Adjust equipment for safety: Lower the bed to the level specified in the person's care plan. Make sure the wheels on the bed are locked. Place the person's method of calling for help within reach. Lower or raise the side rails according to the person's care plan.
19. Clean up your work area.
20. Wash your hands.
21. Report and record.

Skill 9-2
Evaluating a Person's Radial Pulse

PREPARATION

1. Wash your hands.
2. Gather your supplies:
   - Watch with a second hand
   - Pen and paper
3. Knock, greet the person and ensure privacy.
4. Explain the procedure.
5. Adjust equipment for body mechanics and safety: Raise the bed to a comfortable working height. Make sure the wheels on the bed are locked.

PROCEDURE

6. Position the person appropriately:
   - **In bed:** Position the person in Fowler's position (sitting up with the head of the bed elevated) or the supine position (lying on the back). Position the person's arm so that it is resting comfortably on the bed or the person's lap.
   - **In a chair:** Have the person sit with both feet flat on the floor. Position the arm so that it is resting comfortably on the arm of the chair or the person's lap.
7. Gently press your first, second and third fingers over the person's radial artery (located on the inside of the wrist on the same side as the thumb) (Figure 1).

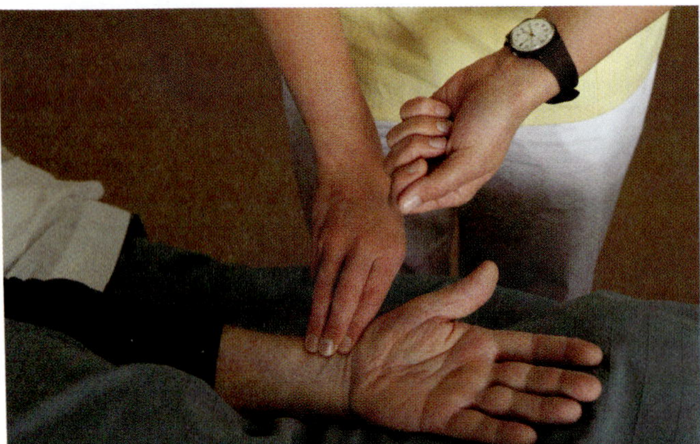

Figure 1

8. Look at your watch. When the second hand reaches the "12," begin counting the pulse. Continue counting for 1 full minute.
9. Note the rhythm and force of the pulse.
10. Write down the person's name, the time, and the pulse rate, rhythm and force.
11. Continue obtaining other vital sign measurements, or follow the completion steps.

COMPLETION

12. Ensure the person's comfort and good body alignment.
13. Adjust equipment for safety: Lower the bed to the level specified in the person's care plan. Make sure the wheels on the bed are locked. Place the person's method of calling for help within reach. Lower or raise the side rails according to the person's care plan.
14. Clean up your work area.
15. Wash your hands.
16. Report and record.

Skill 9-3
Evaluating a Person's Apical Pulse

PREPARATION

1. Wash your hands.
2. Gather your supplies:
   - Watch with a second hand
   - Stethoscope
   - Alcohol wipes
   - Pen and paper
3. Knock, greet the person and ensure privacy.
4. Explain the procedure.
5. Adjust equipment for body mechanics and safety: Raise the bed to a comfortable working height. Make sure the wheels on the bed are locked.

PROCEDURE

6. Position the person appropriately:
   - **In bed:** Position the person in Fowler's position (sitting up with the head of the bed elevated) or the supine position (lying on the back). Position the person's arm so that it is resting comfortably on the bed or the person's lap.
   - **In a chair:** Have the person sit with both feet flat on the floor. Position the arm so that it is resting comfortably on the arm of the chair or the person's lap.
7. Clean the earpieces and diaphragm of the stethoscope with an alcohol wipe. Discard the wipe in a facility-approved waste container.
8. Adjust the top covers and the person's clothing as necessary to expose the apical pulse site (located about 2 to 3 inches to the left of the breastbone, below the left nipple).
9. Put the earpieces of the stethoscope in your ears with the tips facing forward (toward your nose).
10. Warm the diaphragm of the stethoscope by holding it in your hand. Place the diaphragm over the apical pulse site (Figure 1). Hold the diaphragm in place with your fingers, not your thumb.

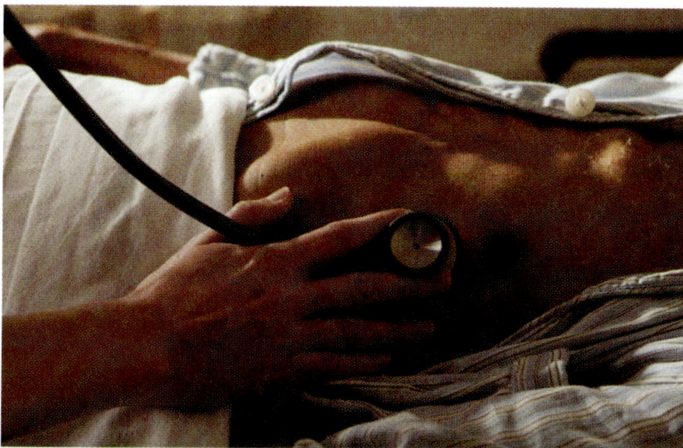

Figure 1

11. Look at your watch. When the second hand reaches the "12," begin counting the pulse. Continue counting for 1 full minute.
12. Note the rhythm and force of the pulse.
13. Write down the person's name, the time, and the pulse rate, rhythm and force.
14. Continue obtaining other vital sign measurements, or follow the completion steps.

COMPLETION

15. Ensure the person's comfort and good body alignment.
16. Adjust equipment for safety: Lower the bed to the level specified in the person's care plan. Make sure the wheels on the bed are locked. Place the person's method of calling for help within reach. Lower or raise the side rails according to the person's care plan.
17. Clean up your work area.
18. Wash your hands.
19. Report and record.

Skill 9-4
Evaluating a Person's Respirations

PREPARATION

1. Wash your hands.
2. Gather your supplies:
   - Watch with a second hand
   - Pen and paper
3. Knock, greet the person and ensure privacy.
4. Explain the procedure.
5. Adjust equipment for body mechanics and safety: Raise the bed to a comfortable working height. Make sure the wheels on the bed are locked.

PROCEDURE

6. Hold the person's wrist as if taking a radial pulse.
7. Look at your watch. When the second hand reaches the "12" and you see the person's chest rise, begin counting the respirations. Remember that one respiration equals one rise and one fall of the chest. Continue counting for 1 full minute.
8. Note the rhythm and depth of the respirations, and whether the person seems to be having any difficulty breathing.
9. Write down the person's name, the time, and the respiratory rate, rhythm and depth.
10. Continue obtaining other vital sign measurements, or follow the completion steps.

COMPLETION

11. Ensure the person's comfort and good body alignment.
12. Adjust equipment for safety: Lower the bed to the level specified in the person's care plan. Make sure the wheels on the bed are locked. Place the person's method of calling for help within reach. Lower or raise the side rails according to the person's care plan.
13. Clean up your work area.
14. Wash your hands.
15. Report and record.

Skill 9-5
Measuring a Person's Blood Pressure

PREPARATION

1. Wash your hands.
2. Gather your supplies:
   - Sphygmomanometer with the correct-size cuff
   - Stethoscope
   - Alcohol wipes
   - Pen and paper
3. Knock, greet the person and ensure privacy.
4. Explain the procedure.
5. Adjust equipment for body mechanics and safety: Raise the bed to a comfortable working height. Make sure the wheels on the bed are locked.

PROCEDURE

6. Position the person appropriately:
   - **In bed:** Position the person in the supine position (lying on the back). Position the person's arm so that it is resting comfortably, palm up, on the bed.
   - **In a chair:** Have the person sit with both feet flat on the floor. Position the arm so that it is fully supported and level with the person's heart.
7. Clean the earpieces and diaphragm of the stethoscope with an alcohol wipe. Discard the wipe in a facility-approved waste container.
8. Turn the screw to the left (down) and squeeze all of the air out of the cuff. Adjust the person's clothing as necessary to expose the upper arm.
9. Locate the person's brachial pulse, on the inside of the elbow (Figure 1).

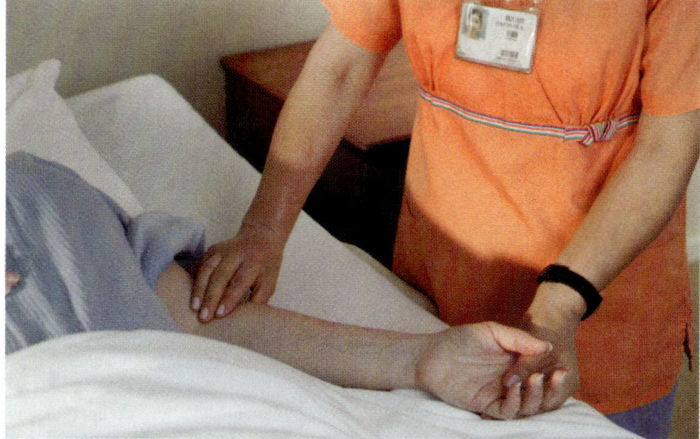

Figure 1

10. Place the cuff on the person's arm, over bare skin, with the arrow directly over the brachial artery. The bottom edge of the cuff should be about 1 inch above the person's elbow. Wrap the cuff around the person's arm snugly and smoothly and secure the cuff. Make sure it is snug enough to stay in place, but not uncomfortably tight (Figure 2).

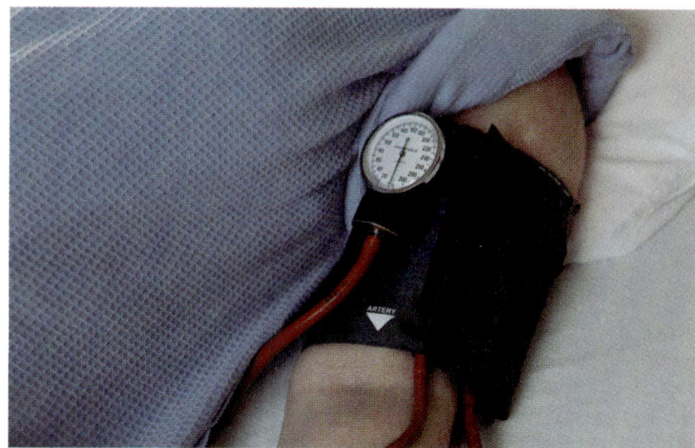

Figure 2

11. Place your fingers on the person's radial pulse, on the wrist.
12. Turn the screw to the right so that the cuff inflates when you pump the bulb. Inflate the cuff by pumping the bulb until you can no longer feel the radial pulse. Look at the gauge and note the reading, which is an estimate of the systolic pressure. Let the air out of the cuff quickly by turning the valve to the left.
13. Put the earpieces in your ears with the tips facing forward (toward your nose). Place the diaphragm of the stethoscope firmly over the person's brachial pulse (Figure 3).

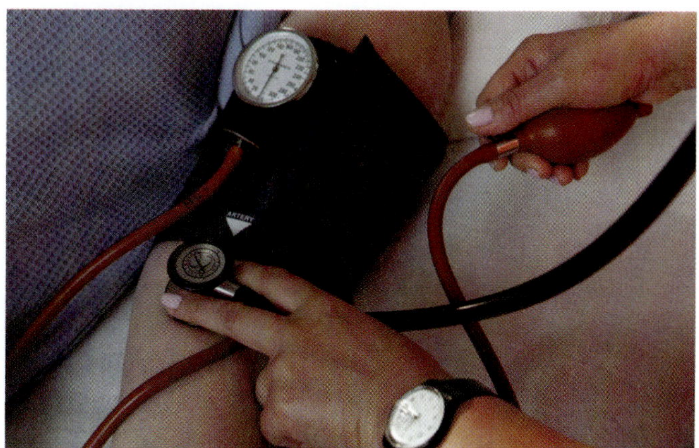

Figure 3

Continued on next page

Skill 9-5
Measuring a Person's Blood Pressure *Continued*

14. Turn the screw to the right (up) and pump the bulb to inflate the cuff to 30 mm Hg above the estimated systolic blood pressure.
15. Turn the screw to the left (down) and let the air out of the cuff slowly (about 2 to 4 mm Hg per second). The reading when you first hear the pulse sound is the *systolic* pressure. Remember this number and continue letting the air out slowly.
16. The reading when the pulse sound stops or changes is the *diastolic* pressure. Remember this number and quickly let out the rest of the air.
17. Write down the person's name, the time and the blood pressure measurement.
18. Remove the cuff from the person's arm.

COMPLETION

19. Ensure the person's comfort and good body alignment.
20. Adjust equipment for safety: Lower the bed to the level specified in the person's care plan. Make sure the wheels on the bed are locked. Place the person's method of calling for help within reach. Lower or raise the side rails according to the person's care plan.
21. Clean up your work area.
22. Wash your hands.
23. Report and record.

Skill 9-6
Measuring a Person's Weight and Height Using an Upright Scale

PREPARATION

1. Wash your hands.
2. Gather your supplies:
   - Upright scale
   - Paper towels
   - Pen and paper
3. Knock, greet the person and ensure privacy.
4. Explain the procedure.
5. Adjust equipment for body mechanics and safety.

PROCEDURE

6. Check the balance of the scale by moving the weights all the way to the left (zero). The pointer should be centered evenly between the top and bottom bars (Figure 1). If the scale is not balanced, notify the nurse.

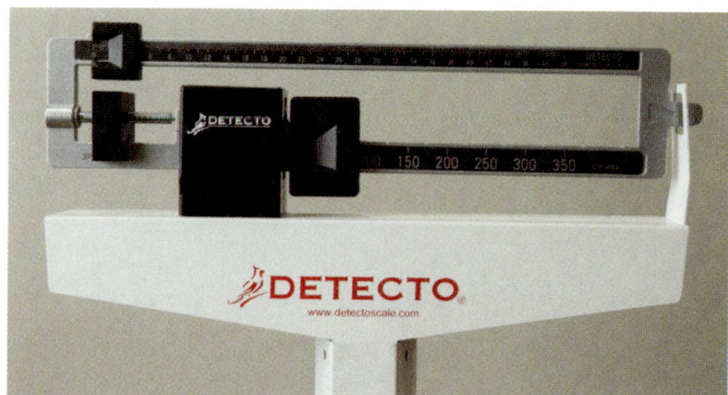

Figure 1

7. Put a paper towel on the scale platform.
8. Assist the person to step onto the scale platform, facing the balance bar (Figure 2).

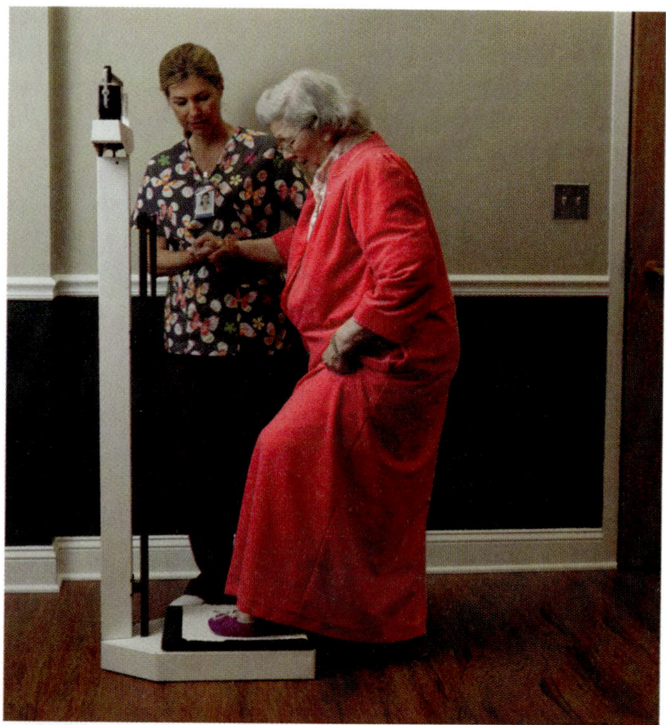
Figure 2

9. The bottom bar is marked in units of 50 pounds. Move the large weight on the bottom bar to the weight that is closest to the person's estimated weight in units of 50 pounds, without exceeding the person's estimated weight. For example, if you think the person weighs about 190 pounds, you would move the bottom weight to the "150" mark.
10. The top bar is marked in units of 1 pound and ¼ pound. Move the small weight on the top bar until the pointer is centered evenly between the top and bottom bars.
11. Add the weight on the top bar to the weight on the bottom bar. This is the person's weight.
12. Write down the person's name, the time and the weight.
13. If you are measuring the person's height as well, assist the person to turn around so that she is facing away from the balance bar.
14. Slide the height scale all the way up and pull out the height rod.

Continued on next page

Skill 9-6
Measuring a Person's Weight and Height Using an Upright Scale
Continued

15. Slide the height rod down until it touches the top of the person's head, and read the number on the height scale (Figure 3). This is the person's height.

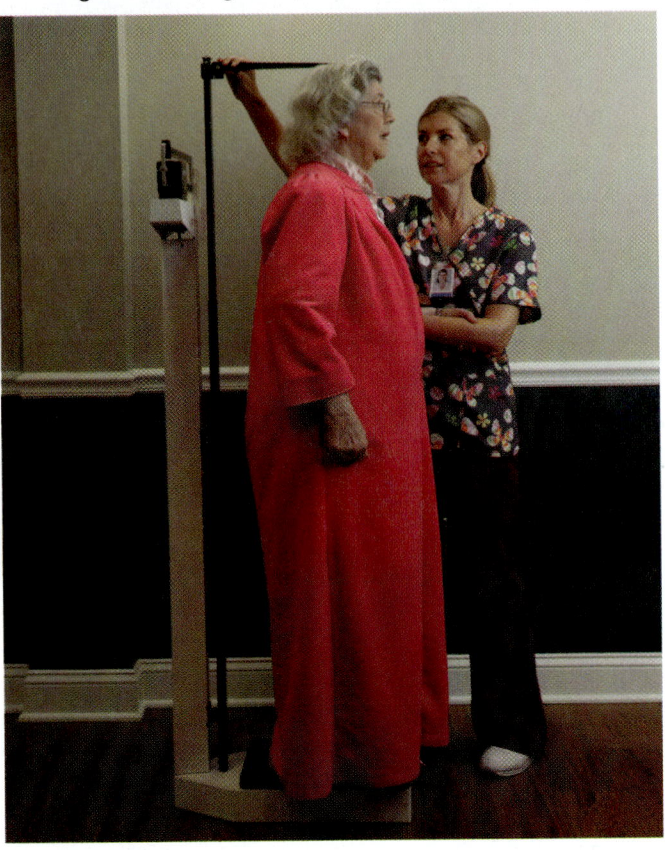

Figure 3

16. Write down the person's height next to her weight.
17. Assist the person to step off the scale.

COMPLETION

18. Ensure the person's comfort and good body alignment.
19. Adjust equipment for safety: Lower the bed to the level specified in the person's care plan. Make sure the wheels on the bed are locked. Place the person's method of calling for help within reach. Lower or raise the side rails according to the person's care plan.
20. Clean up your work area.
21. Wash your hands.
22. Report and record.

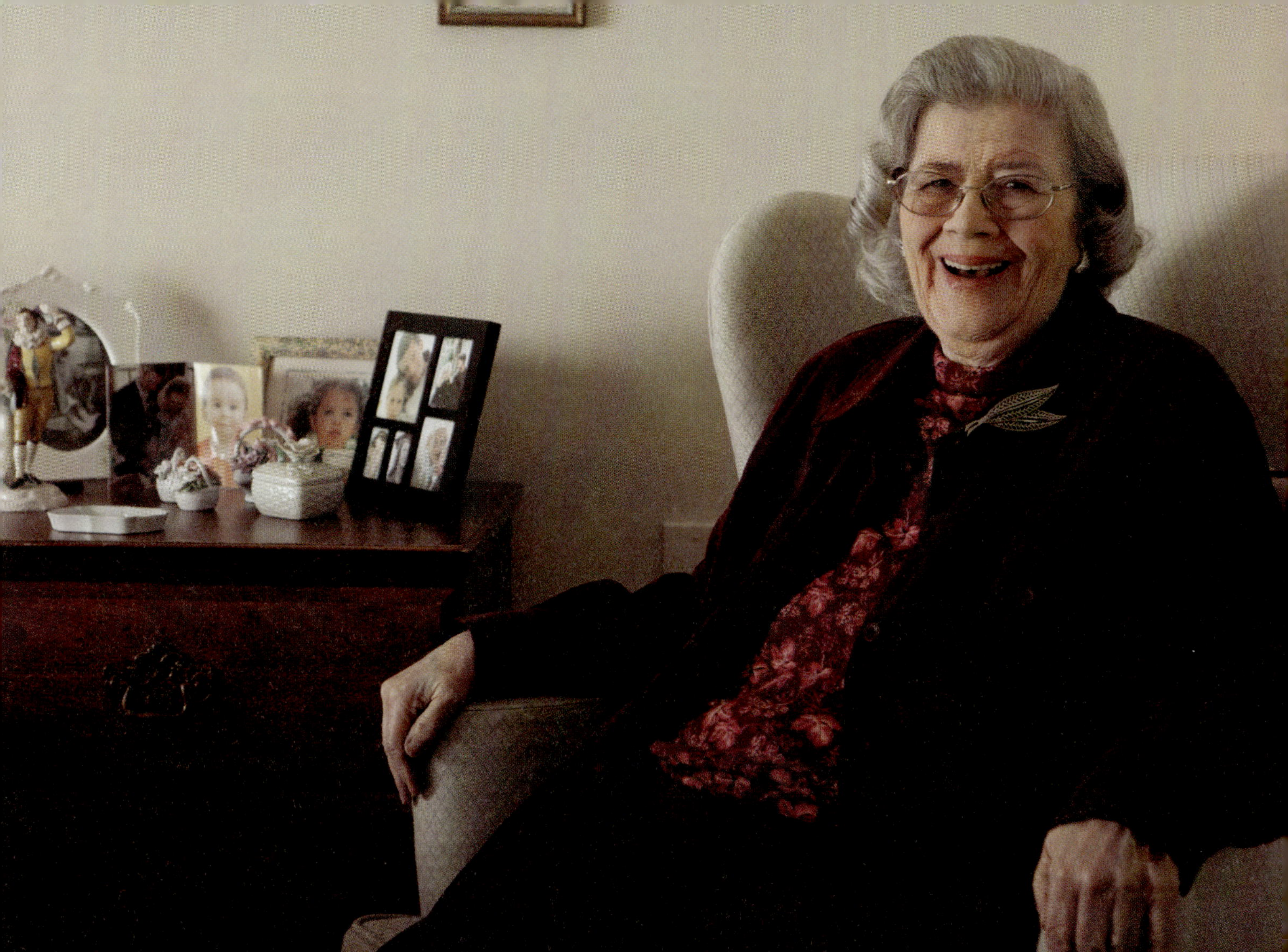

Maintaining a Comfortable Environment

CHAPTER 10

Goals

After reading this chapter, you will have the information needed to:

- Understand the importance of personal items to the person receiving health care.
- Describe environmental conditions that affect a person's comfort, and understand the nurse assistant's role in maintaining an environment that is special, comfortable and safe for the person.
- Describe equipment that is commonly used to furnish a person's room in a health care setting.
- Explain how a properly made bed can contribute to a person's comfort and health.

Continued on next page

Continued from previous page

Goals

- Describe the linens and other supplies that may be used to make a bed.
- Explain measures that are taken when making a bed to prevent the spread of infection.

After practicing the corresponding skills, you will have the information needed to:

- Make an unoccupied and an occupied bed.

Key Terms:

miter **closed bed** **open bed** **surgical bed**

Agnes Ryan shares a room with Louise Wang at Morningside Nursing Home. Mrs. Ryan's part of the room has become home to her. A glass display case filled with cat figurines hangs on the wall near her bed. A quilt, which Mrs. Ryan made many years ago, is folded neatly at the foot of her bed. Mrs. Ryan likes to change the quilt according to the season, so every few months she exchanges the quilt on her bed for another one in her collection. A little stack of books, a pad of paper and pen, an arrangement of silk flowers and a collection of family photos decorate the top of Mrs. Ryan's bedside table. She likes to keep these things arranged in a particular way so that she knows just where they are.

One day as you are helping Mrs. Ryan get ready for physical therapy, you ask her when she started collecting cat figurines. Mrs. Ryan points to a black cat in the center of the top shelf and says, "Do you see that little black cat? It all started with him. My husband, Gerard, gave him to me on Halloween, right after we started dating. He said that contrary to popular belief, he felt the black cat would bring us luck. I guess he was right, since we got married the next year and spent 67 happy years together! After that, Gerard added to my collection over the years. That little calico cat playing with the ball of string next to Blackie? Well, Gerard brought that one back for me from Europe when he came home from the war. Oh, there's a story behind each one of them! My collection used to be much larger, you know. When I came to live here, I had to choose my favorites, because there just wasn't room to bring them all. I gave the rest away to family members and friends who I thought would enjoy them. It was hard to part with them because each one reminded me of Gerard, and I felt like I was giving away a little piece of our life together each time."

Think about your own home. How do the items you keep and display there reflect who you are? Has a visitor to your home ever shown an interest in something that was special to you? How did that make you feel?

Mrs. Ryan said that she had to make hard decisions about what to bring to her new home. Have you ever had to make a decision like that? Was it difficult for you?

As a nurse assistant, how might taking an interest in a person's personal belongings help to strengthen your relationship with that person, and provide better care?

THE PERSON'S SPACE

Emotional Factors That Affect Comfort

Think about the word *home*. What do you picture in your mind when you think of home? Do you think of a favorite, comfortable chair where you sit down after a long, hard day? Do you picture a display of family photographs on the wall, or a special gift that someone gave to you?

Home is your personal space. It is where you live, and where you feel safe and comfortable. For people who are receiving health care, the health care setting becomes their home, either temporarily or permanently. In a hospital, the person's "home space" is usually just part of a room. For a nursing home resident, the person's home space would include her room and common areas, such as the dayroom and dining room. Sometimes the person's own home is modified to become a health care setting, as in home health care. Whether home is a person's own home, a nursing home or a hospital, you help maintain that place so that it is special and personal.

Just as your home and belongings are important to you, the homes and belongings of the people in your care are important to them (Figure 10-1). A person in your care

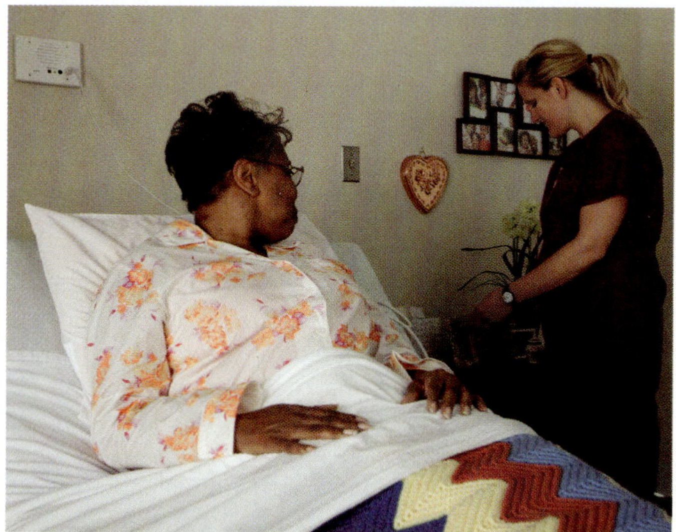

Figure 10-1 Treat the person's personal items with the same care you would treat your own valued possessions.

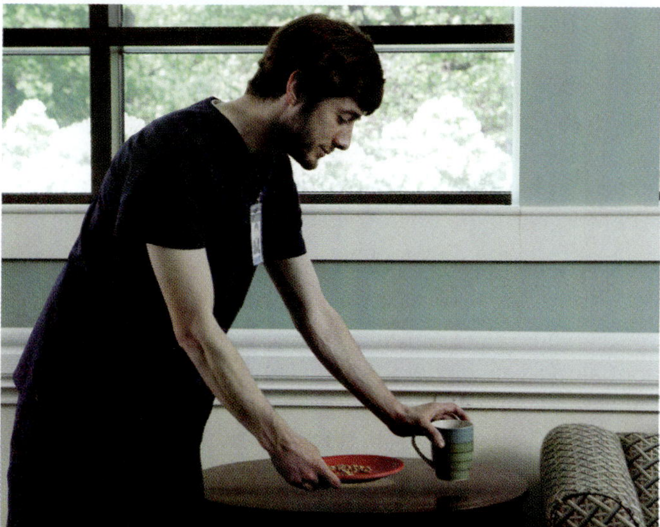

Figure 10-2 A clean, neat environment is essential for controlling infection and odors.

is sensitive about who touches her belongings or comes into her personal space. Show that you respect the person, her home and her belongings by always:

- Knocking and asking permission to enter before entering the person's room.
- Treating the person's personal belongings with the same care you would treat your own.
- Taking care to put items back where you found them if you must move them (for example, to clean).
- Asking the person where to place an item if you are unsure about where it belongs.
- Asking the person about her preferences regarding how her space should be kept.

Physical Factors That Affect Comfort

Displaying personal items that hold special meaning helps us to feel more comfortable and at home in our surroundings. However, physical factors, such as room temperature, lighting and cleanliness, also affect how comfortable we are in a place. To help ensure a comfortable environment for people receiving care, health care facilities establish policies to maintain certain environmental standards.

Cleanliness

As you learned in Chapter 6, cleanliness is essential for preventing the spread of infection. Maintaining a clean environment also helps to prevent odors. All members of the health care team share the responsibility for ensuring a clean environment (Figure 10-2). The housekeeping staff takes care of routine deep cleaning, such as mopping the floors and emptying waste containers. However, as a nurse assistant, you are responsible for making sure that the person's personal space is kept neat and clean (for example, by disposing of disposable items and cleaning and putting away non-disposable equipment after you complete a procedure). You also help maintain cleanliness by ensuring that the person has fresh linens on the bed.

Odor control

Minimizing bad smells, such as those of urine, feces, vomit and body odor, is essential for promoting a pleasant environment. Maintaining a clean environment helps to stop odors from developing. Always empty and clean bedpans, urinals and emesis basins promptly. Also, keep the lids on linen hampers and trash cans closed. Odors can also develop when a person's body, clothing or linens are not clean. These sorts of odors can be prevented by routinely assisting the people in your care with personal care, and replacing the linens on the bed whenever they become wet or soiled, and according to your employer's policy.

Temperature control

We cannot be comfortable if we are too hot or too cold. Loss of body fat is a normal part of aging. As a result, older people tend to become chilled more easily than younger people. People who are ill may also feel chilled. Many health care facilities have individual room-temperature controls. You may find the temperature in the room to be warm because you are busy and moving around, but remember, the temperature is set for the comfort of the person receiving care. You may still need to provide the person with an extra blanket for the bed, a lap blanket or a sweater to help ensure that he is warm enough.

Noise control

Health care facilities can be quite noisy. Equipment beeps. Telephones ring. Staff members, visitors and people receiving care talk to one another. Televisions are turned on. In any busy place, a certain amount of noise is unavoidable. However, an environment that is too noisy can increase stress levels and make it difficult for people to rest and sleep. Because of the impact noise can have on the health and well-being of those receiving care, the noise levels in a facility are often considered when evaluating the quality of care provided by the facility.

You can help to minimize noise by speaking in a normal tone of voice and being mindful of where conversations take place. For example, try to avoid having conversations with other staff members right outside of a person's room. Answer telephones promptly. If you notice that a piece of equipment is squeaky or noisy, make arrangements to have the equipment sent for repair or maintenance.

COMMON FURNISHINGS IN HEALTH CARE SETTINGS

A person's room in a health care setting often contains standard furnishings designed to make it easier to provide care. In a home health setting, the person may rent some of these furnishings, or you may need to make do with furnishings and other items that are already in the home.

Bed

In home health and long-term-care settings, the person may use his own bed, rather than an adjustable bed or a specialty bed.

Adjustable beds

Adjustable beds, or hospital beds, are often used in health care settings because they can be adjusted in different ways to make it easier and safer to provide care, and to promote the comfort of the person in the bed. On an adjustable bed, the entire bed frame can be raised or lowered in relation to the floor. When you are providing care for a person in the bed, you will usually raise the bed to a comfortable working height so that you do not have to bend or stoop. This helps to protect your back. When you are finished providing care, you will lower the bed to the level specified in the person's care plan. When the person sits on the edge of the bed, he should be able to put his feet flat on the floor. This makes it easier and safer for the person to get in and out of the bed.

Adjustable beds also have mattress platforms with "joints" that allow the mattress to be positioned in different ways. For example, you can raise the head of the mattress at the hips so that the person can sit up in bed. You can also raise the mattress under the person's knees, to help prevent the person from sliding down in the bed while he is sitting up (Figure 10-3, A). The mattress should only be raised under the person's knees for a short period of time (for example, while the person eats) because being in this position for an extended period of time can lead to complications such as pressure ulcers. The mattress platform on an adjustable bed also allows the entire mattress to be tilted up or down without bending the person at the waist, so that the person's head is lower than her feet, or vice versa (see Figure 10-3, B and C). The person's primary care provider (a doctor or advanced practice nurse) may order these special positions, called Trendelenburg's

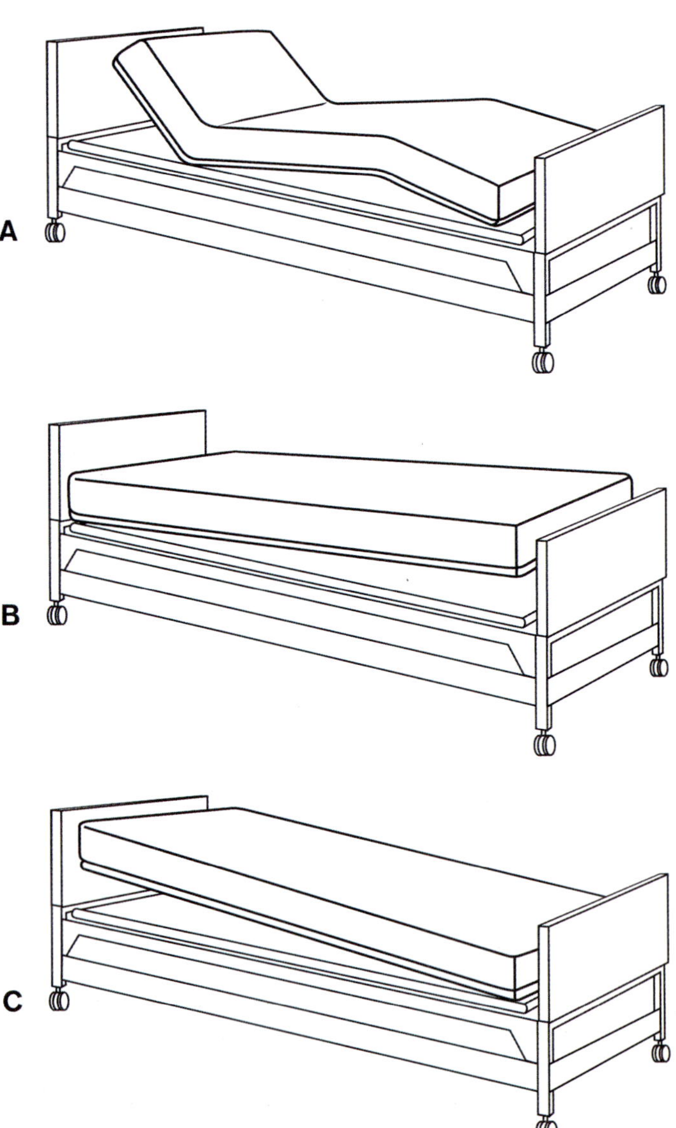

Figure 10-3 The mattress of an adjustable bed can be positioned many different ways. (A) Breaks at the hips and knees raise the head of the mattress and the person's knees to prevent the person from sliding down in the bed while sitting up. (B) In Trendelenburg's position, the entire mattress is tilted so that the head is lower than the feet. (C) Reverse Trendelenburg's position.

position and reverse Trendelenburg's position, respectively, for people with certain medical conditions.

Many adjustable beds in use today are adjusted using an electric control panel. Because the control panel normally is located within the person's reach, the person usually can operate the bed without your assistance. Some adjustable beds are manual, meaning that a series of cranks is used to change the position of the bed or mattress. If you are using a bed with hand cranks, make sure to return the cranks to their correct position after using them. If left out, a person could trip over them or accidentally walk into them, causing injury.

Specialty beds

Specialty beds may be used, depending on the person's specific needs. If you are caring for a person in a specialty bed, make sure the nurse shows you how to operate and care for the bed, if these tasks are within your scope of practice. Examples of specialty beds include:

- **Air-fluidized bed.** This bed has a mattress filled with ceramic beads. A current of air keeps the beads in constant wave-like motion, which helps to relieve pressure on any one area of the body. Air-fluidized beds may be used for people at high risk for pressure ulcers. (Pressure ulcers are discussed in more detail in Chapter 12.)
- **Alternating-pressure bed.** The mattress of this bed has channels that are connected to a pump that alternately fills and empties the channels with air. This type of bed is useful for preventing pressure ulcers and for stimulating circulation.

When caring for a person in a specialty bed, be aware that the edges of the mattresses used on these beds are usually soft and rounded. A person positioned on the edge of the mattress can easily slide off. When the person is in bed, always make sure she is lying in the middle of the mattress (not close to the side). When the person is getting out of the bed, avoid having her sit on the very edge of the mattress (make sure the person has complete support under her thighs).

Over-Bed Table

The over-bed table fits over a bed or a chair to provide a work surface. Wheels allow it to be moved easily from one place to another, and the height is adjustable. The over-bed table is useful for serving meals and for keeping items such as eyeglasses, the television remote, or a water pitcher and glass within the person's reach. You may also use the over-bed table as a place to set up your supplies before carrying out a procedure. Because the over-bed table is considered a clean area, never put dirty items, such as soiled linens or a urinal, on it. If you use the over-bed table as a place to set up your supplies for a procedure, be sure to remove all of your supplies and clean the over-bed table when you are finished with the procedure.

Storage

Equipment and supplies used for personal care, such as washbasins and toiletries, are often stored in the bedside table. The person's room will typically contain a closet, wardrobe or dresser where he can store clothing and other personal items. Remember to ask the person's permission before accessing his storage area or removing anything from it.

Privacy Curtains

Rooms that are shared will have a privacy curtain suspended from a track on the ceiling that can be pulled to separate one half of the room from the other. You should pull the privacy curtain whenever you are assisting a person with care.

Communication Devices

Every person in your care must have a way to call for help. Most health care facilities have a call signal system. A call signal is attached to the bed, within the person's reach. Pushing the button causes a bell to ring and a light to come on over the person's door and at the nurse's station, alerting the staff. A similar device is located in the bathroom.

Make sure that the person understands how to use the call signal system and can operate it. Many of the people you will care for will have some degree of memory loss and will not be able to remember how to use the call signal. Reminding the person over and over simply makes the person anxious, because short-term memory is what the person is lacking. Setting up an alternative way for the person to let you know she needs you is very important. This could be as simple as having the person verbally call out to you, or giving the person a small hand bell or hotel bell to ring. These alternative methods of calling for help also work well in settings that may not have a call signal system, such as the home setting.

BEDMAKING

A clean, fresh bed is important to almost everyone. It is especially important to people who spend most of their time in bed. Nurse assistants are responsible for ensuring that the people in their care have clean, dry linens at all times. The frequency with which you change bed linens depends on how much time the person spends in bed, and it also depends on your employer's policies. In most facilities, linens are routinely changed in the morning, after bathing, grooming and dressing are completed. But the time of day for changing linens also varies according to the needs of the person in your care. One universal rule to follow: Change all linens immediately if they are wet or soiled, because wet, soiled linens can cause skin irritation that can lead to pressure ulcers.

Supplies Used in Bedmaking

Linens

The following types of linens are used to make a bed:

- **Mattress pad.** The mattress pad is a thick, absorbent pad that is used to cushion the mattress. Because the mattress pad is absorbent, it also protects the mattress from becoming soiled. The mattress pad may be flat or fitted. Fitted mattress pads have elastic edges that fit over the mattress to hold the mattress pad in place.
- **Sheets.** A bottom sheet and a top sheet are used to make the bed. Often, in health care facilities, both sheets are flat, although the bottom sheet may be fitted. When a flat sheet is used as a bottom sheet, you must **miter** the corners to hold the sheet in place (Figure 10-4).
- **Blanket.** A blanket is a heavier layer that is added to provide additional warmth.
- **Pillowcase.** A pillowcase is used to cover the pillow and protect it from becoming soiled.
- **Bedspread.** A bedspread is the finishing layer. It covers and protects the linens underneath when the bed is not being used, and provides another layer for warmth when the person is in the bed.

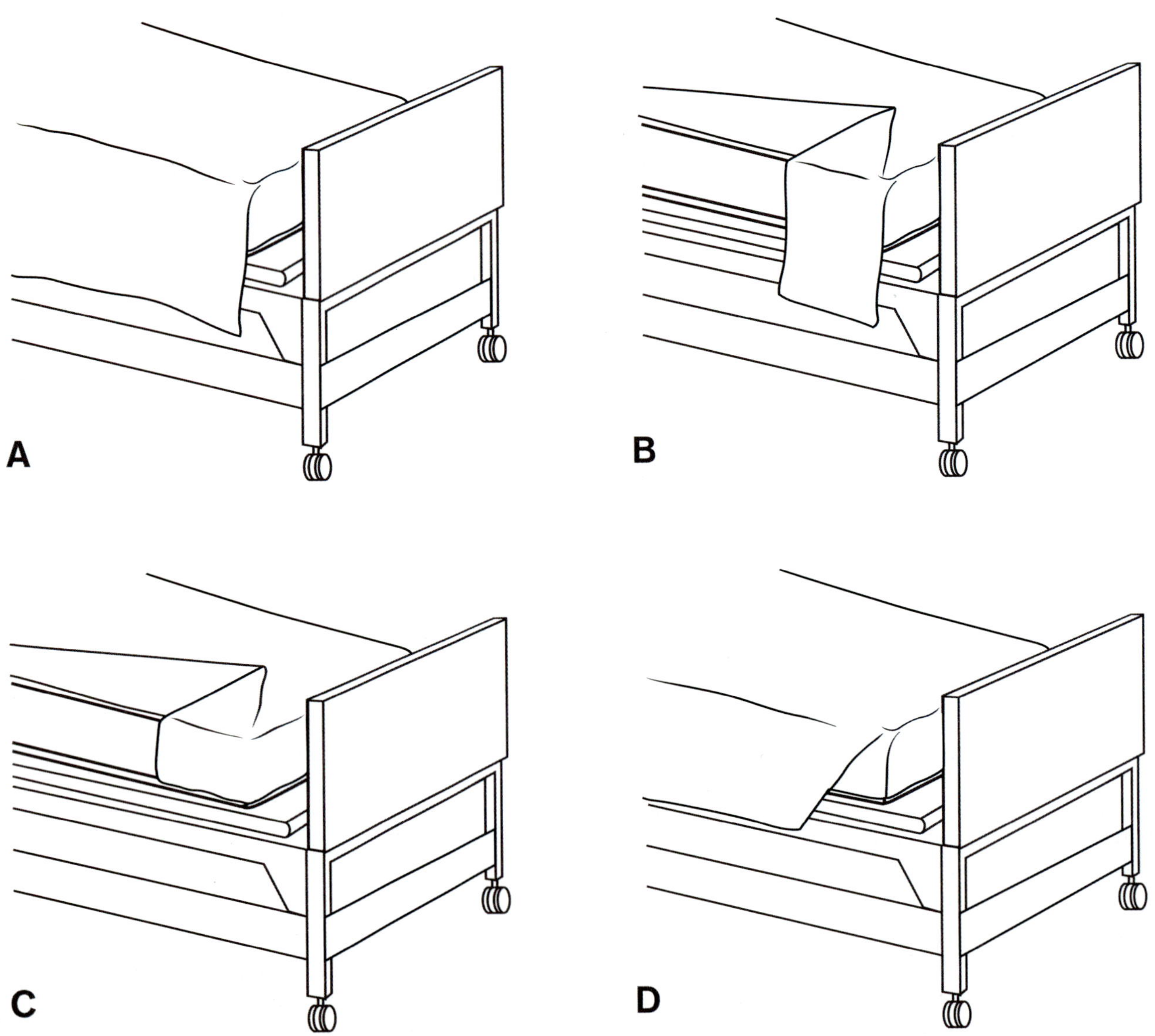

Figure 10-4 Mitering is a way of folding linens to secure them to the bed. To miter a corner: (A) Tuck the sheet under the bottom edge of the mattress. (B) Face the head of the bed with your side next to the bed. With the hand that is next to the bed, lift the edge of the sheet at the side of the bed about 12 inches from the top of the mattress, making a triangle. (C) Lay the triangle on top of the bed, holding the top of the triangle firmly. Tuck the hanging portion of the sheet under the mattress. (D) Bring the sheet back down over the mattress.

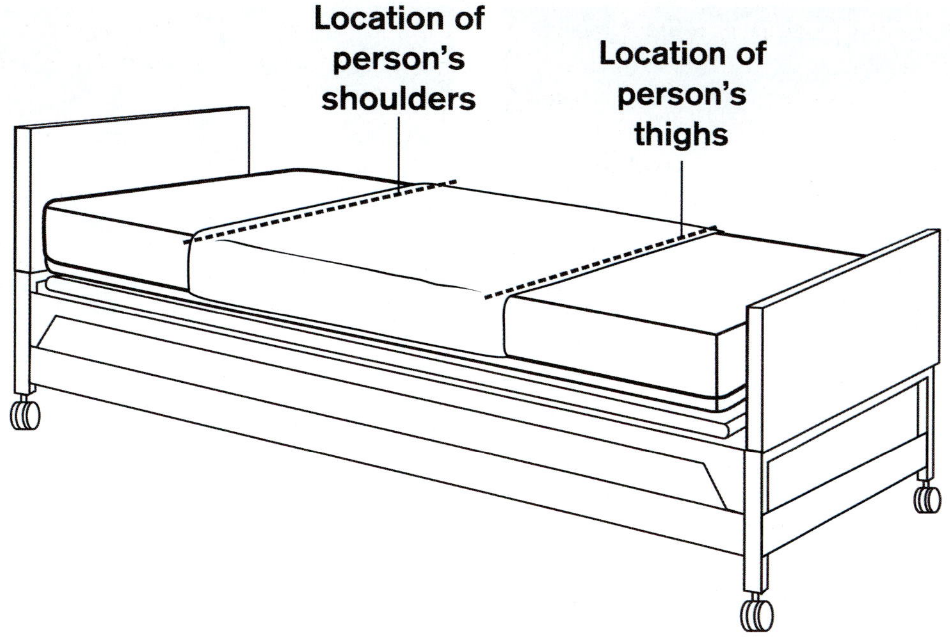

Figure 10-5 A draw sheet may be placed over the bottom sheet. Draw sheets are used when repositioning a person in bed. The draw sheet should extend from the person's shoulders to his thighs.

Other supplies

Depending on the procedure you are performing and the needs of the person, you may need additional supplies for bedmaking as well.

- **Bath blanket.** A bath blanket is a lightweight flannel sheet that is used to provide privacy and warmth when performing personal care procedures (such as a bed bath or linen change with the person still in the bed). The bath blanket is draped over the person to minimize exposure during the procedure.
- **Draw (lift) sheet.** A draw (lift) sheet is a half-sized sheet that is placed over the middle of the bottom sheet and used to assist with repositioning the person in bed. The draw sheet extends from the person's shoulders to her thighs (Figure 10-5). In a home setting, you can make a draw sheet by folding a top sheet in half widthwise.
- **Bed protector.** A bed protector is an absorbent pad that wicks moisture away from the person's body. A bed protector may be placed on top of the bottom sheet when a person is incontinent of urine, has a heavily draining wound or is perspiring heavily.
- **Foam pads.** Solid foam pads or eggcrate foam pads may be placed over the mattress for comfort. These pads can be dangerous, however, because they tend to slip. When making the bed of a person who uses a foam pad, be sure to cover the pad with a sheet and tuck the edges of the sheet in tightly to reduce slipping. Use extra caution when moving the person around in the bed or assisting the person to get out of the bed when one of these pads is in place, because of the tendency of the pad to slip. When the pad becomes soiled, it must be cleaned according to facility policy or replaced.
- **Alternating-pressure pad.** These pads, which are placed over a standard mattress, operate in much the same way as an alternating-pressure bed. An alternating-pressure pad may be used when a person is at high risk for developing pressure ulcers. If an alternating-pressure pad has been ordered for one of the people in your care, the nurse will show you how to set it up. Just as with a foam pad, there is an increased danger of slipping when an alternating-pressure pad is in place.
- **Foot board.** A foot board is a padded board that is placed against the person's feet when she is in bed to keep her feet at right angles to the legs, with the toes pointed upward (Figure 10-6, A). The foot board is used to maintain a position that will prevent "foot drop," a condition that occurs when the toes point downward for an extended period of time and the muscles become weak, making it impossible for the person to bring the foot up into a normal position for walking. Be sure the nurse shows you how to properly position the foot board if one has been ordered for a person in your care.
- **Bed cradle.** A bed cradle is a frame that keeps the top bed linens from rubbing against and putting pressure on the tops of the person's legs, feet and toes. The top linens are placed on the bed over the bed cradle (see Figure 10-6, B).

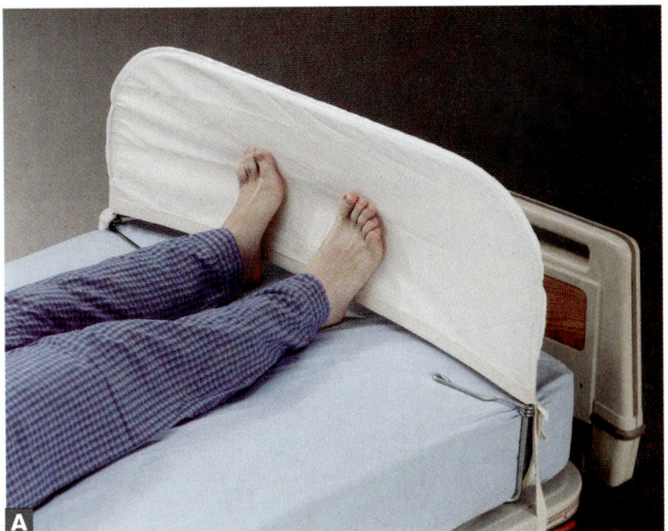

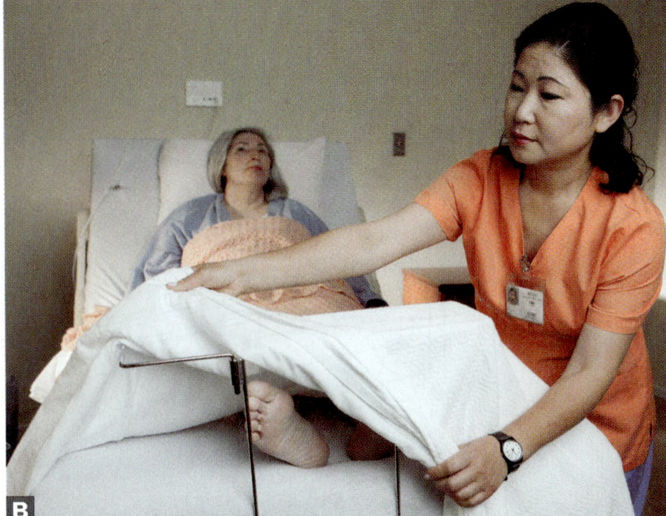

Figure 10-6 Special equipment may be used to lower the person's risk of developing pressure ulcers. (A) A foot board. *Image courtesy of Posey Company; Arcadia, California.* (B) A bed cradle.

How to Make a Bed

Although you may already be familiar with making beds in your own home, making beds in a health care setting is different from the way you perform this task at home. You will make many more beds at work than you do at home, so working efficiently and in a way that reduces strain on your back is important. You must also take infection control measures when making beds in a health care setting.

When making beds in a health care setting, you can save time and energy by:

- Gathering and stacking bed linens in the order in which you use them, so that the mattress pad is on the top.
- Folding reusable linens, such as blankets and spreads, and putting them in a clean place, such as over the back of a chair, until you are ready to put them back on the bed.
- Checking the bed for personal items, such as eyeglasses and dentures, before removing the linens from the bed.
- Making one side of the bed at a time.

In addition to saving time, working on one side of the bed at a time helps prevent you from reaching across the bed, which is important for good body mechanics. Raise the bed to a comfortable working height so that you do not have to stoop and bend. In a home setting, the bed may be low, and you may not be able to raise it. In such situations, you may have to squat or kneel, keeping your upper body erect, to make the bed.

Remember that linens can spread infection. To practice infection control when making a bed, be sure to follow these precautions:

- Take only the linens you need into the person's room. In a hospital or nursing home, once linens have been taken into a person's room, they cannot be used for another person, and they have to be laundered, even if they were not used.
- Keep clean linens on a clean surface, such as the over-bed table or a chair. Never place clean linens on the floor.
- Put soiled linens directly in the linen hamper. Never place soiled linens on the floor.
- Remove and replace linens carefully, without shaking them. Shaking linens causes air currents that may spread dust and microbes around the room.
- Keep linens (clean and soiled) away from your uniform.
- Wear gloves when removing soiled linens from the bed. After removing your gloves, wash your hands before touching the clean linens.

Another difference between making your own beds at home and making beds in a health care setting is that sometimes the person will not be able to get out of the bed while you change the linens. In this situation, you change the linens with the person still in the bed. This is called making an occupied bed. When you are making an occupied bed, never leave the person alone. Because the person will be turned on her side facing away from you as you make the first side of the bed, make sure there is something or someone for the person to hold onto on the side of the bed opposite where you are working. This will prevent you from rolling the person onto the floor by accident while you are working. If the bed has side rails, you can raise the side rail on the opposite side of the bed. If the bed does not have side rails, you will need to get a co-worker to help you, or you could place sturdy high-backed chairs along the opposite side of the bed to give the person something to hold on to.

Bedmaking is an opportunity for you to spend some time in conversation with the person in your care. In addition

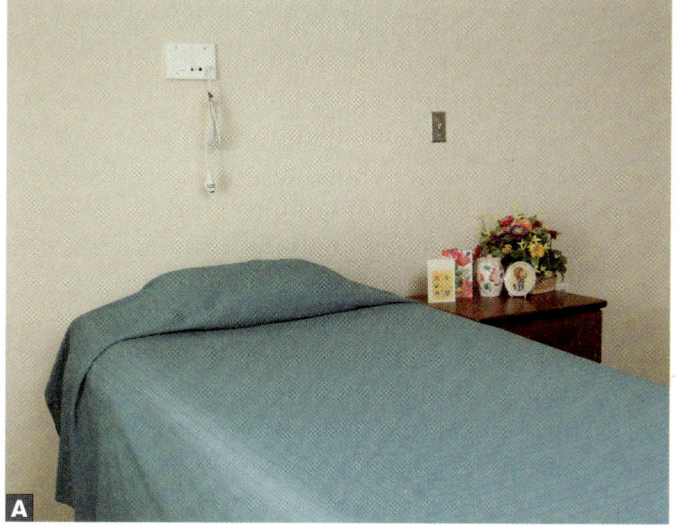

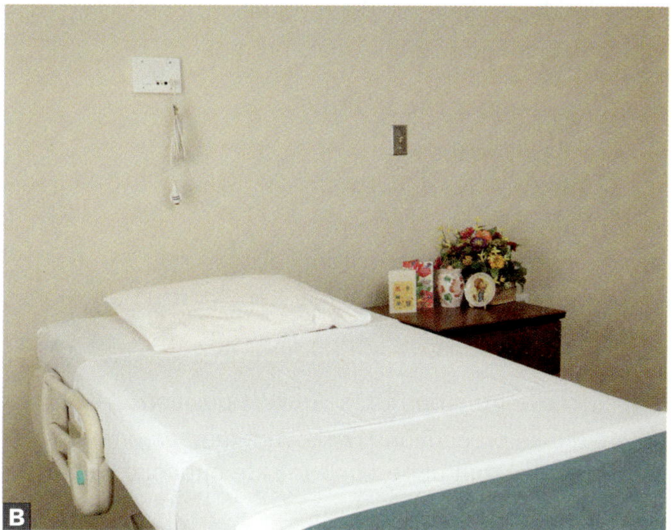

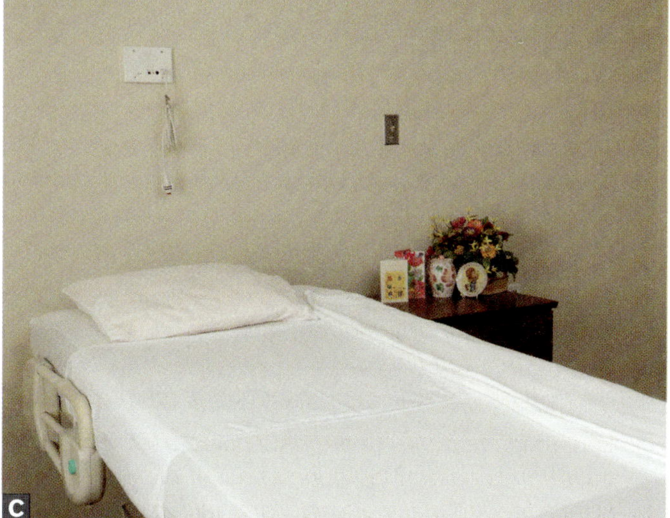

Figure 10-7 Preparing the bed. (A) A closed bed. (B) An open bed. (C) A surgical bed.

to providing a clean, comfortable bed for her, you can use this time to show her that you think she is an important and special person. Skill 10-1 describes how to make an unoccupied bed, and Skill 10-2 describes how to make an occupied bed.

You have been on vacation, and another nurse assistant was filling in for you while you were away. Today is your first day back at work, and you are changing Mrs. Ryan's bed linens. Mrs. Ryan watches you carefully take her quilt off the bed and fold it over the back of the chair, and then she says, "Can you believe that the young lady who was filling in for you put my quilt on the floor while she was making my bed? She didn't even fold it first!"

Why do you think Mrs. Ryan was upset about the way the other nurse assistant handled her quilt?

What other reasons can you think of for folding the quilt neatly and placing it over the back of a chair?

What should you do with the information Mrs. Ryan has given you about the care she received in your absence?

Preparing the Bed for the Person

After you make the bed, you need to prepare it for the person who will be using it. If the person will not be getting back into the bed right away, you may prepare a **closed bed** (Figure 10-7, A). A closed bed is simply a bed that is made, but not occupied. The bedspread is pulled up to cover the linens, protecting them from becoming soiled, and giving the bed a neat appearance. When you know a person will be getting into the bed soon (for example, in the evening before bedtime, or in preparation for a new admission), you will "open" the bed. An **open bed** is one where the bedspread, blanket and top sheet have been folded back toward the bottom of the bed, making it easier for the person to get into the bed (see Figure 10-7, B). Folding the linens back on themselves is called "fanfolding" the linens. A **surgical bed** is a special type of open bed that is prepared for a person who will be arriving on a stretcher. To prepare a surgical bed, the bedspread, blanket and top sheet are fanfolded to the side of the bed, instead of to the bottom (see Figure 10-7, C).

CHECK YOUR UNDERSTANDING

Questions for Review

1. **When making a person's bed, you should:**
   a. Make the bed when it is convenient for you, to improve your efficiency.
   b. Shake the clean linens to get the wrinkles out.

c. Check for personal items left in the bed before removing the soiled linens from the bed.
d. Place the soiled linens on the floor after removing them from the bed.

2. **When making a bed in a health care setting, you should do all of the following except:**
   a. Make one side of the bed at a time.
   b. Carry linens for all of the beds you will be changing that morning with you, so that you do not have to go back and forth to the linen cart.
   c. Wash your hands before handling clean linens.
   d. Hold linens away from your uniform.

3. **What can a nurse assistant do to minimize bad odors in a health care setting?**
   a. Open the windows.
   b. Assist people in their care with personal care, and ensure that they have clean clothes and linens at all times.
   c. Encourage people in their care to wear perfume or cologne.
   d. Nothing; bad odors are unavoidable in health care settings.

4. **When a person is receiving health care, the health care facility becomes the person's home. How do you show respect for the person's home?**
   a. By arranging the person's personal items in a way that you find pleasing
   b. By handling the person's personal items carefully
   c. By encouraging the person to store personal items so that they do not get broken or stolen
   d. All of the above

5. **A person is too ill to get out of bed for meals, so her meals are brought to her room. Which piece of equipment will you use during the meal to make it easier for the person to eat?**
   a. An over-bed table
   b. A bed cradle
   c. A bedside table
   d. A foot board

6. **One of the people in your care is incontinent of urine. When you are changing her bed linens, in addition to the standard linens used to make a bed, you might also gather:**
   a. A bed protector.
   b. An extra bedspread.
   c. A foot board.
   d. A draw sheet.

7. **What measures can you take to minimize noise in a health care setting?**
   a. Be sure to speak loudly so that you do not have to repeat yourself.
   b. Ask people to turn off televisions and radios.
   c. Use personal cell phones instead of the telephone at the nurse's station.
   d. Respond to call signals promptly.

8. **A draw sheet is used to:**
   a. Cushion the mattress.
   b. Provide privacy during personal care procedures.
   c. Protect the linens from soiling.
   d. Assist with repositioning a person in bed.

9. **When making an occupied bed:**
   a. Lower the bed to the lowest position.
   b. Take precautions to prevent the person from rolling out of bed on the side opposite where you are working.
   c. Raise the side rails on both sides of the bed.
   d. Raise the head of the bed.

Questions to Ask Yourself

1. *Mrs. McDay keeps a large, framed picture of her daughter on her bedside table. While making her bed, you need to move the picture to avoid knocking it over. What must you remember to do before leaving the room?*
2. *Mrs. Ross cannot get out of bed, and you have to change her bed linens. What will you do to keep Mrs. Ross safe while you change the linens?*
3. *You notice that one of the new nurse assistants on your unit is gathering linens for all of the beds she is assigned to make at once, and taking the linens from room to room with her. What should you do?*

Skill 10-1
Making an Unocccupied Bed

PREPARATION

1. Wash your hands.
2. Gather your supplies:
   - Pillowcase
   - Top sheet
   - Draw sheet (if needed)
   - Bottom sheet
   - Mattress pad
   - Gloves
3. Knock, greet the person and ensure privacy.
4. Explain the procedure.
5. Adjust equipment for body mechanics and safety: Raise the bed to a comfortable working height. Make sure the wheels on the bed are locked.

PROCEDURE

Task 1: Remove the Dirty Linens

6. Lower the head of the bed so that the bed is flat.
7. Put on the gloves.
8. Check the linens for items the person may have left in the bed. If items were left in the bed, move them to a safe place.
9. Moving around the bed, loosen all of the bed linens.
10. Remove the pillowcase from the pillow, and place it in the linen hamper. Place the pillow on a clean surface.
11. Remove the bedspread. If it is clean and can be reused, fold it and place it on a clean surface. Do the same with the blanket, if it can be reused.
12. Remove the rest of the linens from the bed, rolling them toward the center of the bed so that any soiled areas are contained inside (Figure 1). Place the dirty linens in the linen hamper.
13. Remove and dispose of the gloves. Wash your hands.

Task 2: Place Clean Linens on the First Side of the Bed

14. Put the clean mattress pad on the bed with the center fold in the center of the bed. Unfold the mattress pad. If you are using a fitted mattress pad, fit the elastic corners over the edges of the mattress. If you are using a flat mattress pad, make sure the top edge is even with the head of the mattress.

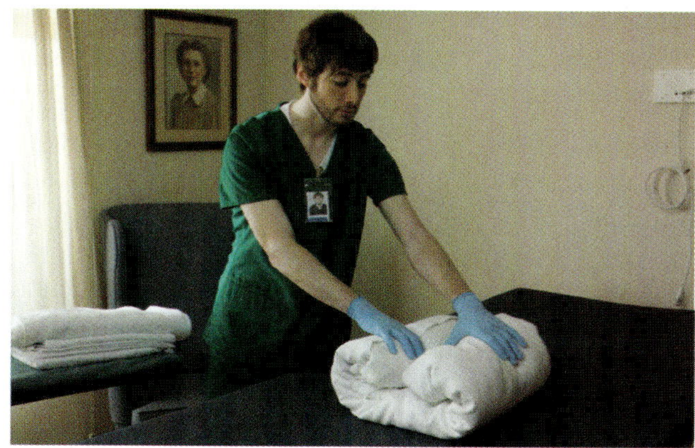

Figure 1

15. Put the clean bottom sheet on the bed. If you are using a fitted sheet, fit the elastic corners over the edges of the mattress. If you are using a flat sheet:
    a. Put the flat sheet on the bed with the center fold in the center of the bed and the bottom edge even with the foot of the mattress. Make sure the sheet is positioned so that when you unfold it, the rough side of the hem stitching at the top of the sheet will be against the mattress. Unfold the sheet.
    b. Tuck the top of the sheet underneath the mattress at the head of the bed.
    c. Miter the top corner. With your palms facing up, continue tucking in the sheet on the side, all the way to the foot of the mattress (Figure 2).

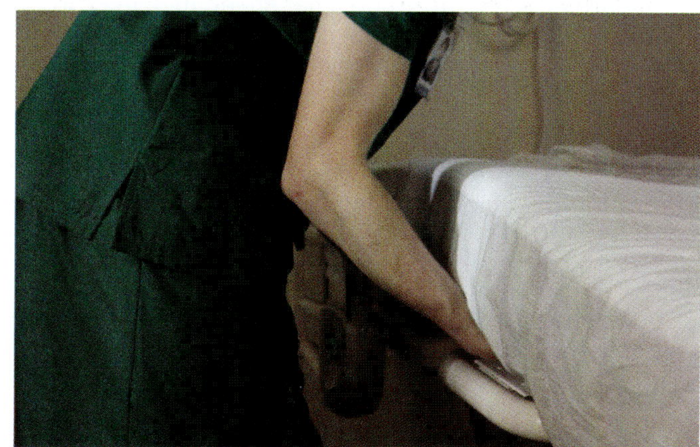

Figure 2

Continued on next page

Skill 10-1
Making an Unocccupied Bed *Continued*

16. If a draw sheet is to be made into the bed, put the draw sheet across the middle of the mattress with the center fold in the center of the bed. Unfold the draw sheet. With your palms facing up, tuck the draw sheet under the mattress, tucking in the middle third first, then the top third and then the bottom third.
17. Put the top sheet on the bed with the center fold in the center of the bed and the top edge even with the head of the mattress. Make sure that the sheet is positioned so that when you unfold it, the rough side of the hem stitching at the top of the sheet will face up. Unfold the sheet.
18. Put the blanket on the bed with the center fold in the center of the bed and the top edge about 6 inches below the head of the mattress. Unfold the blanket.
19. Put the bedspread on the bed with the center fold in the center of the bed. Unfold the bedspread.
20. Together, tuck the top sheet, blanket and bedspread under the foot of the mattress. Miter the corner at the foot of the bed to hold the top sheet, blanket and bedspread in place.

Task 3: Secure the Linens on the Second Side of the Bed

21. Move to the opposite side of the bed.
22. Secure the mattress pad. If you are using a fitted mattress pad, fit the elastic corners over the edges of the mattress. If you are using a flat mattress pad, unfold it the rest of the way and make sure it is aligned properly.
23. Secure the bottom sheet. If you are using a fitted sheet, fit the elastic corners over the edges of the mattress. If you are using a flat sheet, tuck the top of the sheet underneath the mattress at the head of the bed, miter the top corner and, with your palms facing up, tuck in the sheet on the side, all the way to the foot of the mattress.
24. Secure the draw sheet (if used), tucking in the middle third first, then the top third and then the bottom third.
25. Together, tuck the top sheet, blanket and bedspread under the foot of the mattress. Miter the corner at the foot of the bed to hold the top sheet, blanket and bedspread in place.
26. Fold the top of the bedspread down far enough to allow room to cover the pillow.
27. Fold the top sheet down 6 inches over the blanket's edge on each side of the bed to form a neat cuff.

Task 4: Change the Pillowcase and Open or Close the Bed

28. Hold the pillowcase at the center of the bottom seam.
29. Turn the pillowcase inside out, back over the hand that is holding the bottom seam.
30. With the hand that is holding the pillowcase, pick up the pillow at the center of one of the short ends and bring the pillowcase down over the pillow using your other hand (Figure 3). Fit the corners of the pillow into the corners of the pillowcase.

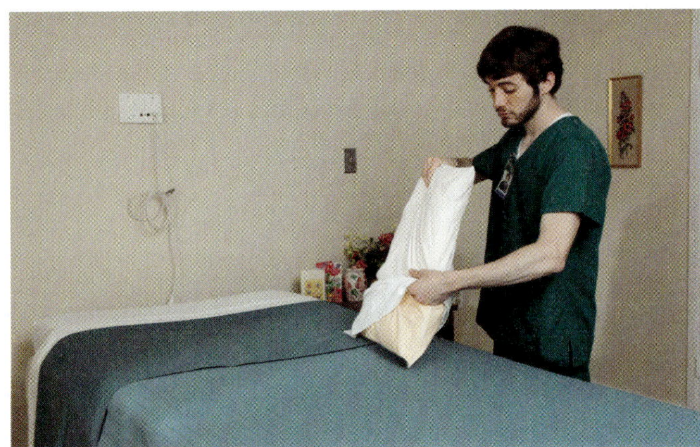

Figure 3

31. Place the pillow at the head of the bed, with the open end of the pillowcase facing away from the door.
32. If the person will be returning to bed shortly, open the bed by fanfolding the top linens to the foot of the bed. If the person will not be returning to bed soon, close the bed by folding the top of the bedspread back over the pillow.

COMPLETION

33. Ensure the person's comfort and good body alignment.
34. Adjust equipment for safety: Lower the bed to the level specified in the person's care plan. Make sure the wheels on the bed are locked. Place the person's method of calling for help within reach.
35. Clean up your work area.
36. Wash your hands.
37. Report and record.

Skill 10-2
Making an Occupied Bed

PREPARATION

1. Wash your hands.
2. Gather your supplies:
   - Pillowcase
   - Top sheet
   - Draw sheet (if used)
   - Bottom sheet
   - Mattress pad
   - Bath blanket
   - Gloves
3. Knock, greet the person and ensure privacy.
4. Explain the procedure.
5. Adjust equipment for body mechanics and safety: Raise the bed to a comfortable working height. Make sure the wheels on the bed are locked.

PROCEDURE

Task 1: Remove and Replace Linens on the First Side of the Bed

6. Lower the head of the bed so that it is as flat as the person can tolerate.
7. Put on the gloves.
8. Remove the bedspread. If it is clean and can be reused, fold it and place it on a clean surface. Do the same with the blanket, if it can be reused.
9. Loosen the top sheet at the foot of the bed. Cover the person and the top sheet with the bath blanket (to provide privacy and warmth). Ask the person to hold the edge of the bath blanket (or tuck the edges under the person's shoulders) while you remove the soiled top sheet and place it in the linen hamper (Figure 1).
10. Help the person roll toward you, onto his side. Raise the side rail and move to the opposite side of the bed (Figure 2).

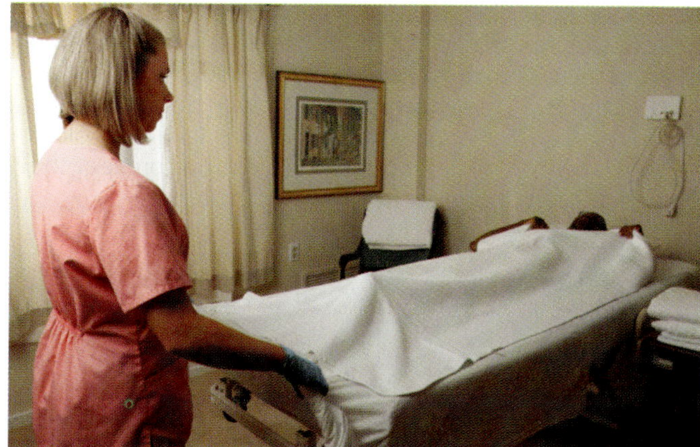

Figure 1

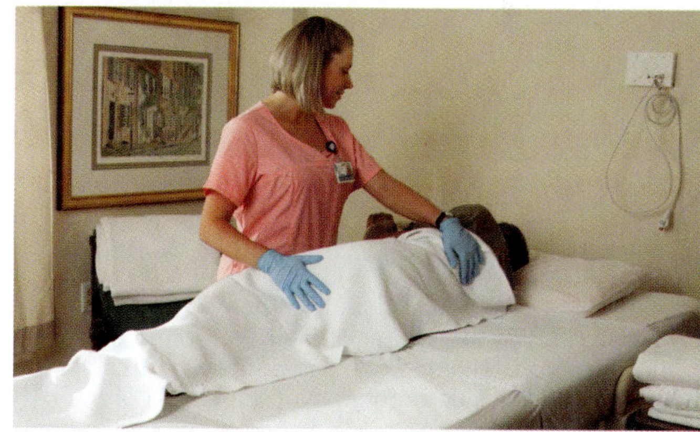

Figure 2

11. Adjust the pillow under the person's head for comfort. Ensure good body alignment and make sure the person is covered with the bath blanket.
12. Check the linens on the side where you are working for items the person may have left in the bed. If items were left in the bed, move them to a safe place.

Continued on next page

Skill 10-2
Making an Occupied Bed *Continued*

13. Loosen the dirty mattress pad, bottom sheet and draw sheet. Fanfold the dirty linens toward the person and tuck them against and slightly under his back (Figure 3). If the linens are soiled with body fluids, tuck a bed protector under the dirty linens and fold it back over them and the person's back to prevent the clean linens from becoming contaminated.

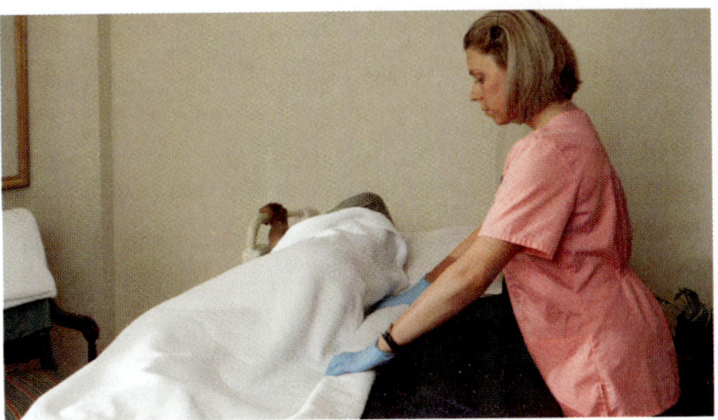

Figure 3

14. Remove and dispose of your gloves.
15. Put the clean mattress pad on the bed with the center fold in the center of the bed. Unfold the mattress pad. If you are using a fitted mattress pad, fit the elastic corners over the edges of the mattress. If you are using a flat mattress pad, make sure the top edge is even with the head of the mattress.
16. Put the clean bottom sheet on the bed. If you are using a fitted sheet, fit the elastic corners over the edges of the mattress. If you are using a flat sheet:
    a. Put the flat sheet on the bed with the center fold in the center of the bed and the bottom edge even with the foot of the mattress. Make sure the sheet is positioned so that when you unfold it, the rough side of the hem stitching at the top of the sheet will be against the mattress. Unfold the sheet.
    b. Tuck the top of the sheet underneath the mattress at the head of the bed.
    c. Miter the top corner. With your palms facing up, continue tucking in the sheet on the side, all the way to the foot of the mattress.
17. If a draw sheet is to be made into the bed, put the draw sheet across the middle of the mattress with the center fold in the center of the bed. Unfold the draw sheet. With your palms facing up, tuck the draw sheet under the mattress, tucking in the middle third first, then the top third and then the bottom third.
18. Fanfold the opposite side of the clean linens toward the person.
19. Flatten the fanfolded linens as much as possible. Help the person roll toward you, over the fanfolded linens.
20. Adjust the pillow under the person's head for comfort. Ensure good body alignment and make sure the person is covered with the bath blanket.
21. Raise the side rail and move to the opposite side of the bed.

Task 2: Remove and Replace Linens on the Second Side of the Bed

22. Lower the side rail on the side where you are working.
23. Put on a clean pair of gloves.
24. Check the linens on the side where you are working for items the person may have left in the bed. If items were left in the bed, move them to a safe place.
25. Loosen and remove the soiled linens and place them in the linen hamper.
26. Remove and dispose of your gloves.
27. Pull the clean, fanfolded mattress pad toward you until it is completely unfolded. If you are using a fitted mattress pad, fit the elastic corners over the edges of the mattress. If you are using a flat mattress pad, make sure it is aligned properly.
28. Pull the clean, fanfolded bottom sheet toward you until it is completely unfolded. If you are using a fitted sheet, fit the elastic corners over the edges of the mattress. If you are using a flat sheet, tuck the top of the sheet underneath the mattress at the head of the bed, miter the top corner, and with your palms facing up, tuck in the sheet on the side, all the way to the foot of the mattress.

29. Pull the clean, fanfolded draw sheet toward you until it is completely unfolded. With your palms facing up, tuck the draw sheet under the mattress, tucking in the middle third first, then the top third and then the bottom third (Figure 4).

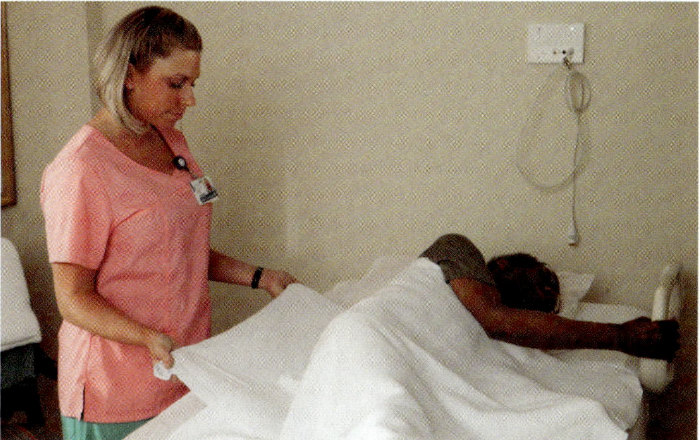

Figure 4

30. Help the person roll onto his back in the center of the bed. Adjust the pillow under the person's head for comfort. Ensure good body alignment and make sure the person is covered with the bath blanket.
31. Put the top sheet over the person with the center fold in the center of the bed and the top edge even with the head of the mattress. Make sure that the sheet is positioned so that when you unfold it, the rough side of the hem stitching at the top of the sheet will face up.
32. Have the person hold the clean top sheet in place while you remove the bath blanket from underneath. Place the bath blanket in the linen hamper.

Task 3: Change the Pillowcase

33. Remove the pillow from under the person's head.
34. Remove the pillowcase from the pillow, and place it in the linen hamper.
35. Hold the clean pillowcase at the center of the bottom seam.
36. Turn the pillowcase inside out, back over the hand that is holding the bottom seam.
37. With the hand that is holding the pillowcase, pick up the pillow at the center of one of the short ends and bring the pillowcase down over the pillow using your other hand. Fit the corners of the pillow into the corners of the pillowcase.
38. Place the pillow under the person's head, with the open end of the pillowcase facing away from the door.

Task 4: Tuck in the Top Linens and Make a Toe Pleat

39. Put the blanket on the bed with the center fold in the center of the bed and the top edge about 6 inches below the head of the mattress. Unfold the blanket.
40. Put the bedspread on the bed with the center fold in the center of the bed and the top hem even with the head of the mattress. Unfold the bedspread.
41. Together, tuck the top sheet, blanket and bedspread under the foot of the mattress. Miter the corners at the foot of the bed to hold the top sheet, blanket and bedspread in place.
42. Fold the top of the bedspread down far enough to allow room to cover the pillow.
43. Fold the top sheet down 6 inches over the blanket's edge on each side of the bed to form a neat cuff.
44. Standing at the foot of the bed, grasp both sides of the top covers about 18 inches from the foot of the bed. Pull the top covers up and toward the foot of the bed, making a 3- to 4-inch fold (called a toe pleat) across the foot of the bed (Figure 5).

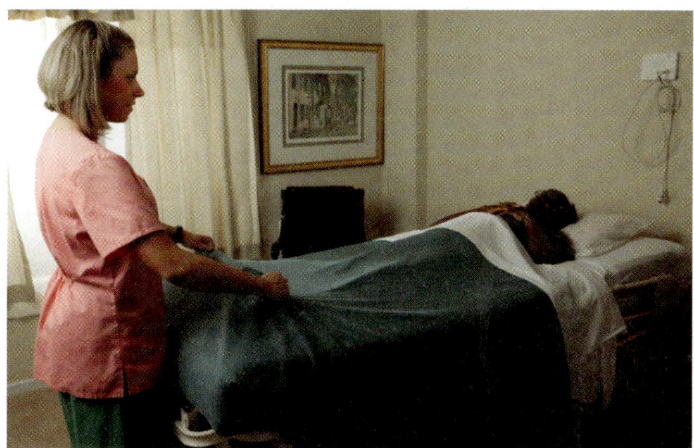

Figure 5

COMPLETION

45. Ensure the person's comfort and good body alignment.
46. Adjust equipment for safety: Lower the bed to the level specified in the person's care plan. Make sure the wheels on the bed are locked. Place the person's method of calling for help within reach. Lower or raise the side rails according to the person's care plan.
47. Clean up your work area.
48. Wash your hands.
49. Report and record.

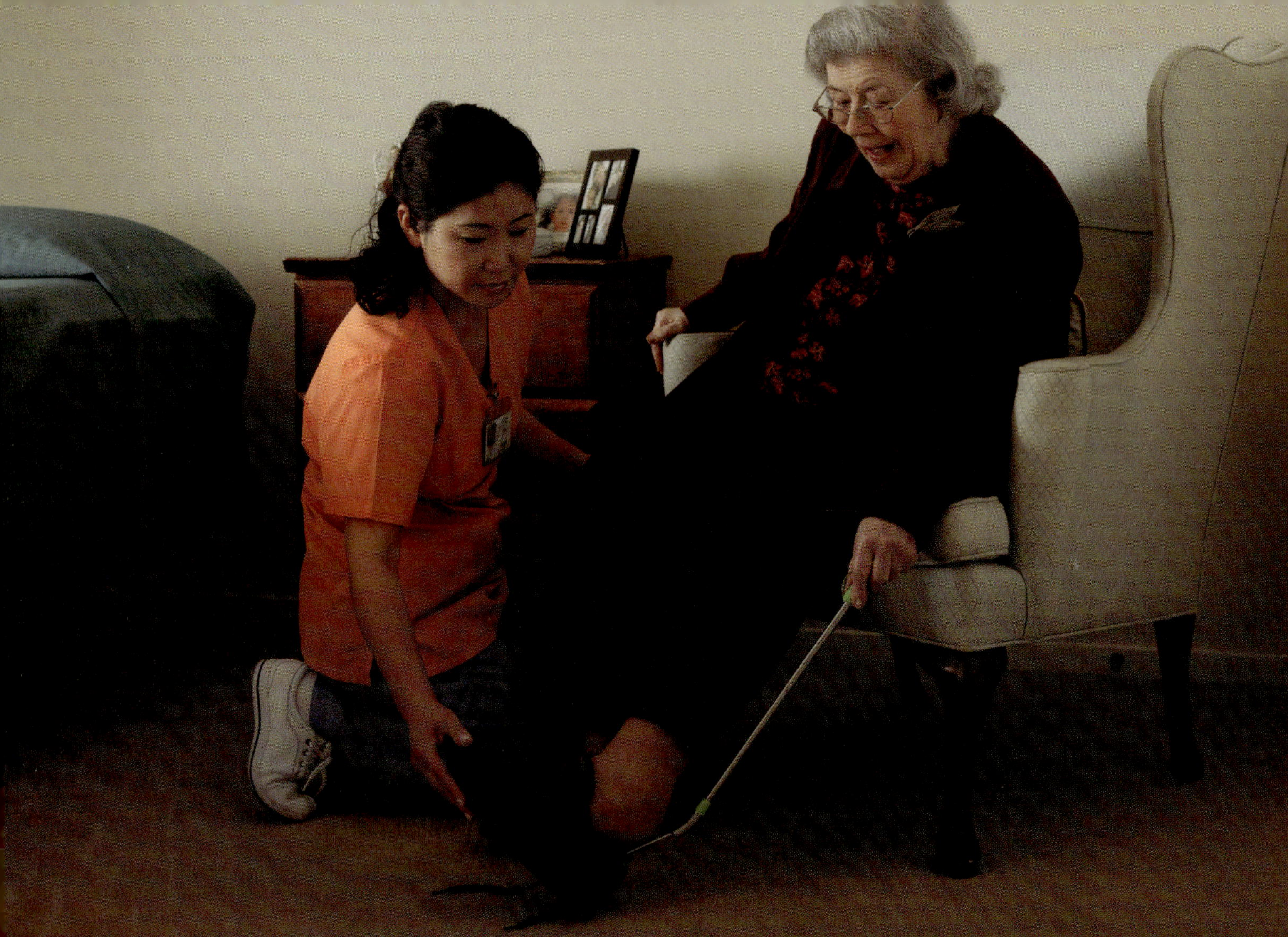

CHAPTER

11 Providing Restorative Care

Goals

After reading this chapter, you will have the information needed to:

- Explain the goals of restorative care.
- Describe the nurse assistant's role in providing restorative care.
- Promote independence and self-care.
- Help a person to be active.

After practicing the corresponding skills, you will have the information needed to:

- Help a person walk with and without a cane, crutches and a walker.
- Help a person with passive range-of-motion exercises.

Key Terms:

restorative care (rehabilitation nursing)

immobility

atrophy

contracture

ambulation

range-of-motion exercises

transfer (gait) belt

Today you arrive for your shift at Morningside Nursing Home promptly at 6:45 a.m. After clocking in and putting your personal belongings in your locker, you report to the supervising nurse to find out which residents you will be caring for today. Your first responsibility will be to help your residents with early morning care in preparation for breakfast. You decide to start with Mrs. Winnie Steele and Mrs. Dorothy Winesap, roommates in Room 120. Mrs. Steele, who is 72 years old, has chronic heart failure. Because her weak and damaged heart struggles to pump oxygen-rich blood throughout her body, Mrs. Steele becomes tired and short of breath very easily. As a result, she must stop what she is doing frequently to rest and catch her breath. However, you know that Mrs. Steele can do a great deal for herself if she is allowed to take her time and go at her own pace. Mrs. Winesap, her roommate, fell and broke her hip just after her 95th birthday. Mrs. Winesap is not allowed to stand up and bear weight on her hip for several more weeks; as a result, she requires a great deal of assistance with toileting and dressing. After greeting the roommates and helping Mrs. Steele into the bathroom so that she can use the toilet and brush her teeth, you turn your attention to helping Mrs. Winesap use a fracture pan (a special type of bedpan often used for people with broken hips). In this way, while you are helping Mrs. Winesap, you can still keep an eye on Mrs. Steele and be available to offer assistance if she needs it.

GOALS OF RESTORATIVE CARE

The people in your care require nursing care because they are ill, injured or very frail. Because of physical disability, mental disability or both, their ability to care for themselves is decreased. One of the primary goals of the nursing staff is to help people maintain the abilities they still have, and to help them regain (to the greatest extent possible) the abilities they have lost. This kind of caregiving is called **restorative care** or **rehabilitation nursing.** Restorative care helps a person become as fully functional and independent as possible, which increases the person's ability to enjoy life.

Practicing the principles of restorative care is important with all of the people in your care, no matter where you work. However, if you work in a facility that receives Medicare funding, providing restorative care is a particularly important part of your job. To meet Omnibus Budget Reconciliation Act (OBRA) requirements, the health care staff must identify each person's risk factors for functional decline (loss of abilities), and take appropriate steps to maintain the person's existing abilities and prevent any future loss of abilities from occurring. Providing restorative care is essential to achieving these goals.

THE NURSE ASSISTANT'S ROLE IN PROVIDING RESTORATIVE CARE

Restorative care is primarily carried out by the nursing staff. As a nurse assistant, you play a critical role in providing restorative care. This is a very important and essential part of your job, because you are the member of the health care team who will spend the most time with the person each day. As you carry out your daily responsibilities, you will provide restorative care by encouraging and helping the person to do as much for herself as she is able, and by providing care according to the person's care plan (Figure 11-1). Much of the physical care you provide, such as repositioning people and helping them to get out of bed and walk, is essential for helping the people in your care to maintain or regain their physical health, strength and abilities. In addition, when you encourage a person to do something for himself (instead of just doing it for him), you help to maintain the person's physical abilities as well as his sense of independence, which is important for the person's dignity and emotional health.

Some of the people in your care will need to learn new ways to do old things so that they can do as much for themselves as possible. Another important aspect of providing restorative care is encouraging and helping those in your care to practice these new skills. Often, the person will work with other members of the health care team (such as a physical therapist, occupational therapist or speech therapist) to learn these new skills, but you will be responsible for helping the person to practice the skills on an ongoing basis (Figure 11-2). For example, a physical therapist may teach a person how to walk with a walker, but you will be responsible for encouraging the person to use the walker, and making sure that she is using the walker correctly.

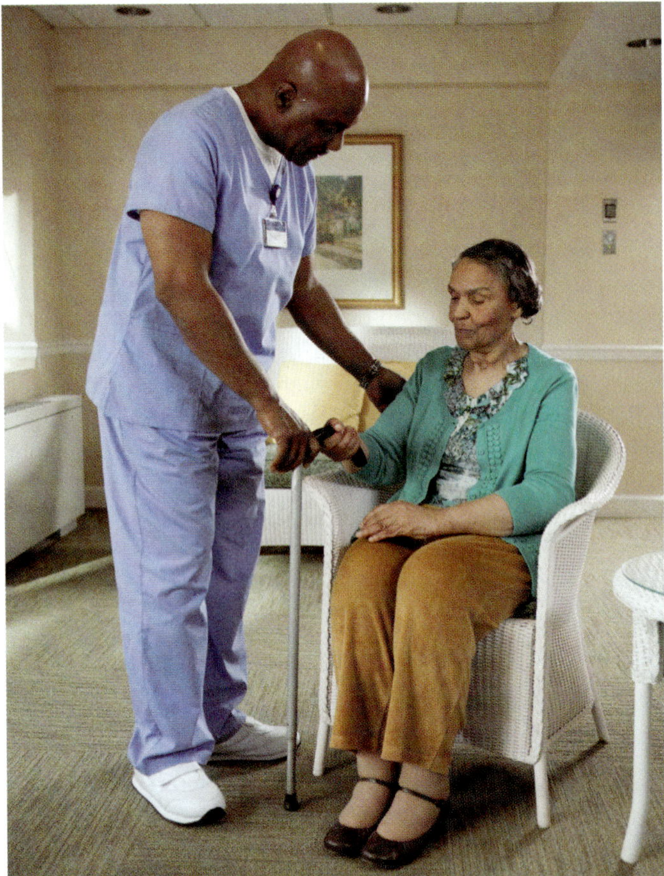

Figure 11-1 Enabling the resident by ensuring that her cane is within reach gives her the power to be more independent.

Seeing positive results from restorative care can take a long time. A key part of your job is observing and reporting even the smallest changes in a person's abilities. What you observe depends on the goals that are written in the person's care plan. You may have to watch to see how far the person walks, how much she eats or how far she can bend a joint. It is important to note changes in the person's abilities in measurable terms, such as distance, amount, or length of time. Also take note of how much effort it took for the person to complete the task. Listen to the person's comments, and observe physical signs, such as sweating, difficulty catching the breath, or the number of times the person must stop and rest before continuing. Always remember to report and record the restorative care that you provide, and your observations about the person's progress or setbacks. This information helps the other health care team members adjust the person's care plan as necessary. In facilities that receive Medicare funding, accurate documentation is also essential for ensuring that the person continues to be eligible for therapy and other services as needed, and that the facility receives proper reimbursement for the services provided.

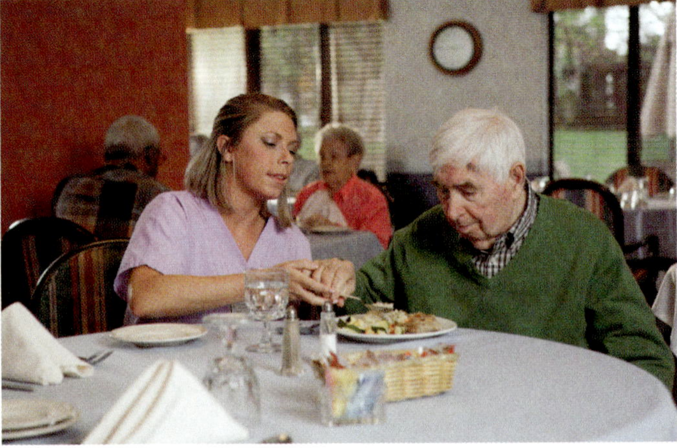

Figure 11-2 Nurse assistants help the people in their care to practice new skills that they are learning in therapy.

Guidelines for providing restorative care are given in Box 11-1.

PROMOTING INDEPENDENCE

Helping a person to keep or achieve his best level of independence is an important goal of restorative

Box 11-1 Nurse Assistant DO's and DON'Ts

Providing Restorative Care

DO follow the person's care plan.

DO recognize what the person can do for herself, and encourage her to do it.

DO emphasize the person's abilities, rather than her disabilities.

DO focus on the whole person, not just the affected part of her body. Consider the person's emotional needs as well as her physical ones.

DO help the person set realistic goals.

DON'T offer false encouragement, or compare the person to others. Each person is an individual.

DO be patient.

DON'T rush the person through tasks. Give the person enough time to complete the task independently.

DO recognize and celebrate even the smallest successes.

DO ask the therapist or nurse to show you how to best help the person practice new skills or use new assistive devices correctly.

DO report and record the restorative care you provide and your observations regarding the person's abilities, using measurable terms.

care. Remember that promoting independence is one of the five principles of care. Think about how it would make you feel to have to depend on another person to help you with routine activities, like dressing, eating or bathing. Would you feel like a burden? Would you feel ashamed that you need help doing things that other people are able to do easily on their own? Would it frustrate you to have to arrange your schedule around when someone else is available to help you? Most people, even people who are ill, injured or elderly, have an emotional need to do as much for themselves as possible, for as long as possible. The ability to act independently is important for a person's self-esteem and sense of dignity. Doing things for oneself is also important for a person's physical health. Activity strengthens and inactivity weakens.

As a nurse assistant, you will help to promote independence by allowing the people in your care to provide for their own personal care as much as they are able (Figure 11-3). By encouraging the person to do as much for himself as possible, you help increase his self-esteem and sense of purpose. Explain what you want the person to do in a way that he can understand, and review the steps if necessary. Make sure the person has the supplies he needs to complete the task. Many people use assistive devices to make it easier for them to complete certain tasks independently (Figure 11-4). If the person uses an assistive device for a certain task, make sure it is within reach. Reassure the person that you are available to help if necessary, but encourage him to do as much for himself as possible. Remember to be patient. The person will require more time to complete the task and may need to try several times before successfully completing a step. Resist the urge to complete the task for the person. It is better to allow him the opportunity to succeed and feel the sense of accomplishment that comes with success. Of course, if the person is becoming very frustrated or seems overly exhausted, it is appropriate to step in and help him to complete the task. Always notice and comment on small successes. If you say, "Mr. Lightfoot, you were able to eat everything on your tray but dessert today, and last week you could only get halfway through your meal before getting tired!" he will probably want to try to eat the entire meal without any help by next week. Sharing your observations about the progress he has made encourages him to keep trying to improve.

Many of the people in your care will be receiving therapy to learn new skills to help increase their independence. For example, the occupational therapist may teach the person how to use an assistive device for eating, or the physical therapist may teach the person how to use an assistive device for walking. You continue that teaching by encouraging the person to use her new skills, and by making sure that she is performing the skills correctly. Prompting is a communication technique that can be used to remind a person what to do without actually telling her. If a person hesitates to do something that you know she can do, it is better to prompt her than to do it for her. For example, suppose a person is about to stand up by herself and use her walker. The walker should be in front of her when she stands up, but it is to the left of where she is going to stand. By asking the person if her walker is where she wants it, you remind her that it is not in the right place and give her the chance to move the walker into the correct position before proceeding. If the person seems to get stuck while completing the task and gives you a questioning look, do not assume that the person does not know what to do. She may just be worried about doing the task incorrectly in front of you. Help by asking, "What do you think you should do next?" The person may tell you and then go on with the task. If necessary, tell her what step should come next, but encourage her to complete the task independently.

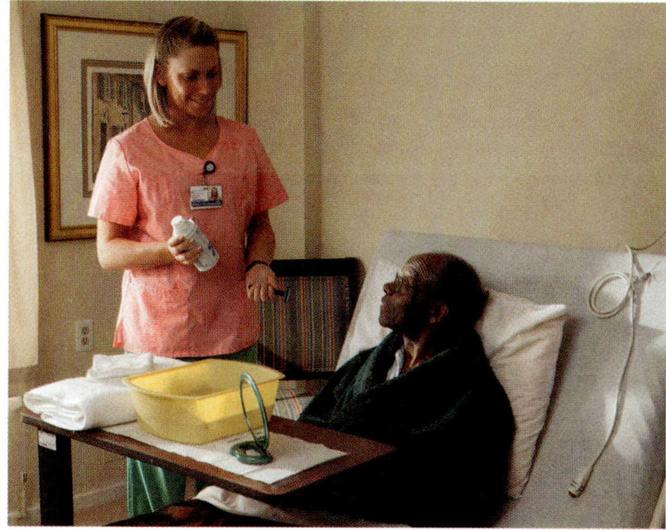

Figure 11-3 An important part of providing restorative care is helping the person to be as independent as possible. This man can shave himself if someone brings him the necessary supplies.

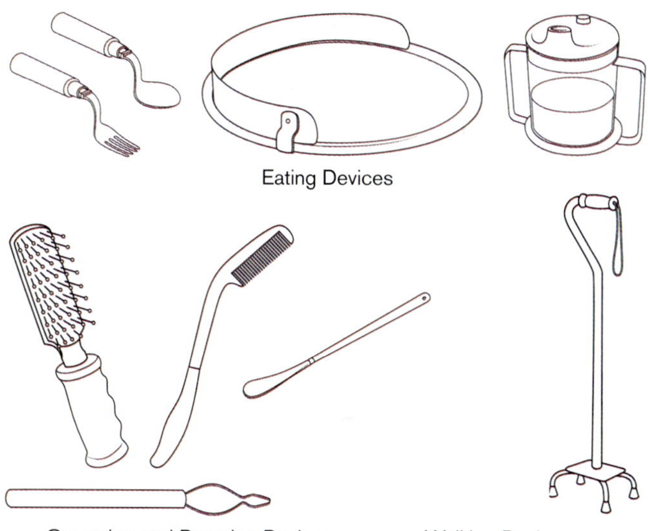

Figure 11-4 Assistive devices can help people remain independent.

Although Mrs. Steele tires very easily, she likes to choose her own clothes and dress herself as much as possible. Today, Mrs. Steele has selected a pair of slacks, a sweater set and a necklace. She has put on her slacks and the short-sleeved sweater, but she is having trouble with the cardigan. She is sitting on the edge of the bed and is clearly very tired. It has taken a lot of energy for her to use the toilet, brush her teeth, choose her outfit and begin dressing. You are almost finished helping Mrs. Winesap when Mrs. Steele says, "Honey, would you be a sweetheart and just help me with these sleeves?" You are almost finished in Room 120 and would like to finish helping your other four assigned residents get ready for breakfast. You know that the easiest and quickest thing to do would be just to finish dressing Mrs. Steele in her cardigan, but instead, you say, "Of course! Here, let me help you." You hold up the cardigan for her and ask her to put one arm in. Before continuing with the other arm, Mrs. Steele needs to stop and rest, but after about a minute she is able to put her other arm in the sleeve. Then you fasten her necklace for her and help her to apply lipstick. You say, "Mrs. Steele, I'm so proud of how much you were able to accomplish on your own today! I hardly had to help you at all!" Mrs. Steele looks up at you and smiles weakly. She says, "I've done things for myself my whole life. I don't want to stop now."

Nurse assistants are taught to always put the client first. By allowing Mrs. Steele to complete most of her personal care by herself while you helped Mrs. Winesap, did you neglect your responsibilities toward Mrs. Steele? Why or why not?

You decided to help Mrs. Steele finish putting on her cardigan herself, instead of just putting the cardigan on her. Was the extra time it took to help Mrs. Steele put on the cardigan herself worth it? Why or why not?

Mrs. Steele's condition, heart failure, is terminal (that is, it cannot be cured, and eventually, it will probably cause her death). Do you think it is important to provide restorative care for a person who has a terminal condition? Why or why not?

PROMOTING MOBILITY

Another major goal of restorative care is helping the person to maintain or achieve her best level of mobility. If we cannot move, it becomes much more difficult to do things for ourselves and to remain independent. In addition, the ability to move is important for our physical and emotional health.

Have you ever heard the expression "Use it or lose it"? This condition really can happen. **Immobility**, or the state of not moving, can cause many physical and emotional problems (Figure 11-5). For example:

Continued on page 146

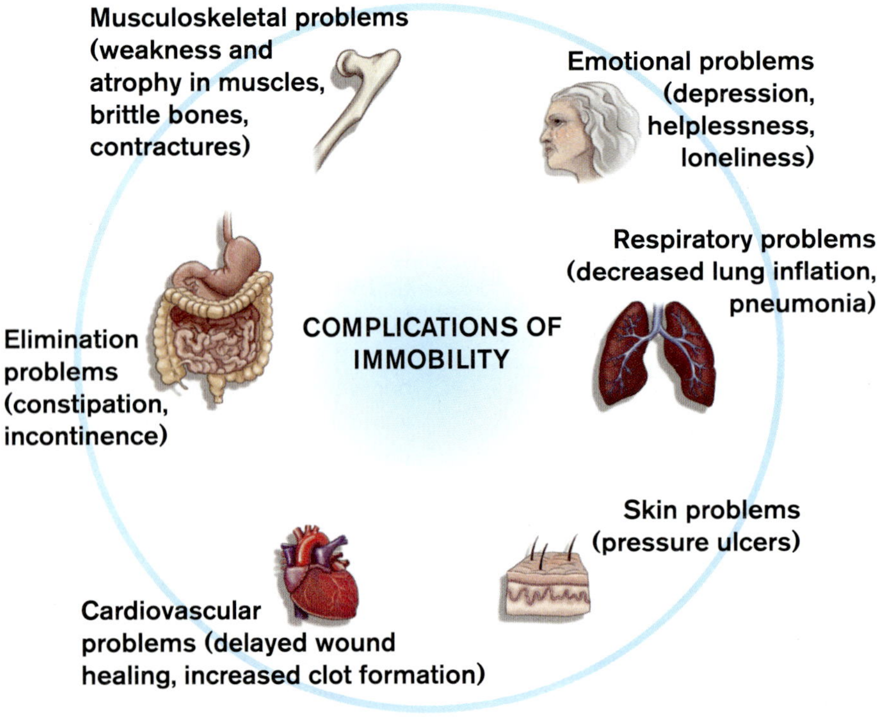

Figure 11-5 Immobility can cause physical and emotional problems.

Table 11-1 **Assistive Devices for Walking**

Assistive Device	Used By	Ensuring Proper Fit	Guidelines for Proper Use
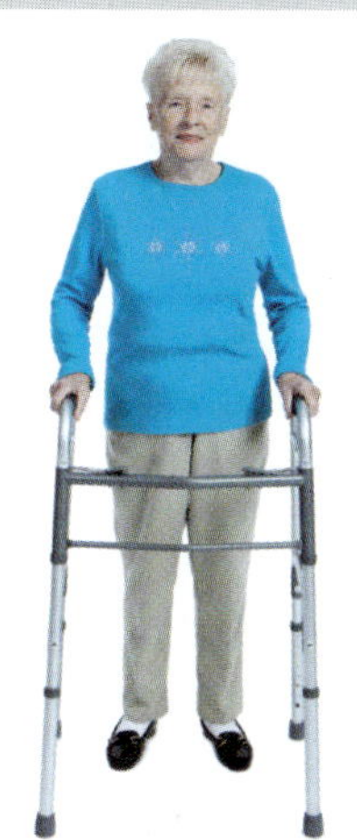 Walker	A person who can bear weight but needs support on both sides	The top of the walker frame should be even with the person's hip bones.	■ Make sure the walker is directly in front of the person. ■ Make sure the person places his hands on the walker's handgrips, stands erect and slightly flexes his elbows. ○ **Pick-up walker:** Have the person lift the walker and put it down about 6 inches forward and then step or hop into it. ○ **Four-wheeled or semi-wheeled walker:** Have the person roll the walker forward about 6 inches and then step into it. ■ Encourage the person to walk normally, looking ahead, while using the walker.
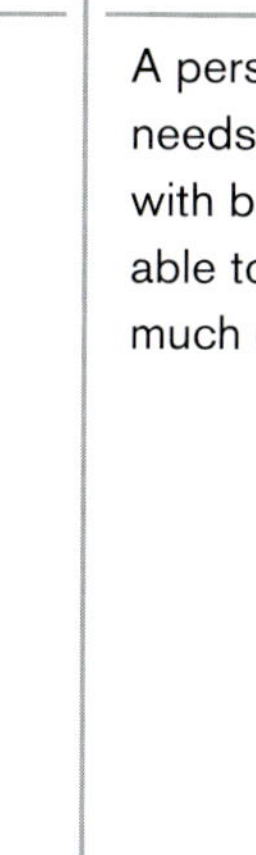 Cane	A person who needs assistance with balance but is able to walk without much difficulty	The top of the cane should be even with the person's hip bone.	■ Make sure the person holds the cane handle with the hand opposite the weak leg and stands erect, with his elbow slightly flexed. ■ Position yourself on the person's weaker side. ■ Have the person move the cane forward about 6 to 11 inches. Make sure the tip of the cane is firmly on the floor. ■ Have the person use the cane for support while standing on the stronger side and moving the weaker leg forward until it is even with the cane. Next, the person moves the stronger leg forward, ahead of the cane and the weaker leg. ■ Encourage the person to look ahead while using the cane.
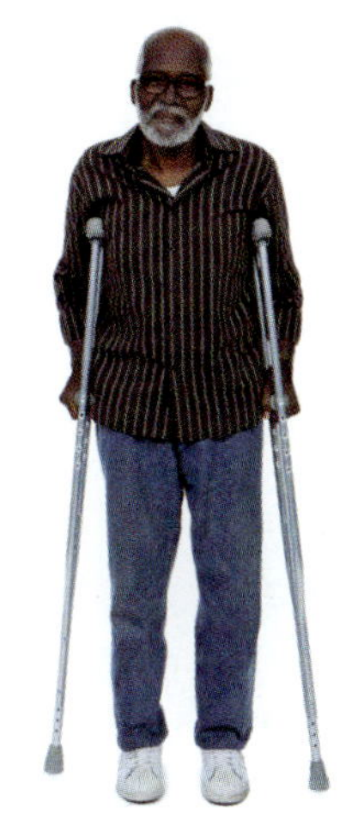 Crutches	A person who cannot use one leg or when both legs are weak and need support	The top of the crutches should rest against the person's sides (not in the person's armpits).	■ Make sure the person stands erect, supporting his weight on the handgrips and gripping the crutches between the chest and the inside of the upper arms. ■ Have the person move both crutches forward along with the weaker leg, and then bring the strong leg up to meet the crutches. ■ Encourage the person to look ahead while using the crutches.

- **Musculoskeletal problems**. Bones lose calcium and become brittle. Muscle mass decreases (a condition called **atrophy**), and strength is lost. Holding a joint in the same position for too long can cause the tendons to shorten and become stiff, resulting in loss of motion in the joint. This is called a **contracture**. Bend your wrist so that your palm moves toward the inside of your arm. This position is similar to that of a contracture that affects the wrist. Imagine what it would be like to try to eat, dress and go to the bathroom with your hand bent in this position.
- **Respiratory problems.** Lying down for long periods of time decreases the person's ability to fully inflate the lungs with each breath, which allows secretions to pool in the lungs and puts the person at risk for pneumonia.
- **Cardiovascular problems.** Inactivity slows circulation. As a result, healing is delayed and dangerous blood clots can form.
- **Skin problems.** Pressure ulcers can develop. Pressure ulcers are painful, difficult-to-heal sores that can be fatal. You will learn more about pressure ulcers in Chapter 12.
- **Elimination problems.** A lack of activity causes food to move more slowly through the intestines, putting the person at risk for constipation. Immobility can also lead to incontinence (an inability to control the release of urine or feces).
- **Emotional problems.** Depression and feelings of helplessness, anger and loneliness can occur.

As a nurse assistant, you help a person stay active and mobile with **ambulation** (walking) and **range-of-motion exercises** (exercises that help to keep joints functional by moving them in a systematic way).

Helping a Person to Walk

Encouraging the people in your care who can walk to do so several times a day has many important health benefits, even if the person only goes a short distance at a time. Some people will only need your assistance to remain safe and steady on their feet while they are walking. Others will use an assistive device, such as a cane, a walker or crutches, to walk (Table 11-1). For many people, the use of an assistive device allows the person to walk independently.

Dizziness is common when a person sits up after being in bed for awhile. Before assisting a person to walk, allow her to sit on the edge of the bed for several minutes before standing up. If the dizziness does not pass after several minutes, help the person to lie back down and report the dizziness to the nurse. The person may also become dizzy after she has been walking for awhile. If this occurs, or if the person becomes sweaty, short of breath or complains of pain, help her to sit down and rest. Some people may begin to fall quite suddenly while they are walking, especially if they are weak, ill or unsteady on their feet. Do not try to stop a fall; doing so may injure you and the person. Instead, use the technique shown in Box 11-2 to minimize injury to the person and to yourself if the person begins to fall while you are assisting her with walking.

A **transfer (gait) belt** is a wide, webbed belt that is placed around the person's waist when you are assisting the person to walk. The transfer belt allows you to support the person by giving you a safe place to put your hands (Figure 11-6). Many employers will require you to use a transfer belt when helping a person to stand, walk or transfer (for example, from the bed to a chair), unless the person has a medical condition that makes using a transfer belt unsafe. A transfer belt should not be used for people with certain medical conditions, including recent abdominal, chest or back surgery; severe respiratory problems; or severe cardiac problems. When putting a transfer belt on a person, make sure that it is snug without being too tight. You should be able to slip two fingers between the person's body and the belt.

Guidelines for helping a person to walk safely are given in Box 11-3. Skill 11-1 describes step by step how to help a person to walk.

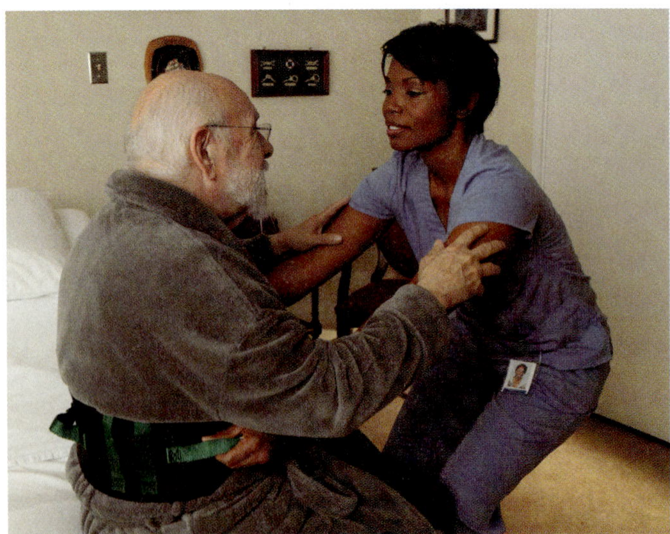

Figure 11-6 A transfer belt gives you a safe place to grasp when helping a person to stand up and move from one place to another.

Box 11-2 **Minimizing Injury When a Person Starts to Fall While Walking**

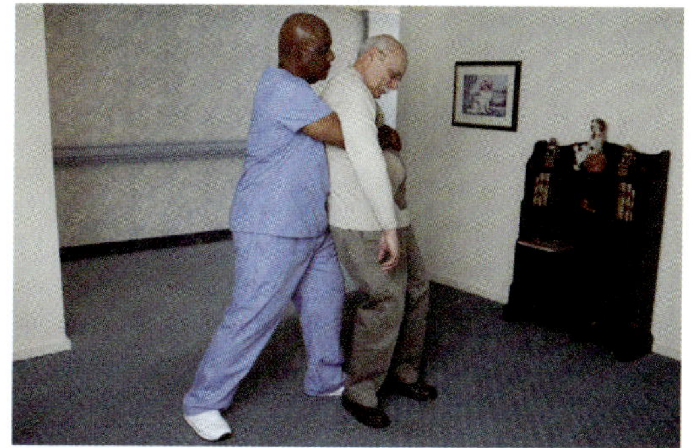

Put your arms around the person's waist or under his arms, and hug the person's torso close to your body.

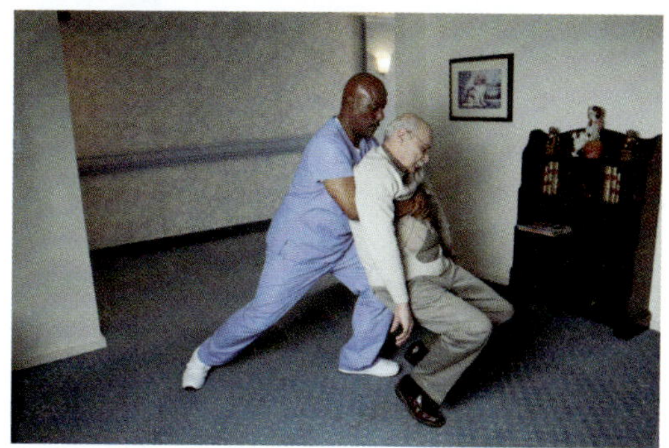

Bend your knees and lower the person slowly to the floor by sliding him down your leg.

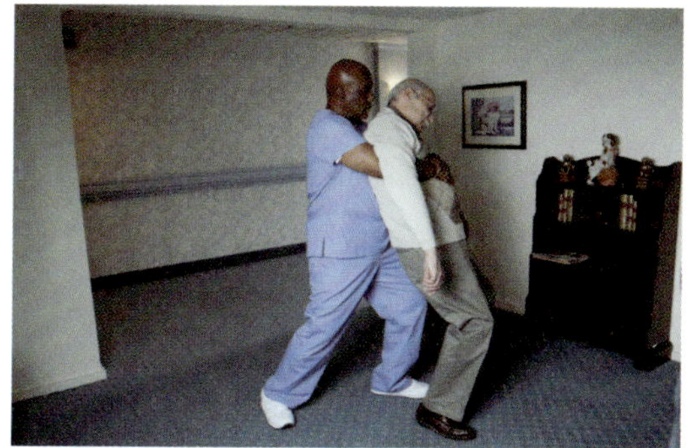

Place one foot behind the other to widen your base of support.

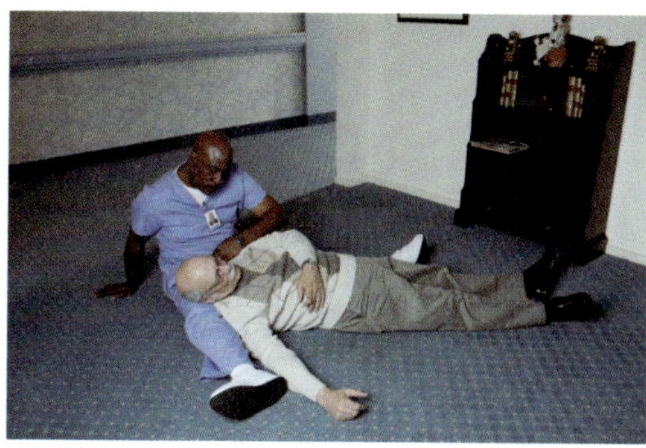

Lower yourself to the floor and sit beside the person. Call for help. While waiting for help to arrive, stay with the person. Provide reassurance and make the person comfortable.

Box 11-3 Nurse Assistant DO's and DON'Ts

Helping a Person to Walk

DO make sure the person is wearing footwear. The person's shoes or slippers should fit well and have nonskid soles.

DO use a transfer belt, unless the person has a condition that makes the use of a transfer belt dangerous (for example, recent abdominal, chest or back surgery; severe respiratory problems; or severe cardiac problems).

DON'T hold onto the person's arm. Instead, grasp the transfer belt.

DO allow the person to sit on the edge of the bed for several minutes before standing up to walk, if the person has been lying down in bed.

DO handle medical equipment, such as an IV bag and tubing or a urinary catheter drainage bag and tubing, appropriately so that treatment is not disrupted and the person is not harmed as you help her walk. An IV bag should always be higher than the IV entry site. A urinary catheter drainage bag and tubing should always be lower than the bladder. Make sure tubing is properly secured so that it does not become a tripping hazard.

DO make sure you know the proper way to use the person's assistive device for walking, if the person uses one. Watch the person's technique and correct any errors.

DO make sure the assistive device is in good working order. Rubber tips on canes, crutches or walkers that are missing, worn or cracked should be replaced. Frames on walkers should be secure.

DO watch the person carefully for signs of fatigue, dizziness or pain.

DO gradually increase the distance the person walks to help build confidence.

Table 11-2 **Common Medical Terms Used To Describe Movement**

Term	Defintion
Flexion	Bending
Extension	Straightening
Abduction	Moving away from the body
Adduction	Moving toward the body
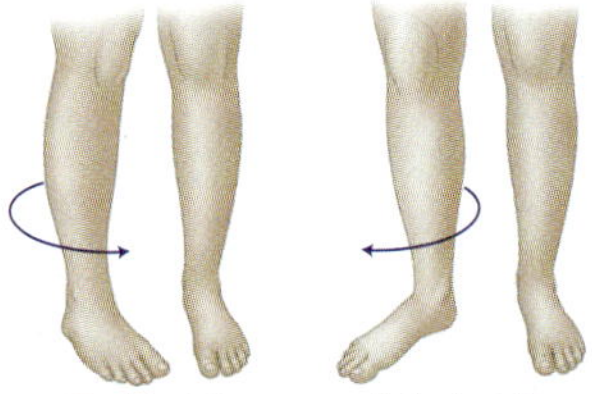 Rotation	Moving in a circular motion along a fixed point or axis
Pronation	Turning the palm downward
Supination	Turning the palm upward
Radial Deviation	Bending the wrist toward the thumb (the side where the radius bone is located)
Ulnar Deviation	Bending the wrist toward the little finger (the side where the ulna bone is located)
Dorsiflexion	Bending the ankle so that the toes point up
Plantar Flexion	Bending the ankle so that the toes point down
Inversion	Turning the ankle inward
Eversion	Turning the ankle outward

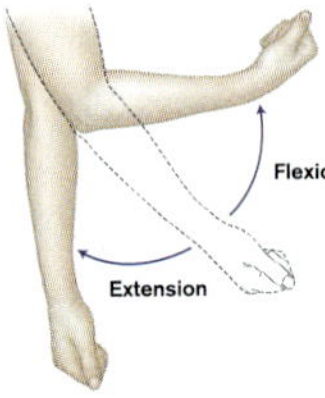

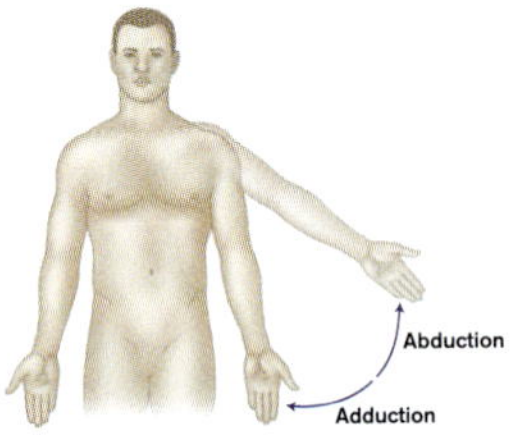

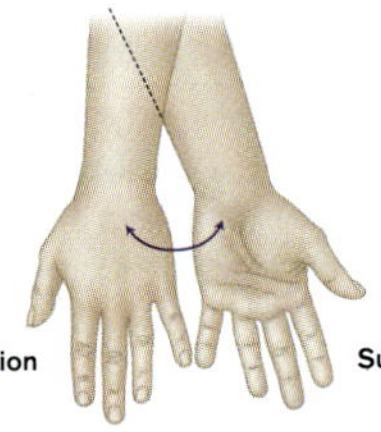

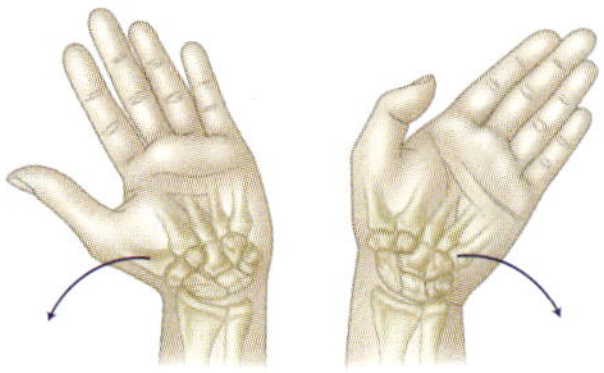

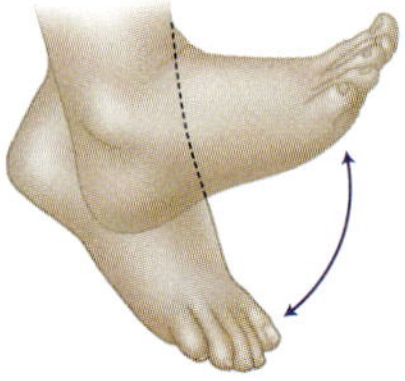

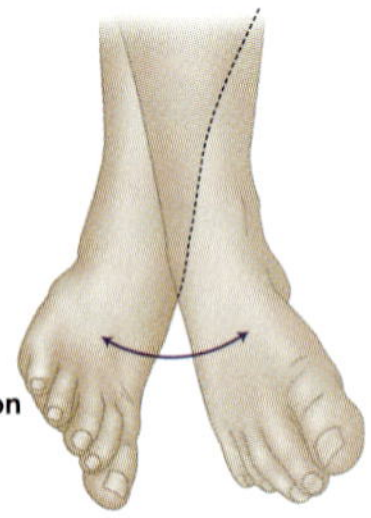

Box 11-4 Nurse Assistant DO's and DON'Ts

Assisting with Range-of-Motion Exercises

DO follow the person's care plan, and exercise only the joints specified on the care plan.

DO work in a systematic manner.

DO use good body mechanics.

DO move each joint slowly, gently and smoothly.

DO support the joint during the movement.

DON'T move the joint further than the person can tolerate.

DO pay attention to verbal and nonverbal expressions of pain. If the person has pain, stop the movement and report your observations to the nurse.

While you are helping Mrs. Winesap with her early morning care, she says to you, "I am so tired of lying in this bed all day! I can't wait until I'm able to be up and on my feet again!" You know that Mrs. Winesap is not allowed to bear weight on her healing hip right now, but later on in her recovery she will begin to walk again using an assistive device.

Once Mrs. Winesap's doctor has approved a change to weight-bearing status, which assistive device for walking would you expect the physical therapist to recommend for Mrs. Winesap?

When Mrs. Winesap has progressed enough in therapy to walk without the physical therapist present, what will you look for when you are helping her to use the assistive device to ensure that she is safe and using the device properly?

Helping a Person with Range-of-Motion Exercises

To remain functional, joints must be used and put through their normal range of motion. Normally, the activities we do every day are enough to keep our joints healthy and functioning well. However, when a person has an injury or condition that prevents normal activity, range-of-motion exercises may be used to keep the joints flexible and mobile. Range-of-motion exercises put the joint through its maximal extent of movement (that is, the joint's range of motion) and are important for preventing contractures from developing. Common medical terms used to describe movement are defined in Table 11-2.

Range-of-motion exercises may be *active* (done independently by the person), *active-assisted* (done by the person with help from a caregiver), or *passive* (done by a caregiver for the person). When you are helping a person with range-of-motion exercises, you should only move the joint as far as is comfortable for the person. Be aware that range of motion differs from person to person. It may even differ within the same person, depending on the time of day. For example, a person who has arthritis may not have much range of motion in the early morning because of joint pain. But in the late morning, after her bath and after she has taken her pain medication, she may have more range of motion.

Range-of-motion exercises may be ordered for one joint, several joints or all joints. Always check the person's care plan. When assisting a person with range-of-motion exercises, work in a systematic manner, beginning at the top of the person's body and working your way down. Do all of the exercises on one side of the body, and then repeat them on the other side. Box 11-4 contains general guidelines for assisting a person with range-of-motion exercises, and Skill 11-2 provides step-by-step instructions for assisting with passive range-of-motion exercises.

CHECK YOUR UNDERSTANDING

Questions for Review

1. **The nursing staff provides what kind of care to help people maintain or achieve their best possible level of functioning?**
   a. Physical therapy
   b. Occupational therapy
   c. Restorative care
   d. Personal care

2. **A stroke has made it difficult, but not impossible, for Mrs. Klein to feed herself. To best assist Mrs. Klein, you would:**
   a. Feed Mrs. Klein yourself so that her food does not get cold.
   b. Place Mrs. Klein's meal tray on her over-bed table, and then leave the room.
   c. Let Mrs. Klein feed herself for 5 minutes, and then finish feeding her the rest of the meal.
   d. Encourage Mrs. Klein to use the assistive device the occupational therapist gave to her for eating.

3. **Inactivity can cause:**
   a. Atrophied muscles.
   b. Blindness.
   c. Arthritis.
   d. All of the above.

4. **Mrs. Clymer has arthritis and needs to do range-of-motion exercises. When you go to her room to help her, she says that she cannot do them today because she hurts too much. The best way to respond is to say:**
   a. "You need to do them because the doctor ordered them. Let's just do them and get them over with."
   b. "If we do them quickly, we'll finish up faster."
   c. "Okay, we'll do them tomorrow."
   d. "It's so important for you to do these exercises to keep your joints flexible. Let's try to do them very slowly, and you can let me know when you need to rest or stop."

5. **You are helping Mr. Grey to walk to the bathroom when he suddenly starts to fall. What should you do?**
   a. Grab Mr. Grey's arm to keep him from falling.
   b. Assist Mr. Grey to sit in a chair or on the floor.
   c. Hug Mr. Grey's body close to yours and use good body mechanics to lower him gently to the floor.
   d. Call for the nurse so that she can check Mr. Grey for injuries.

6. **Mrs. Ward has emphysema, a lung disease that makes it difficult for her to breathe. As a result, she becomes winded and tired very easily. To make it easier for her to walk and to help her maintain her current level of independence, the physical therapist has recommended that she use an assistive device for walking. Which type of assistive device would be most appropriate for Mrs. Ward?**
   a. Crutches
   b. A cane
   c. A transfer belt
   d. A wheeled walker

7. **As part of providing restorative care, nurse assistants are responsible for which of the following?**
   a. Helping the person practice what he or she has been taught in therapy
   b. Providing support and encouragement
   c. Reporting and recording the restorative care that was provided and what the person was able to achieve, using measurable terms
   d. All of the above

8. **Which of the following people is a candidate for receiving restorative care?**
   a. Mrs. O'Leary, who is 98 years old and blind
   b. Mr. Dunlap, who has had several toes amputated (surgically removed) due to complications of diabetes
   c. Mrs. Singer, who has multiple sclerosis, a progressive neurologic disease with no cure
   d. All of the above

9. **Mrs. Garcia, who is recovering from a broken hip, is upset because she couldn't reach the end of the hallway today. "Yesterday I walked twice as far with this stupid thing!" she says, and angrily pushes her walker away. What can you say to help her feel better?**
   a. "I'm sure you'll be back on your feet and have no need for the walker soon!"
   b. "I know you can do it! Why, just last week Mrs. Reynolds made it all the way down the hall and back."
   c. "Yes, you made it all the way to the end of the hall yesterday, and you made it almost that far today. You're doing great! Healing from a broken hip takes a long time, and I'm really pleased with how much you've been able to do already."
   d. "I'll talk to the physical therapist. Maybe he can help you with the walker."

Questions to Ask Yourself

1. *Mr. Rivera had a stroke, which resulted in left-side paralysis. What suggestions do you have for Mr. Rivera to help him increase his activity?*
2. *Mr. Roberts, one of your home care clients, has severe Parkinson's disease. Because his hands shake so much, he struggles to eat. You are responsible for making sure Mr. Roberts eats lunch. You know that with time and encouragement, he*

can eat independently using adaptive devices for eating. One day, Mr. Roberts' wife says to you, "You are so patient! I just don't have that kind of patience. For me, it's just easier to feed him his dinner every night." How would you respond?

3. *Ms. Jones is unsteady on her feet and very afraid of falling. She wants you to take her to the bathroom in her wheelchair. What do you think would be the best thing for you to do?*
4. *How can you help maintain independence for a person who needs to use a walker?*
5. *How can you help maintain good body mechanics for someone who uses a cane to walk?*
6. *Name some of the body parts that are exercised when you help someone with passive range-of-motion exercises. Why are these exercises important for providing restorative care?*
7. *Ever since he developed severe arthritis in his hands, Mr. Hudson has lost weight. "I'm just not as hungry as I used to be," he tells you at lunch. One day you overhear Mr. Hudson telling his roommate that he doesn't want to be a burden to anyone. What can you do to make sure Mr. Hudson receives adequate nutrition and maintains his independence?*

Skill 11-1
Helping a Person to Walk

PREPARATION

1. Wash your hands.
2. Gather your supplies:
   - Transfer belt, if you are using one
   - The person's walker, cane or crutches (if the person uses an assistive device)
   - The person's robe, and slippers or shoes
3. Knock, greet the person and ensure privacy.
4. Explain the procedure.
5. Adjust equipment for body mechanics and safety: Lower the bed to the level specified in the person's care plan. Make sure the wheels on the bed are locked.

PROCEDURE

6. If the person has been lying down in bed, allow her to sit on the edge of the bed with her feet flat on the floor for at least 2 minutes before continuing. Some dizziness is common when a person sits up after being in bed for a while. See if the dizziness passes in 2 minutes. If it does not pass, if it gets worse, if she becomes sweaty or short of breath, or if she is in any pain, help the person to lie back down and report your observations to the nurse.
7. Help the person put on the robe and footwear. Put the transfer belt on the person.
8. If necessary, help the person to stand up: Stand facing the person, and either grasp the transfer belt on the back side of her waist with your palms up or, if you are not using a transfer belt, put your arms underneath the person's arms and place your hands on her shoulder blades. Place your toes against the person's toes and bend your knees so that they rest against, or near, her knees. Have the person lean forward, toward you. Tell the person that on the count of 3 she can push down on the bed or chair with her hands while you assist her to a standing position. On the count of 3, straighten your legs, helping to lift the person to a standing position.
9. If the person is using an assistive device for walking, make sure it is positioned properly. If the person is using a walker, it should be positioned directly in front of her. If the person uses a cane, make sure she is holding it in the hand opposite her weak leg.
10. Stand slightly behind the person on the person's weaker side. Grasp the transfer belt on the back side of the person's waist, with your palms up (Figure 1).

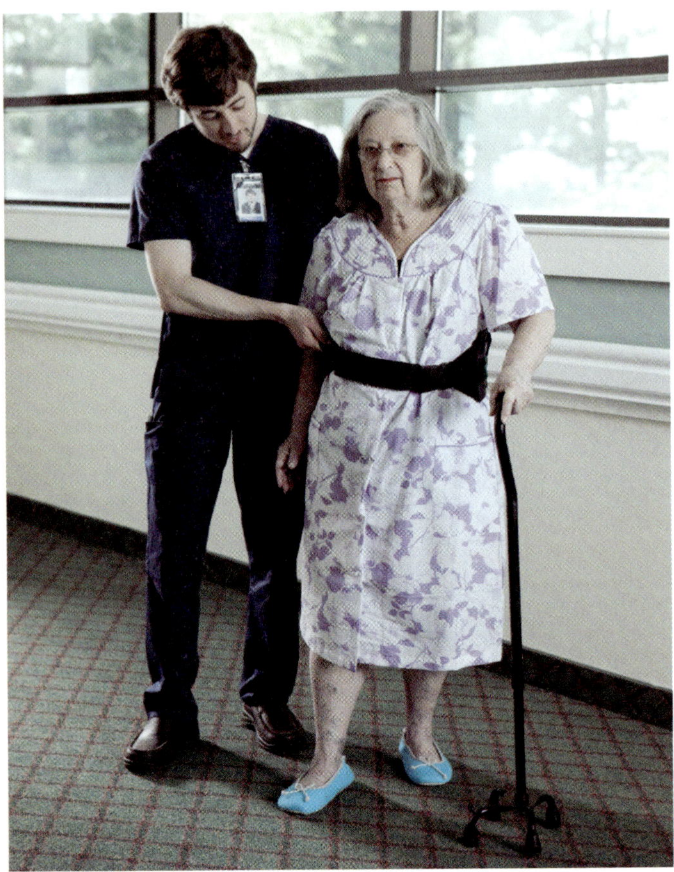

Figure 1

11. Starting on the same foot as the person, walk on her weaker side and a little behind.

COMPLETION

12. Ensure the person's comfort and good body alignment.
13. Adjust equipment for safety: Lower the bed to the level specified in the person's care plan. Make sure the wheels on the bed are locked. Place the person's method of calling for help within reach. Lower or raise the side rails according to the person's care plan.
14. Clean up your work area.
15. Wash your hands.
16. Report and record.

Skill 11-2
Helping a Person with Passive Range-of-Motion Exercises

PREPARATION

1. Wash your hands.
2. Gather your supplies.
3. Knock, greet the person and ensure privacy.
4. Explain the procedure.
5. Adjust equipment for body mechanics and safety: Raise the bed to a comfortable working height. Make sure the wheels on the bed are locked.

PROCEDURE

6. Lower the head of the bed as low as the person can tolerate. Make sure the person is in the supine position (lying on the back) and in good body alignment.

Task 1: Exercise the Shoulder

7. With one hand, hold the person's wrist and put your other hand under the elbow. Provide this support throughout the following motions.
8. **Flexion and extension.** With the person's arm by his side and the palm down, raise the person's arm straight up and then move it alongside the ear (Figure 1A). Then lower the arm to the person's side. Repeat 5 times.

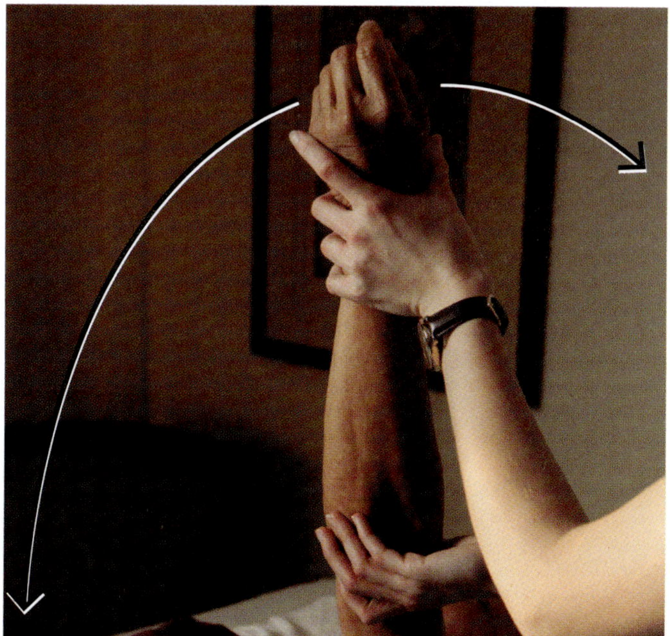

Figure 1A

9. **Abduction and adduction.** With the person's arm by his side and the palm up, move the person's arm out away from the body (Figure 1B). Then return the arm to the person's side. Repeat 5 times.

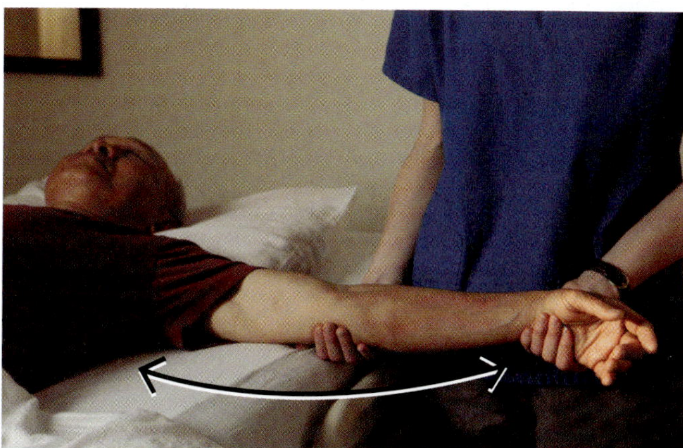

Figure 1B

10. **Horizontal abduction and adduction.** Hold the person's arm out away from the body with the palm up. Bend the elbow, touching the person's hand to the opposite shoulder (Figure 1C). Then straighten the person's elbow, returning the hand to its original position. Repeat 5 times.

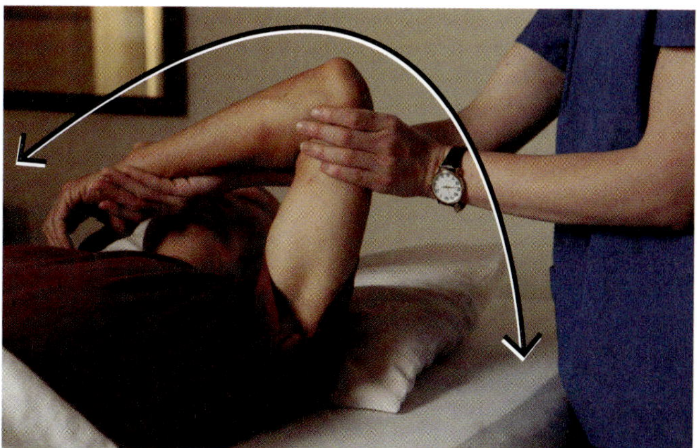

Figure 1C

11. **Rotation.** Bend the person's arm and position the elbow so that it is at the same height as the shoulder. Move the hand up toward the person's head and then down (Figure 1D). Repeat 5 times.

Continued on next page

Skill 11-2
Helping a Person with Passive Range-of-Motion Exercises *Continued*

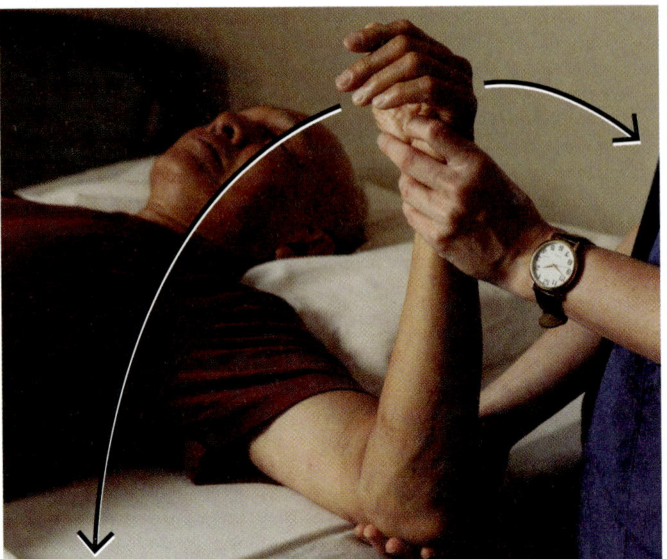

Figure 1D

Task 2: Exercise the Elbow

12. With one hand, hold the person's wrist and put your other hand under the elbow. Provide this support throughout the following motions.
13. **Flexion and extension.** With the person's arm by his side with the palm up, bend the person's arm at the elbow so that the hand moves toward the shoulder on the same side (Figure 2A). Then straighten the arm back down to the hip. Repeat 5 times.

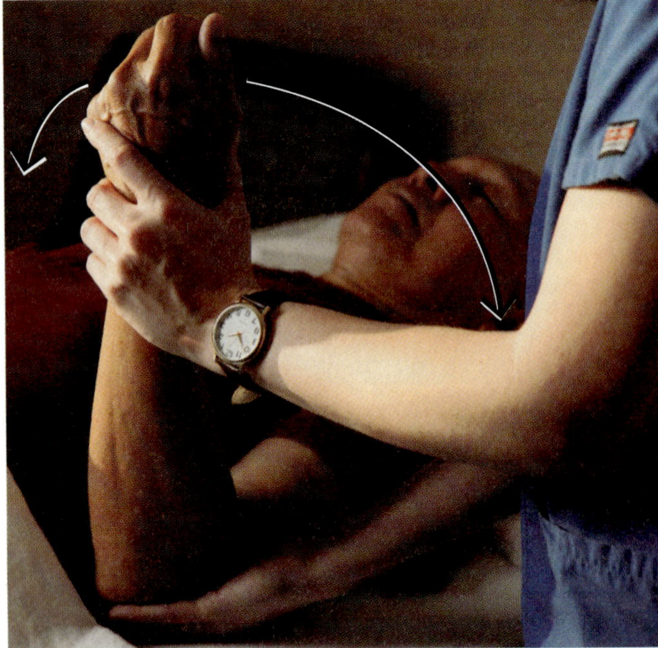

Figure 2A

14. **Pronation and supination.** Bend the person's elbow so that the forearm is at a right angle to the bed. Gently turn the person's hand so that the palm is facing the foot of the bed. Then turn the hand so that the palm is facing the head of the bed (Figure 2B). Repeat 5 times.

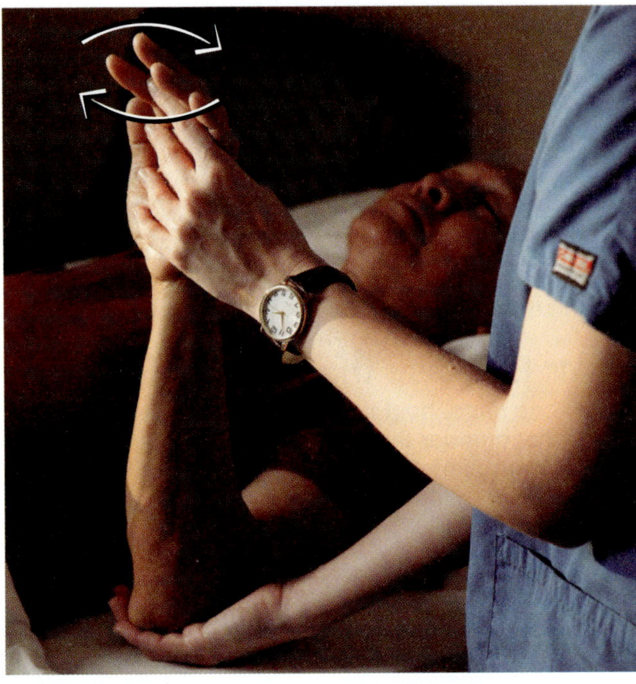

Figure 2B

Task 3: Exercise the Wrist

15. Hold the person's wrist with the palm down with one hand and the person's fingers with your other hand. Provide this support throughout the following motions.
16. **Flexion and extension.** Bend the person's elbow so that the forearm is at a right angle to the bed. Bend the wrist to move the person's hand forward, and then straighten the wrist to move the hand backward (Figure 3A). Repeat 5 times.

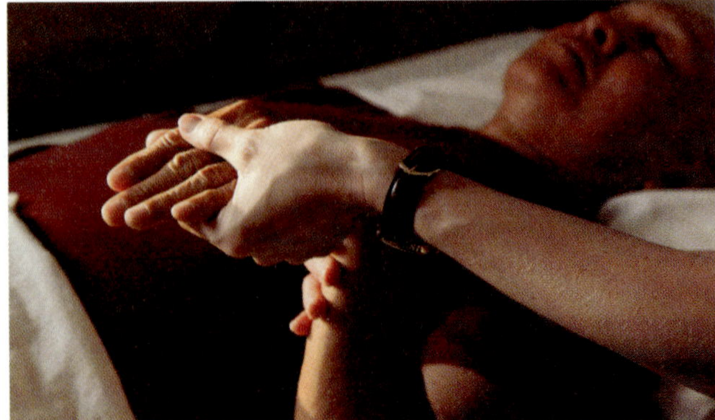

Figure 3A

17. **Radial and ulnar deviation.** With the person's hand still raised off the mattress, gently tilt the person's hand toward the thumb. Then tilt the hand the other way, toward the person's little finger (Figure 3B). Repeat 5 times.

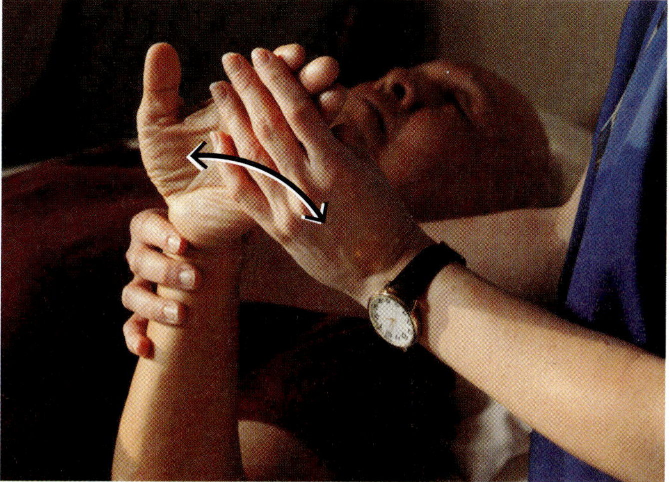

Figure 3B

Task 4: Exercise the Fingers and Thumb

18. Raise the person's hand off the mattress. Hold the person's wrist with one hand and the fingers with your other hand. Provide this support throughout the following motions.

19. **Flexion and extension.** Bend each of the fingers (one at a time) and the thumb to touch the palm (Figure 4A). Then extend each of the fingers (one at a time) and the thumb. Repeat 5 times.

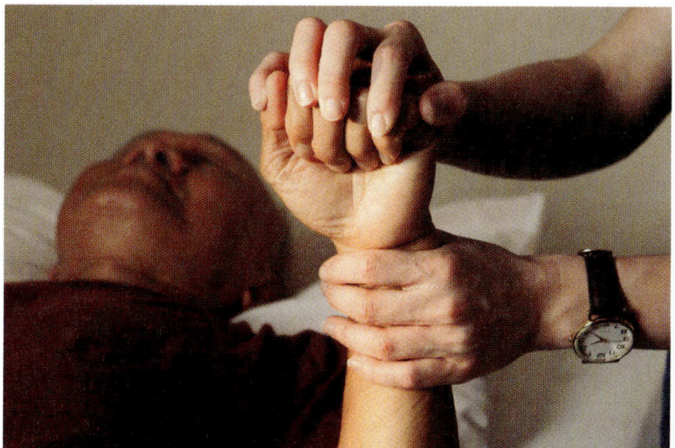

Figure 4A

20. **Abduction and adduction.** Hold the person's thumb and index finger together in one of your hands. With the other hand, spread the middle finger away from the index finger. Move the middle finger to the index finger and hold the middle finger, index finger and thumb together. Move the ring finger away from the other three fingers (thumb, index and middle), then back to them (Figure 4B). Hold all four fingers. Move the little finger away from the other four fingers (thumb, index, middle and ring), then back to them. Now work in the other direction. Hold the little finger and ring finger together and move the middle finger away and back. Complete with the index finger and thumb. Repeat 5 times.

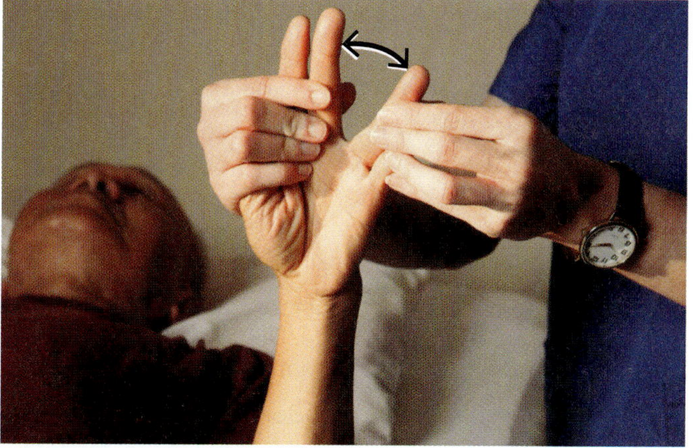

Figure 4B

21. **Thumb flexion and extension.** Bend the person's thumb in toward the palm, and then return it to its natural position (Figure 4C). Repeat 5 times.

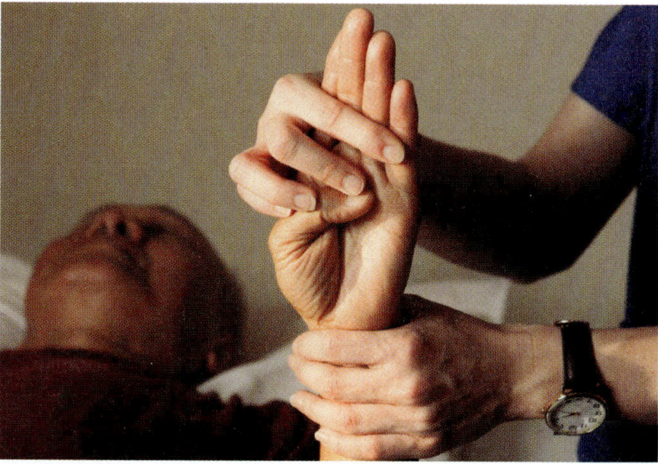

Figure 4C

Continued on next page

Skill 11-2
Helping a Person with Passive Range-of-Motion Exercises *Continued*

22. **Thumb opposition.** Touch the tip of the thumb to each finger (Figure 4D). Repeat 5 times.

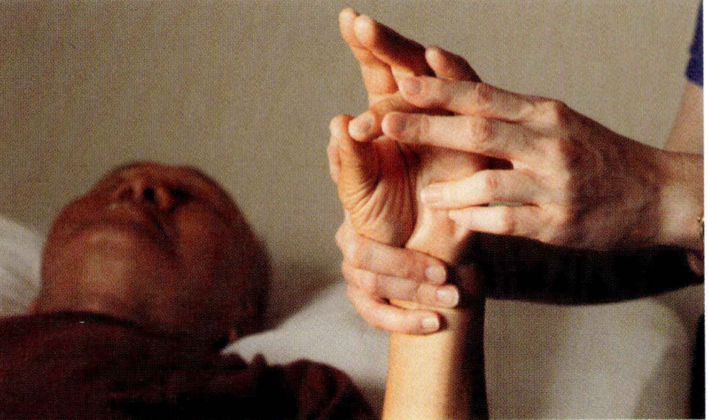

Figure 4D

Task 5: Exercise the Hip and Knee

23. Put one hand under the person's knee and your other hand under the ankle. Provide this support throughout the following motions.
24. **Flexion and extension.** Bend the person's knee and move it up toward the head to flex the knee and hip (Figure 5A), then straighten the person's knee, extending the knee and hip. Lower the person's leg to the bed. Repeat 5 times.

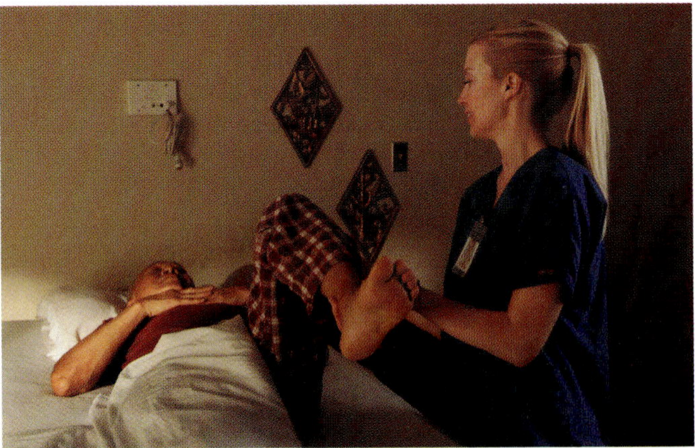

Figure 5A

25. **Abduction and adduction.** Move the person's leg out away from his body (Figure 5B). Then return the leg to the person's side. Repeat 5 times.

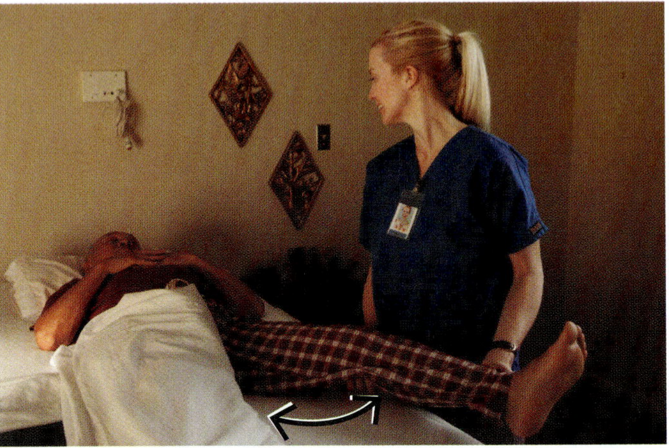

Figure 5B

26. **Hip rotation.** Keeping the person's leg straight, turn the leg inward and then outward to rotate the hip (Figure 5C). Repeat 5 times.

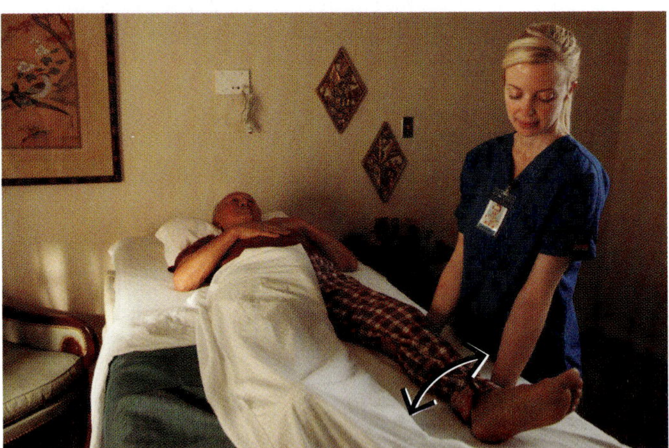

Figure 5C

Task 6: Exercise the Ankle

27. Put one hand under the person's ankle and grasp the foot with your other hand. Provide this support throughout the following motions.

28. **Dorsiflexion and plantar flexion.** Gently push the person's foot backward toward his head and then forward toward the mattress (Figure 6A). Repeat 5 times.

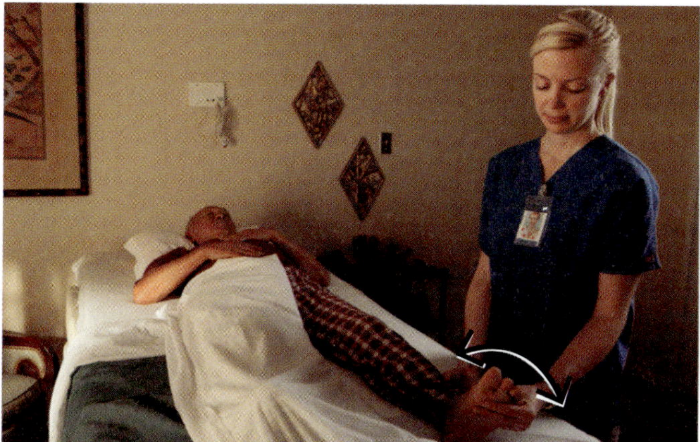

Figure 6A

29. **Inversion and eversion.** Turn the person's foot inward and then outward (Figure 6B). Repeat 5 times.

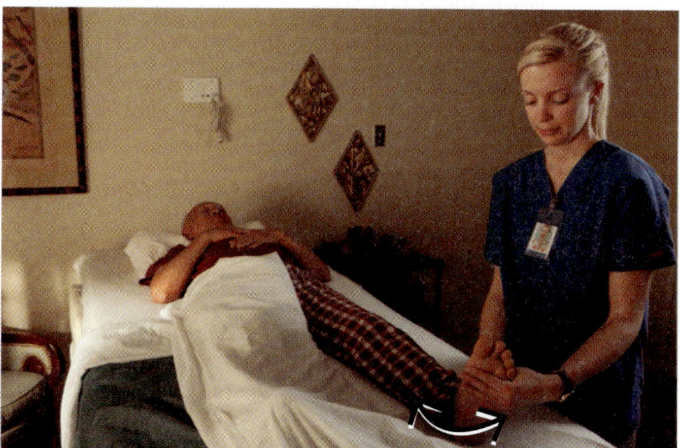

Figure 6B

Task 7: Exercise the Toes

30. Put one hand under the person's foot. Provide this support throughout the following motions.
31. **Flexion and extension.** Place your other hand on the top of the foot, over the toes. Curl the toes downward and then straighten them (Figure 7A).

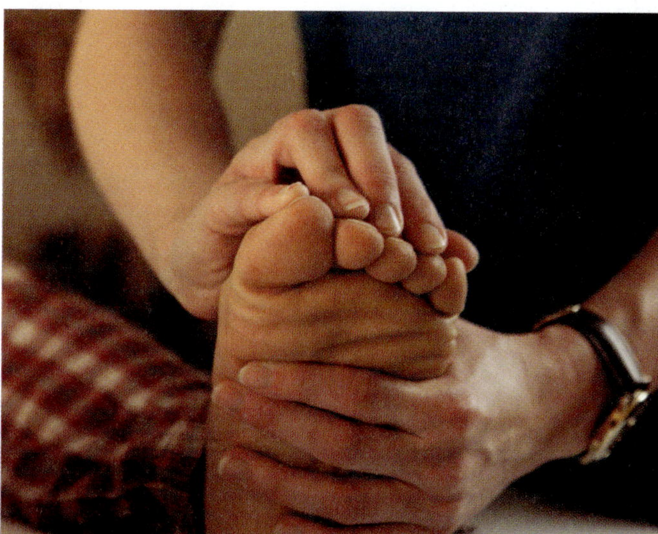

Figure 7A

32. **Abduction and adduction.** Starting with the big toe and the one next to it, hold the two toes together and move the middle toe away from them (Figure 7B). Continue spreading the toes in the same way you spread the fingers in Task 4, Step 20. Repeat 5 times.

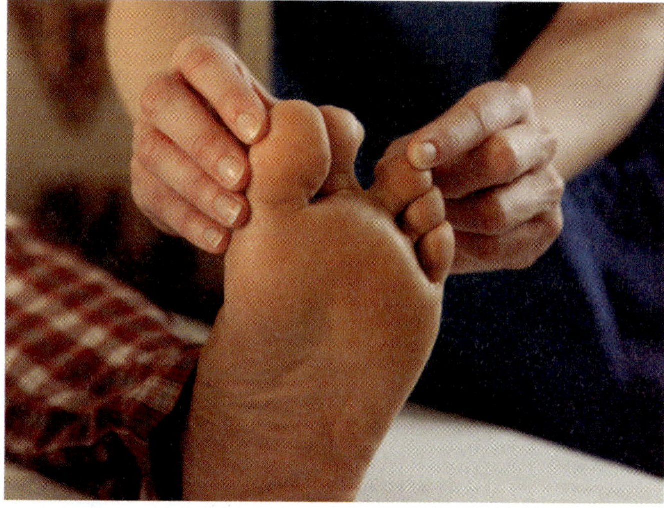

Figure 7B

COMPLETION

33. Ensure the person's comfort and good body alignment.
34. Adjust equipment for safety: Lower the bed to the level specified in the person's care plan. Make sure the wheels on the bed are locked. Place the person's method of calling for help within reach. Lower or raise the side rails according to the person's care plan.
35. Clean up your work area.
36. Wash your hands.
37. Report and record.

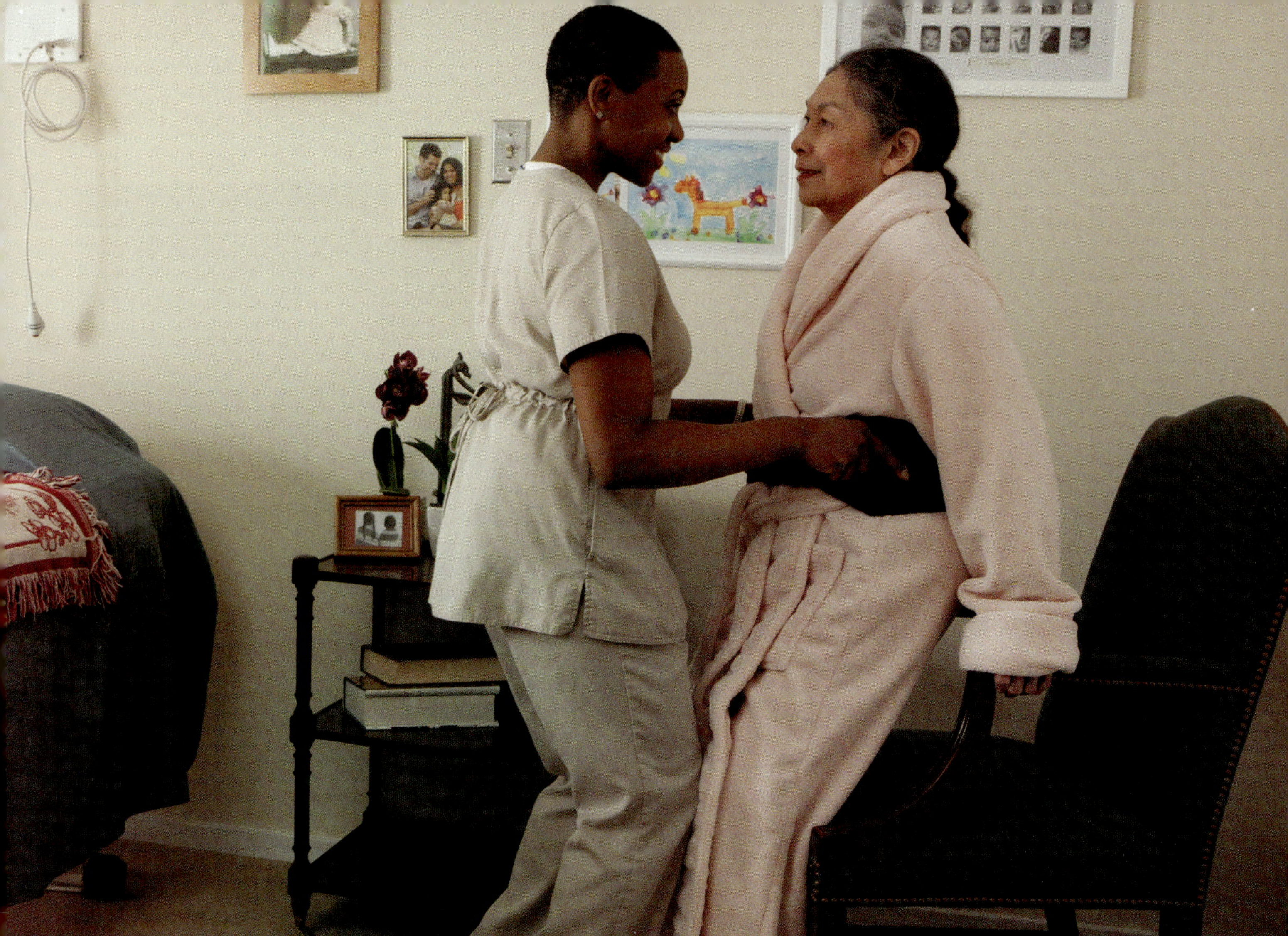

CHAPTER

12 Assisting with Positioning and Transferring

Goals

After reading this chapter, you will have the information needed to:

- Explain factors that put people at risk for developing pressure ulcers.
- Describe the role frequent repositioning plays in helping to prevent pressure ulcers.
- Describe basic positions that are often used in the health care setting.
- Explain the importance of good body alignment for the people in your care.
- Protect your safety and the safety of those in your care when you position or transfer them.

After practicing the corresponding skills, you will have the information needed to:

- Reposition a person in bed or a chair.
- Transfer a person from a bed to a chair, and from a chair to a bed.
- Use a mechanical lift to transfer a person from a bed to a chair.

Key Terms:

pressure ulcer
bony prominences
skin breakdown
friction
shearing
supine position
Fowler's position
low Fowler's position
high Fowler's position
side-lying (lateral) position
modified side-lying position
Sims' position
prone position
logrolling

You have been providing care for 78-year-old Victor Rivera since he was transferred from the hospital to Morningside Nursing Home several weeks ago. An earlier stroke left him paralyzed on his left side and incontinent of urine and stool. The stroke also affected Mr. Rivera's ability to speak, chew and swallow.

Because of his paralysis, Mr. Rivera is unable to move much by himself. So every day, according to his care plan, you help him change position at least every 2 hours. By changing his position and relieving pressure on certain parts of his body, you help provide comfort and help prevent pressure ulcers from developing on his dry, fragile skin. When Mr. Rivera's wife comes to visit every day, she helps by gently rubbing lotion into his skin.

This morning, when you first check on Mr. Rivera, you notice that he has been positioned on his side for sleeping. But he has moved his unaffected leg, which has caused the pillow that was between his knees to shift out of position, so his knees have been lying against each other. As you reposition him, you check the inner surfaces of his knees and notice a red spot on each knee. You report the condition of Mr. Rivera's skin to the nurse.

Like Mr. Rivera, many of the people in your care will have difficulty changing positions, moving from one place to another, or both. As you learned in Chapter 11, immobility puts a person at risk for many serious complications. In addition, remaining in one position for too long is very uncomfortable. As a nurse assistant, you will help to prevent complications of immobility and promote comfort by assisting those in your care to reposition themselves and to transfer (that is, move from one place to another).

PRESSURE ULCERS

Pressure ulcers are one of the most serious complications of immobility. A **pressure ulcer** is a sore that develops when part of a person's body presses against a hard surface (such as a mattress or the seat of a chair) for a long period of time. Pressure ulcers usually develop over **bony prominences** (parts of the body where there is only a thin layer of fat and muscle between the skin and the bone or cartilage underneath). Examples of these areas include the back of the head, shoulder blades, elbows, hips, coccyx (tailbone), knees, ankles and heels (Figure 12-1). When a person stays in one position too long, the weight of his body squeezes the tissue between the bone and the surface he is resting on, which slows down blood flow to the area. Because the tissue is not getting enough oxygen and nutrients, it starts to die. This loss of healthy, intact skin, called **skin breakdown**, can lead to a pressure ulcer.

Friction and shearing injuries can also lead to skin breakdown, putting a person at risk for developing a pressure ulcer. **Friction** occurs when two surfaces rub against each other. Friction injuries can occur when the skin rubs against another surface, such as the bed linens, or when skin rubs against skin (for example, under folds of skin in very overweight people, under the breasts, or where the buttocks meet the thighs). Medical devices, such as catheter tubing or a nasal cannula (the device used to deliver oxygen through the nose), can also cause friction injuries when they rub against the skin. **Shearing** occurs when a surface moves one way against another surface that offers resistance, causing a dragging effect. Shearing injuries can occur when a person is pulled across the bed instead of lifted. Because the bed offers resistance, the person's body does not move easily across the sheets, and the

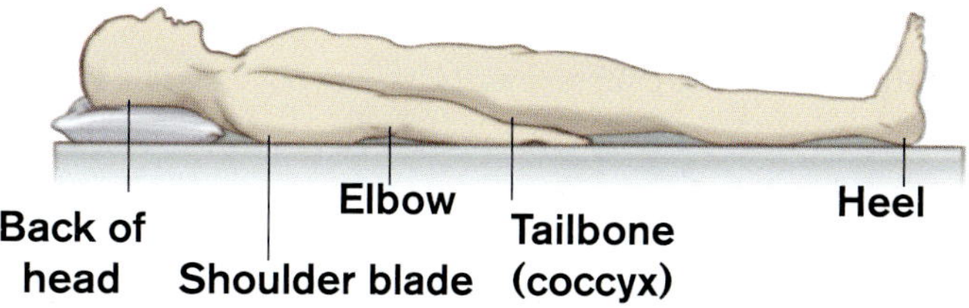

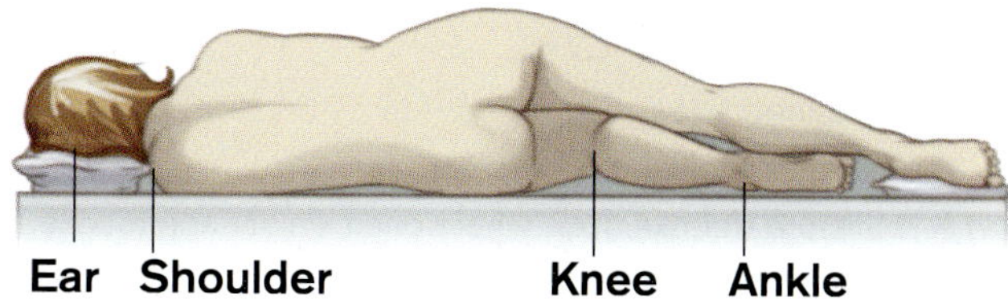

Figure 12-1 A pressure ulcer can form on *any* part of the body. Common sites of pressure ulcer formation are shown here.

top layer of skin is pulled in a direction opposite the underlying layers, leading to injury.

Pressure ulcers develop in stages (Box 12-1) and can be very difficult to treat, especially in the later stages. Pressure ulcers are extremely painful for the person, and they can lead to the person's death. For these reasons, every effort must be made to prevent a pressure ulcer from forming in the first place.

Observations Into Action!

The following may be early signs of a pressure ulcer and should be reported to the nurse right away. Your ability to identify a pressure ulcer in the early stages can make all the difference!

- **A reddened or darkened area that does not return to normal within a few minutes when the pressure is relieved**
- **A white, pale or shiny area**
- **An area that feels hot or cool to the touch, or is painful**

In addition to immobility, many of the people in your care will have other risk factors for developing pressure ulcers (Box 12-2). As a nurse assistant, you will play a very important role in helping to keep the person's skin healthy and prevent pressure ulcers (Table 12-1, Figure 12-2). Closely observing the person's skin for signs of excessive pressure and skin breakdown while you are providing care and reporting your observations to the nurse can help prevent a pressure ulcer in the early stages from getting worse. You also help to prevent pressure ulcers by regularly helping the people in your care to reposition themselves, if they cannot do this independently.

When you report the reddened areas on Mr. Rivera's knees to the nurse, she thanks you and says that she will go check on Mr. Rivera right away. She says, "Mr. Rivera has so many risk factors for developing pressure ulcers—it's great that you are paying such close attention to the condition of his skin. We'll keep a close eye on those areas, and I'll take another look at Mr. Rivera's care plan to make sure we are doing everything we can to protect his skin and lower his risk for developing a pressure ulcer."

Why could Mr. Rivera easily develop pressure ulcers? Give three reasons.

What are some of the actions to help prevent pressure ulcers that you would expect to see listed on Mr. Rivera's care plan?

Box 12-1 **Stages of Pressure Ulcer Development**

Stage 1. An area is red, pale or dark, and the normal color does not return within a few minutes of relieving the pressure. The area may be firmer, softer, warmer, cooler or more painful than the surrounding tissue. Detection may be more difficult in people with darker skin.

Stage 2. The area may look like a shallow, open ulcer with pink or red exposed tissue at the bottom. Sometimes, instead of looking like an ulcer, the area looks like a blister.

Stage 3. More tissue is lost. The fat that lies beneath the skin may be visible.

Stage 4. A deep crater forms. Muscle or bone may be visible.

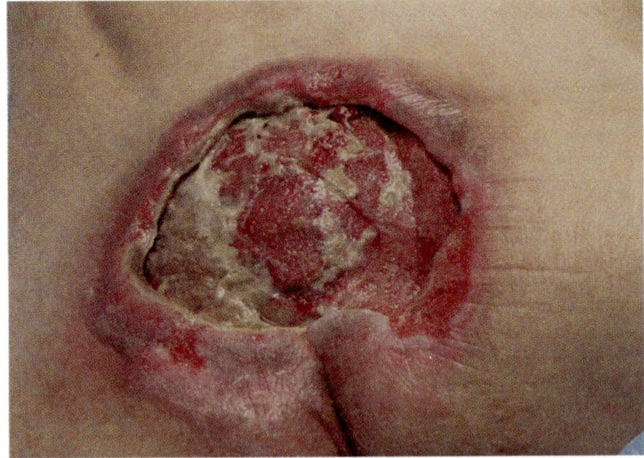

Stage 4 pressure ulcer. *Image © B. Slaven/Custom Medical Stock Photo, Inc., 2012.*

Box 12-2 **Risk Factors for Pressure Ulcer Development**

- Immobility
- Advanced age
- Fragile, dry skin
- Moisture (for example, where one skin surface touches another, or where skin is in contact with soiled linens or clothes)
- Poor nutrition
- Poor hydration (not enough fluid intake)
- Poor circulation (for example, as a result of cardiovascular disease)
- Poor oxygenation (for example, as a result of respiratory disease)

Table 12-1 **Protecting the Person's Skin**

To Prevent This...	Do This...
Direct Pressure	■ Change the person's position according to the person's care plan and at least every 2 hours. ■ Observe and report immediately any reddened, pale or darkened areas of the skin. ■ Make sure the person is in good body alignment. Use appropriate positioning aids when needed. ■ Use pressure-reducing devices (for example, pressure-reducing mattress pads, heel and elbow protectors) as ordered to relieve pressure and protect skin. ■ If the person uses hair pins or barrettes to style the hair, make sure these items are removed when the person's head is resting on a pillow.
Friction and Shearing Injuries	■ Get help when moving the person—be sure to lift the person's body all the way off the mattress. ■ Elevate the head of the bed no more than 30 degrees (except when a person is eating or has difficulty breathing). This will keep the person from sliding down in bed. Avoid leaving the person in Fowler's position for any length of time. ■ Make a tight, neat, wrinkle-free bed. ■ Prevent medical equipment from rubbing against the person's body. ■ Pad supportive devices (such as splints). ■ Ensure that shoes and socks fit correctly.
Skin-to-Skin Contact	■ Check for skin changes under skin folds, especially under breasts, and under the folds of skin on people who are overweight. ■ Position the person so that air circulates around the person's arms and legs to keep skin from touching skin.
Moisture	■ Wash, rinse and dry the person's skin thoroughly, especially in areas where skin meets skin. ■ Check people with incontinence at least every 2 hours and keep their skin, clothing and linens clean and dry. ■ Cover a vinyl chair with a pad or sheet. ■ Have the person wear moisture-absorbing clothes made from natural fabrics such as cotton.
Poor Circulation	■ Elevate the person's arms and legs. ■ Provide gentle massage. ■ Observe the person's skin frequently and report any changes to the nurse.
To Improve This...	**Do This...**
Nutrition and Hydration	■ Encourage the person to eat a well-balanced diet. ■ Encourage the person to drink an adequate amount of fluids.
Mobility	■ Reposition the person often. ■ If the person is able, assist the person with transferring out of bed and walking.

PRESSURE ULCER PREVENTION

Providing good skin care

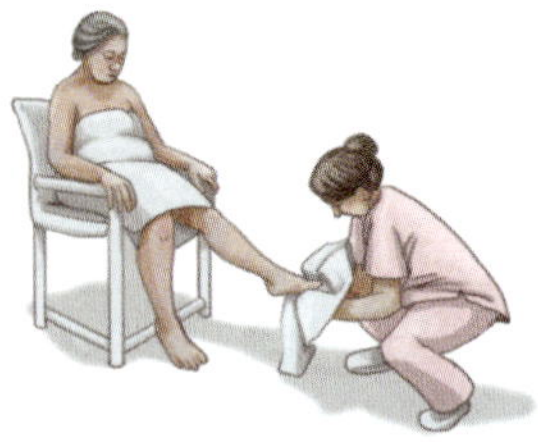

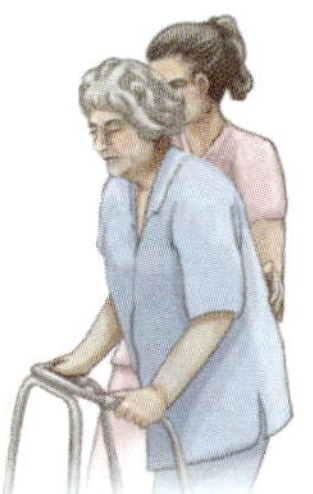

Encouraging movement

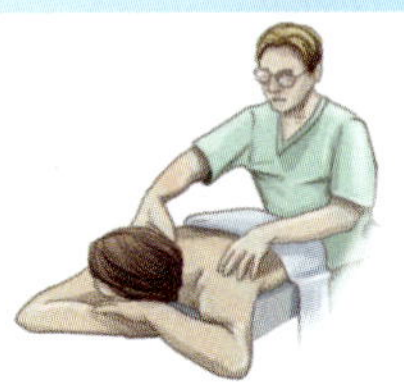

Observing for signs of skin breakdown

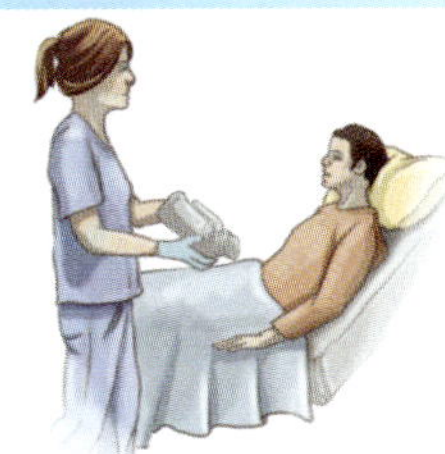

Assisting with regular toileting and providing perineal care

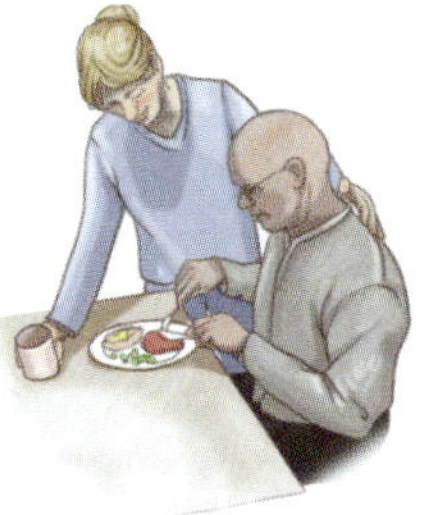

Encouraging good nutrition and fluid intake

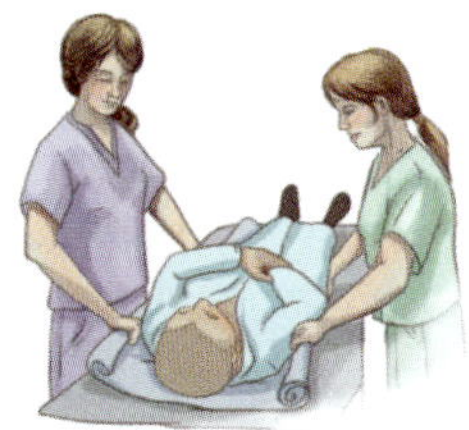

Assisting with repositioning and avoiding friction and shearing injuries

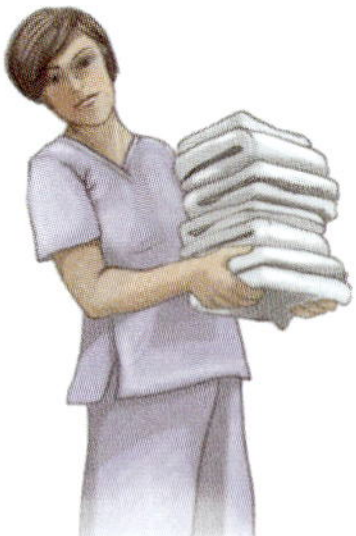

Ensuring clean, dry, wrinkle-free linens

Figure 12-2 Nurse assistants do many things to lower a person's risk for developing pressure ulcers.

ASSISTING WITH POSITIONING

Many of the people in your care will need your help to change positions and maintain good body alignment. In Chapter 7, you learned how maintaining good body alignment can help to reduce strain on your joints and muscles and prevent you from injuring yourself on the job. Good body alignment is important for those in your care, too. It is essential for comfort, and it helps to prevent complications such as contractures and pressure ulcers.

Helping people to reposition themselves and ensuring good body alignment are major responsibilities of the nurse assistant. Some people will only need to be encouraged to change their position, and checked to make sure they are in good body alignment. Other people, such as those who are confused, weak, frail, in pain, paralyzed or unconscious, will need more help from you. To check the alignment of a person who is lying in bed, imagine a line starting at the person's nose, continuing through the person's belly button, and ending between the person's feet. The line should be straight (Figure 12-3, A). When a person is sitting in a chair, his back and buttocks should rest against the back of the chair. His feet should rest flat on the floor (or the footrests of a wheelchair), and his knees should be level with his hips (see Figure 12-3, B). Many people will have a tendency to lean to the side or slump when they are in bed or sitting in a chair. To help the person maintain good body alignment, you may need to support parts of the body with rolled towels or pillows (Figure 12-4). Special positioning aids, such as foam wedges, may also be ordered for the person to help keep the body in proper alignment.

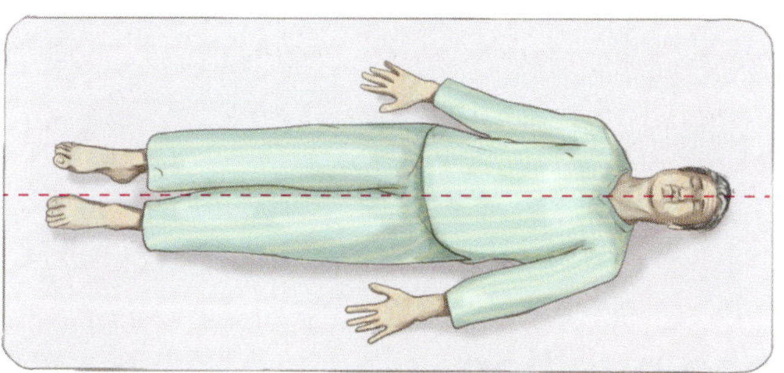

A

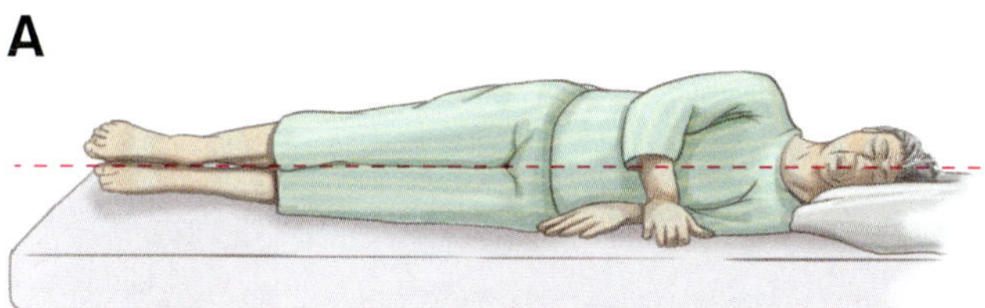

B

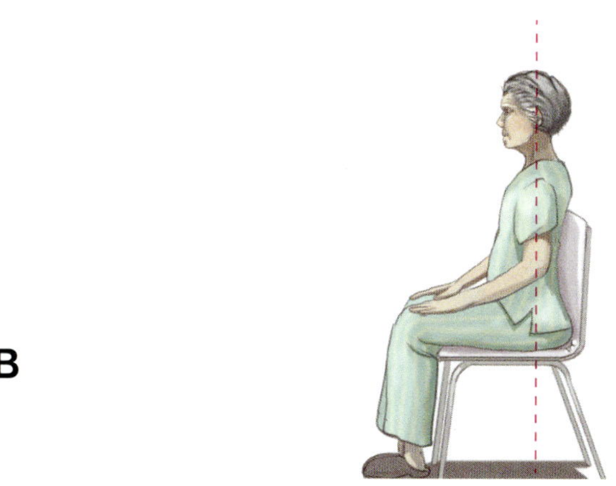

Figure 12-3 Proper body alignment is as important for those in your care as it is for you. (A) When a person is lying in bed, the spine should be straight. (B) When a person is seated in a chair, the back and buttocks should be positioned against the chair, the feet should be resting flat on the floor (or on the footrests of a wheelchair) and the knees should be level with the hips.

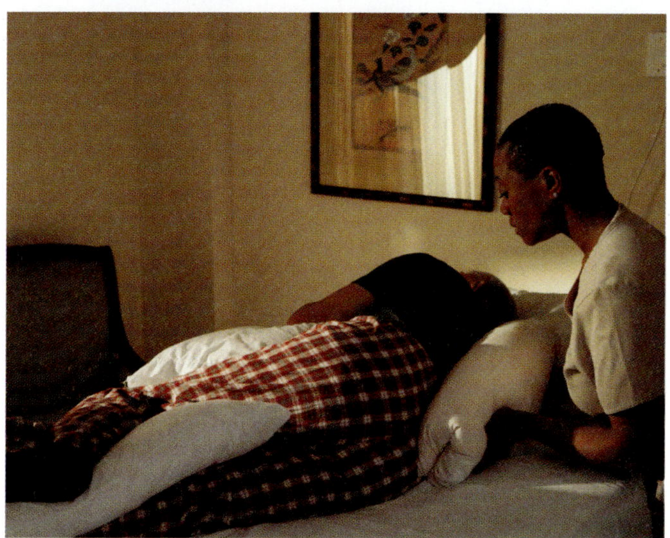

Figure 12-4 You may need to use positioning aids such as pillows, rolled towels or blankets, or devices made specifically for the purpose of providing support, to help the person maintain good body alignment.

Basic Positions

In the health care setting, several basic positions are used. A person may be positioned a certain way during a procedure, or to make an activity, such as eating, easier and safer. People who are unable to change positions easily on their own will have an individualized schedule for repositioning. This schedule will be part of the person's care plan. The schedule uses a sequence of positions to ensure that no single area is under pressure for too long. This is essential for reducing the person's risk for developing pressure ulcers. Basic positions that are commonly used in the health care setting are shown in Figure 12-5 and described in the sections that follow.

Supine position

In the **supine position**, the bed is flat. The person is on her back, with her head supported by a pillow. A small pillow or rolled towel is used to support the small of the back. The person's arms are extended at her sides, with her palms down. If the person's arms are paralyzed or weak, they should be supported with small pillows. The person's thighs extend in a straight line from her hips. If the person's feet tend to roll outward, rolled towels or pillows can be placed against the outer thighs to keep the legs in alignment. A foot board may be used to prevent foot drop and keep the toes pointing upward. To keep pressure off the heels, a small pad may be placed under the person's calves and ankles.

Fowler's position

In **Fowler's position**, the person is in the supine position, but the head of the bed is raised 45 degrees so that the person is sitting up in bed. There are two variations of Fowler's position: **low Fowler's position** (also called semi-Fowler's position), where the head of

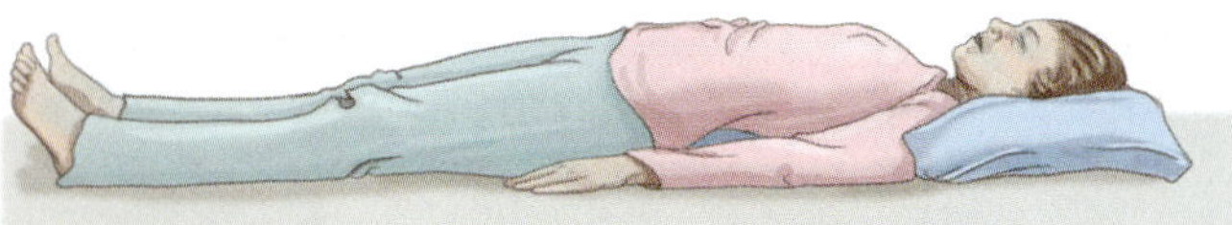

Supine position

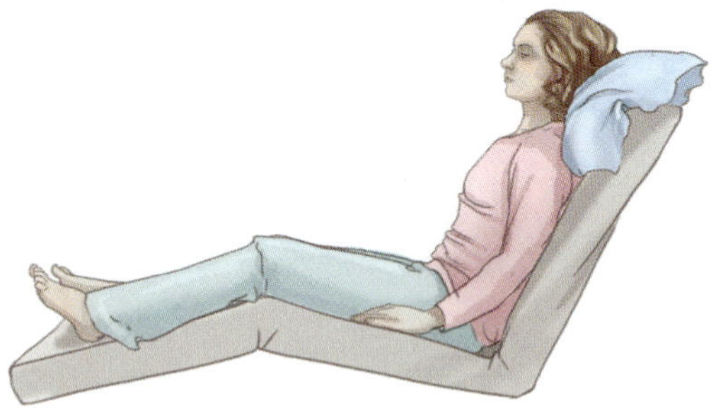

Fowler's position
45°

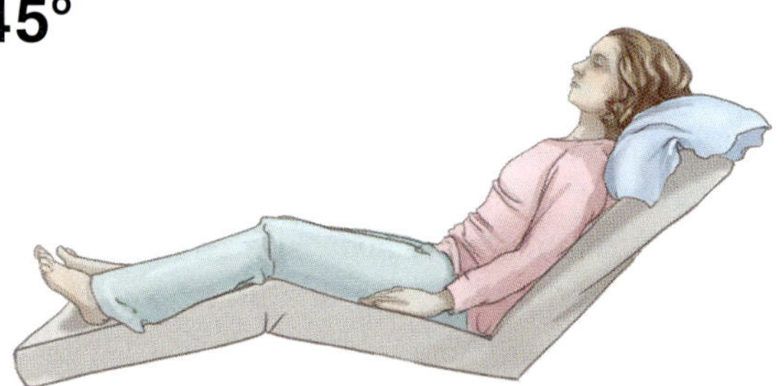

Low Fowler's position
30°

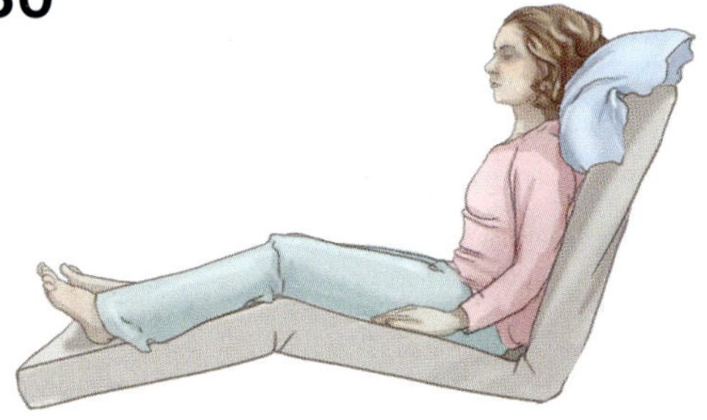

High Fowler's position
90°

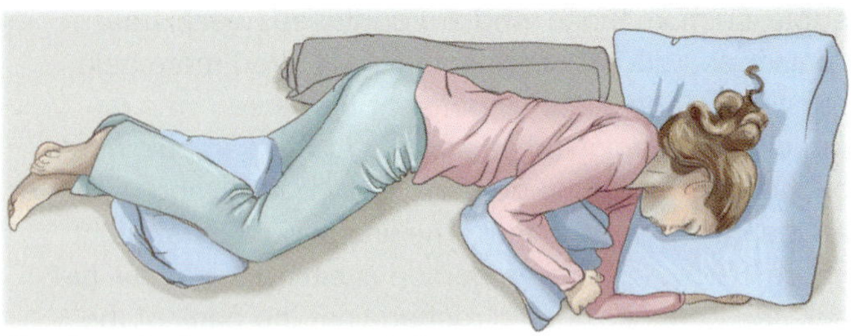

Side-lying position

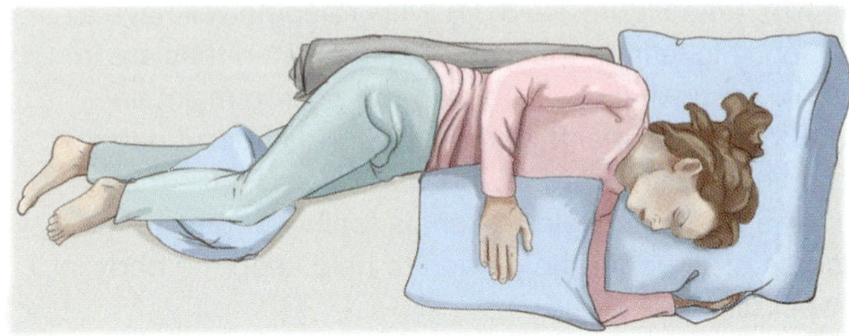

Modified side-lying position

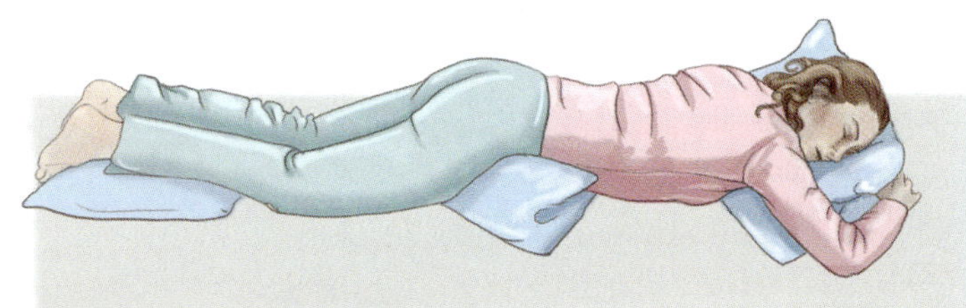

Prone position

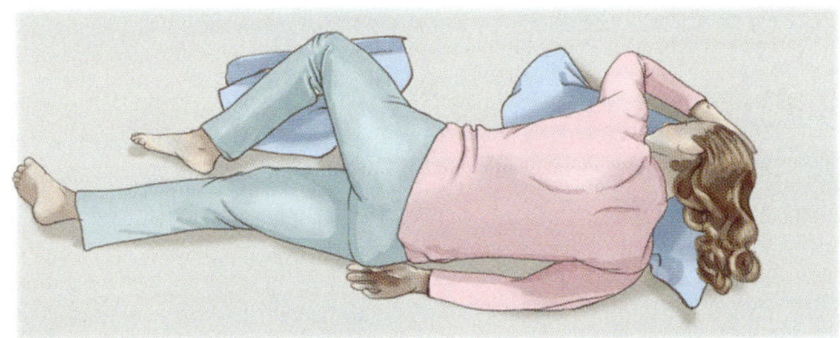

Sims' position

Figure 12-5 Basic positions used in the health care setting.

the bed is raised only 30 degrees, and **high Fowler's position**, where the head of the bed is raised 90 degrees. If the person is in an adjustable bed, the bed may be raised under the person's knees to prevent him from sliding down in the bed. Alternatively, a small pillow or folded blanket can be placed under the person's knees. As in the supine position, positioning aids should be used as necessary to support the arms, legs and feet.

Fowler's position should only be used for short periods of time (for example, when the person is eating in bed). Leaving a person in Fowler's position for too long puts the person at risk for shearing injuries, because the person will tend to slide down in the bed. Fowler's position also places a great deal of pressure on the person's tailbone, which can lead to pressure ulcer formation.

Side-lying (lateral) position

In the **side-lying (lateral) position**, the person is lying on her side, with her head supported by a pillow. The lower arm is positioned so that the person is not lying on it, and the top arm is supported on a pillow. A rolled blanket or towel is placed along the back to keep the person in the proper position. The bottom leg is straight, and the top knee is bent. A pillow is placed lengthwise between the lower legs to support the knee and ankle and prevent the legs from resting on each other.

The **modified side-lying position** is a variation of the side-lying position. In the modified side-lying position, a pillow is placed along the person's back, and the person is tilted slightly backward to lean onto the pillow. This helps to relieve pressure on the hip. The modified side-lying position is frequently part of the sequence of positions used in a repositioning schedule. For example, the person may move from the left modified side-lying position (left side down) to the supine or low Fowler's position, and then to the right modified side-lying position (right side down).

Sims' position

Sims' position is an exaggerated side-lying position that is used for procedures such as taking a rectal temperature or giving an enema. In Sims' position, the person is almost lying on his stomach. His head is turned to the side. The top leg is bent at the knee and supported by a pillow, and the top arm is bent at the elbow, with the hand near the face and supported by a pillow. The bottom leg is straight and the bottom arm is positioned so that the hand is near the person's hips. Make sure the person is not lying on the arm.

Prone position

In the **prone position**, the person lies on his stomach, with his head turned toward the side. The head is supported with a small pillow. The arm the person is facing is bent at a 90-degree angle, with the hand placed palm-down near the person's head. The other arm is extended straight along his side. A folded blanket or small pillow is tucked underneath the person's lower abdomen or pelvis to give the person's chest room to expand when the person breathes. A pillow is placed under the person's shins to raise the person's toes off the bed. The prone position is not used often because many people find it uncomfortable. If the prone position has been ordered for a person (or the person prefers the prone position), ask the nurse to help you assist the person into the prone position.

Helping a Person to Change Position in a Bed or a Chair

Before repositioning a person in bed, it is important to know the person's capabilities and plan the move accordingly. Always encourage the person to help you as much as possible with the move. This is important for the person's self-esteem and sense of independence. Equipment such as a trapeze that hangs over the bed (Figure 12-6) or a raised side rail that the person can grasp may increase the person's ability to assist with the move. Also consider whether or not you will need help from a co-worker to move the person safely. Two people can lift or move someone more easily than one person can. Generally, if a person is much heavier or larger than you are, or very ill or injured, it is best to ask a co-worker to help you with repositioning the person. Just remember to return the favor! Guidelines for repositioning people safely are given in Box 12-3.

ELDER CARE NOTE. Elderly skin is very fragile and thin, and it can rip or tear very easily. Whenever you are repositioning an elderly person (or providing any other type of hands-on care), handle the person carefully to avoid damaging the person's skin.

Many different skills are used for repositioning a person in bed or a chair:

- **Lifting a person's head and shoulders.** To adjust a pillow or help a person sit up in bed (for example, to readjust her clothing), you will have to lift the person's head and shoulders off the bed. This is described in Skill 12-1.
- **Moving a person up in bed.** A person who is sitting up in bed may slide down toward the end of the bed. To ensure good body alignment and to keep the person comfortable, you will need to move the person up in bed. Skills 12-2, 12-3 and 12-4 describe different ways of moving a person up in bed, depending on the situation, the person's ability to help, and whether or not you have help from a co-worker.
- **Moving a person to the side of the bed.** The first step of many procedures is to move the person to the side of the bed. For example, if you want to turn

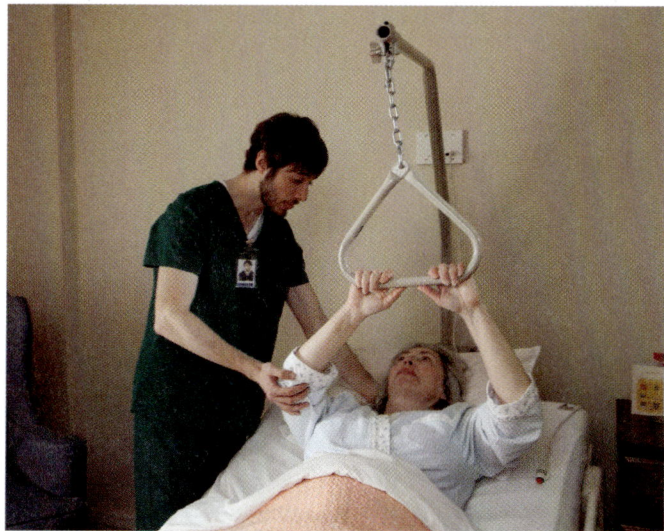

Figure 12-6 A trapeze enables people to change positions by themselves or with some assistance.

Box 12-3 Nurse Assistant DO's and DON'Ts

Repositioning People

DO be familiar with the person's care plan. Not all positions are allowed for every person.

DO plan how you will reposition the person and what you need to accomplish the move safely (for example, help from a co-worker, special equipment).

DO tell the person how you are going to reposition him, even if the person is unconscious. As you move through the steps, explain each step as you come to it.

DO tell the person what he can do to help make the move easier, and encourage the person to help as much as possible.

DO give clear directions to the people who are helping you (that is, the person receiving care, your co-worker or both).

DO use good body mechanics to protect your back. Raise the bed to a comfortable working height.

DO make sure the brakes on the bed are locked.

DO use a draw (lift) sheet to lift, rather than pull, the person into position. This helps to prevent friction and shearing injuries.

DO be careful while you are repositioning the person not to pull out medical devices that may be in place, such as catheter tubing or an IV line.

DO protect the person's dignity by not exposing her body unnecessarily while you are moving her.

DO smooth the bed linens and the person's clothes after repositioning the person. Lying on wrinkles can cause skin breakdown, putting the person at risk for pressure ulcers.

DO make sure the person is comfortable, that his body is in proper alignment and that he is supported as needed by pillows or other positioning aids.

a person onto his side in bed, first you will need to move him to the side of the bed so that he is in the center of the bed when you are finished repositioning him. Skill 12-5 describes how to move a person to the side of the bed if you are working alone. Skill 12-6 describes how to move a person to the side of the bed when you have help.

- **Turning a person onto her side in bed.** Skill 12-7 describes how to turn a person onto her side in bed. **Logrolling** is the method used to turn a person onto her side in bed when her spine must be kept in alignment throughout the move. Skill 12-8 explains how to logroll a person.
- **Repositioning a person in a chair.** A person who is seated in a chair may slide down in the chair over time. Skill 12-9 explains how to move the person back up in the chair for proper body alignment.

You return to Mr. Rivera's room to prepare him for breakfast. He is lying on his right side in a modified side-lying position, with a rolled blanket supporting his back. He has a pillow between his knees to reduce strain on his upper hip and to prevent pressure on his knees and ankles. His paralyzed arm rests on a pillow. You ask a co-worker to help you position Mr. Rivera in high Fowler's position for eating. You roll him onto his back, move him up in bed, and elevate the head of his bed so that he can sit up and eat. After breakfast, you collect Mr. Rivera's meal tray and tell him it will soon be time for his personal care. He shakes his head and, with effort, tells you that he wants to rest. Although you had planned to start your day by providing personal care for Mr. Rivera, you observe that he seems tired, and you adjust your schedule to meet his needs. Because he has just eaten, you lower the head of the bed to low Fowler's position and make him comfortable.

In about 15 minutes, you return to Mr. Rivera's room to help him with his bath. To perform this personal care procedure, you lower the head of the bed and put him in a supine position. During the bath you need to turn him onto his side to wash his back and give him a backrub. Because of his paralysis, he finds it difficult to position himself but is able to help turn with his unaffected side.

As you reposition Mr. Rivera in his bed to make it easier to accomplish various tasks throughout the day, what will you do to ensure Mr. Rivera's safety, as well as your own?

What skills will you use?

ASSISTING WITH TRANSFERRING

To transfer means to move from one place to another (for example, from the bed to a chair). As when repositioning a person in bed or a chair, you will need to plan the safest way to transfer the person and make arrangements for help or special equipment (such as a mechanical lift or standing-assist device) as needed. When planning a transfer, knowledge about the person's mobility and level of independence can help you determine how much the person will be able to help with the transfer. Questions to consider include:

- Can the person support all of his weight on one leg or both legs?
- Is one side stronger than the other?
- Can the person maintain his sense of balance?
- Does the person have vision problems?
- Is the person able to hear and respond to verbal instructions?
- Does the person have pain when he moves?
- Is the person afraid of being moved?
- Has the person ever suddenly refused to cooperate?
- Does the person behave in a predictable way?

When assisting a person who can bear weight, a transfer belt is used unless the person has a medical condition that makes it dangerous to use a transfer belt (see Chapter 11). During the transfer, you grasp the transfer belt to support the person, rather than the person's clothing or arms. Remember that the transfer belt is a support device, not a lifting device! A person who cannot bear any weight at all or who is very heavy will need to be transferred using a mechanical lift (Figure 12-7). There are many different types of mechanical lifts. Although they all work in generally the same way, make sure you have been trained specifically in how to use the lift at your facility before using it.

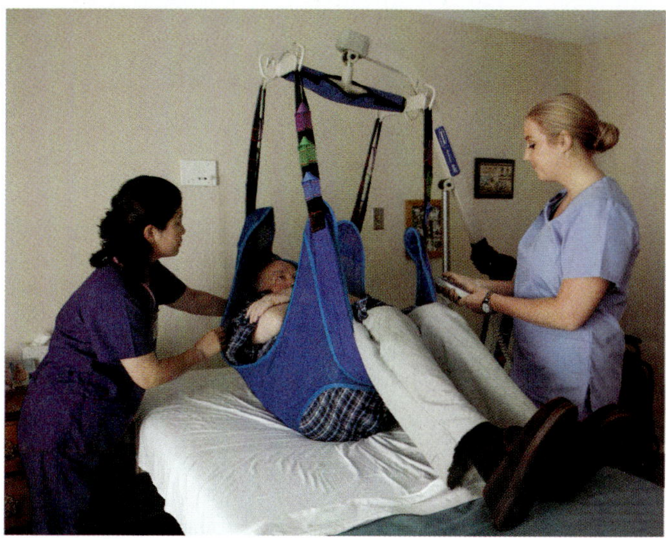

Figure 12-7 A mechanical lift is the safest way to assist a person who is heavy or unable to bear weight with transferring.

General guidelines for completing transfers safely are given in Box 12-4. Skill 12-10 describes how to assist a person with transferring from a bed to a chair, and Skill 12-11 describes how to assist a person with transferring from a chair to a bed. If the person is usually predictable but may not be consistent about helping to bear his own weight, you will want to ask a co-worker to help you with the transfer. Skill 12-12 describes how to use a mechanical lift to transfer a person. Use a mechanical lift according to your employer's policy and the person's

Box 12-4 Nurse Assistant DO's and DON'Ts

Transferring People

DO plan the transfer and identify what you need to accomplish the transfer safely (for example, help from a co-worker, special equipment). Move furniture out of the way, if necessary, and plan the transfer so that the person is leading with her strongest side.

DO tell the person how you are going to transfer him, even if he is unconscious. As you move through the steps, explain each step as you come to it.

DO tell the person what he can do to help make the transfer easier, and encourage the person to help as much as possible.

DO give clear directions to the people who are helping you (that is, the person receiving care, your co-worker or both).

DO use good body mechanics to protect your back. Get as close as possible to the person. Use a good base of support, keep the person close, keep your back straight and lift smoothly, without jerking or twisting.

DO lower the bed to its lowest height and make sure the brakes on the bed and the wheelchair are locked.

DO make sure the person is wearing footwear. The person's shoes or slippers should fit well and have nonskid soles.

DO use a transfer belt, unless the person has a condition that makes the use of a transfer belt dangerous (for example, recent abdominal, chest or back surgery; severe respiratory problems; or severe cardiac problems).

DO allow the person to sit on the edge of the bed for several minutes before continuing with the transfer. Dizziness is common when a person sits up after being in bed for awhile. If the person is dizzy and the dizziness does not pass, do not continue with the transfer.

DON'T rush the person. Ask the person if she is ready to stand up before continuing with the transfer.

DON'T allow the person to put her arms around your neck during the transfer. Instead, have the person place her hands on your arms for support.

DON'T use a mechanical lift until you have been properly trained in its use.

care plan. For many people, being moved in a lift is very frightening, so be sure to reassure the person throughout the procedure.

After his bath, Mr. Rivera agrees that he would like to get out of bed and sit in the chair by his bed. His mobility is limited because of his left-sided paralysis, but he can balance himself with assistance and can support his own weight.

What do you consider before getting Mr. Rivera out of bed and into the chair? Which type of transfer method should you use?

CHECK YOUR UNDERSTANDING

Questions for Review

1. **What is the *first* sign of a pressure ulcer?**
   a. A reddened area on the skin
   b. A fever
   c. An open sore
   d. Bleeding
2. **To avoid damaging the skin of a person who is unable to move without help, you should reposition him:**
   a. Whenever you can fit him into your schedule.
   b. At least every 4 hours.
   c. According to the schedule in the person's care plan.
   d. When you come to work and before you go home.
3. **When planning to move a person, some of the things you must know are:**
   a. Whether the person is permitted to move (per the person's care plan).
   b. Whether the person has risk factors for pressure ulcers.
   c. How recently the person ate.
   d. The person's mobility, level of independence and ability to help.
4. **In which position is the head of the bed raised 30 degrees?**
   a. Supine
   b. Modified side-lying
   c. Prone
   d. Low Fowler's
5. **Mr. Klein is in the side-lying (lateral) position. Where will you place positioning aids to ensure good body alignment?**
   a. Under Mr. Klein's knees
   b. Between Mr. Klein's lower legs and against his back
   c. Against his outer thighs
   d. Against his feet
6. **Miss Singleton is at risk for developing pressure ulcers. Which piece of equipment will you use when repositioning her to help prevent friction and shearing that can lead to skin breakdown and put her at further risk for pressure ulcers?**
   a. A foot board
   b. A bed cradle
   c. A draw sheet
   d. A wheelchair
7. **You are helping Mr. Lipkin transfer from his bed to a wheelchair. What should you do to ensure Mr. Lipkin's safety during the transfer?**
   a. Allow him to place his arms around your neck.
   b. Use a draw (lift) sheet.
   c. Allow him to rest on the edge of the bed before continuing with the procedure.
   d. Raise the bed to a comfortable working height and unlock the wheels on the bed and wheelchair.

Questions to Ask Yourself

1. *Mrs. Karmody has been sitting in a chair watching television for the past 2 hours. When you come to help her change position, she wants to lie on her back and sleep. What should you do?*
2. *Mr. Eller, who is paralyzed on his right side, is sitting in a chair next to his bed. Every time you look into his room, he has slumped over to his weaker side. What could you do to position him properly and maintain his alignment?*
3. *Mrs. Hillman, who weighs 200 pounds, begins to stand up from the chair where she is sitting. Knowing that she often gets dizzy without warning, you offer to help her, but she insists that she is able to stand up by herself. What safety precautions should you take to prevent potential injury? How many people are needed to help Mrs. Hillman transfer safely?*
4. *Mrs. Romano is sitting in the chair in her room while her niece is visiting. When Mrs. Romano says she wants to get back into her bed, her niece says that she will help her. You offer to help, but the niece says she can do it by herself. What should you do?*

Skill 12-1
Lifting a Person's Head and Shoulders off the Bed

PREPARATION

1. Wash your hands.
2. Gather your supplies.
3. Knock, greet the person and ensure privacy.
4. Explain the procedure.
5. Adjust equipment for body mechanics and safety: Raise the bed to a comfortable working height. Make sure the wheels on the bed are locked.

PROCEDURE

6. Face the head of the bed and position your feet so that one foot is about 12 inches in front of your other foot.
7. If the person can help, ask him to place his arm that is nearer to you under your arm and to hold on behind your shoulder.
8. Place your arm that is nearer to the person under his closest arm and behind his shoulder. Place your arm that is farthest from the person under his upper back and shoulders (Figure 1).

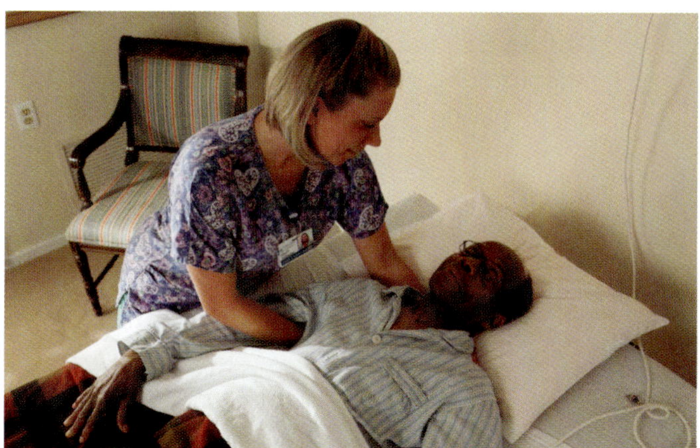

Figure 1

9. Raise the person's head and shoulders off the bed by shifting your weight toward the foot of the bed (Figure 2). Remember not to twist when you lift. Ask the person to assist you as much as he can by helping to support himself with his free hand.

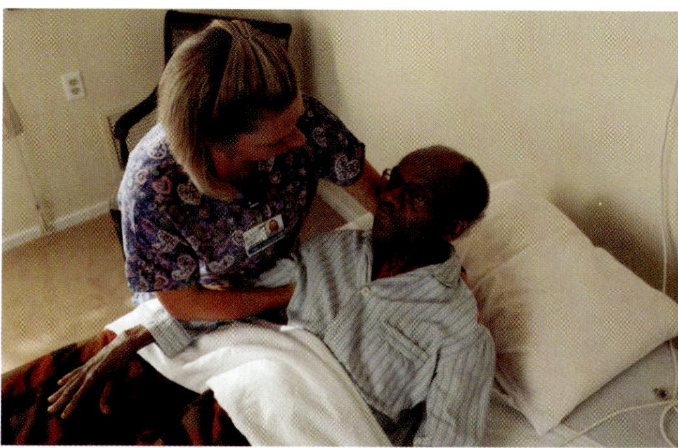

Figure 2

10. Use your hand that is under the person's shoulders to readjust the pillow, and then help the person lie back down.

COMPLETION

11. Ensure the person's comfort and good body alignment.
12. Adjust equipment for safety: Lower the bed to the level specified in the person's care plan. Make sure the wheels on the bed are locked. Place the person's method of calling for help within reach. Lower or raise the side rails according to the person's care plan.
13. Clean up your work area.
14. Wash your hands.
15. Report and record.

Skill 12-2
Moving a Person Up in Bed (One Nurse Assistant)

PREPARATION

1. Wash your hands.
2. Gather your supplies.
3. Knock, greet the person and ensure privacy.
4. Explain the procedure.
5. Adjust equipment for body mechanics and safety: Raise the bed to a comfortable working height. Make sure the wheels on the bed are locked.

PROCEDURE

6. Lower the head of the bed as low as the person can tolerate. Ask the person to lift his head, or if he is unable, gently lift his head and remove the pillow. Place the pillow against the headboard.
7. Face the head of the bed and position your feet so that one foot is about 12 inches in front of your other foot (Figure 1). Bend your hips and knees so that your upper back remains straight.

Figure 1

8. Prepare the person to help with the move.
   - **Option A:** Ask the person to bend his knees and place his feet firmly on the bed. Then ask him to place his hands palm side down on the bed. Place one arm under his shoulders and one hand under his thighs (Figure 2A). Ask the person to help by pushing against the bed with his hands and feet on your count of 3.

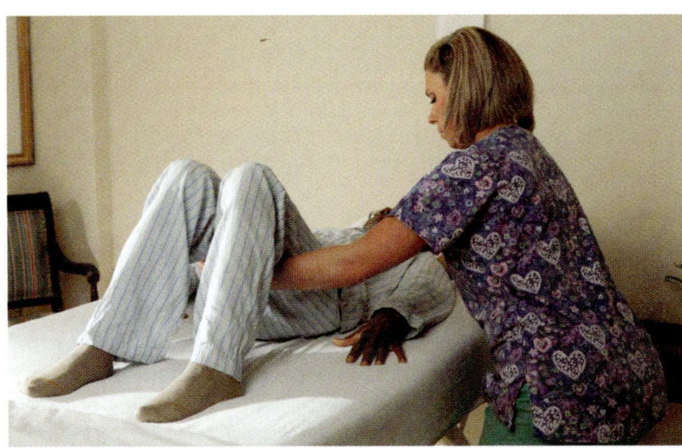

Figure 2A

   - **Option B:** If the person is able, ask him to grasp a trapeze (Figure 2B). Ask the person to assist you by pulling himself up on your count of 3.

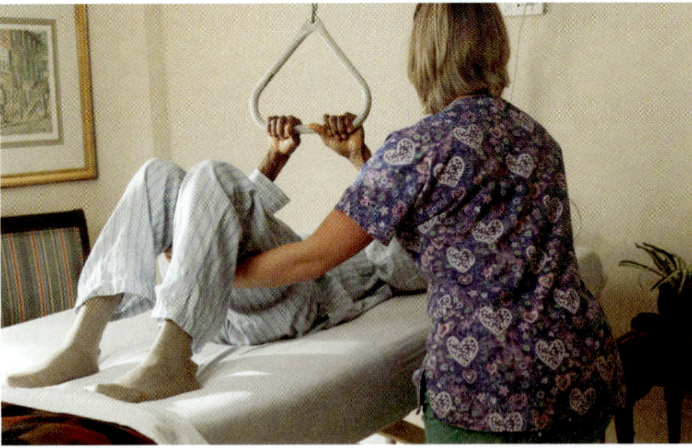

Figure 2B

9. Tell the person to get ready to move on your count of 3.
10. On your count of 3, shift your weight onto the foot nearest the headboard, moving the person up toward the head of the bed.
11. Help the person lift his head and replace the pillow.

COMPLETION

12. Ensure the person's comfort and good body alignment.
13. Adjust equipment for safety. Lower the bed to the level specified in the person's care plan. Make sure the wheels on the bed are locked. Place the person's method of calling for help within reach. Lower or raise the side rails according to the person's care plan.
14. Clean up your work area.
15. Wash your hands.
16. Report and record.

Skill 12-3
Moving a Person Up in Bed Using a Draw Sheet (Two Nurse Assistants)

PREPARATION

1. Wash your hands.
2. Gather your supplies:
   - Draw sheet, if one is not already on the bed
3. Knock, greet the person and ensure privacy.
4. Explain the procedure.
5. Adjust equipment for body mechanics and safety: Raise the bed to a comfortable working height. Make sure the wheels on the bed are locked.

PROCEDURE

6. Ask your co-worker to stand as close to the bed as possible on one side of the bed while you stand on the other side. Review the procedure with your co-worker.
7. Lower the head of the bed as low as the person can tolerate. If a draw sheet is not already on the bed, position one under the person now. Make sure the person is in the *center* of the bed.
8. Ask the person to lift his head, or if he is unable, gently lift his head and remove the pillow. Place the pillow against the headboard.
9. Face the head of the bed and position your feet so that one foot is about 12 inches in front of your other foot. Bend your hips and knees so that your upper back remains straight. Your co-worker does the same.
10. Loosen the draw sheet on each side of the bed and roll it toward the side of the person. Your co-worker does the same.
11. With your palms up and your hands close to the person's body, grasp the rolled draw sheet with both hands, placing one hand at the person's shoulders and the other at the person's hips (Figure 1). Your co-worker does the same.

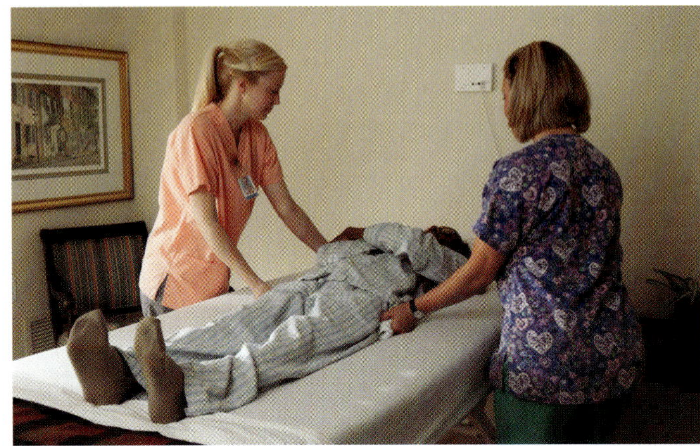

Figure 1

12. Tell the person that if he is able to help, he should bend his knees and push up with his feet at your count of 3. Tell your co-worker that on your count of 3, together you will move the person to the top of the bed by lifting up and moving the draw sheet toward the head of the bed.
13. On your count of 3, both you and your co-worker shift your weight onto the foot nearest the headboard, moving the person up toward the head of the bed by lifting and moving the draw sheet. Lift smoothly, without jerking, and lift the person high enough off the bed so that he does not slide along the bottom sheet. Keep your elbows as close to your body as you can to avoid straining your back.
14. Help the person lift his head and replace the pillow.
15. Retuck or remove the draw sheet.

COMPLETION

16. Ensure the person's comfort and good body alignment.
17. Adjust equipment for safety: Lower the bed to the level specified in the person's care plan. Make sure the wheels on the bed are locked. Place the person's method of calling for help within reach. Lower or raise the side rails according to the person's care plan.
18. Clean up your work area.
19. Wash your hands.
20. Report and record.

Skill 12-4

Moving a Person Up in Bed Using a Draw Sheet (One Nurse Assistant)

NOTE: This procedure can only be performed with a bed that does not have a headboard.

PREPARATION

1. Wash your hands.
2. Gather your supplies:
   - Draw sheet, if one is not already on the bed
3. Knock, greet the person and ensure privacy.
4. Explain the procedure.
5. Adjust equipment for body mechanics and safety: Raise the bed to a comfortable working height. Make sure the wheels on the bed are locked.

PROCEDURE

6. Loosen the draw sheet on both sides of the bed.
7. Lower the head of the bed as low as the person can tolerate. If a draw sheet is not already on the bed, position one under the person now. Make sure the person is in the *center* of the bed.
8. Ask the person to lift his head, or if he is unable, gently lift his head and remove the pillow. Place it alongside the person or on a chair.
9. Stand at the center of the head of the bed (facing the foot of the bed) and position your feet so that one foot is about 12 inches in front of your other foot.
10. Roll the draw sheet close to the person's head and shoulders. With your palms up, grasp the rolled draw sheet with both hands, on either side of the person's head (Figure 1). Ask the person to bend his knees if he is able and place his feet flat against the bed so that he can help push up.

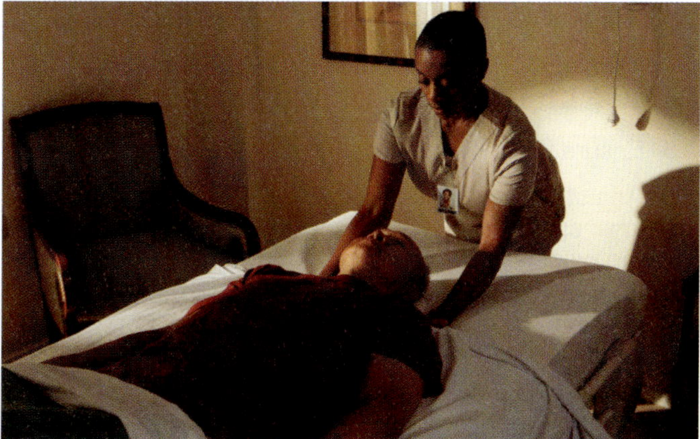

Figure 1

11. Bend your hips and knees so that your upper back remains straight.
12. Tell the person to get ready to move on your count of 3. On your count of 3, rock backward, moving the person up toward the head of the bed by lifting and moving the draw sheet.
13. Help the person lift his head and replace the pillow.
14. Retuck or remove the draw sheet.

COMPLETION

15. Ensure the person's comfort and good body alignment.
16. Adjust equipment for safety: Lower the bed to the level specified in the person's care plan. Make sure the wheels on the bed are locked. Place the person's method of calling for help within reach. Lower or raise the side rails according to the person's care plan.
17. Clean up your work area.
18. Wash your hands.
19. Report and record.

Skill 12-5

Moving a Person to the Side of the Bed (One Nurse Assistant)

PREPARATION

1. Wash your hands.
2. Gather your supplies.
3. Knock, greet the person and ensure privacy.
4. Explain the procedure.
5. Adjust equipment for body mechanics and safety: Raise the bed to a comfortable working height. Make sure the wheels on the bed are locked.

PROCEDURE

6. Lower the head of the bed as low as the person can tolerate. Ask the person to lift her head, or if she is unable, gently lift her head and remove the pillow. Place the pillow against the headboard.
7. Face the bed and position your feet so that one foot is about 12 inches in front of your other foot. Bend your hips and knees so that your upper back remains straight.
8. Ask the person to cross her arms over her chest.
9. Place one of your arms under the person's neck and shoulders and the other arm under the person's upper back. On your count of 3, rock backward and lift the person's upper body toward you (Figure 1).

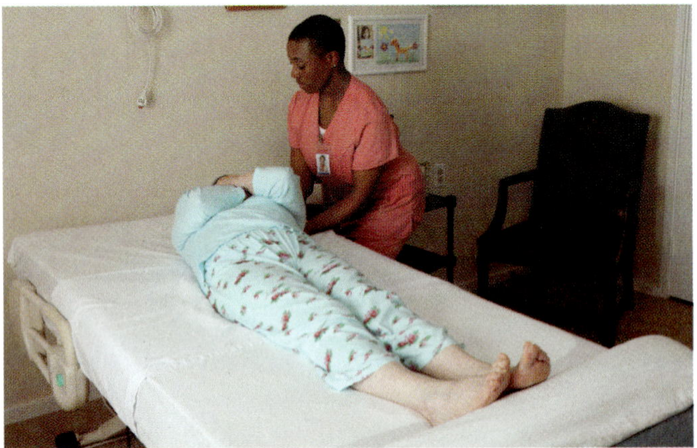

Figure 1

10. Reposition your hands, placing one hand under the person's waist and the other under her thighs (Figure 2). Using the same motion, count to 3 and rock backward, lifting the person's lower body toward you.
11. Finally, reposition your hands under the person's calves and feet and, on your count of 3, move the person's lower legs toward you so that the person is in proper body alignment (Figure 3).

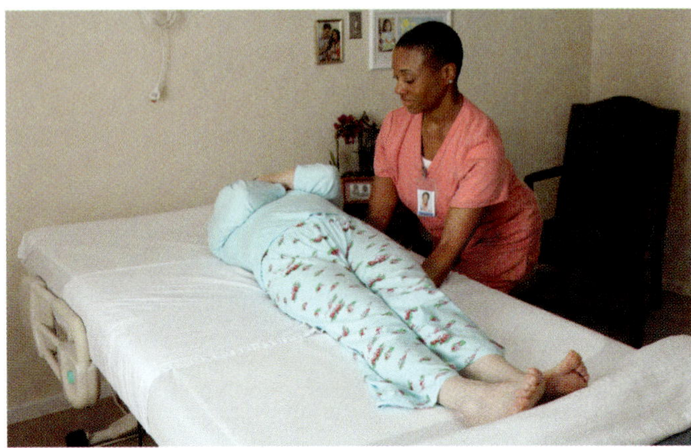

Figure 2

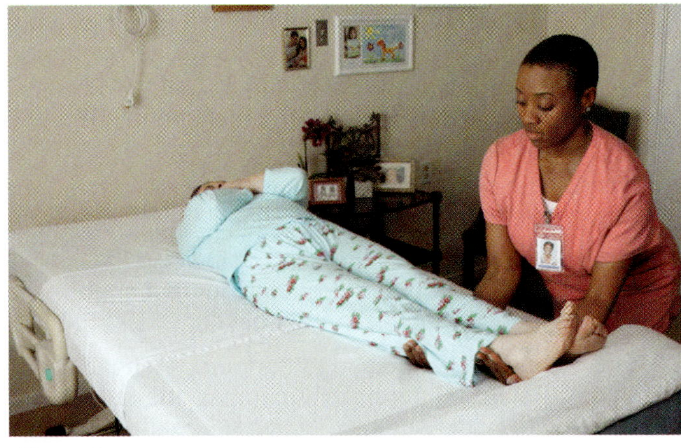

Figure 3

12. Moving the person to the side of the bed is usually the first step in another procedure. Continue with the other procedure as planned.

COMPLETION

13. Ensure the person's comfort and good body alignment.
14. Adjust equipment for safety: Lower the bed to the level specified in the person's care plan. Make sure the wheels on the bed are locked. Place the person's method of calling for help within reach. Lower or raise the side rails according to the person's care plan.
15. Clean up your work area.
16. Wash your hands.
17. Report and record.

Skill 12-6
Moving a Person to the Side of the Bed (Two Nurse Assistants)

PREPARATION

1. Wash your hands.
2. Gather your supplies:
   - Draw sheet, if one is not already on the bed
3. Knock, greet the person and ensure privacy.
4. Explain the procedure.
5. Adjust equipment for body mechanics and safety: Raise the bed to a comfortable working height. Make sure the wheels on the bed are locked.

PROCEDURE

6. Ask your co-worker to stand on one side of the bed while you stand on the other side. Review the procedure with your co-worker.
7. Lower the head of the bed as low as the person can tolerate. If a draw sheet is not already on the bed, position one under the person now.
8. Ask the person to lift her head, or if she is unable, gently lift her head and remove the pillow. Place the pillow against the headboard.
9. Face the side of the bed and position your feet so that one foot is about 12 inches in front of your other foot. Bend your hips and knees so that your upper back remains straight. Your co-worker does the same.
10. Loosen the draw sheet on each side of the bed and roll it toward the side of the person. Your co-worker does the same.
11. With your palms up and your hands close to the person's body, grasp the rolled draw sheet with both hands, placing one hand at the person's shoulders and the other at the person's hips (Figure 1). Your co-worker does the same.

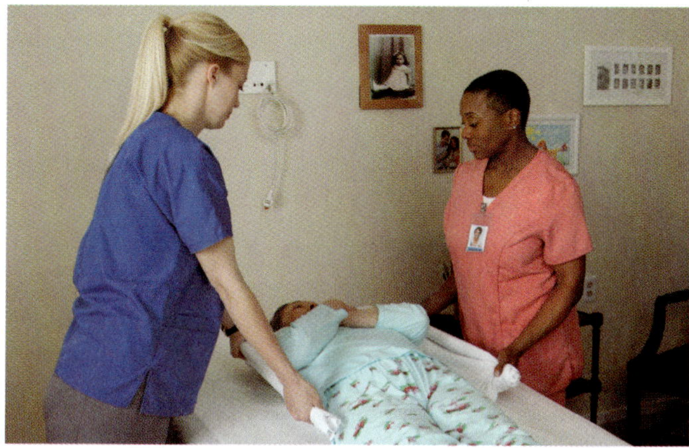

Figure 1

12. Tell your co-worker that on your count of 3, together you will move the person by lifting up and moving the draw sheet toward your co-worker's side of the bed.
13. On your count of 3, shift your weight from your back foot to your front foot, while your co-worker shifts her weight from her front foot to her back foot. Move the person toward your co-worker's side of the bed by lifting and moving the draw sheet. Lift smoothly, without jerking, and lift the person high enough off the bed so that she does not slide along the bottom sheet. Keep your elbows as close to your body as you can to avoid straining your back.
14. Moving the person to the side of the bed is usually the first step in another procedure. Continue with the other procedure as planned.

COMPLETION

15. Ensure the person's comfort and good body alignment.
16. Adjust equipment for safety: Lower the bed to the level specified in the person's care plan. Make sure the wheels on the bed are locked. Place the person's method of calling for help within reach. Lower or raise the side rails according to the person's care plan.
17. Clean up your work area.
18. Wash your hands.
19. Report and record.

Skill 12-7
Turning a Person onto Her Side (One or Two Nurse Assistants)

PREPARATION

1. Wash your hands.
2. Gather your supplies:
   - Draw sheet, if one is not already on the bed
   - Blanket or towel
   - Two or three extra pillows
3. Knock, greet the person and ensure privacy.
4. Explain the procedure.
5. Adjust equipment for body mechanics and safety: Raise the bed to a comfortable working height. Make sure the wheels on the bed are locked.

PROCEDURE

6. If a co-worker is assisting you, ask your co-worker to stand on one side of the bed while you stand on the other side. Review the procedure with your co-worker.
7. Lower the head of the bed as low as the person can tolerate. If a draw sheet is not already on the bed, position one under the person now.
8. Ask the person to lift her head, or if she is unable, gently lift her head and remove the pillow. Place the pillow against the headboard.
9. Move the person to the side of the bed nearest you (see Skills 12-5 or 12-6).
10. Tell the person that she can help you by crossing her arms over her chest and crossing her ankles toward the direction that you are turning her. For example, if the person is turning onto her left side, cross her right ankle over her left (Figure 1).

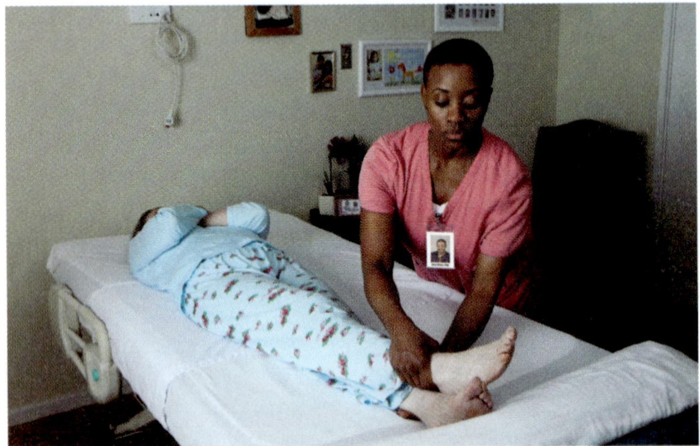

Figure 1

11. Turn the person onto her side.
    - **Option A:** If you are working alone, stand on the side of the bed toward which the person is turning. Face the side of the bed and position your feet so that one foot is about 12 inches in front of your other foot. Bend your hips and knees so that your upper back remains straight. Place one hand on the person's far shoulder and the other hand on her upper thigh (Figure 2A). Roll the person toward you by transferring your weight from your front foot to your back foot.

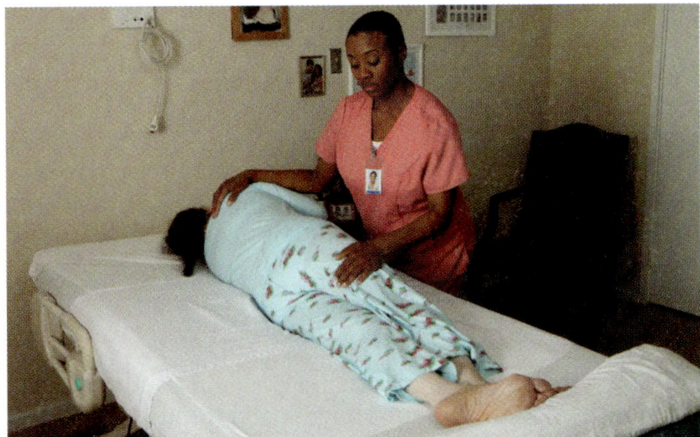

Figure 2A

    - **Option B:** If you are working with a co-worker, your co-worker grasps the draw sheet and rolls it close to the side of the person's body. Grasping the rolled-up draw sheet with palms up and using a broad base of support, your co-worker counts to 3, lifts the draw sheet, and rolls the person toward you onto her side (Figure 2B). You help to roll the person toward you by transferring your weight from your front foot to your back foot.

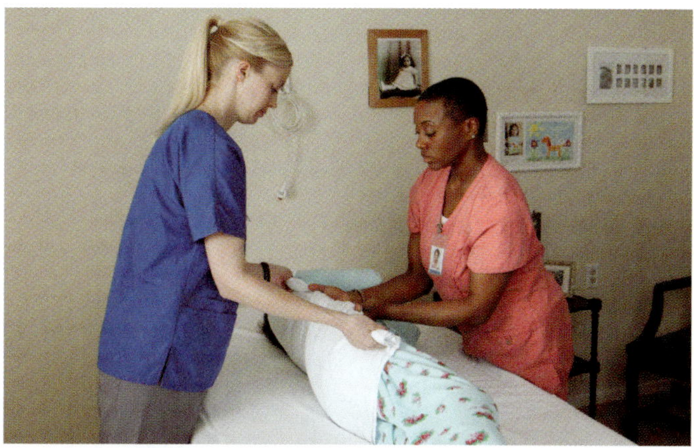

Figure 2B

12. Make sure the person is not lying on her lower arm. Help the person lift her head and replace the pillow. If the person will be remaining in the side-lying position, place a second pillow under the person's top arm and a third pillow lengthwise between the person's lower legs. (The bottom leg should be straight and the top leg slightly bent.) Place a rolled towel or blanket, or another pillow, along the person's back.
13. Retuck or remove the draw sheet.

COMPLETION

14. Ensure the person's comfort and good body alignment.
15. Adjust equipment for safety: Lower the bed to the level specified in the person's care plan. Make sure the wheels on the bed are locked. Place the person's method of calling for help within reach. Lower or raise the side rails according to the person's care plan.
16. Clean up your work area.
17. Wash your hands.
18. Report and record.

Skill 12-8
Turning a Person Using a Logrolling Technique

PREPARATION

1. Wash your hands.
2. Gather your supplies:
   - Blanket or towel
   - Two or three extra pillows
3. Knock, greet the person and ensure privacy.
4. Explain the procedure.
5. Adjust equipment for body mechanics and safety: Raise the bed to a comfortable working height. Make sure the wheels on the bed are locked.

PROCEDURE

6. Stand with your co-worker on the same side of the bed.
7. Lower the head of the bed as low as the person can tolerate.
8. Place your hands under the person's head and shoulders, and have your co-worker place his hands under the person's hip and legs (Figure 1).

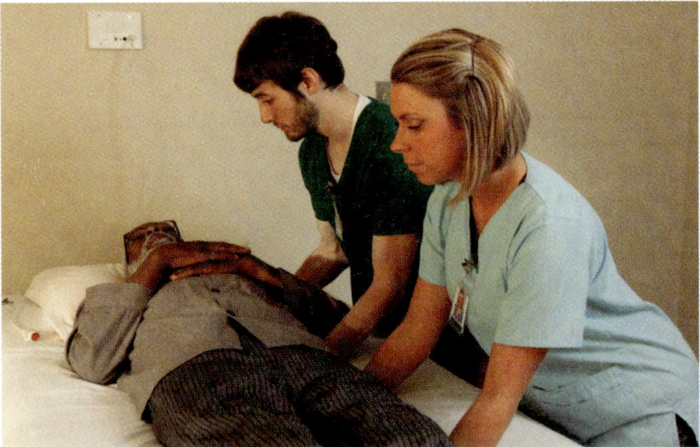

Figure 1

9. Face the side of the bed and position your feet so that one foot is about 12 inches in front of your other foot. Bend your hips and knees so that your upper back remains straight. Your co-worker does the same.
10. On your count of 3, both of you rock backwards, transferring your weight to the back foot to move the person toward the side of the bed (Figure 2).

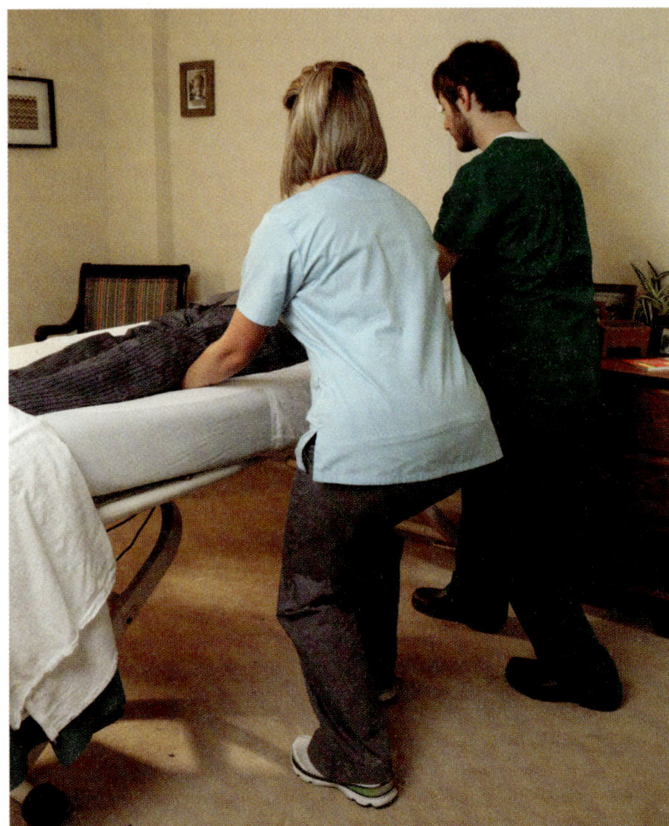

Figure 2

11. Raise the side rail and move to the opposite side of the bed.
12. Place a pillow lengthwise between the person's lower legs. Cross the person's arms over his chest. If the person is turning onto his right side, place his right arm on top. If the person is turning onto his left side, place his left arm on top.

13. Place your hands on the person's far shoulder and hip, and have your co-worker place his hands on the person's far hip and calf (Figure 3).

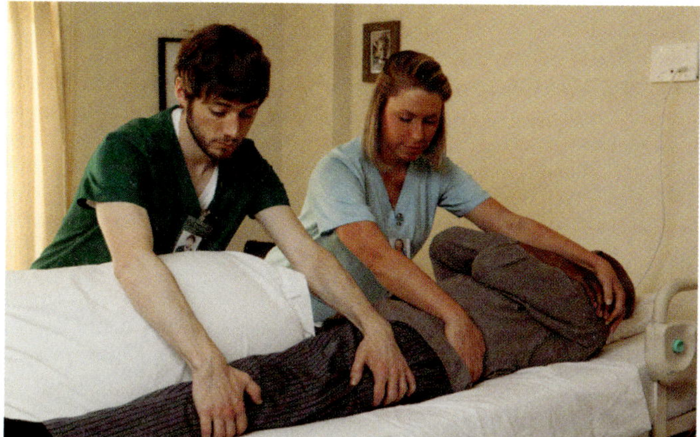

Figure 3

14. On your count of 3, roll the person toward you, keeping his head, back and legs in a straight line (Figure 4).

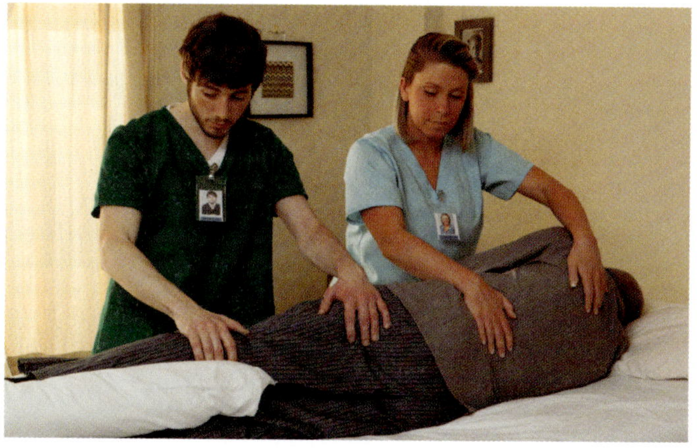

Figure 4

15. Make sure the person is not lying on his lower arm. Place a small pillow or folded blanket under the person's head, if allowed. Leave the pillow between the person's legs in place. Place another pillow under the person's top arm and a third along the person's back.

COMPLETION

16. Ensure the person's comfort and good body alignment.
17. Adjust equipment for safety: Lower the bed to the level specified in the person's care plan. Make sure the wheels on the bed are locked. Place the person's method of calling for help within reach. Lower or raise the side rails according to the person's care plan.
18. Clean up your work area.
19. Wash your hands.
20. Report and record.

Skill 12-9
Repositioning a Person in a Chair (Two Nurse Assistants)

PREPARATION

1. Wash your hands.
2. Gather your supplies:
   - Transfer belt
3. Knock, greet the person and ensure privacy.
4. Explain the procedure.
5. Adjust equipment for body mechanics and safety: If the person is in a wheelchair, remove or fold back the footrests and lock the brakes.

PROCEDURE

6. Put the transfer belt on the person.
7. Stand as close as possible to the back of the chair, facing the person's back.

   To give yourself a broad base of support, place one leg against the back of the chair, and place your other leg about 12 inches behind the first. Bend your knees.
8. Ask your co-worker to kneel on one knee close to the person's legs and place an arm under the person's knees (Figure 1).

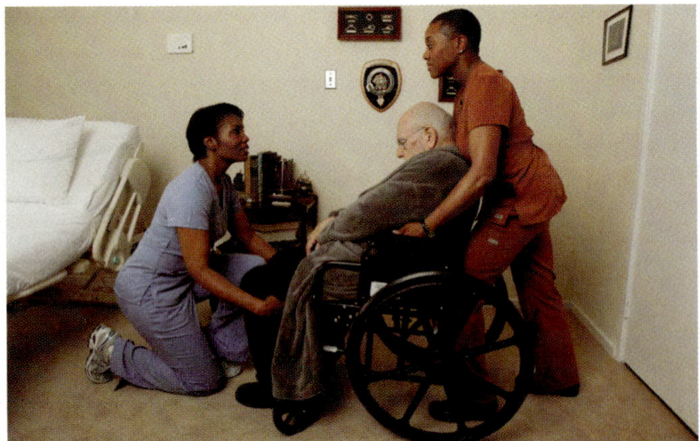

Figure 1

9. Support the person's head against your chest or one shoulder, and grip the transfer belt firmly with your palms up.
10. Tell the person and your co-worker that on your count of 3 you are going to move the person back.
11. On your count of 3, your co-worker slightly lifts the person's legs and guides them toward the back of the chair, while you lift the person's upper body by slowly straightening your legs (Figure 2). Make sure the person's back and buttocks are resting against the back of the chair. Place his feet on the footrests, if used.

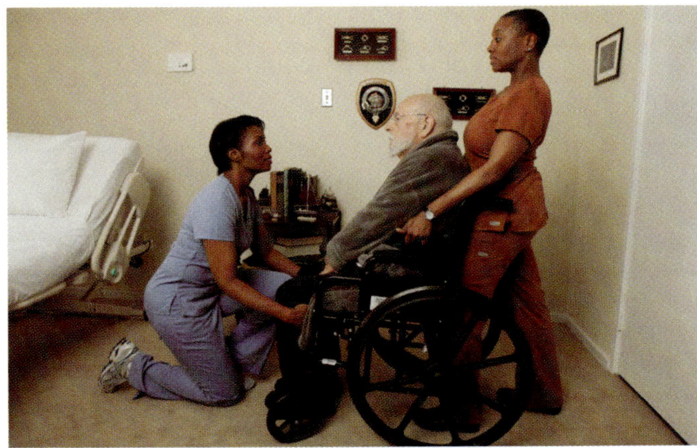

Figure 2

COMPLETION

12. Ensure the person's comfort and good body alignment.
13. Adjust equipment for safety: If the person is in a wheelchair, make sure the wheels on the wheelchair are locked. Place the person's method of calling for help within reach.
14. Clean up your work area.
15. Wash your hands.
16. Report and record.

Skill 12-10
Transferring a Person from the Bed to a Chair (One or Two Nurse Assistants)

PREPARATION

1. Wash your hands.
2. Gather your supplies:
   - Transfer belt
   - Wheelchair or chair
   - The person's robe and slippers or shoes
3. Knock, greet the person and ensure privacy.
4. Explain the procedure.
5. Adjust equipment for body mechanics and safety. Lower the bed to its lowest position. Make sure the wheels on the bed are locked.

PROCEDURE

6. Place the chair against the bed on the person's stronger side so that it faces the foot of the bed. If you are using a wheelchair, remove or fold back the footrests and lock the brakes.
7. Raise the head of the bed so that the person is almost in a sitting position.
8. Face the side of the bed, and position your feet so that one foot is about 12 inches in front of your other foot. With your knees bent and back straight, put one of your arms across the person's upper back and the other arm under his thighs. On your count of 3, pivot your feet to turn the person toward you so that he is sitting on the edge of the bed (Figure 1).

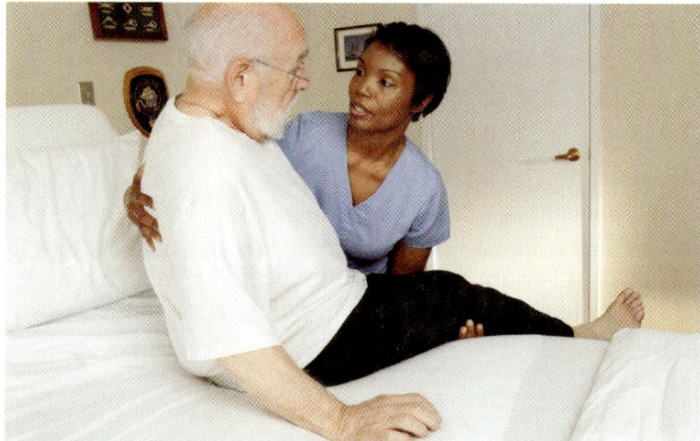

Figure 1

9. Allow the person to sit on the edge of the bed with his feet flat on the floor for at least 2 minutes before continuing. Some dizziness is common when a person sits up after being in bed for a while. See if the dizziness passes in 2 minutes. If it does not pass, if it gets worse, if he becomes sweaty or short of breath, or if he is in any pain, help the person to lie back down and report your observations to the nurse.
10. Help the person put on the robe and footwear. Put the transfer belt on the person.
11. Prepare the person to stand up.
    - **Option A:** Grasp the transfer belt on the back side of the person's waist (Figure 2A).

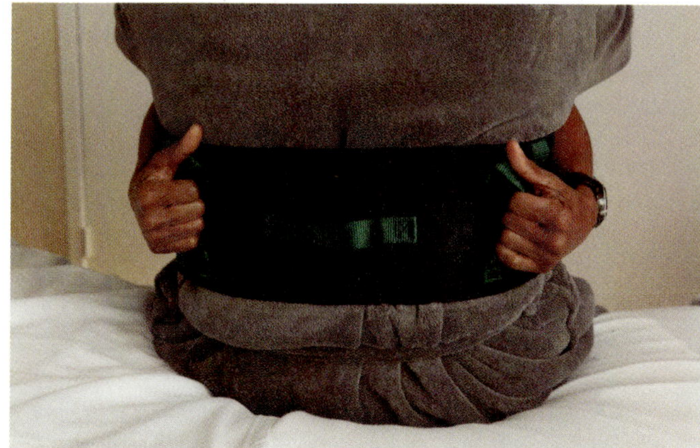

Figure 2A

    - **Option B:** If you are not using a transfer belt, put your arms underneath the person's arms, and place your hands on his shoulder blades (Figure 2B).

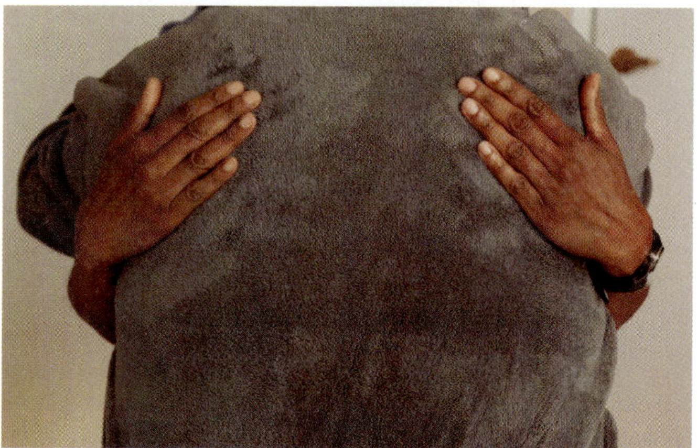

Figure 2B

Continued on next page

Skill 12-10
Transferring a Person from the Bed to a Chair (One or Two Nurse Assistants) *Continued*

- **Option C:** If you have help from a co-worker, have your co-worker grasp one side of the transfer belt on the back side of the person's waist, while you grasp the other. Alternatively, each of you can place one arm underneath the person's arm, resting your hand on the person's shoulder blade.

12. Block the person's lower extremities to prevent him from slipping. To do this, face the person, placing your feet "toe-to-toe." Turn your toes slightly outward to create a supportive base, and position your foot closest to the chair farther back than the other foot. Bend your knees deeply so that they rest against or near the person's knees (Figure 3). Have the person lean forward toward you. If you are working with a co-worker, each of you blocks one of the person's feet.

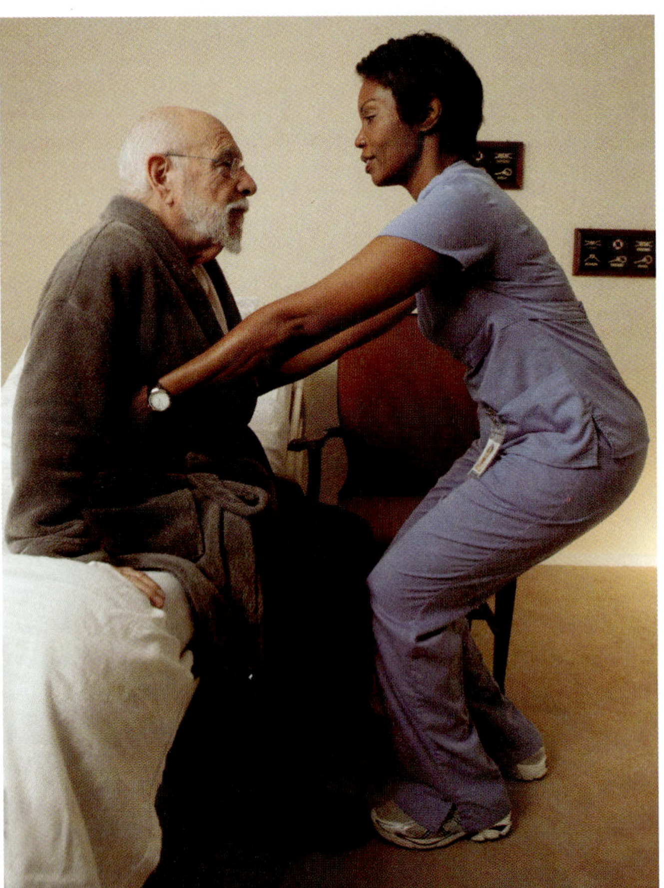

Figure 3

13. Tell the person that on your count of 3, he can push down on the bed with his hands while you assist him to a standing position. On your count of 3, straighten your legs, helping to lift the person to a standing position (Figure 4).

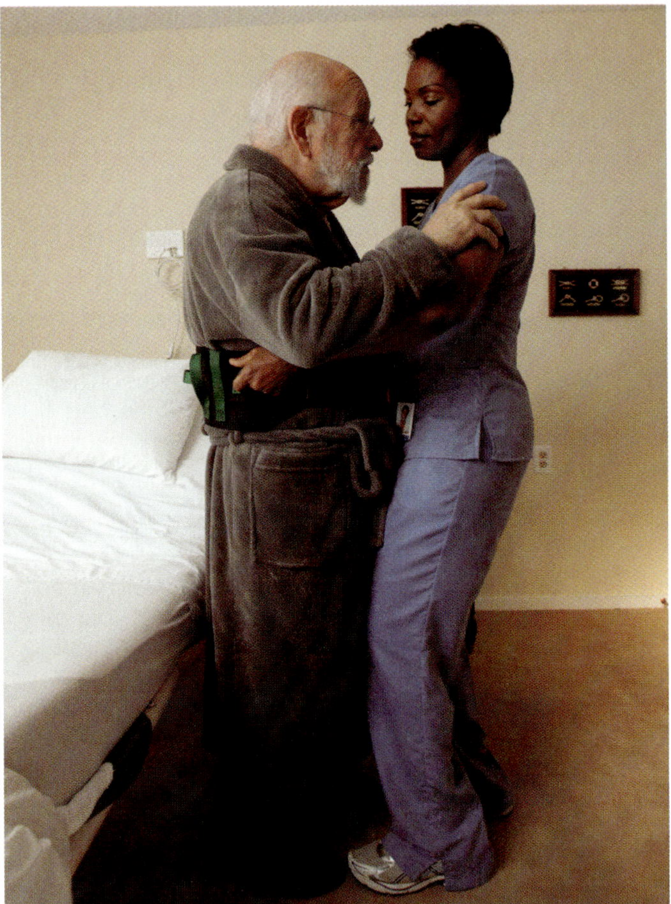

Figure 4

14. Tell the person to place his arms on your upper arms or shoulders to steady himself during the move. Taking small steps, together, pivot around until the person is right in front of the chair. Ask the person to tell you when he can feel the chair against the back of his legs (Figure 5).

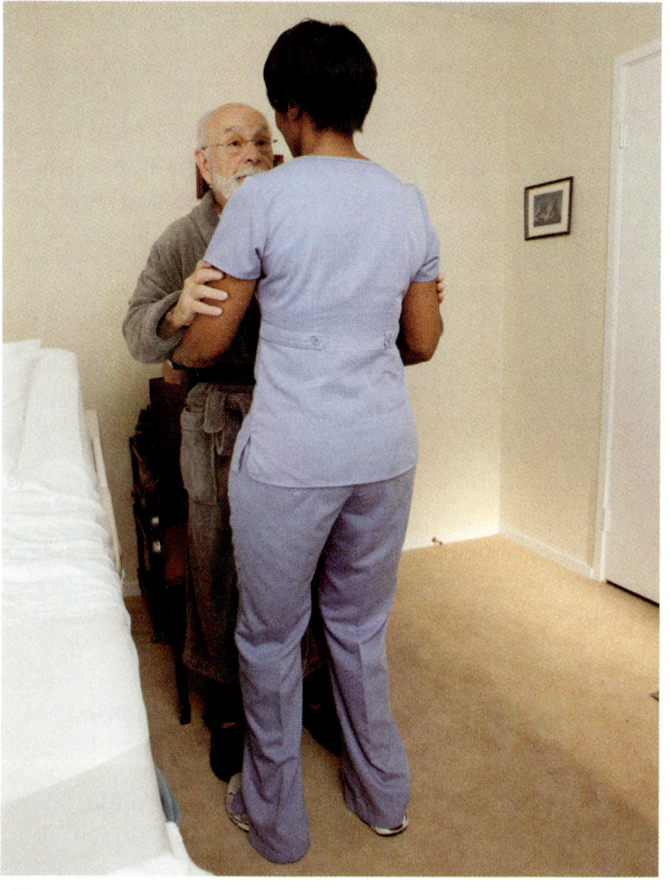

Figure 5

15. Help the person to feel for the arms of the chair, one arm at a time, while keeping your other arm around his waist for support. Put your head to the person's side closest to the chair so that you can keep the chair in sight during the move. Lower the person into the chair by bending your knees and keeping your back straight (Figure 6).

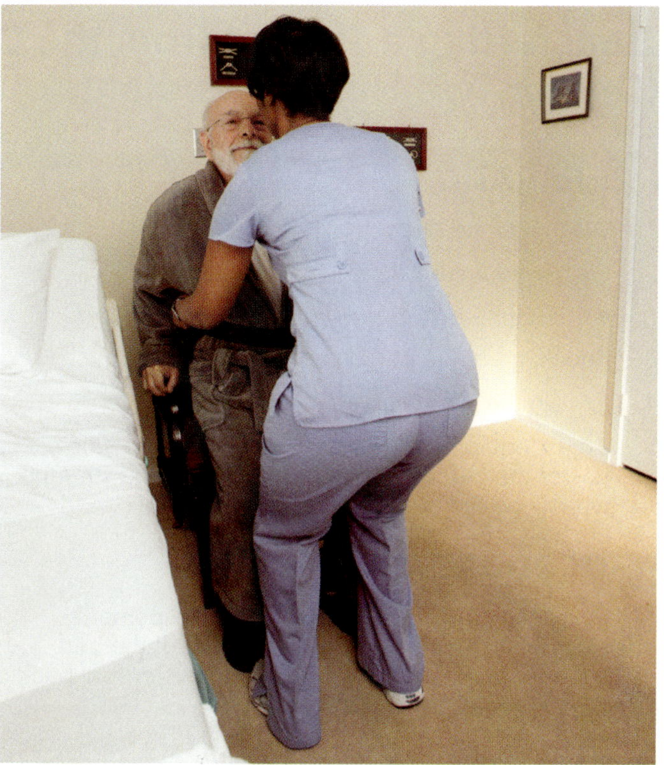

Figure 6

16. Assist the person to position himself in the chair so that his back is against the back of the chair. Place his feet on the footrests, if used.
17. Remove the transfer belt.

COMPLETION

18. Ensure the person's comfort and good body alignment.
19. Adjust equipment for safety: If the person is in a wheelchair, make sure the wheels on the wheelchair are locked. Place the person's method of calling for help within reach.
20. Clean up your work area.
21. Wash your hands.
22. Report and record.

Skill 12-11

Transferring a Person from the Chair to a Bed (One or Two Nurse Assistants)

PREPARATION

1. Wash your hands.
2. Gather your supplies:
    - Transfer belt
3. Knock, greet the person and ensure privacy.
4. Explain the procedure.
5. Adjust equipment for body mechanics and safety: Lower the bed to its lowest position. Make sure the wheels on the bed are locked.

PROCEDURE

6. Place the chair against the bed on the person's stronger side so that it faces the foot of the bed. If the person is in a wheelchair, remove or fold back the footrests and lock the brakes.
7. Raise the head of the bed.
8. Put the transfer belt on the person.
9. Face the person and position your feet so that one foot is about 12 inches in front of your other foot. Help the person move to the front of the seat so that she is able to place her feet flat on the floor.
10. Prepare the person to stand up.
    - **Option A:** Grasp the transfer belt on the back side of the person's waist.
    - **Option B:** If you are not using a transfer belt, put your arms underneath the person's arms and place your hands on her shoulder blades.
    - **Option C:** If you have help from a co-worker, have your co-worker grasp one side of the transfer belt on the back side of the person's waist, while you grasp the other. Alternatively, each of you can place one arm underneath the person's arm, resting your hand on the person's shoulder blade.
11. Block the person's lower extremities to prevent her from slipping. To do this, face the person, placing your feet "toe-to-toe." Turn your toes slightly outward to create a supportive base, and position your foot closest to the chair farther back than the other foot. Bend your knees deeply so that they rest against or near the person's knees. Have the person lean forward toward you. If you are working with a co-worker, each of you blocks one of the person's feet.
12. Tell the person that on your count of 3, she can push down on the arms of the chair with her hands while you assist her to a standing position. On your count of 3, straighten your legs, helping to lift the person to a standing position.
13. Tell the person to place her arms on your upper arms or shoulders to steady herself during the move. Taking small steps, together, pivot around until the person is in front of the bed. Ask the person to tell you when she can feel the bed against the back of her legs.
14. Help the person to sit on the edge of the bed. Put your head to the person's side closest to the bed so that you can keep the bed in sight during the move. Lower the person onto the bed by bending your knees and keeping your back straight.
15. Remove the transfer belt, the person's robe and the person's footwear.
16. Move the wheelchair out of the way.
17. With your knees bent and back straight, put one of your arms across the person's upper back and the other arm under her thighs. On your count of 3, pivot your feet to turn the person so that she is lying on the bed.

COMPLETION

18. Ensure the person's comfort and good body alignment.
19. Adjust equipment for safety: Make sure the wheels on the bed are locked. Place the person's method of calling for help within reach. Lower or raise the side rails according to the person's care plan.
20. Clean up your work area.
21. Wash your hands.
22. Report and record.

Skill 12-12
Using a Mechanical Lift to Transfer a Person (Two Nurse Assistants)

PREPARATION

1. Wash your hands.
2. Gather your supplies:
   - Mechanical lift
   - Sling in the correct size for the person
   - Wheelchair or chair
   - The person's robe, and her slippers or shoes
3. Knock, greet the person and ensure privacy.
4. Explain the procedure.
5. Adjust equipment for body mechanics and safety: Raise the bed to a comfortable working height. Make sure the wheels on the bed are locked.

PROCEDURE

6. Place the chair against the bed on the person's stronger side so that it faces the foot of the bed. If you are using a wheelchair, remove or fold back the footrests and lock the brakes.
7. Ask your co-worker to stand on one side of the bed while you stand on the other side. Review the procedure with your co-worker.
8. Detach the sling from the lift and fanfold half of it.
9. Roll the person toward you and place the fanfolded part of the sling along his back, making sure it is smooth for comfort (Figure 1A). Make sure the top of the sling is under the person's shoulders and the bottom is at the person's knees. Roll the person over the fanfolds, toward your co-worker and onto the flat part of the sling. Pull the fanfolded sling toward you until it is completely unfolded (Figure 1B). Help the person lie flat.

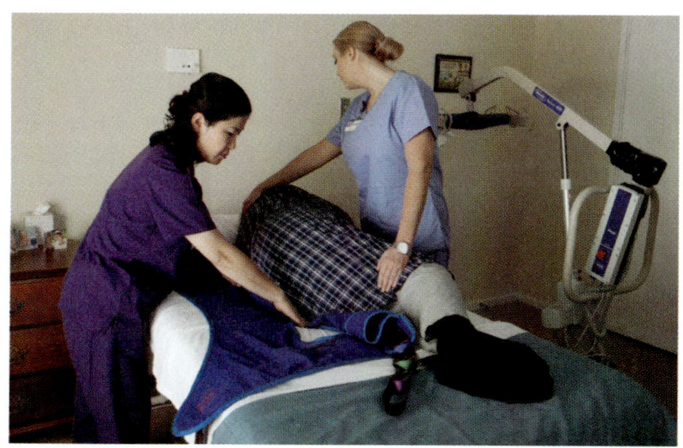

Figure 1A

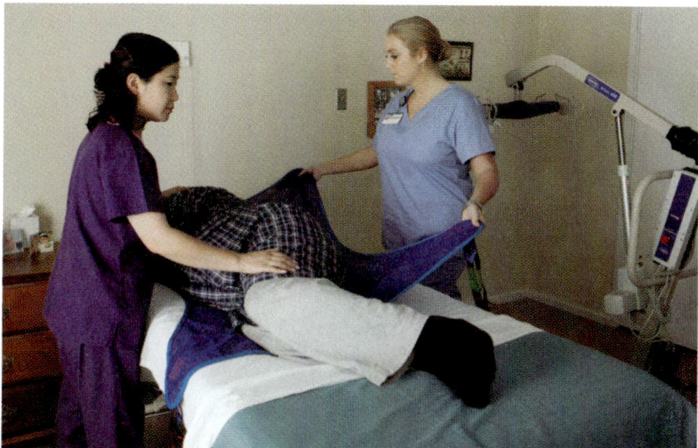

Figure 1B

Note: *You can help the person put on his bathrobe while he is turning from side to side. Make sure the person's clothing is wrinkle-free. Put the person's footwear on at this time too.*

10. Wheel the lift into place over the person. Spread the legs of the lift so that they are in their widest position to provide a wide base of support during the move. Lock the brakes on the lift.
11. Attach the sling to the mechanical lift according to the manufacturer's instructions (Figure 2).

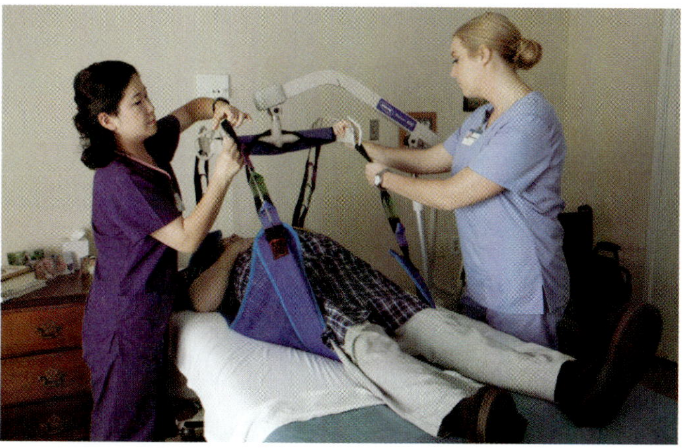

Figure 2

Continued on next page

Skill 12-12
Using a Mechanical Lift to Transfer a Person (Two Nurse Assistants) *Continued*

12. Tell the person he may place his arms across his chest or grasp the straps or chains. Use the crank, handle or electronic control on the lift to slowly lift the person from the bed (Figure 3).

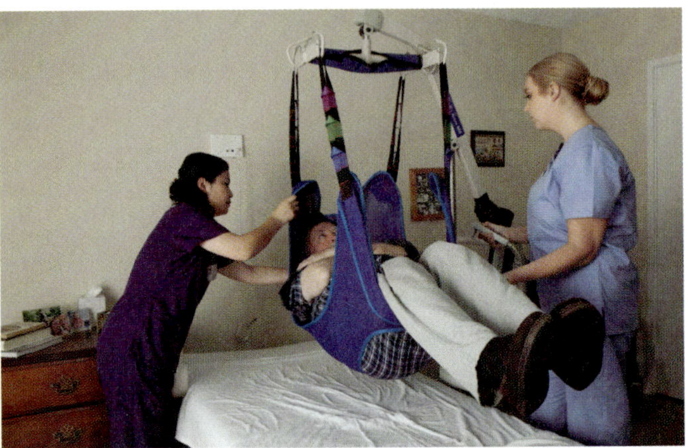

Figure 3

13. Release the brakes on the lift and move the lift away from the bed to the chair. Your co-worker makes sure that the person's body does not come in contact with the lift as you move him into position over the chair (Figure 4).

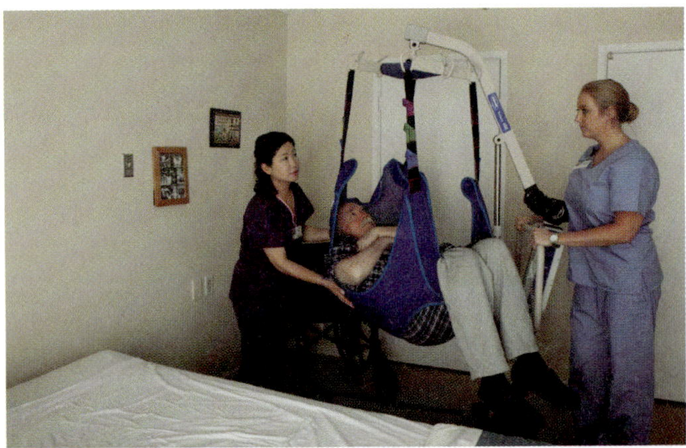

Figure 4

14. Lock the brakes on the lift. While you slowly lower the person into the chair, your co-worker guides and steadies the person so that he is properly seated in the chair (Figure 5). Make sure the person's back and buttocks are resting against the back of the chair. Place his feet on the footrests, if used.

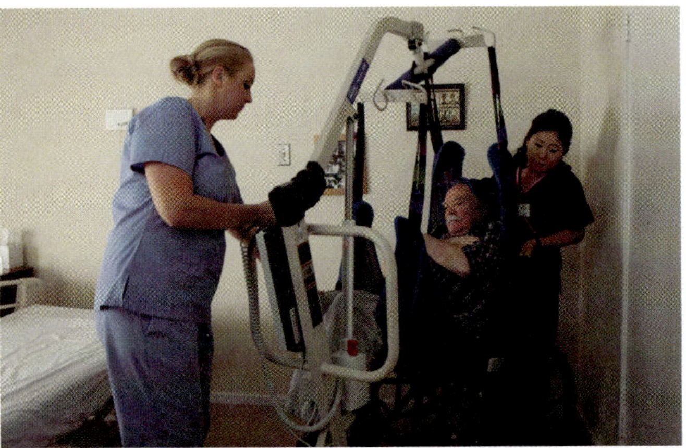

Figure 5

15. Remove the sling from the lift. You may keep the sling under the person, in preparation for using the lift to move the person back to the bed later. Make sure the fabric of the sling is wrinkle-free.

COMPLETION

16. Ensure the person's comfort and good body alignment.
17. Adjust equipment for safety: If the person is in a wheelchair, make sure the wheels on the wheelchair are locked. Place the person's method of calling for help within reach.
18. Clean up your work area.
19. Wash your hands.
20. Report and record.

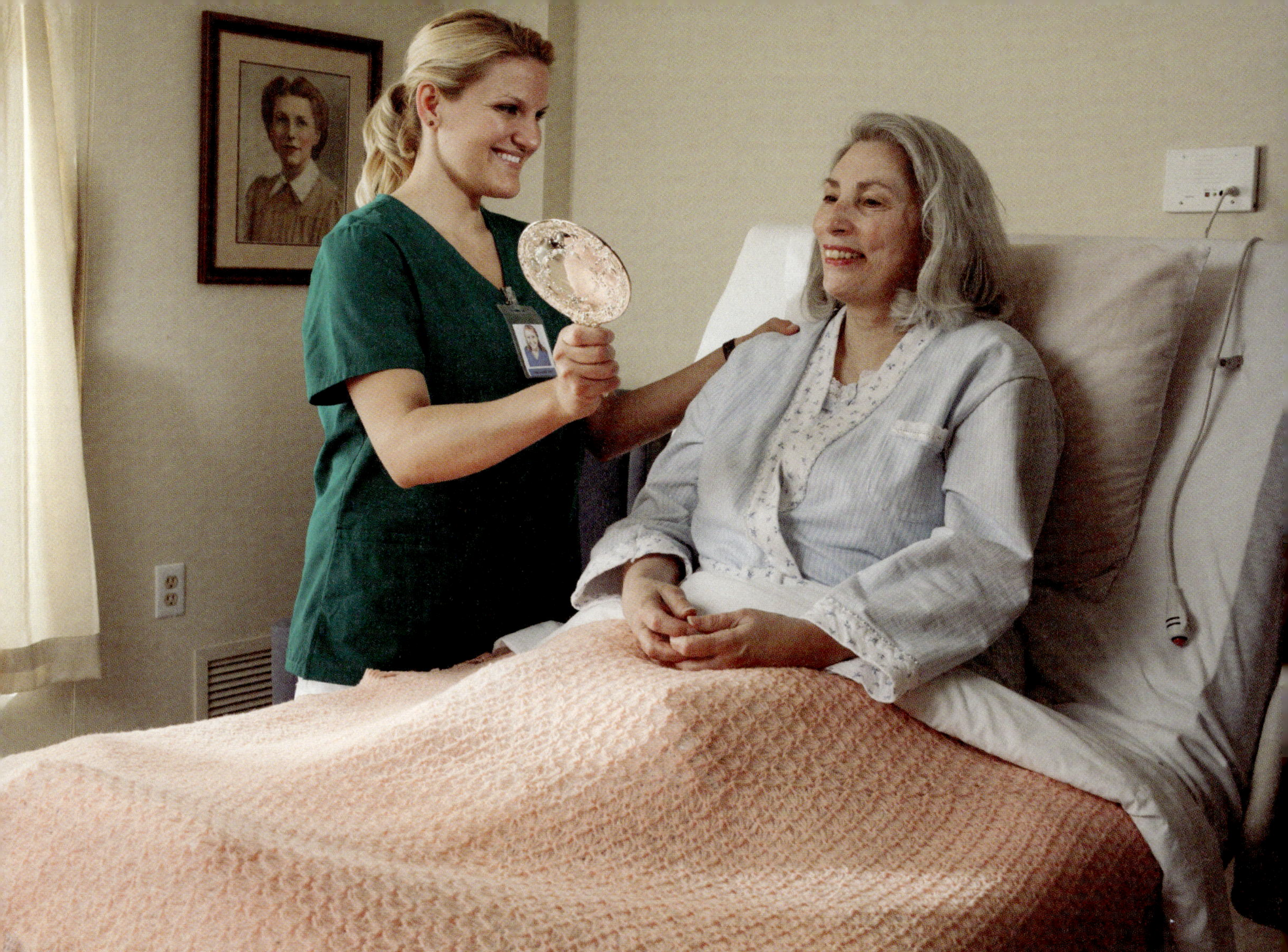

Assisting with Personal Cleanliness and Grooming

CHAPTER 13

Goals

After reading this chapter, you will have the information needed to:

- Understand how personal care can affect a person's physical and emotional health.
- Incorporate the five principles of care when assisting a person with personal care.
- List observations that should be reported when assisting a person with personal care.
- Explain why mouth care is important, and describe when mouth care should be provided.
- Explain how to maintain the hair.
- Explain how to assist a person with shaving, and describe safety measures that should be observed.

Continued on next page

Continued from previous page

- Explain general principles to follow when assisting a person with dressing or undressing.
- Explain how to assist a person with maintaining vision and hearing aids.
- Explain why hand care and foot care are important.
- Explain general principles to follow when assisting a person with perineal care.
- Explain the benefits of bathing.
- Explain the benefits of a back rub.

Goals

After practicing the corresponding skills, you will have the information needed to:

- Assist a person with natural teeth, a person with dentures and an unconscious person with mouth care.
- Brush and comb a person's hair.
- Wash a person's hair in bed.
- Assist a person with shaving using a safety razor and an electric razor.
- Assist a person to dress and undress.
- Assist a person to insert and remove an in-the-ear hearing aid.
- Assist a person with hand and foot care.
- Assist a person with perineal care.
- Give a person a complete bed bath.
- Assist a person with a shower or tub bath.
- Give a person a back rub.

Key Terms:

aspiration
depilatory
cuticles
hangnail
ingrown toenail
podiatrist
perineal care
circumcision

Whenever you see Mrs. Winnie Steele, one of your residents at Morningside Nursing Home, you are always impressed by how nice she looks and the care she takes with her appearance. Even though heart failure has slowed her down considerably and made even the most routine tasks challenging for her, she still makes the effort needed to maintain her appearance. Mrs. Steele has olive skin and black hair, which she has professionally washed and styled every Wednesday at Morningside's hair salon. She favors sweater sets in bright jewel tones, such as emerald green, turquoise blue and ruby red, paired with white or black dress slacks. Every day, she chooses jewelry or a scarf to accessorize her outfit perfectly, and she never leaves her room without first applying her signature shade of lipstick.

As a nurse assistant, you will help the people in your care with the activities necessary for maintaining personal cleanliness and a neat, well-cared-for appearance. Personal cleanliness (hygiene), which is achieved through regularly washing the body and hair and brushing the teeth, is important for both physical and emotional health. These activities help to keep the skin, hair and mouth healthy by removing infection-causing microbes. In addition, keeping the body and mouth clean prevents odors, which is important for self-esteem. Grooming activities, such as dressing, shaving, and styling the hair, help to maintain a neat appearance and are also important for maintaining a person's emotional health. When you help a person with personal hygiene and grooming activities, you help the person feel confident and attractive. A person who feels confident and attractive is more likely to socialize with others, and feel better about himself or herself in general. Think about how you felt on a day when you knew you looked your best, versus how you felt on a day when you had to rush through your normal personal care activities!

The way we appear to others says a lot about who we are and how we view ourselves. The decisions we make that affect our outward appearance, such as how we choose to style our hair or what clothes we choose to wear, are deeply personal because they are so closely tied to our self-image and self-esteem. Cultural and religious beliefs can influence the decisions a person makes about his or her outward appearance. So can the person's feelings about his or her own sexuality. Many of the people in your care will need your help to maintain personal cleanliness and a neat appearance. However, this does not mean that they have given up the desire to make their own decisions concerning hygiene and grooming. When you are assisting with personal care, always try to find out the person's preferences and honor them.

In health care facilities, activities related to personal hygiene and grooming usually take place at predictable times (Table 13-1). Scheduling of these activities is necessary because they must be accomplished in addition to other routine events throughout the day, such as meals, therapy sessions and social events. It is still possible, however, to take an individual's preferences into account when scheduling these activities. For example, some people may prefer to bathe in the evening instead of in the morning. It is important to try and accommodate the person's preferences as much as possible when scheduling care. Also, be aware that often, care related to personal hygiene and grooming is provided outside of the regularly scheduled time. For example, if a person spills food on her blouse while eating, you will help her to change her blouse after the meal.

Illness or disability can make it difficult for a person to maintain her normal personal care routines. For many people, it can be difficult or embarrassing to accept help with activities of such a private, personal nature. Imagine what it would feel like to have a stranger brush your teeth, bathe you, comb your hair and dress you. Be sensitive to the person's feelings, and remember to provide restorative care by encouraging the person to do as much for himself as he is able. This is important for the person's self-esteem and sense of independence.

Table 13-1 **Scheduling of Routine Personal Care and Grooming Activities**

Type of Care	When It Is Provided	What It Includes
Early Morning Care	After the person wakes up, in preparation for breakfast	Toileting Mouth care Washing the face and hands Brushing the hair Dressing
Morning Care	After breakfast, in preparation for the rest of the day	Toileting Mouth care Bathing Washing and styling the hair Shaving Dressing Bedmaking
Afternoon Care	Before and after lunch and dinner, in preparation for these meals and other activities, such as visiting hours or social events	Toileting Mouth care Washing the face and hands Brushing the hair
Evening Care	Before bed	Toileting Mouth care Washing the face and hands Changing into sleepwear Back rub

Today, Mrs. Steele's daughter is coming to take her mother to afternoon tea at a local hotel. Mrs. Steele is excited about seeing her daughter. She tells you that she has decided to wear a purple dress, because it looks nice with a scarf her daughter gave her for her birthday. While you are helping Mrs. Steele with her early morning care, she reminds you that her daughter is coming today and asks if you can help her get ready before her daughter arrives at 2:00. She says she is going to need help changing clothes, tying the scarf and styling her hair. You have a busy day ahead, but you tell Mrs. Steele that you will come by around 1:15 to help her get ready for her daughter's visit.

If you were a visitor to Morningside Nursing Home and saw Mrs. Steele in the common area, what opinions would you form about her well-being and the care she is receiving?

You agree to spend a little extra time to help Mrs. Steele get ready for the outing with her daughter. Why is this important? Do you think Mrs. Steele would enjoy the visit with her daughter as much if her hair weren't styled the way she likes it, or if she was wearing an outfit she didn't pick out herself? Why or why not?

MOUTH CARE

When you get up in the morning, how does your mouth feel? What do your teeth feel like after you eat a meal? Part of your responsibility in assisting with personal care is to help provide mouth care, also called *oral hygiene*. Mouth care includes care of the teeth, gums, tongue, lips and soft parts of the inside of the mouth, such as the cheeks and the roof of the mouth.

Good oral hygiene is necessary to keep the mouth and the body healthy. Regular brushing and flossing helps to remove plaque, a sticky, colorless layer of bacteria that forms on the teeth. Sugars and starches in the food we eat cause the bacteria in plaque to grow. These bacteria can cause bad breath odors. In addition, they produce acids, which destroy the outer surface of the tooth, leading to tooth decay. If plaque is not removed by brushing the teeth, it hardens into tartar. Tartar can cause gum irritation and infection, as well as tooth decay and loss. The same bacteria that cause gum inflammation and infection can also cause inflammation and infection in other parts of the body, putting the person at risk for heart disease, stroke and other serious conditions. In addition to removing harmful bacteria, regular mouth care also helps to keep the tissues of the oral cavity moist. A dry mouth is uncomfortable and can alter the taste of food and beverages, making them less appealing.

ELDER CARE NOTE. Good mouth care is important for people of all ages, but it is especially important for older people. Saliva helps to keep bacteria from sticking to the surfaces of the teeth. However, as we age, saliva production decreases, leading to a dry mouth. Medications that older people commonly take, such as those used to treat high blood pressure, can also decrease saliva production. In addition to allowing plaque to build up faster, a dry mouth is uncomfortable and can make food less appealing. For these reasons, regular mouth care is particularly important for the older people in your care.

At minimum, assist those in your care with mouth care:

- Every morning
- Every evening
- After each meal
- Every 2 hours, if the person is unconscious, on "nothing by mouth" (NPO) status, on oxygen therapy or breathes through the mouth (all of these conditions can cause the mouth to become dry and uncomfortable)
- After the person vomits

Assistive devices, such as toothbrushes with built-up handles or electric toothbrushes, may enable some people to provide for their own mouth care independently (Figure 13-1). Others will need varying amounts of assistance from you to ensure that they receive the proper mouth care. When assisting with mouth care, follow standard precautions, and take the opportunity to observe for changes that could indicate a health problem.

Observations Into Action!

Whenever you assist a person with mouth care, observe for changes in the person's mouth that could be a sign of a problem. Report any of the following to the nurse:

- **Swollen, red or tender gums**
- **Bleeding gums**
- **White patches**
- **Sores**
- **Painful or sensitive areas**
- **Ill-fitting or broken dentures**
- **Bad breath that does not go away**

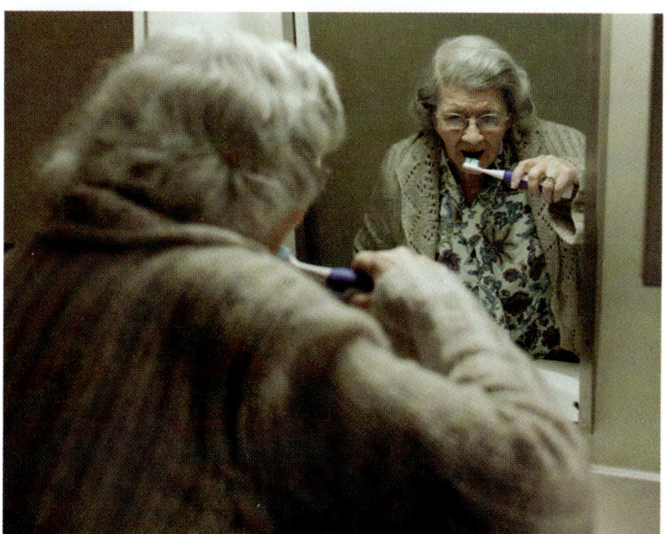

Figure 13-1 Some people may be able to manage their own mouth care, if you set them up with the necessary supplies.

Mouth Care for a Person with Natural Teeth

Natural teeth are cared for using a soft-bristled toothbrush, toothpaste and dental floss. The soft bristles of the toothbrush remove plaque and food particles from the teeth and tongue and stimulate circulation in the gums, which helps keep them healthy. The toothbrush should be replaced every 3 to 4 months, or when it begins to show wear. A toothbrush with worn or frayed bristles does not properly clean the teeth and may injure the gums. Unless instructed otherwise, use a toothpaste that contains fluoride (a chemical that helps to strengthen the tooth enamel and prevent tooth decay). In some regions of the United States where the water contains high levels of fluoride, dentists may recommend using toothpaste that does not contain fluoride. After brushing, dental floss is used to remove plaque and food particles from between the teeth. Waxed dental floss slides between the teeth more easily than unwaxed dental floss does. Before flossing a person's teeth, check with the nurse or review the person's care plan to see whether there are any restrictions or special precautions to be considered. For example, some people taking certain medications may bleed excessively if their teeth are flossed. Skill 13-1 describes step by step how to provide mouth care for a person with natural teeth.

Mouth Care for a Person with Dentures

Many people have dentures (false teeth). Complete (full) dentures replace all of the top teeth or all of the bottom teeth. Partial dentures replace only a few teeth. Wearing dentures decreases gum shrinkage after teeth have been removed and maintains the shape of the mouth. With dentures in place, it is easier for the person to chew food properly and speak clearly.

Keeping the soft tissues of the person's mouth healthy and the dentures clean is important for health and also makes it more likely that the person will want to wear the dentures. Dentures are cleaned by brushing them with a special toothpaste made for dentures. Some people may also soak their dentures in a denture-cleansing solution as part of their denture-cleaning routine. Dentures that have been soaking in a denture-cleansing solution should be brushed and thoroughly rinsed before placing them in the person's mouth. A soft mouth sponge is used to clean the soft tissues of the mouth after the dentures are removed for cleaning. Caring for the soft tissues of the person's mouth keeps the tissue healthy and helps to ensure that the dentures continue to fit properly.

Dentures are removed for cleaning and, ideally, for at least 8 hours every day (usually overnight) to rest the gums. However, some people may prefer to wear their dentures at all times and only remove them for cleaning. When the person is not wearing the dentures, they should be stored in a labeled denture cup in water or denture-cleansing solution to prevent warping. Always handle a person's dentures carefully, so that they do not chip or break. Also, take care not to lose the person's dentures. Dentures are expensive and time-consuming to replace, because they are custom-made for the person. To make it easier to return dentures to their owner should they be misplaced in a health care setting, many dentists label the dentures with the person's initials or some other identification code when they are made. Denture-labeling kits are also available and can be used if the dentures were not labeled at the time of manufacture.

Skill 13-2 describes step-by-step how to provide mouth care for a person with dentures.

Mouth Care for a Person Who Is Unconscious

An unconscious person is not able to respond to her environment and will be totally reliant on you for mouth care. People who are unconscious breathe through their mouths, which causes drying of the soft tissues of the mouth and leads to the build-up of mucus and other secretions on the teeth and tongue. You must provide mouth care for an unconscious person every 2 hours throughout the day and night to remove these secretions and prevent the mouth from becoming excessively dry.

When providing mouth care for a person who is unconscious, elevate the head of the bed (if allowed) and turn the person's head to the side to allow fluids to run out of the mouth instead of down the person's throat. This is important to prevent **aspiration** (inhalation of fluids or other foreign materials into the lungs). Aspiration can lead to pneumonia. Use a mouth sponge to clean the soft tissues of the person's mouth and a soft-bristled toothbrush moistened with water or a mixture of mouthwash and water to clean the person's teeth. Remember to tell the person what you are doing as you are doing it. Even though the person cannot respond to you, he may be aware that something is being done to him. Skill 13-3 describes step-by-step how to provide mouth care for a person who is unconscious.

HAIR CARE

Hair care, which includes washing, brushing, combing and styling the hair, is necessary to keep the hair and scalp healthy, and to maintain a neat appearance. Washing the hair (shampooing) removes dirt, oil and bacteria from the hair and scalp. Brushing, combing and styling the hair helps to prevent painful tangles from forming and provides for a neat appearance. Many long-term care facilities have salons where residents can go to have their hair professionally cut, washed and styled. Many residents will choose to take advantage of this service, but you will be responsible for helping the person with hair care in between visits to the salon.

People often have strong preferences regarding what products are used to care for their hair. For example, some people may prefer a certain type of shampoo, or like to use a conditioning rinse in addition to shampoo. People of African descent, who often have very curly hair and dry scalps, may use oils, creams or lotions to make the hair easier to comb and to moisturize the scalp. These products are usually applied to the scalp after shampooing and then massaged into the scalp and hair. When assisting a person with hair care, find out what products the person likes to use, and honor those preferences as much as possible.

Brushing, Combing and Styling the Hair

A comb with widely spaced, blunt teeth is used to remove tangles from wet or dry hair. A brush is used on dry hair to neaten the appearance of the hair. To prevent hair from breaking and to detangle the ends, start brushing or combing from the ends of the hair, working toward the scalp, and work in small sections. If the hair is very tangled, wet the hair and apply conditioner before combing, and then wash and rinse the hair after you have removed all the tangles. Remember to comb and brush hair gently so that you do not pull it out. With age, hair becomes drier and more fragile. In addition, some medications and medical treatments cause hair to become brittle or fall out.

When styling a person's hair, be sure to ask about the person's preferences and follow them as closely as you can. For example, most people have a preferred side for parting their hair. Provide the person with a mirror, so that she can see what you are doing. If you must make decisions about how to style a person's hair for the person, choose an age-appropriate, attractive style. Some people with very curly hair may find it easier to keep their hair tangle-free if it is braided. Check with the person to make sure that she wants her hair braided. If she does, be careful not to braid the hair too tightly, because hair tends to draw tighter as it dries and may pull too tightly on the scalp.

Skill 13-4 explains the procedure for brushing and combing a person's hair.

Shampooing the Hair

Shampooing cleans the scalp and hair and stimulates blood flow to the scalp. Many people find it very relaxing to have the head and scalp gently massaged as part of the shampoo, and having clean hair can help a person to feel better in general.

How often the hair is washed varies from person to person. Older people tend to have drier skin and hair and are usually less active than younger people, so they may only need to wash their hair once or twice a week. People with oily skin and hair or people who are very active may need to wash their hair every day. Take into account the person's preferences and your employer's policies when working out a schedule for shampooing the person's hair. Also, be aware that sometimes an unscheduled shampoo can help a person to feel better (for example, if the person is feverish and the hair has become sweaty).

Shampooing is often accomplished in the shower or tub while bathing. If the person is unable to get out of bed, his hair can be washed while he is in the bed using a shampoo tray (a device that funnels the water into a wash basin placed on a chair or the floor beside the bed) (Figure 13-2, A). If a shampoo tray is not available (for example, in the home setting), one can be improvised using a large plastic trash bag. Place a rolled towel inside the bag. Twist it into a C shape. Place the person's head in the center of the C. Drape the sheet or bag toward the side of the bed so that water drains into a washbasin placed on a chair. Skill 13-5 describes step-by-step how to wash a person's hair in bed using a shampoo tray. A shampoo cap can also be used to wash a person's hair in bed (see Figure 13-2, B). The cap, which contains a rinse-free cleanser, is placed over the person's hair, and the hair and scalp are massaged through the cap to remove dirt and oils.

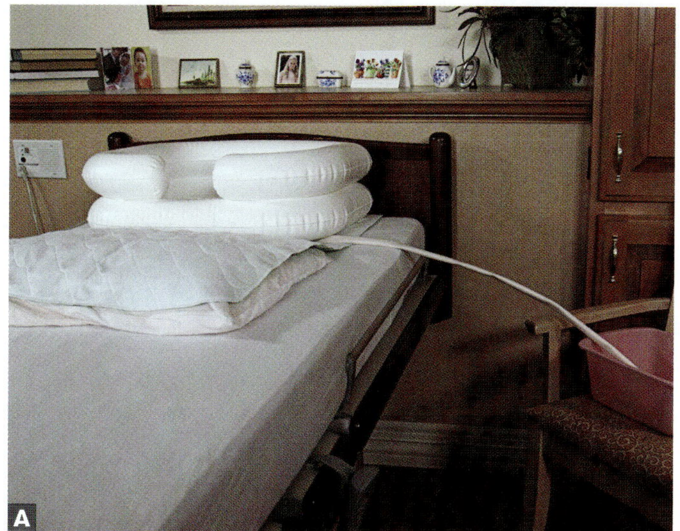

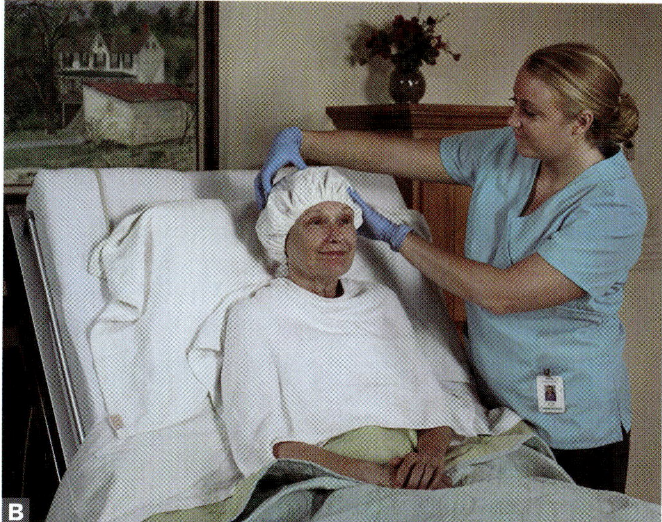

Figure 13-2 A person's hair can be washed in bed using (A) a shampoo tray or (B) a shampoo cap.

Observations Into Action!

Whenever you assist a person with hair care, observe for unusual conditions. Report any of the following to the nurse:

- **Sores on the person's scalp**
- **Unusual flaking or dandruff**
- **Excessive hair loss**
- **Tangles that cannot be removed**

SHAVING

Shaving is done to remove unwanted hair from the body. Many men shave their faces daily, either in the morning or at bedtime, to remove facial hair. Skill 13-6 describes how to help a man to shave his face. Women may shave leg and underarm hair. This type of shaving is most easily done at bath time.

Removal of unwanted hair can be accomplished in a variety of ways. A safety razor is used with warm water and shaving cream, gel or soap. An electric razor is used after applying a pre-shave lotion. Men who have very curly beards may prefer not to shave, but to use a **depilatory** cream or powder to chemically dissolve and remove facial hair. Many women also use a depilatory product to remove unwanted leg, underarm or facial hair.

Shaving with a Safety Razor

When using a safety razor, it is easy to nick the skin, causing bleeding. Because people with certain medical disorders or who are taking certain medications can bleed excessively if they are cut, check the person's care plan or ask the nurse before assisting a person to shave with a safety razor. For people with conditions that can cause them to bleed excessively, an electric razor is usually preferred.

Before helping a person to shave using a safety razor, inspect the skin for moles or other raised areas. Shave carefully around these areas to avoid scraping or cutting them, which could cause bleeding. Apply shaving cream, gel or soap to soften the hair and help the razor glide over the skin. Many men will prefer to finish the shave by applying aftershave lotion, which has a nice scent and helps to soothe the skin. The alcohol in most aftershave lotions also acts as an antiseptic and can help to stop bleeding from small nicks or cuts. If a nick or cut does occur while shaving, report this to the nurse.

Always take standard precautions when helping a person to shave with a safety razor. Because blood particles may be left on the razor blade and can spread infection, make sure each person has his own safety razor. When the blade on a safety razor becomes dull, it is more likely to nick the person's skin. Depending on the type of safety razor, the entire unit may be disposable, or you may just need to replace the blade. Always handle razors and blades carefully to avoid nicking yourself, and dispose of them properly in a sharps container. To store a safety razor between uses, place it blade-end down in a container without recapping it. You may accidentally cut yourself if you attempt to recap the razor.

Shaving with an Electric Razor

An electric razor lifts the hair away from the skin before slicing it off with the blade. Thus, an electric razor carries a lower risk of cutting or nicking the skin and is preferred for people with blood-clotting disorders and those who are taking medications that affect the blood's ability to clot. Applying a pre-shave lotion can help to soften the hairs and may result in a smoother shave when using an electric razor.

Electric razors are small appliances, so remember to take the same precautions when using them that you would with any electrical appliance. Inspect the razor before using it to make sure that the cord is not frayed and that it is operating normally. If the razor is malfunctioning (for example, it stops and starts, or is making a strange sound), do not use it. Check with the nurse before using an electric razor in a room where a person is receiving oxygen therapy, because an electrical spark could ignite a fire. (It may be safe to use a battery-operated or rechargeable electrical razor in these circumstances, but check with the nurse first.) To keep the razor in good working order, take it apart and clean it after each use.

DRESSING AND UNDRESSING

Clothing changes occur several times throughout the day. At minimum, people usually change clothing in preparation for the day ahead and in preparation for sleep. In addition, whenever an article of clothing becomes soiled or wet, it must be changed.

Many people will be able to dress and undress with minimal assistance from you. Assistive devices such as shoehorns, buttoning aids and zipper pulls can help a person function more independently with dressing and undressing. So can choosing clothing that is easier for the person to put on and take off. For example, pants with elastic waistbands may be easier for a person to manage than pants with zippers, buttons or ties.

For some people who are receiving health care, it can be very difficult to make the effort required to get dressed each day. However, it is important to encourage them to do so, unless they are very ill. Getting dressed every day helps people to maintain their sense of identity and purpose. Encourage the person to do as much as he can, and provide help as needed.

It is also important to allow people to make their own decisions about what they want to wear (Figure 13-3). If the person has trouble making decisions, limit the number of choices, but still allow the person to choose. When helping a person select clothing, consider:

- The person's preferences.
- The person's physical capabilities.
- What the person will be doing that day.
- The weather and the season.

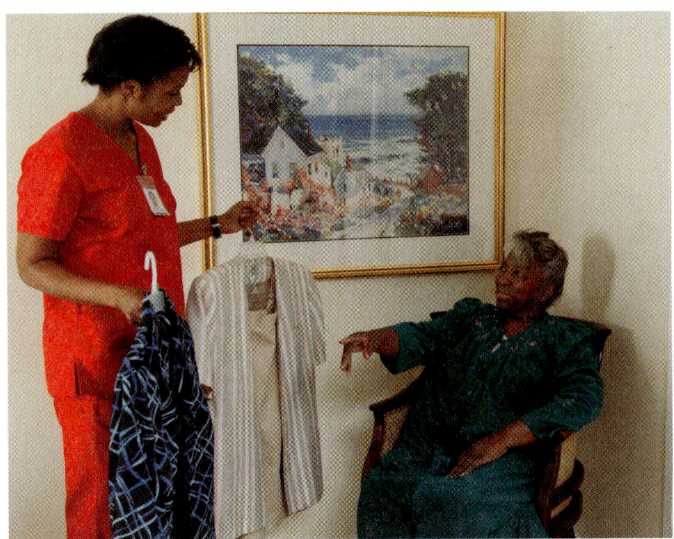

Figure 13-3 Allow the people in your care to choose what clothing they will wear whenever possible.

Clothing should fit properly and be in good condition. If you notice that an article of clothing is stained, ripped, torn, missing buttons or in need of alterations to make it fit properly, talk to the nurse so that arrangements can be made to have the clothing cleaned, altered, repaired or replaced.

Skill 13-7 describes how to help a person to put on and take off clothing. Sometimes there will be special circumstances that you must take into account when helping a person to dress. When helping a person with a weak, paralyzed or injured arm or leg to dress, put the garment on the affected arm or leg first. Then, do the opposite when you are helping the person to undress: Remove the garment from the affected arm or leg last.

Some people will be required to wear compression stockings. These stockings, which are made of tight-fitting elastic, compress (squeeze) the veins in the legs. Compressing the veins in the legs helps to return blood to the heart, preventing complications such as blood clots. Because they are so tight, these stockings can be very difficult for a person to put on independently. Skill 13-8 describes how to assist a person with putting on compression stockings. These stockings must be put on before the person gets out of bed in the morning. If the person has been standing, have her sit in a chair with the legs elevated for 15 minutes before putting on the stockings. Compression stockings usually have an opening across the top of the toes. This opening is so that you can check the person's toes for changes that might suggest poor circulation to the toes, such as a bluish color or coldness. Check the person's circulation hourly. If you note that the toes are pale, blue or cold, or the person complains of numbness or tingling in the feet, report these signs and symptoms to the nurse.

At 1:15, you go to Mrs. Steele's room as promised. She has gotten the dress and scarf she wants to wear out of the closet and laid them on the bed. You pull the privacy curtain, and help Mrs. Steele sit on the edge of the bed and get out of the clothes she is wearing. While you are helping Mrs. Steele get ready, you chat with her about her daughter and about how excited she is for this visit. Mrs. Steele is able to put her slip on by herself, but she needs your help pulling her stockings up. After you help her with her stockings, Mrs. Steele pulls the dress over her head, and you help her zip it up the back. Next, you arrange the scarf around her neck and tie it the way you know she likes it tied. You smile and say, "Here's a hand mirror, Mrs. Steele. Did I get it right?" Mrs. Steele checks the mirror, smiles back and says, "It's perfect, dear." You hand Mrs. Steele her hair brush and say, "Let me hold the mirror for you while you brush your hair. We messed it up a bit when we pulled that dress over your head." Mrs. Steele brushes her hair, and then you help her to put her shoes on. Just then, Mrs. Steele's daughter knocks and calls out, "Mom? OK if I come in?" You pull back the privacy curtain and open the door. "Mom, you look beautiful as always," says Mrs. Steele's daughter as she enters the room. "Are you all ready to go?"

Why do you think it is important for Mrs. Steele's daughter to see her mother looking "beautiful as always"? Do you think she would be concerned if there were a change in Mrs. Steele's usual neat, well-cared-for appearance? Why or why not?

What are some of the advantages of talking with the people in your care while you assist them with personal care?

VISION AND HEARING AIDS

Many of the people in your care will use vision aids (such as eyeglasses or contact lenses), hearing aids or both. These devices help the person interact with others and are therefore important to the person's overall quality of life. Although prosthetic (false) eyes do not help the person to see, they are important for helping the person maintain his or her appearance, and in that respect are important to the person's self-esteem and quality of life.

Eyeglasses

Eyeglasses are worn to correct vision problems. Encourage the people in your care who have glasses to wear them, especially when they are out of bed. This is important for safety.

Eyeglasses are expensive and it can be inconvenient to replace them if they become broken or lost, so always handle them carefully. When the person is not wearing them, they should be stored in their case. The person may need help keeping the glasses clean. Clean the glasses with soap and water or eyeglass-cleaning wipes, which are moistened with a cleansing agent meant specifically for cleaning eyeglasses. If soap and water are used to clean the glasses, dry them with a soft, clean cloth to avoid scratching the lenses.

! Observations Into Action!

When a person in your care wears eyeglasses, report any of the following observations to the nurse:

- **The person does not seem to be seeing well with the eyeglasses.**
- **The person states that the eyeglasses are "not working as well as they used to."**
- **The eyeglasses pinch or rub the person's nose or ears, or slip down the person's nose.**
- **The eyeglasses are in need of repair.**

Contact Lenses

Contact lenses are placed directly on the eye to correct vision. Some contact lenses are worn once and discarded, while others need to be cleaned daily. The solutions used to clean and store contact lenses vary, depending on the type of lens. If you need to help a person maintain his contact lenses, be sure you know what products to use. Because contact lenses are placed directly on the eye, it is very important to maintain them properly. A damaged or dirty contact lens can scratch the eye or cause an infection. Always wash your hands before handling a person's contact lenses.

Prosthetic (False) Eyes

A person who has had an eye removed due to illness or disease may choose to wear a prosthetic (false) eye. Prosthetic eyes are custom-made for the person and can be very expensive to replace. If a person in your care has a prosthetic eye and needs help caring for it, the nurse will show you how to assist the person with removing, cleaning and re-inserting the prosthesis. As with contact lenses, it is important to care for the prosthetic eye properly to prevent injury to the eye socket and eyelid. Always handle a prosthetic eye carefully, and with clean hands.

Hearing Aids

A person with impaired hearing may use a hearing aid. Hearing aids are battery-operated devices worn in or behind the ear to make sounds louder. Some of the people in your care may need help inserting or removing their hearing aids, and keeping them clean. Skill 13-9 describes how to insert and remove an in-the-ear hearing aid. You may also need to help the person to keep the hearing aid clean. Follow the manufacturer's instructions for cleaning. Make sure the person keeps an extra battery on hand, so that the battery can be replaced promptly when necessary.

Like other assistive devices, hearing aids are expensive to replace if they are lost or damaged. Moisture and hair care products (such as hair spray) can damage a hearing aid, so help the person to insert the hearing aid *after* providing hair care. Store the hearing aid in its case, and out of reach of children, pets and confused adults who might mistake the battery for something that can be swallowed.

HAND AND FOOT CARE

Hand and foot care involves cleaning and caring for the skin of the hands and feet, and keeping the nails trimmed and smooth. Many people who are receiving health care need help caring for their hands and feet. Skill 13-10 describes how to provide hand and foot care.

Caring for the Hands

You will help the people in your care to wash their hands before meals, after using the bathroom and whenever else it may seem necessary. Assisting with care for the fingernails is done as needed. Keeping the fingernails trimmed and smooth helps to prevent the person from accidentally scratching herself. Keeping the skin of the hands moisturized promotes comfort and helps to keep the **cuticles** (the skin along the edges of the nails) from becoming ragged and torn. **Hangnails** (ragged and torn cuticles) are painful and unsightly, and can become infected.

Soaking the nails in warm water softens them and makes them easier to trim. For this reason, nail care is often done following a bath or shower. However, you can assist a person with nail care any time by bringing a small basin of warm water to the bedside.

Equipment used when providing nail care includes:

- Nail clippers (used to trim the nails).
- An emery board (used to smooth rough edges).
- An orange stick (a wooden stick with an angled edge that is used to push the cuticles back and clean underneath the nails).

Trimming the person's fingernails may not be within your scope of practice. Even if trimming the fingernails is within your scope of practice, it may not be permitted with certain people (such as those who have diabetes or other conditions that can impair circulation and sensation). Check with the nurse or consult the person's care plan to make sure that you are allowed to trim the person's fingernails before doing so. If you are allowed to trim the nails, cut them straight across so that the edge of the nail extends slightly beyond the tip of the finger (Figure 13-4). Then, smooth the edges of the nails using the emery board.

Observations Into Action!

Assisting with hand care gives you a good opportunity to observe for changes that could be a sign of a medical problem. Report any of the following observations to the nurse:

- **Reddened or discolored areas**
- **Sores**
- **Hangnails**
- **Badly torn nails**
- **Nails that have an odd shape or are unusually thick**
- **Nail beds that are blue or pale, instead of pink**

Caring for the Feet

The feet have a large number of sweat glands. Washing and drying the feet and changing the socks regularly are important for comfort and to control odor. Keeping the nails trimmed and the edges smooth makes wearing footwear more comfortable.

Many of the people in your care will not be mobile enough to care for their own feet. In addition, many will have conditions such as diabetes that affect circulation and sensation in the feet. In a person with poor circulation and sensation in the feet, a small injury such

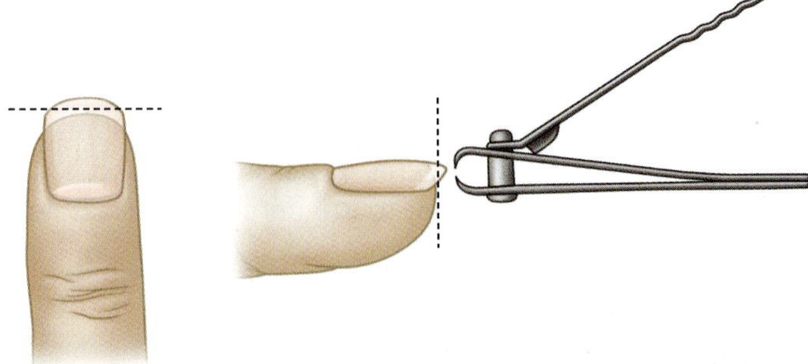

Figure 13-4 If trimming the person's fingernails is within your scope of practice, trim the nail straight across so that the nail extends slightly beyond the fingertip.

as a blister or an **ingrown toenail** can lead to a serious infection. (An ingrown toenail occurs when the toenail is trimmed too short and the edge curls down and grows into the neighboring skin.) Because sensation is impaired in the foot, the person may not even be aware of the injury.

With age, the toenails become thicker and more difficult to cut. In addition, many people have conditions such as diabetes that can make even a small injury to the foot very dangerous. Because it is easy to injure the person by trimming the toenails too short or nicking the skin around the toenail, and because such injuries can have serious consequences, trimming a person's toenails is usually outside of the scope of practice for a nursing assistant. Instead, a doctor who specializes in care of the feet (called a **podiatrist**) or a nurse is usually responsible for trimming the person's toenails.

Your responsibilities with regard to foot care include caring for the skin of the feet by washing the feet, drying them well, and applying lotion to avoid dryness and cracking. Foot care is often carried out during bath time, but it may also be done independent of a bath. While you are providing foot care, you will have an opportunity to inspect the feet for injuries or other problems. Report any unusual conditions to the nurse.

Observations Into Action!

Assisting with foot care gives you a good opportunity to observe for changes that could be a sign of a medical problem. Report any of the following:

- **Reddened or discolored areas**
- **Sores or blisters**
- **Breaks in the skin between the toes**
- **Toenails that need trimming**
- **Ill-fitting socks or shoes**

PERINEAL CARE

Perineal care is the cleansing of the area between the legs, including the genitals and the anus (Figure 13-5). Perineal care is provided during a bath or shower, but it may also be provided any time it is needed. For example, a person who is incontinent of urine or feces will need perineal care after each episode of incontinence. Urine and feces are very irritating to the skin and if not removed, they can lead to skin breakdown. Also, removing urine and feces from the skin is necessary to prevent odor and protect the person's dignity and self-esteem.

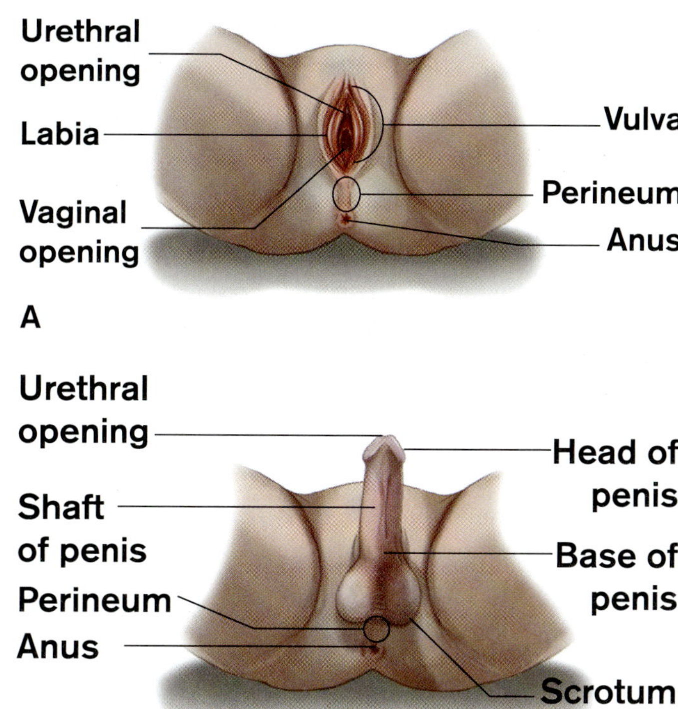

Figure 13-5 During perineal care, the genitals, perineum and anal region are cleansed. (A) Female anatomy. (B) Male anatomy.

When providing perineal care, it is especially important to take steps to protect the person's dignity and privacy. Always ask the person's permission first, and explain what you are going to do using words the person can understand. For example, you can say, "I'm going to clean the area between your legs now." Use a bath blanket to cover the person so that only the perineal area is exposed. Allow the person to provide for his or her own perineal care to the greatest extent possible.

Assisting a person with perineal care may also be embarrassing for you. Although these feelings are normal, if the person senses that you are embarrassed or uncomfortable, he or she will likely become embarrassed or uncomfortable, too. A straightforward, professional approach can help to put the person at ease. Think about how you would feel if you were unable to provide for your own perineal care. Would you feel better about the situation if the person helping you was kind, competent and professional?

Practice proper infection-control measures when providing perineal care. Wear gloves, because contact with body fluids is likely. Also, use proper technique for washing, rinsing and drying to avoid contaminating clean areas of the person's body with microbes from dirtier areas. The digestive tract contains microbes that are passed from the body with feces, through the anus. It is important not to contaminate other parts of the body, such as the urethra or vagina, with these

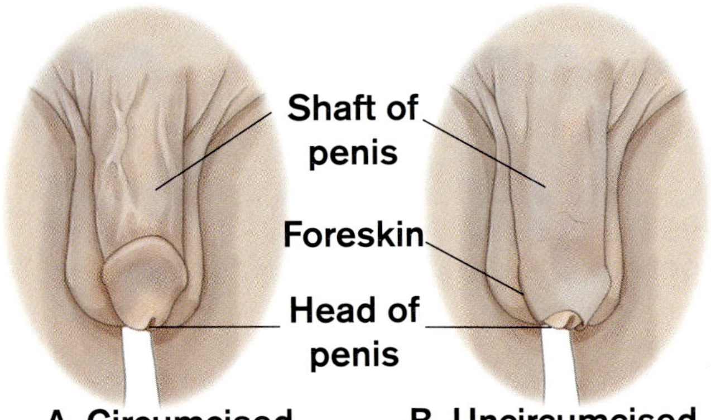

Figure 13-6 A man may be (A) uncircumcised or (B) circumcised.

microbes, because they can cause an infection if they are introduced into parts of the body where they do not normally live. When assisting a person with perineal care, wipe from front to back (that is, from the genitals to the anus; see Figure 13-5). Cleaning in this direction avoids contaminating the urethral opening (and the vaginal opening in women) with bacteria from the anal area.

Men may be uncircumcised or circumcised (Figure 13-6). **Circumcision** is the surgical removal of the foreskin (the fold of skin that covers the head of the penis). When providing perineal care for an uncircumcised man, you must pull the foreskin back to wash, rinse and dry the head of the penis. Always return the foreskin to its natural position after you are finished washing, rinsing and drying the head of the penis.

Skill 13-11 describes how to provide perineal care.

Observations Into Action!

Providing perineal care gives you a good opportunity to observe for changes that could be a sign of a medical problem. Report any of the following:

- **Redness or swelling**
- **Discharge**
- **Foul odor**
- **Person seems to be experiencing pain or discomfort during the procedure, or states that the procedure is painful or uncomfortable**

SKIN CARE

Bathing does a lot for a person: It refreshes and relaxes; eliminates body odor; removes dirt, oils and dead skin cells; and stimulates blood flow (circulation) through the body. Good blood flow to the skin helps to keep the skin healthy. A back rub, which is often provided as part of the bath, stimulates blood flow to the skin as well.

When and how a person chooses to bathe can be influenced by factors such as the person's culture, religious beliefs or long-standing habits. Always make an effort to accommodate a person's preferences for bathing.

Bathing

Have you ever had to be bathed by another person? If so, how did you feel? Was the person who bathed you sensitive to your feelings? When you are assisting a person to bathe, be aware that the person may be embarrassed about needing help. Encourage the person to complete as much of the bath as he or she can independently, and take measures to keep the person warm and protect his or her modesty.

When you are scheduling bath times, take into account the person's preferences as well as your employer's policies. Be aware that the people in your care do have the right to refuse a bath. However, if this happens too frequently, you will need to talk to the nurse because regular bathing is necessary for good hygiene.

Close attention is needed to prevent accidents when bathing. Water on hard bathroom surfaces can be very slippery. Make sure that showers and tubs have nonskid mats and surfaces and that grab bars are tightly fastened to the wall. To prevent burns, check the temperature of shower or bath water by using a bath thermometer (Figure 13-7). The temperature should be between 105° F and 115° F. If a thermometer is not available, use the inside of your wrist to check the temperature of the water.

Observations Into Action!

Assisting with bathing gives you a good opportunity to observe the person for changes that could be a sign of a medical problem. Report any of the following:

- **The person refuses the bath**
- **Reddened areas of skin**
- **Sores or bruises**
- **Signs of physical abuse (such as burn marks or bruises in unusual places)**
- **Changes in mental status (such as confusion in a person who is not normally confused)**

Assisting a person with a bed bath

A complete bed bath involves bathing all parts of a person's body while she is in bed. A partial bed bath involves bathing only the face, hands, axillae (armpits), perineal area, back

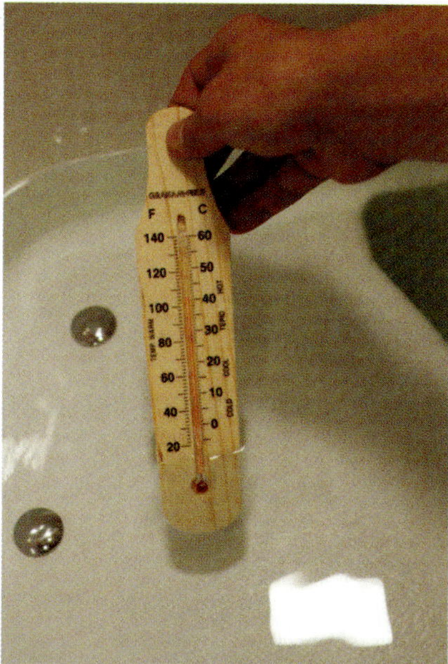

Figure 13-7 Always check the temperature of the water before allowing the person to get in the bathtub or shower.

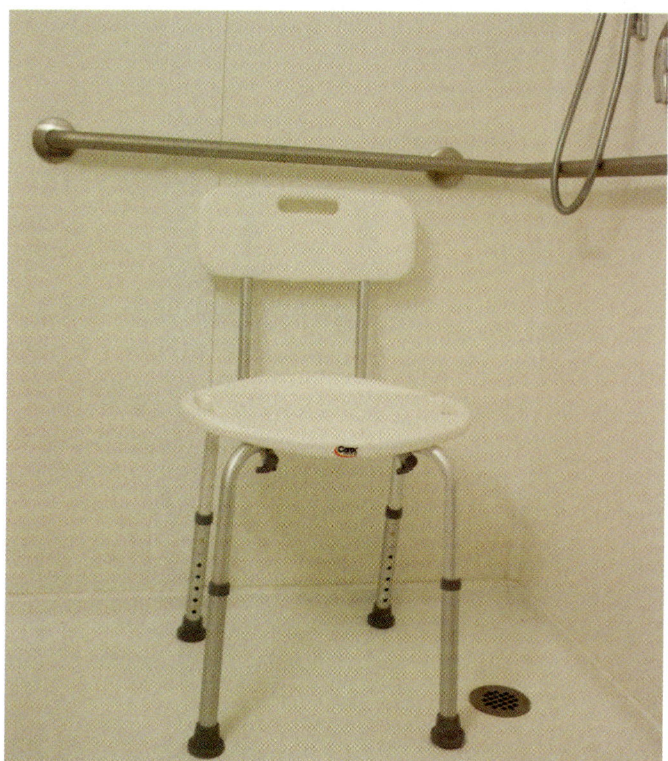

Figure 13-8 A shower chair should be used for a person who is weak or unsteady on her feet.

and buttocks. A partial bath may be given on days when a complete bath is not scheduled. A partial bath can also be a useful compromise when the person refuses a complete bath. When assisting with a bed bath, help the person maintain her independence by discussing with her how she can help. A person may be able to help only by washing her face, but any amount of self-care is good. If the person has more ability, you may suggest that she do her own perineal care. In this case, hand her the washcloth and provide privacy for her, after making sure she is safe. Skill 13-12 describes how to assist a person with a complete bed bath.

Assisting a person with a shower or tub bath

People who are able to get out of bed will take a shower or a tub bath.

Shower stalls in health care facilities are usually large enough to accommodate a shower chair, so that the person can sit down while showering (Figure 13-8). A shower chair should be used if the person is not reliably steady on his feet.

You may see several different types of bathtubs in use in a health care facility. Walk-in tubs have a door that swings open so that the person can easily enter the tub without stepping over a high edge (Figure 13-9). Some tubs may be equipped with a lift device that the person sits on to be lowered into the tub. If using a standard bathtub (for example, in a person's home), make sure that the person can get in and out of the tub safely. The person should be:

- Predictable.
- Able to bear all or most of his own weight.
- Able to stand on one foot and lift the other foot over the edge of the tub with minimal assistance.
- Able to lower his body into the tub.

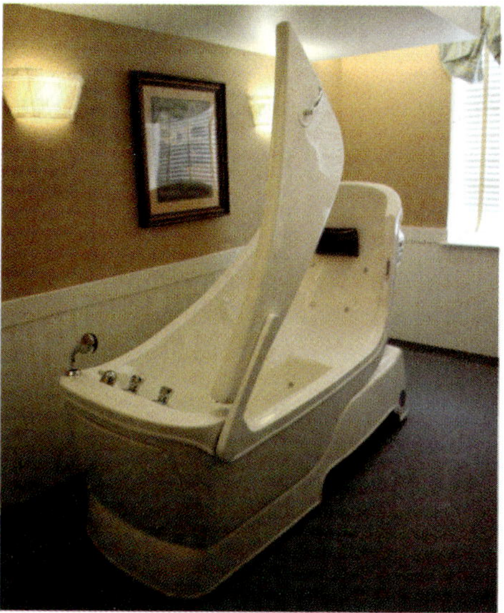

Figure 13-9 Bathtubs in health care facilities are often modified to allow easier access for the person.

For some people, a whirlpool bath may be ordered. A whirlpool bath is given in a special type of bathtub called a hydrotherapy tub. The hydrotherapy tub circulates the water, massaging and improving blood flow to the skin during the bath. Often the water temperature is a bit warmer than it would be for a regular bath. If you are required to assist a person with a whirlpool bath, the nurse or physical therapist will show you how to operate the tub and tell you how hot the water should be and how long the person should remain in the tub. A person may become faint or dizzy while taking a whirlpool bath because the bath increases blood flow to the skin and away from the brain. Never leave a person alone during a whirlpool bath, and observe carefully for signs of dizziness or fainting.

Skill 13-13 describes how to help a person with a shower or tub bath.

Back Rub

Back rubs promote blood flow to the skin and can be very relaxing for the person. Often a back rub is provided as part of the bed bath. Alternatively, you may give a person a back rub before bed to help the person relax and sleep better. During a back rub, you can also check the person's skin for reddened areas or other changes that could signal the beginning of a pressure ulcer.

Before giving a back rub, consult with the nurse or check the person's care plan. Back rubs are not allowed for people with certain conditions, such as those who are recovering from back surgery. Skill 13-14 describes how to give a back rub.

CHECK YOUR UNDERSTANDING

Questions for Review

1. **When you help a person with mouth care:**
   a. Use a stiff toothbrush to clean the teeth thoroughly.
   b. First rinse the person's mouth with plain water.
   c. Rinse the person's mouth with full-strength mouthwash after brushing.
   d. Rinse the person's mouth with diluted mouthwash before and after mouth care.

2. **When providing mouth care for an unconscious person, you should:**
   a. Position the person in a supine position.
   b. Use a lot of water to clean the person's mouth thoroughly.
   c. Turn the person's head to the side.
   d. Remain silent, because the person cannot hear you talk.

3. **When giving a person a complete bed bath and shampoo, do all of the following except:**
   a. Inspect the person's skin for injuries or changes in condition.
   b. Ensure that the water temperature is 140° F.
   c. Keep the person well covered.
   d. Cover the person's eyes with a washcloth while shampooing.

4. **What should you do when you finish using a disposable safety razor to shave someone?**
   a. Recap the razor. Put it in the person's drawer.
   b. Do not recap the razor. Put it in the person's drawer.
   c. Do not recap the razor. Put it in the sharps container.
   d. Do not recap the razor. Put it in a plastic bag and put the bag in a waste container.

5. **Mr. Upchurch is paralyzed on his right side. How will you help him put on a button-down shirt?**
   a. Button the shirt and pull it over Mr. Upchurch's head, then help him to put his arms through the sleeves.
   b. Help Mr. Upchurch put on the right sleeve first, then the left.
   c. Help Mr. Upchurch put on the left sleeve first, then the right.
   d. Mr. Upchurch cannot wear a button-down shirt.

6. **Mr. Boyer is a new resident at Morningside Nursing Home. When you tell him that usually residents are assisted with bathing three times a week in the morning, Mr. Boyer tells you that he prefers to bathe before bed. How should you respond?**
   a. Tell Mr. Boyer that he must follow the facility's policies now.
   b. Tell Mr. Boyer that he can choose which mornings he would like to have his bath.
   c. Explain to Mr. Boyer that it is very difficult to make exceptions to the rules, but you will try to accommodate him.
   d. Tell Mr. Boyer that you will be glad to make bathing part of his evening care routine.

7. **Which of the following observations should be reported when assisting a person with foot care?**
   a. The person's toenails need to be cut.
   b. A blister is forming on the person's heel.
   c. The person complains that his shoes hurt his feet.
   d. All of the above

8. **Which of the following responsibilities is usually outside of the nurse assistant's scope of practice?**
   a. Providing perineal care
   b. Trimming a person's toenails
   c. Helping a woman to shave her legs
   d. Helping a person with a paralyzed, weak or injured arm or leg to change clothes

9. **Which of the following statements about assisting a person to dress and undress is true?**
   a. There is no need to provide privacy, because the person's body is exposed frequently for care procedures, and the person must get used to it.
   b. Most people do not care what they wear, so it is best to just choose an outfit for the person.
   c. Assistive devices and smart clothing choices can help a person be more independent with dressing and undressing.
   d. A person who does not want to get dressed should be allowed to remain in pajamas all day.

10. **Which of the following is a benefit of hair care?**
   a. It helps to massage the scalp.
   b. It helps to keep hair tangle-free.
   c. It is important for the person's self-esteem and dignity.
   d. All of the above

11. **When assisting a person with a shower, you should:**
   a. Encourage the person to do as much for himself as he is able.
   b. Use a shower chair if the person is unsteady on his feet.
   c. Take measures to provide privacy and warmth.
   d. All of the above

Questions to Ask Yourself

1. *Mrs. Jaskowitz is right-handed, but because of her stroke, she is not able to use her right hand to grip the toothbrush. How should you help Mrs. Jaskowitz brush her teeth?*
2. *Mr. Randal is unconscious. What should you talk about while you provide mouth care for him?*
3. *You are bathing Mrs. Feld when Mr. Lloyd, a confused resident from down the hall, walks into the room. He tries to enter the privacy curtain, but cannot seem to find the opening immediately. What should you do?*
4. *You walk by Mrs. Kitzmiller's room while a new nurse assistant is styling her hair. You have assisted Mrs. Kitzmiller before and you know she likes to wear her hair in a bun. The new nurse assistant is putting it in pigtails. What should you do?*
5. *Because of a problem with his leg, Mr. Wingard has been having bed baths without a shampoo for 11 days. He likes to wash his hair only in the shower. Today the nurse has asked you to make sure his hair is washed. How should you do this?*
6. *Mrs. Lanver wants to help dress herself, but she is very slow. What can you do to increase her independence and maintain her dignity?*

Skill 13-1
Brushing and Flossing a Person's Teeth

PREPARATION

1. Wash your hands.
2. Gather your supplies:
   - Towel
   - Gloves
   - Protective eyewear and a gown (optional; use if blood may splash or spray)
   - Paper towels
   - Toothbrush
   - Toothpaste
   - Emesis basin
   - Cup
   - Floss pick or dental floss
   - Mouthwash
   - Lip balm or petroleum jelly and cotton-tipped applicator
3. Knock, greet the person and ensure privacy.
4. Explain the procedure.
5. Adjust equipment for body mechanics and safety: Raise the bed to a comfortable working height. Make sure the wheels on the bed are locked.

PROCEDURE

6. Cover the over-bed table with the paper towels and arrange your supplies. In the cup, prepare a solution of half water and half mouthwash.
7. Position the person in high Fowler's position.
8. Unfold the towel. Place it across the person's chest.
9. Put on the gloves and any other personal protective equipment.
10. Give the person a mouthful of the mouthwash mixture to rinse his mouth. Hold the emesis basin under the person's chin to catch the liquid (Figure 1). Dry the person's mouth and chin using the towel.

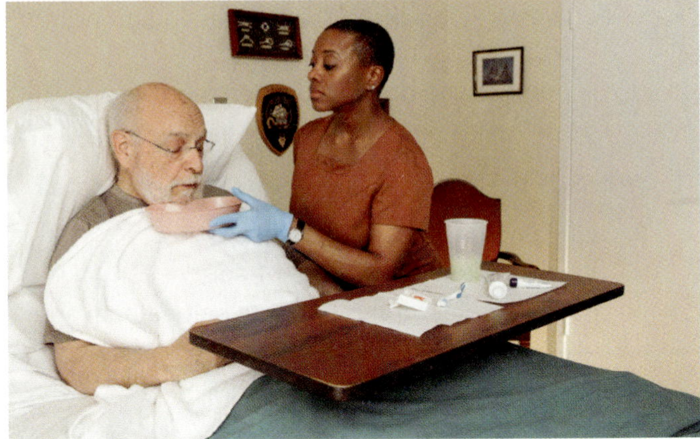

Figure 1

11. Wet the toothbrush by pouring mouthwash solution over it.
12. Put toothpaste on the wet brush.
13. Brush the upper teeth and gums:
    - Starting at the back of the mouth, place the toothbrush on the outer surface of the upper teeth at a 45-degree angle (Figure 2). Gently brush the outer surface of each tooth, using short back-and-forth (tooth-wide) strokes.

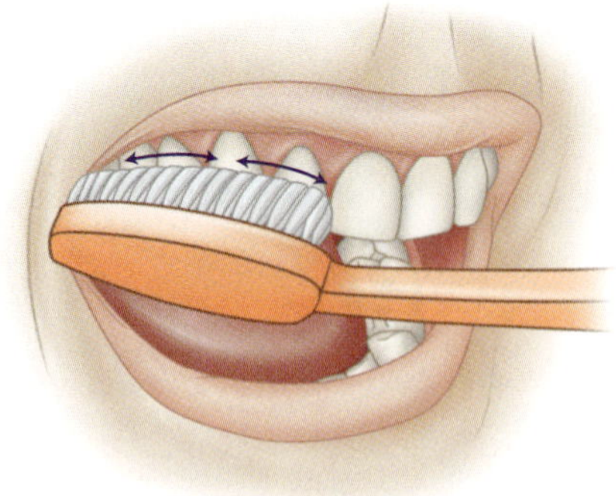

Figure 2

- Next, clean the chewing surfaces of the upper teeth, moving from one side of the mouth to the other and using the same short, back-and-forth strokes. (Figure 3).

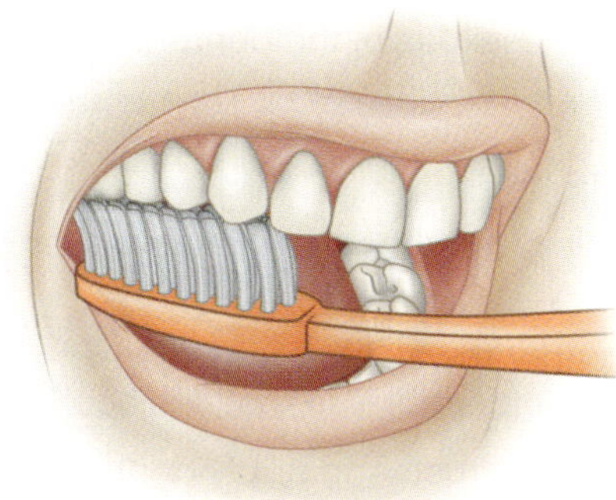

Figure 3

- Finally, put the brush vertically against the inside surfaces of the front upper teeth and brush with a gentle up-and-down motion (Figure 4).

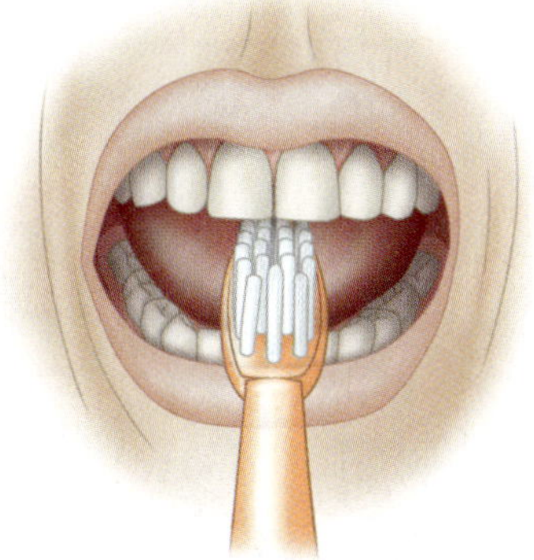

Figure 4

14. Brush the lower teeth and gums in the same way.
15. Brush the tongue.
16. Give the person a mouthful of the mouthwash mixture to rinse his mouth. Hold the emesis basin under the person's chin to catch the liquid. Dry the person's mouth and chin using the towel.
17. Floss the person's teeth.
    - **Floss pick.** Starting between the two front teeth, hold the handle of the floss pick and slide the floss carefully between the teeth. Hold the floss against the tooth and scrape the side of the tooth, moving the floss away from the gum. Repeat with the next tooth, moving from the front of the mouth to the back of the mouth on one side and then the other side. Then repeat for the lower teeth.
    - **Dental floss.** Break off about 18 inches of floss from the dispenser. Wrap most of the floss around the middle fingers of both hands, leaving 1 inch of floss between your hands. Stretch the floss tightly between your thumbs and index fingers (Figure 5). Starting between the two front teeth, slide the floss carefully between the teeth. Hold the floss against the tooth and scrape the side of the tooth, moving the floss away from the gum. After you floss each tooth, unwrap a clean 1-inch section of floss from your finger and wrap the soiled floss around the other finger. Floss from the front of the mouth to the back of the mouth on one side and then the other side. Then repeat for the lower teeth.

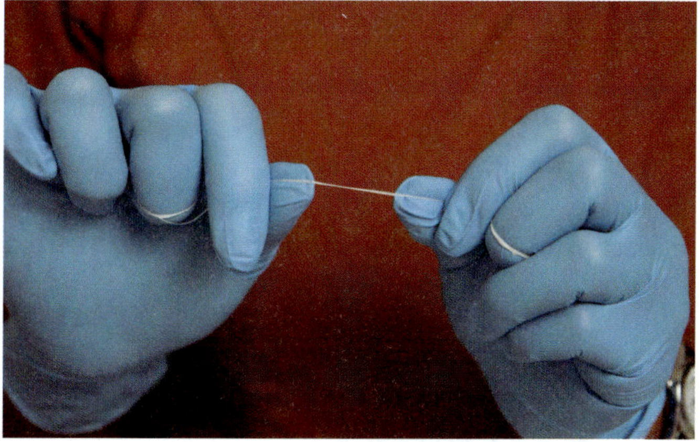

Figure 5

18. Give the person a mouthful of the mouthwash mixture to rinse his mouth. Hold the emesis basin under the person's chin to catch the liquid.
19. Dry the person's mouth and chin with the towel, and place the towel in the linen hamper.
20. Encourage the person to apply lip balm or petroleum jelly to the lips. Assist the person as needed.
21. Remove and dispose of your gloves.

COMPLETION

22. Ensure the person's comfort and good body alignment.
23. Adjust equipment for safety: Lower the bed to the level specified in the person's care plan. Make sure the wheels on the bed are locked. Place the person's method of calling for help within reach. Lower or raise the side rails according to the person's care plan.
24. Clean up your work area.
25. Wash your hands.
26. Report and record.

Skill 13-2
Providing Denture Care

PREPARATION

1. Wash your hands.
2. Gather your supplies:
   - Washcloth
   - Towel
   - Gloves
   - Paper towels
   - Cup
   - Emesis basin
   - Denture cup
   - Disposable mouth sponges
   - Regular toothpaste, toothbrush and dental floss if the person has some natural teeth
   - Denture brush or toothbrush
   - Denture toothpaste
   - Mouthwash
   - Lip balm or petroleum jelly and cotton-tipped applicator
3. Knock, greet the person and ensure privacy.
4. Explain the procedure.
5. Adjust equipment for body mechanics and safety: Raise the bed to a comfortable working height. Make sure the wheels on the bed are locked.

PROCEDURE

6. Cover the over-bed table with the paper towels and arrange your supplies. In the cup, prepare a solution of half water and half mouthwash.
7. Position the person in high Fowler's position.

Task 1: Remove the Denture

8. Unfold the towel. Place it across the person's chest.
9. Put on the gloves.
10. Have the person remove her denture and put it in the emesis basin. If the person needs assistance removing the denture, grasp the denture firmly with your thumb and index finger and use a rocking motion to gently remove the denture and put it in the emesis basin. A person may wear more than one denture (for example, one to replace the upper teeth and one to replace the lower teeth). If necessary, repeat to remove the other denture.

Task 2: Clean the Denture

11. Take the emesis basin, the denture cup, the washcloth, the denture brush or toothbrush, the denture toothpaste and the denture-cleansing tablet (if used) to the sink.
12. Line the sink with the washcloth or several paper towels.
13. Using a paper towel, turn on the faucet and adjust the water temperature so that it is cool.
14. Wet the toothbrush and apply denture toothpaste.
15. Allow the sink to fill halfway with cool water.
16. If the person has more than one denture, clean one denture at a time. Remove one denture from the emesis basin and hold it in the palm of your hand over the sink. Use the toothbrush to clean all surfaces of the denture, using circular movements (Figure 1).

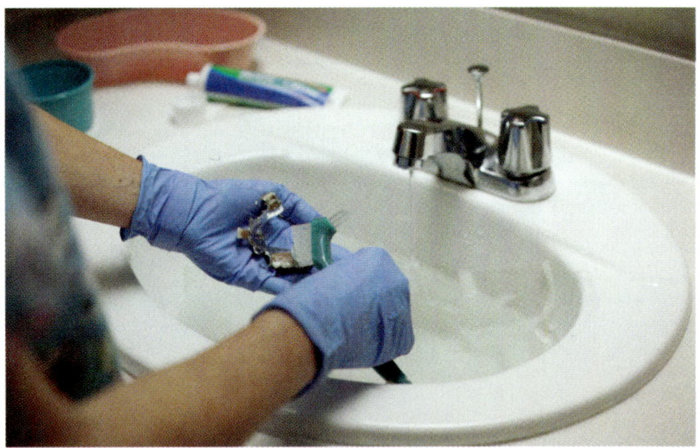

Figure 1

17. Rinse the denture thoroughly under cool, running water and place it in the denture cup.
18. Repeat steps 16 and 17 with the other denture.
19. If the person will not be putting the denture back in the mouth right away, add enough cool water to the denture cup to cover the denture. Add a denture-cleansing tablet, if used, and replace the lid.
20. Turn off the faucet with a paper towel.

Task 3: Provide Care for the Person's Mouth

21. Take the denture cup and the emesis basin back to the person's bedside.
22. Give the person a mouthful of the mouthwash mixture to rinse her mouth. Hold the emesis basin under the person's chin to catch the liquid. Dry the person's mouth and chin with the towel.
23. Help the person clean the roof of the mouth, the inside of the cheeks, the gums, under the tongue, and the lips with mouth sponges dipped in the mouthwash mixture (Figure 2). If the person has any natural teeth, help her brush and floss them.

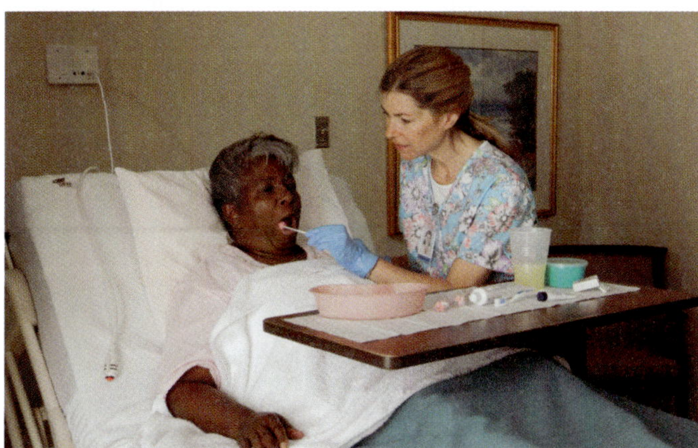

Figure 2

24. Give the person a mouthful of the mouthwash mixture to rinse her mouth. Hold the emesis basin under the person's chin to catch the liquid. Dry the person's mouth and chin with the towel.
25. Have the person put the denture back in the mouth. If the person needs assistance, grasp the denture with your gloved thumb and index finger and guide it into place. If the person is not returning the denture to the mouth right away, make sure the denture cup is within the person's easy reach.
26. Dry the person's mouth and chin with the towel, and place the towel in the linen hamper.
27. Encourage the person to apply lip balm or petroleum jelly to the lips. Assist the person as needed.
28. Remove and dispose of your gloves.

COMPLETION

29. Ensure the person's comfort and good body alignment.
30. Adjust equipment for safety: Lower the bed to the level specified in the person's care plan. Make sure the wheels on the bed are locked. Place the person's method of calling for help within reach. Lower or raise the side rails according to the person's care plan.
31. Clean up your work area.
32. Wash your hands.
33. Report and record.

Skill 13-3

Providing Mouth Care for an Unconscious Person

PREPARATION

1. Wash your hands.
2. Gather your supplies:
   - Two towels
   - Gloves
   - Gauze squares
   - Tongue depressor
   - Tape
   - Paper towels
   - Cup
   - Disposable mouth sponges
   - Toothbrush
   - Mouthwash
   - Lip balm or petroleum jelly and cotton-tipped applicator
3. Knock, greet the person and ensure privacy.
4. Explain the procedure.
5. Adjust equipment for body mechanics and safety: Raise the bed to a comfortable working height. Make sure the wheels on the bed are locked.

PROCEDURE

6. Cover the over-bed table with the paper towels and arrange your supplies. In the cup, prepare a solution of half water and half mouthwash.
7. Position the person in high Fowler's position. Turn the person's head toward you.
8. Unfold one towel. Place it across the person's chest. Place the other towel under the person's head.
9. Put on the gloves.
10. Place the emesis basin on the towel near the person's cheek.
11. Pad the tongue depressor by wrapping the end in gauze and securing the gauze with tape.
12. Without using force, gently separate the person's upper and lower teeth. To do this, cross the middle finger and thumb of one hand. Put the thumb against the person's top teeth and the middle finger against her lower teeth and gently push the finger and thumb apart to open the jaw (Figure 1).

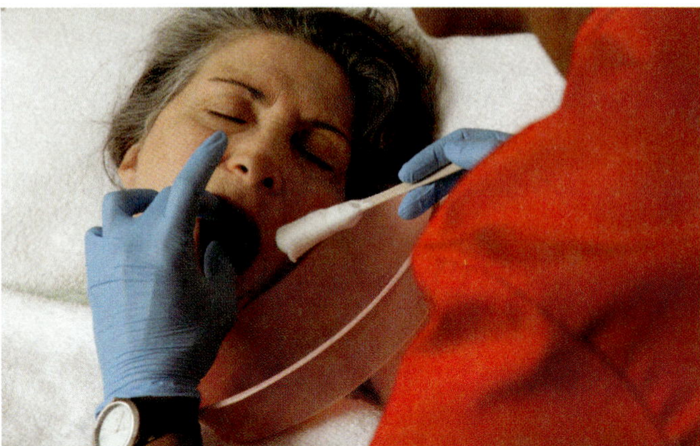

Figure 1

13. Insert the padded tongue depressor between the upper and lower teeth at the back of the mouth to hold the person's mouth open (Figure 2).

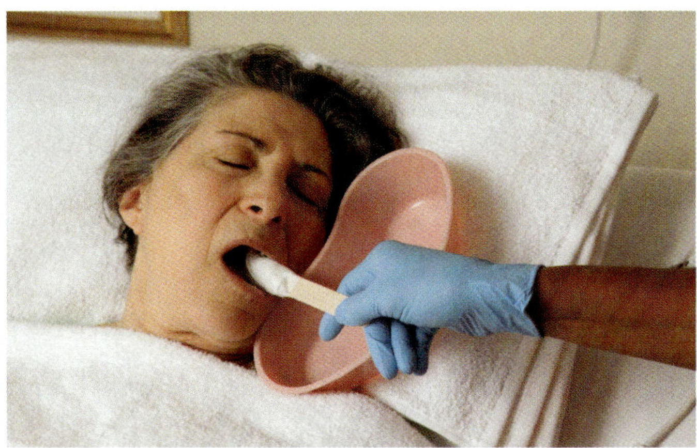

Figure 2

14. Clean the roof of the mouth, the inside of the cheeks, the gums, under the tongue, and the lips with mouth sponges dipped in the mouthwash mixture. Wrap a gauze square around your finger or use a mouth sponge to remove thick mucus or secretions.
15. Use a toothbrush moistened with diluted mouthwash to clean the person's teeth.
16. Apply lip balm or petroleum jelly to the person's lips.
17. Remove and dispose of your gloves.
18. Lower the head of the bed.

COMPLETION

19. Ensure the person's comfort and good body alignment.
20. Adjust equipment for safety: Lower the bed to the level specified in the person's care plan. Make sure the wheels on the bed are locked. Place the person's method of calling for help within reach. Lower or raise the side rails according to the person's care plan.
21. Clean up your work area.
22. Wash your hands.
23. Report and record.

Skill 13-4
Brushing and Combing a Person's Hair

PREPARATION

1. Wash your hands.
2. Gather your supplies:
   - Comb and brush
   - Towel
   - Mirror
   - Paper towels
3. Knock, greet the person and ensure privacy.
4. Explain the procedure.
5. Adjust equipment for body mechanics and safety: Raise the bed to a comfortable working height. Make sure the wheels on the bed are locked.

PROCEDURE

6. Cover the over-bed table with the paper towels and arrange your supplies.
7. Position the person in high Fowler's position. If the person cannot tolerate having the head of the bed raised, you can comb her hair while she is lying in the supine position by turning her head to one side, and then to the other.
8. Place the towel over the person's shoulders (or under the shoulders if the person is in bed).
9. If the person wears glasses, remove them. Remove any hairpins or other styling aids from the hair.
10. Comb or brush the hair gently, beginning at the ends, and work up in sections to the scalp (Figure 1).

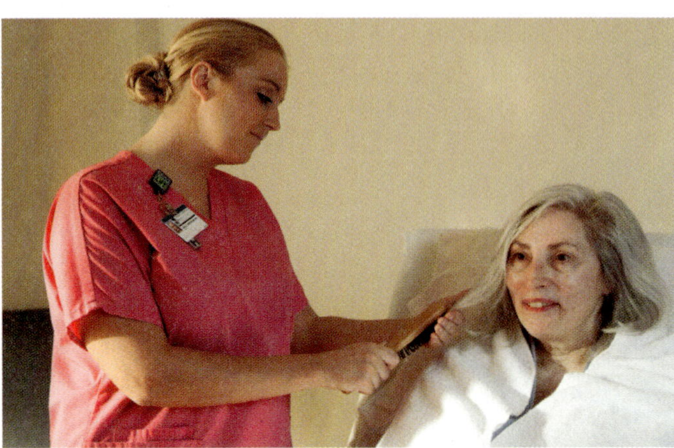

Figure 1

11. Style the person's hair the way she likes it.
12. Give the person the hand mirror so that she can see the way her hair is styled.

COMPLETION

13. Ensure the person's comfort and good body alignment.
14. Adjust equipment for safety: Lower the bed to the level specified in the person's care plan. Make sure the wheels on the bed are locked. Place the person's method of calling for help within reach. Lower or raise the side rails according to the person's care plan.
15. Clean up your work area.
16. Wash your hands.
17. Report and record.

Skill 13-5
Shampooing a Person's Hair in Bed

PREPARATION

1. Wash your hands.
2. Gather your supplies:
   - Towels
   - Washcloth
   - Gloves (optional)
   - Paper towels
   - Bed protector
   - Shampoo tray
   - Two wash basins
   - Paper cup
   - Bath thermometer
   - Shampoo and other desired hair care products
   - Comb and brush
3. Knock, greet the person and ensure privacy.
4. Explain the procedure.
5. Adjust equipment for body mechanics and safety: Raise the bed to a comfortable working height. Make sure the wheels on the bed are locked.

PROCEDURE

6. Cover the over-bed table with the paper towels and arrange your supplies. Fill one of the wash basins with warm water. Use the bath thermometer to verify that the water temperature is between 105° F and 115° F. Place the wash basin on the over-bed table. Place a chair close to the head of the bed, and place the empty wash basin on the chair.
7. Position the person in high Fowler's position. Remove any pins or clips from the hair. Brush or comb the hair to remove any tangles.
8. Lower the head of the bed as low as the person can tolerate.
9. Assist the person to raise her head and shoulders off the pillow. Reposition the pillow under the person's shoulders. Cover the head of the bed and the pillow with a bed protector, and place the shampoo tray on the bed protector. Gently lower the person's head and shoulders so that the person's head is resting on the shampoo tray. Make sure the runoff from the shampoo tray is directed into the wash basin on the chair.
10. Place a towel across the person's chest. Ask the person to hold the washcloth over her eyes (Figure 1). Put on the gloves, if you are using them.

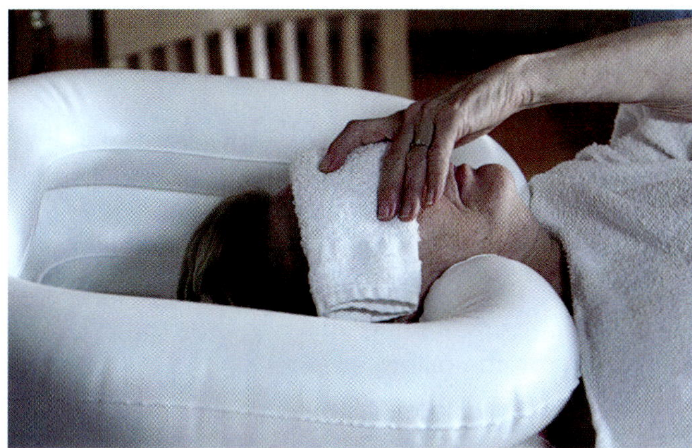

Figure 1

11. Wet the hair with cups of water from the wash basin until it is fully wet.
12. Apply a small amount of shampoo to the hair and massage the scalp with your fingertips, starting at the hairline and working toward the back of head, until the scalp is completely lathered.
13. Rinse the person's hair with cups of water from the wash basin until all shampoo is removed (Figure 2).

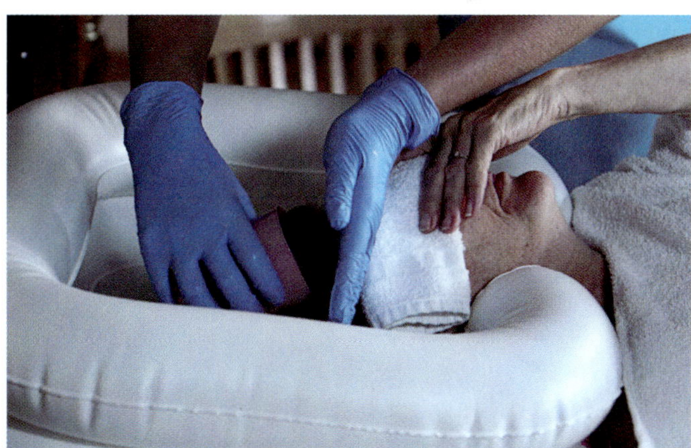

Figure 2

Continued on next page

Skill 13-5
Shampooing a Person's Hair in Bed *Continued*

14. Apply conditioner if the person likes to use it. Work the conditioner through the hair with your fingertips. Rinse the hair until the conditioner is removed.
15. Unfold a clean, dry towel and dry the hair. Wrap the person's head in the towel.
16. Assist the person to raise her head and shoulders. Remove the shampoo tray and bed protector. Reposition the pillow under the person's head. Gently lower the person's head and shoulders so that the person's head is resting on the pillow.
17. Remove and dispose of your gloves, if used.
18. Raise the head of bed so that the person is almost in a sitting position. Comb the person's hair to remove tangles. Dry and style the hair as the person prefers.
19. Replace any wet linens.

COMPLETION

20. Ensure the person's comfort and good body alignment.
21. Adjust equipment for safety: Lower the bed to the level specified in the person's care plan. Make sure the wheels on the bed are locked. Place the person's method of calling for help within reach. Lower or raise the side rails according to the person's care plan.
22. Clean up your work area.
23. Wash your hands.
24. Report and record.

Skill 13-6
Helping a Man to Shave

PREPARATION

1. Wash your hands.
2. Gather your supplies:
   - Towel
   - Washcloths
   - Gloves
   - Paper towels
   - Wash basin
   - Bath thermometer
   - Soap (optional)
   - Aftershave lotion (optional)

Safety razor:

- Safety razor
- Shaving cream, gel or soap

Electric razor:

- Electric razor
- Pre-shave lotion

3. Knock, greet the person and ensure privacy.
4. Explain the procedure.
5. Adjust equipment for body mechanics and safety: Raise the bed to a comfortable working height. Make sure the wheels on the bed are locked.

PROCEDURE

6. Cover the over-bed table with the paper towels and arrange your supplies. Fill the wash basin with warm water. Use the bath thermometer to verify that the water temperature is between 105° F and 115° F. Place the wash basin on the over-bed table.
7. Position the person in high Fowler's position.
8. Unfold the towel. Place it across the person's chest.
9. Put on the gloves.
10. Inspect the area to be shaved for moles, birthmarks or sores.
11. Assist the person in washing his face with soap (optional) and warm water. Remove soap, if used, with a wet washcloth.
12. If the person is using a safety razor, assist him in applying shaving cream, gel or soap to his face. If the person is using an electric razor, assist him to apply pre-shave lotion.
13. Assist the person with shaving, if needed. Shave one side of the face first and then the other.
    - **Safety razor:** With the fingers of one hand, hold the person's skin on the cheek tight as you use the razor to shave downward, in the direction that the hair grows (Figure 1A). Shave both cheeks, rinsing the razor often in the washbasin. Use shorter strokes around the person's chin and lips. To shave the neck, have the person tip his head back. Pull the skin tight and shave the neck, moving the razor up toward the chin.

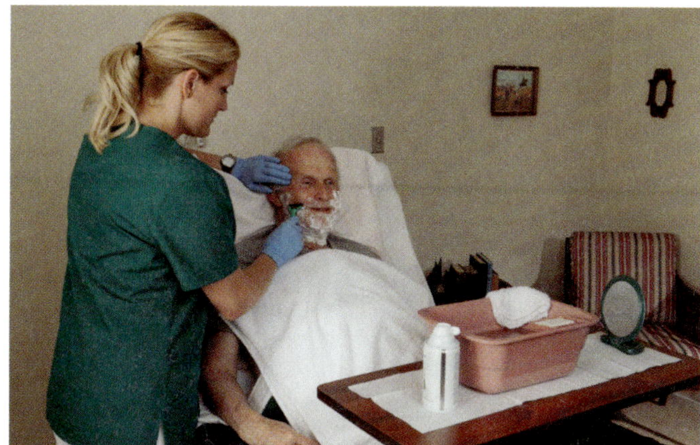

Figure 1A

    - **Electric razor:** With the fingers of one hand, hold the person's skin tight as you use the razor to shave as the manufacturer suggests, usually in a circular motion (Figure 1B).

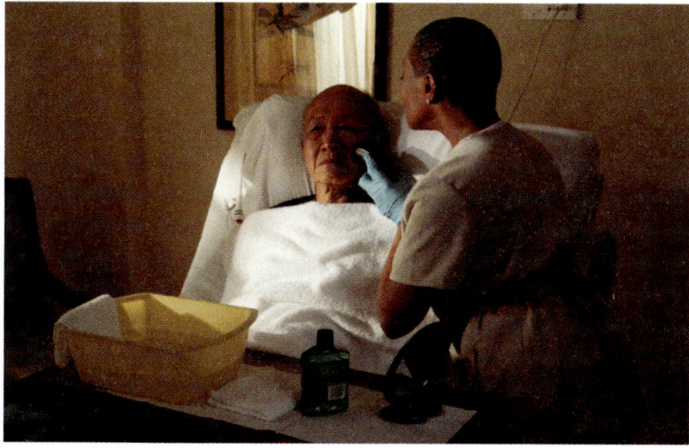

Figure 1B

Continued on next page

Skill 13-6
Helping a Man to Shave *Continued*

14. Use the wet washcloth to rinse the person's face.
15. Dry the person's face with the towel, and place the towel in the linen hamper.
16. Give the person a hand mirror so that he can inspect the shaved area.
17. Assist the person to apply aftershave lotion (optional).
18. Remove and dispose of your gloves.

COMPLETION

19. Ensure the person's comfort and good body alignment.
20. Adjust equipment for safety: Lower the bed to the level specified in the person's care plan. Make sure the wheels on the bed are locked. Place the person's method of calling for help within reach. Lower or raise the side rails according to the person's care plan.
21. Clean up your work area.
22. Wash your hands.
23. Report and record.

Skill 13-7
Helping a Person to Change Clothes

PREPARATION

1. Wash your hands.
2. Gather your supplies:
   - Bath blanket
   - Clean clothes
3. Knock, greet the person and ensure privacy.
4. Explain the procedure.
5. Adjust equipment for body mechanics and safety: Raise the bed to a comfortable working height. Make sure the wheels on the bed are locked.

PROCEDURE

Task 1: Assist the Person with Undressing

6. Lower the head of the bed as low as the person can tolerate.
7. Cover the person and the top sheet with the bath blanket (to provide privacy and warmth). Ask the person to hold the edge of the bath blanket (or tuck the edges under the person's shoulders) while you fold the top linens down to the bottom of the bed.
8. Help the person remove her clothing.
   - **Tops that pull over the head:** Undo any fasteners, such as buttons or zippers. Help the person remove her strong arm from the top first, then her weak arm, by sliding the sleeves down the arms. Gather the top around the person's neck. Assist the person to raise her head and shoulders off the pillow (Figure 1). Remove the top by lifting it over the person's head. (If the person cannot lift her head and shoulders from the pillow, turn the person onto her side and remove her arm from the sleeve on that side. Repeat the process on the other side, and then turn the person back into the supine position.)
   - **Tops that fasten in the front:** Undo any fasteners, such as buttons or zippers. Assist the person to raise her head and shoulders off the pillow. Help the person to remove her strong arm from the top first, then her weak arm, by sliding the sleeves down the arms.
   - **Bottoms:** Undo any fasteners, such as buttons or zippers. Ask the person to bend her knees and place her feet firmly on the bed, so that she can raise her hips off the bed. Reach under the bath blanket and slide the pants down over the hips (Figure 2). (If the person cannot raise her hips off the bed, turn the person onto her side and pull the pants over the buttocks and hip on that side. Repeat the process on the other side, and then turn the person back into the supine position).

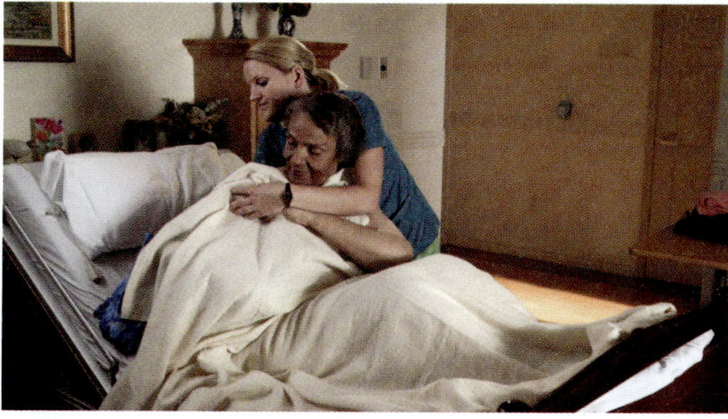
Figure 1

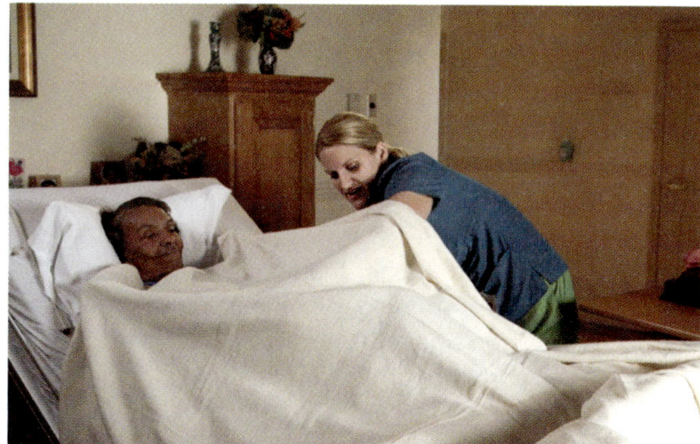
Figure 2

Task 2: Assist the Person with Dressing

9. Help the person put on undergarments.
   - **Underpants:** Gather the leg opening to the waistband. Help the person place her weak foot through the leg opening first, then her strong

Continued on next page

Skill 13-7
Helping a Person to Change Clothes *Continued*

foot, and slide the underpants up the person's legs as far as they will go. Ask the person to bend her knees and place her feet firmly on the bed, so that she can raise her hips off the bed. Reach under the bath blanket and pull the underpants over her hips. (If the person cannot raise her hips off the bed, turn the person onto her side and pull the underpants over the hips and buttocks on that side. Repeat the process on the other side, and then turn the person back into the supine position.)

- **Bra:** Help the person place her weak arm through the strap of the bra, then her strong arm. Slide the straps onto the person's shoulders, and adjust the cups of the bra so that they cover the person's breasts. Assist the person to raise her head and shoulders off the pillow and fasten the bra in the back (Figure 3).

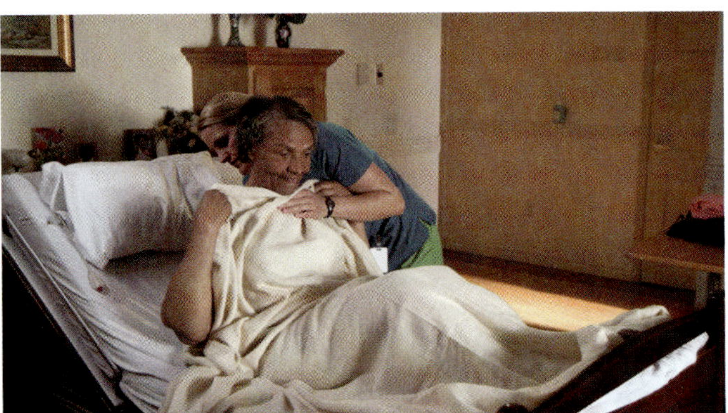

Figure 3

- **Undershirt:** Gather the hem of the undershirt to the neck opening. Slip the undershirt over the person's head. Assist the person to put her weak arm through the arm opening, then her strong arm (Figure 4). Assist the person to raise her head and shoulders off the pillow and pull the undershirt down.

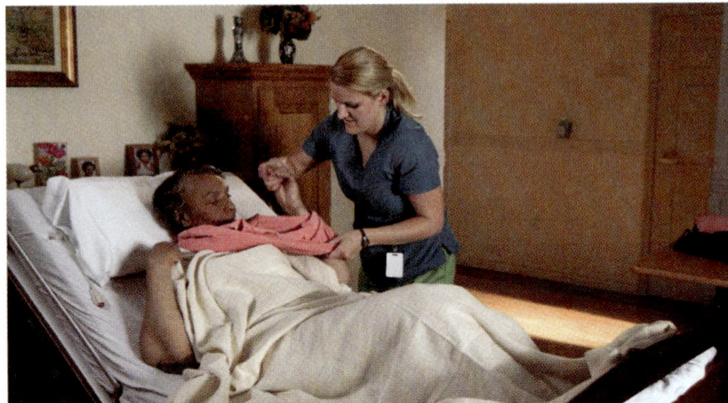

Figure 4

10. Help the person to put on outerwear.
    - **Pants:** Use the same technique used for putting on underpants. Fasten any fasteners, such as zippers or hooks.
    - **Tops that fasten in the front:** Face the person and put your hand through the wrist opening of the top. Hold the person's hand and slip the sleeve off your hand and onto the person's arm (Figure 5). Adjust the sleeve so it sits properly on the person's shoulder. Assist the person to raise her head and shoulders off the pillow and bring the top around the person's back. Assist the person to place her other arm in the sleeve. Fasten any fasteners, such as zippers or buttons.

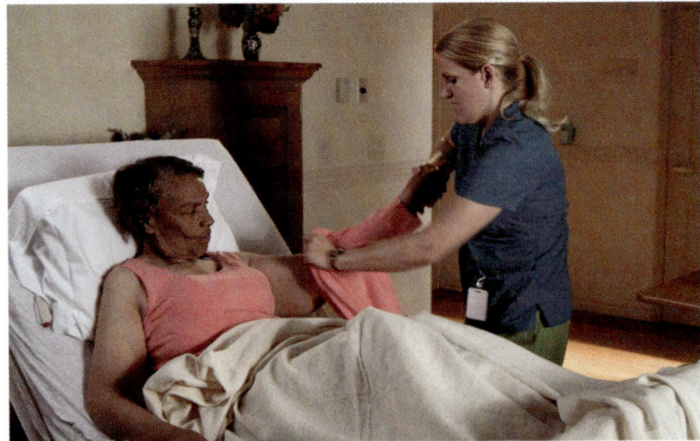

Figure 5

- **Tops that fasten in the back:** Face the person and put your hand through the wrist opening of the top. Hold the person's hand and slip the sleeve off your hand and onto the person's arm. Adjust the sleeve so it sits properly on the person's shoulder. Repeat on the other side. Assist the person to raise her head and shoulders off the pillow so that you can fasten the top in the back.

11. Help the person put on footwear.
    - **Socks or stockings:** Gather the opening of the sock or stocking to the toe. Guide the person's foot into the sock or stocking, adjusting the sock or stocking so that it fits properly on the foot. Pull the sock or stocking up the leg, smoothing any wrinkles.
    - **Shoes or slippers:** Loosen any laces. Guide the person's foot into the shoe or slipper, and tie the laces or secure other fasteners.

COMPLETION

12. Ensure the person's comfort and good body alignment.
13. Adjust equipment for safety: Lower the bed to the level specified in the person's care plan. Make sure the wheels on the bed are locked. Place the person's method of calling for help within reach. Lower or raise the side rails according to the person's care plan.
14. Clean up your work area.
15. Wash your hands.
16. Report and record.

Skill 13-8
Helping a Person to Put On Compression Stockings

PREPARATION

1. Wash your hands.
2. Gather your supplies:
   - Compression stockings in the correct size
3. Knock, greet the person and ensure privacy.
4. Explain the procedure.
5. Adjust equipment for body mechanics and safety: Raise the bed to a comfortable working height. Make sure the wheels on the bed are locked.

PROCEDURE

6. Lower the head of the bed as low as the person can tolerate.
7. Adjust the top covers and the person's clothing as necessary to expose one leg at a time.
8. Turn one stocking inside out down to the heel (Figure 1).

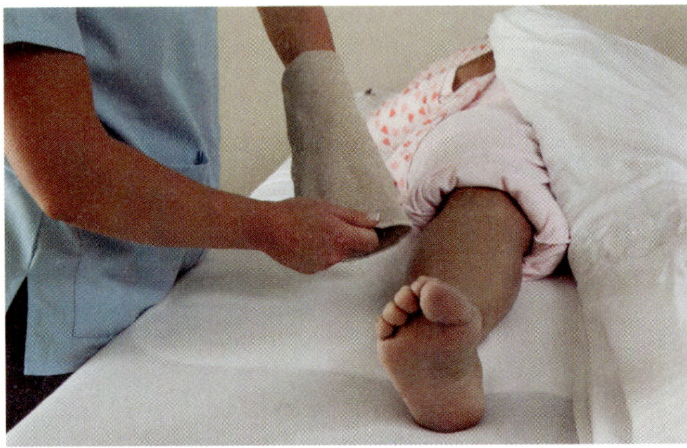

Figure 1

9. Hold the stocking so that when you place it on the person's foot, the toe opening is facing up or down, according to the manufacturer's instructions. Slide the foot of the stocking over the person's toes, foot and heel (Figure 2). Make sure the opening is positioned properly across the person's toes and that the stocking fits smoothly over the heel.

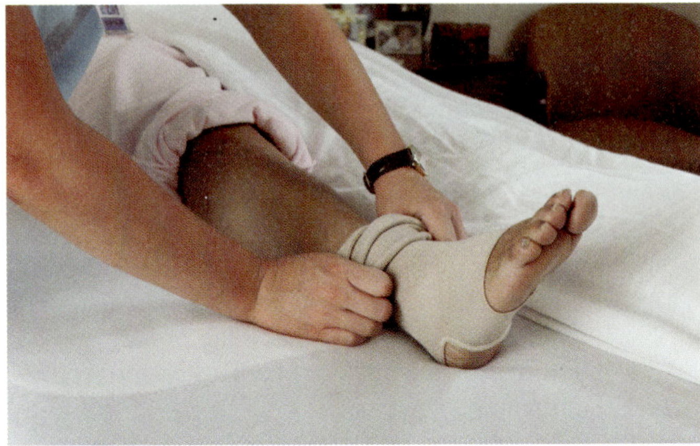

Figure 2

10. Slide the rest of the stocking up the person's leg, smoothing out any wrinkles (Figure 3).

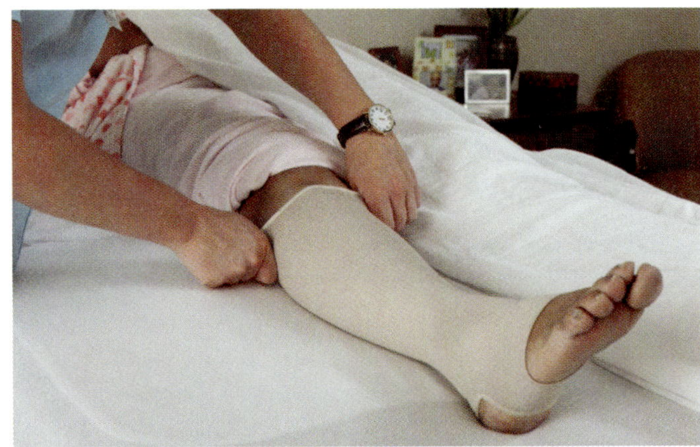

Figure 3

11. Cover the person's leg, and apply the second stocking to the other leg.

COMPLETION

12. Ensure the person's comfort and good body alignment.
13. Adjust equipment for safety: Lower the bed to the level specified in the person's care plan. Make sure the wheels on the bed are locked. Place the person's method of calling for help within reach. Lower or raise the side rails according to the person's care plan.
14. Clean up your work area.
15. Wash your hands.
16. Report and record.

Skill 13-9

Inserting and Removing an In-The-Ear Hearing Aid

PREPARATION

1. Wash your hands.
2. Gather your supplies.
3. Knock, greet the person and ensure privacy.
4. Explain the procedure.
5. Adjust equipment for body mechanics and safety: Raise the bed to a comfortable working height. Make sure the wheels on the bed are locked.

PROCEDURE

6. Help the person into a comfortable position that allows you to easily access the person's ear.

Task 1: Insert the Hearing Aid

7. Make sure the hearing aid is turned off and the volume is turned down.
8. Inspect the person's ear canal for excessive ear wax. If necessary, gently wipe the ear canal with a warm, wet washcloth, and then dry.
9. Gently place the narrow end of the hearing aid in the person's ear canal, and then rotate the hearing aid so that it follows the curve of the ear. While using one hand to gently pull down on the person's earlobe, use the other hand to gently push up and in to seat the hearing aid properly in place.
10. Turn the hearing aid on and adjust the volume until the person can hear you.

Task 2: Remove the Hearing Aid

11. Turn the hearing aid off.
12. While using one hand to gently pull the top of the person's ear up, use the other hand to gently lift the hearing aid up and out of the ear canal.
13. Place the hearing aid in its case.

COMPLETION

14. Ensure the person's comfort and good body alignment.
15. Adjust equipment for safety: Lower the bed to the level specified in the person's care plan. Make sure the wheels on the bed are locked. Place the person's method of calling for help within reach. Lower or raise the side rails according to the person's care plan.
16. Clean up your work area.
17. Wash your hands.
18. Report and record.

Skill 13-10
Providing Hand and Foot Care

PREPARATION

1. Wash your hands.
2. Gather your supplies:
   - Washcloth
   - Towel
   - Bed protector
   - Emesis basin (hand care) or wash basin (foot care)
   - Bath thermometer
   - Nail clippers
   - Orange stick
   - Emery board (nail file)
   - Soap
   - Lotion
   - Paper towels
   - Gloves (optional)
3. Knock, greet the person and ensure privacy.
4. Explain the procedure.
5. Adjust equipment for body mechanics and safety: If the person will be staying in the bed, raise the bed to a comfortable working height. If the person will be getting out of bed, lower the bed to the level specified in the person's care plan. Make sure the wheels on the bed are locked.

PROCEDURE

6. Cover the over-bed table with the paper towels and arrange your supplies. Fill the emesis basin or wash basin with warm water. Use the bath thermometer to verify that the water temperature is between 105° F and 115° F. Place the wash basin or emesis basin on the over-bed table.
7. Help the person to transfer from the bed to a chair, or to sit on the edge of the bed. Alternatively, position the person in high Fowler's position.
8. Put on the gloves, if you are using them.
9. Help the person to soak her hands or feet.
   - **Hand care:** Position the emesis basin within the person's reach. Help the person put her fingertips in the basin. Soak the fingertips in the water for 5 minutes (Figure 1).

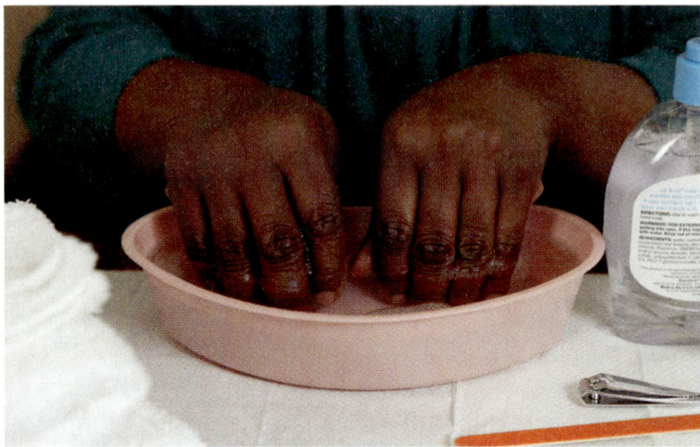

Figure 1

   - **Foot care:** Place the bed protector on the floor or the mattress near the person's feet. Place the wash basin on the bed protector, and help the person put her feet in the basin. Soak the feet in the water for 5 minutes.
10. Wet the washcloth and apply soap. Lift the person's hand or foot from the water, one at a time. Wash the hand or foot, pushing the cuticles back gently with the washcloth (Figure 2). Use the orange stick to gently clean underneath the person's nails. Wipe the orange stick on the towel after cleaning under each nail.

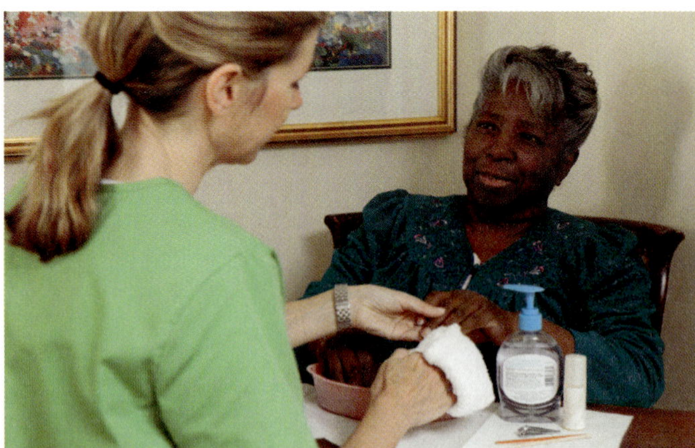

Figure 2

11. Rinse the person's hands or feet.
12. Dry the person's hands or feet thoroughly, including between the fingers and toes.

13. Care for the nails.
    - **Hand care:** If you are permitted to do so, use nail clippers to trim the person's fingernails so that the nail extends slightly beyond the tip of the finger. Trim the nails straight across, and then shape and smooth the edges with the emery board.
    - **Foot care:** Note whether or not the nails need to be trimmed. Also inspect the condition of the skin on the person's feet, including in between the toes.
14. Massage the person's hands or feet with lotion. Begin with the fingers or toes and move upward toward the wrists or ankles. Do *not* massage the person's legs.
15. Remove and dispose of your gloves, if used.

COMPLETION

16. Ensure the person's comfort and good body alignment.
17. Adjust equipment for safety: Lower the bed to the level specified in the person's care plan. Make sure the wheels on the bed are locked. Place the person's method of calling for help within reach. Lower or raise the side rails according to the person's care plan.
18. Clean up your work area.
19. Wash your hands.
20. Report and record.

Skill 13-11
Providing Perineal Care

PREPARATION

1. Wash your hands.
2. Gather your supplies:
   - Washcloths
   - Towels
   - Bath blanket
   - Bed protector
   - Wash basin
   - Bath thermometer
   - Soap
   - Paper towels
   - Gloves
   - Clean clothing
   - Clean linens (if needed)
3. Knock, greet the person and ensure privacy.
4. Explain the procedure.
5. Adjust equipment for body mechanics and safety: Raise the bed to a comfortable working height. Make sure the wheels on the bed are locked.

PROCEDURE

6. Cover the over-bed table with the paper towels and arrange your supplies. Fill the wash basin with warm water. Use the bath thermometer to verify that the water temperature is between 105° F and 115° F. Place the wash basin on the over-bed table.
7. Lower the head of the bed as low as the person can tolerate.
8. Cover the person and the top sheet with the bath blanket (to provide privacy and warmth). Ask the person to hold the edge of the bath blanket (or tuck the edges under the person's shoulders) while you fold the top linens down to the bottom of the bed.
9. Put on the gloves.
10. Help the person to remove soiled clothing.
11. Have the person bend her knees and spread her legs as much as possible.
12. Have the person raise her buttocks off the bed, and place a bed protector under the person's hips. If providing perineal care for a woman, elevate the woman's pelvis by placing a bedpan or a folded towel or bath blanket under her buttocks.
13. Adjust the bath blanket as needed so that only the perineal area is exposed.
14. Wet the washcloth and make a mitt with it by:
    - Holding a corner of the washcloth between your thumb and fingers.
    - Wrapping the rest of the washcloth around your hand and holding it with your thumb.
    - Folding the cloth over your fingers and tucking it under the fold in your palm.
15. Put soap on the washcloth mitt.
16. Wash the perineal area.
    - **Female:** Separate the labia with one hand. Place the washcloth mitt at the top of the vulva and stroke downward, toward the anus. Clean the middle, then one side, then the other side, using a clean part of the mitt for each stroke (Figure 1A). Using a clean wet washcloth, form another mitt and rinse the perineal area in the same manner as you washed it. Dry the perineal area with a clean towel, using the same steps as you did when washing and rinsing. Remove the bedpan or the folded towel or bath blanket.

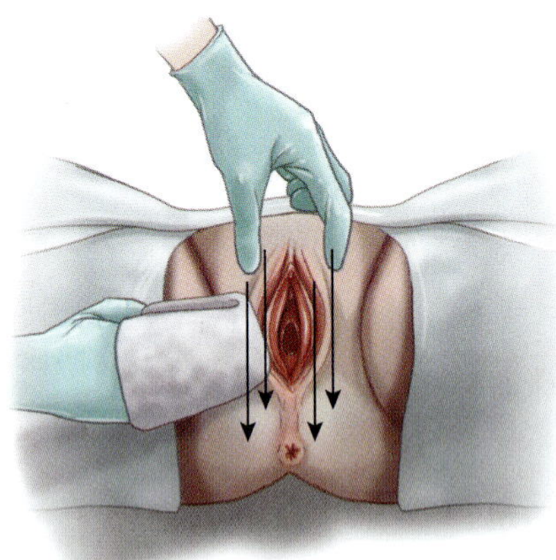

Figure 1A

    - **Male:** Hold the man's penis in one hand. If the man is uncircumcised, retract the foreskin. Moving from the urethral opening outward, wash the penis using a circular motion, starting with the tip and moving down to the base (Figure 1B). Using a clean wet washcloth, form another mitt and rinse the penis in the same manner as you washed it. Dry the penis with a clean towel, using the same steps as you did when washing and rinsing. If the man is uncircumcised, return the foreskin to its natural position. Wash, rinse and pat dry the scrotum and perineum.

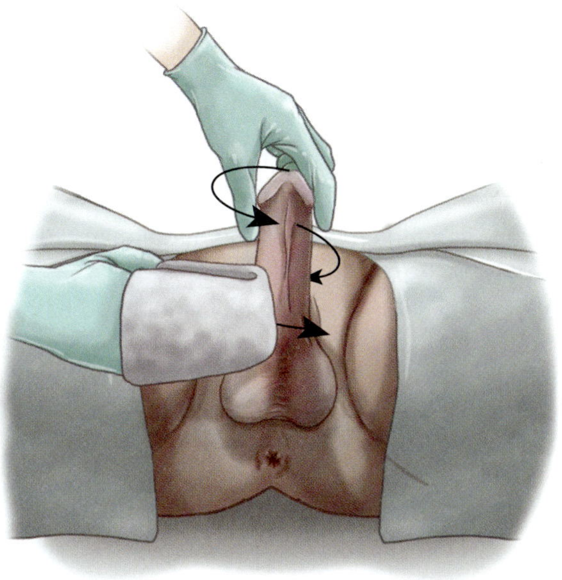

Figure 1B

17. Help the person turn onto one side so that his or her back is facing you.
18. Wet another washcloth, form a mitt and apply soap. Using your other hand, separate the buttocks. Moving from the genitals toward the anus (front to back), wash one side, then the other side, and then the middle, using a different part of the washcloth for each stroke (Figure 2). Using a clean wet washcloth, form another mitt and rinse the anal area in the same manner as you washed it. Dry the anal area with a clean towel, using the same steps as you did when washing and rinsing.

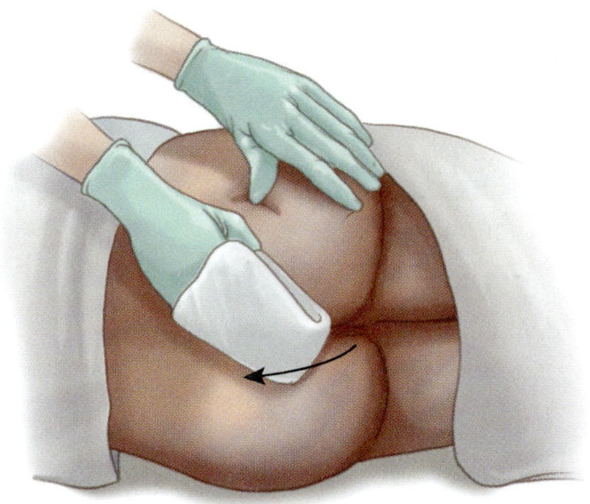

Figure 2

19. Remove the bed protector.
20. Remove and dispose of your gloves.
21. Help the person back into the supine position.
22. Help the person to put on clean clothing.
23. If the linens are soiled or wet, change the linens.
24. Pull up the top linens and remove the bath blanket.

COMPLETION

25. Ensure the person's comfort and good body alignment.
26. Adjust equipment for safety: Lower the bed to the level specified in the person's care plan. Make sure the wheels on the bed are locked. Place the person's method of calling for help within reach. Lower or raise the side rails according to the person's care plan.
27. Clean up your work area.
28. Wash your hands.
29. Report and record.

Skill 13-12

Helping a Person with a Complete Bed Bath

PREPARATION

1. Wash your hands.
2. Gather your supplies:
   - Washcloths
   - Towels
   - Bath blanket
   - Bed protector
   - Wash basin
   - Bath thermometer
   - Soap
   - Paper towels
   - Gloves
   - Clean clothing
   - Lotion (optional)
   - Deodorant or antiperspirant (optional)
   - Clean linens (if needed)
3. Knock, greet the person and ensure privacy.
4. Explain the procedure.
5. Adjust equipment for body mechanics and safety: Raise the bed to a comfortable working height. Make sure the wheels on the bed are locked.

PROCEDURE

6. Cover the over-bed table with the paper towels and arrange your supplies. Fill the wash basin with warm water. Use the bath thermometer to verify that the water temperature is between 105° F and 115° F. Place the wash basin on the over-bed table.
7. Lower the head of the bed as low as the person can tolerate.
8. Help the person move closer to the side of the bed where you are working.
9. Remove and fold the bedspread and blanket for reuse. Cover the person and the top sheet with the bath blanket (to provide privacy and warmth). Ask the person to hold the edge of the bath blanket (or tuck the edges under the person's shoulders) while you fold the top linens down to the bottom of the bed.
10. Put on the gloves.
11. Help the person to remove soiled clothing.

Task 1: Wash the Person's Face, Neck and Ears

12. Place a towel on top of the bath blanket, across the person's chest. This helps to keep the bath blanket dry while you wash the person's face, neck and ears.
13. Wet the washcloth and make a mitt with it by:
    - Holding a corner of the washcloth between your thumb and fingers.
    - Wrapping the rest of the cloth around your hand and holding it with your thumb.
    - Folding the cloth over your fingers and tucking it under the fold in your palm.
14. Without using soap, use the washcloth to bathe the eye farther from you. Begin at the inner corner of the eye, near the nose. Then move the washcloth across the eye to the outer corner. Use the towel to dry the eye. Use the opposite end of the mitt and towel to bathe and dry the other eye (Figure 1).

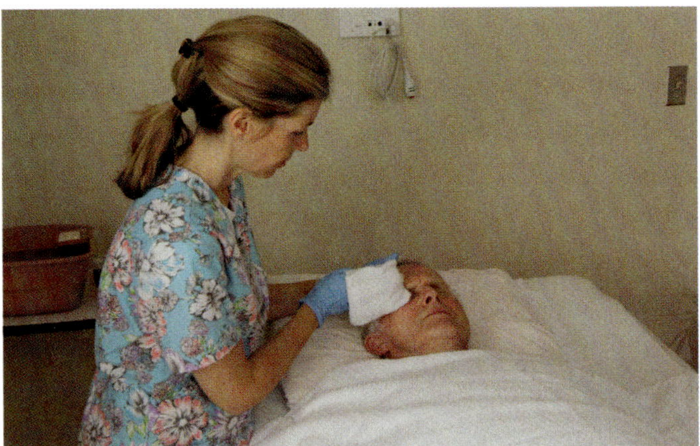

Figure 1

15. Using soap sparingly, wash, rinse and dry the person's face, neck and ears.

Task 2: Wash the Person's Arms and Hands

16. Fold back the bath blanket to expose the person's arm that is farther from you. Place the towel lengthwise under the arm.
17. Wash, rinse and dry the shoulder, arm and underarm (axilla). Use the towel that was under the arm to dry the shoulder, arm and underarm.

18. Place a bed protector on the mattress near the person's hand, and place the wash basin on the bed protector. Place the person's hand in the wash basin. Wash, rinse and dry the person's hand.
19. Recover the person's arm with the bath blanket.
20. Fold back the bath blanket on the person's arm that is nearer to you. Place the towel lengthwise under the arm.
21. Wash, rinse and dry the shoulder, arm, axilla and hand as in steps 17 and 18 (Figure 2).

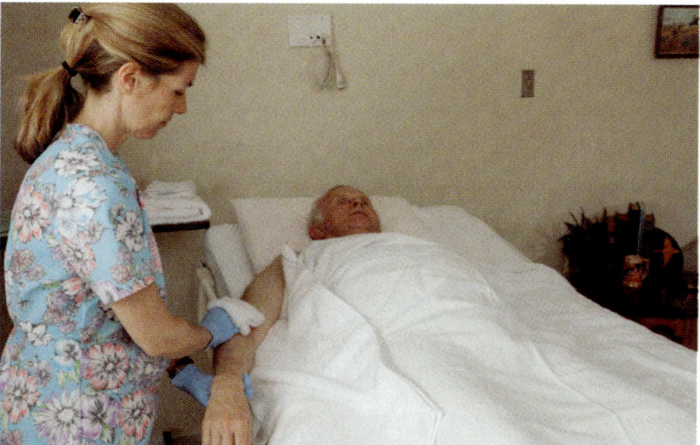

Figure 2

22. Remove the towel from under the arm, and cover the arm with the bath blanket.

Task 3: Wash the Person's Chest and Abdomen

23. Place the towel on top of the bath blanket, over the person's chest and abdomen (stomach).
24. Reach under the towel that is over the bath blanket and fold the bath blanket down to the person's pubic area without exposing it. Leave the towel in place so that the person is not completely exposed.
25. Fold back the towel to expose the side of the person's chest that is farther from you. Wash, rinse and dry the person's chest. Inspect under the person's breast and skin folds as you work.
26. Dry the person's skin completely. Re-cover the chest with the towel.
27. Fold back the towel to expose the side of the person's chest that is nearer to you.
28. Wash, rinse and dry the chest as in steps 25 and 26 (Figure 3).

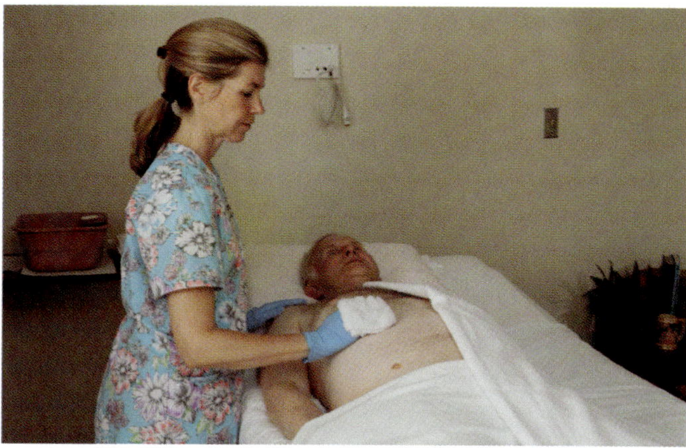

Figure 3

29. Wash, rinse and dry the person's abdomen in the same manner as the chest, doing the farther side first, and then the nearer side.
30. Pull the bath blanket back up to cover the chest and abdomen, and remove the towel from underneath.
31. Change the water if it becomes too soapy or cool.

Task 4: Wash the Person's Legs and Feet

32. Fold the bath blanket away from the person's leg that is farther from you. Place the towel lengthwise under the leg.
33. Wash, rinse and dry the leg. Use the towel that was under the leg to dry it.
34. Place a bed protector on the mattress near the person's foot, and place the wash basin on the bed protector. Place the person's foot in the wash basin. Wash, rinse and dry the person's foot.
35. Re-cover the person's leg with the bath blanket.
36. Fold back the bath blanket on the person's leg that is nearer to you. Place the towel lengthwise under the leg.
37. Wash, rinse and dry the leg and foot as in steps 33 and 34 (Figure 4).

Continued on next page

Skill 13-12

Helping a Person with a Complete Bed Bath *Continued*

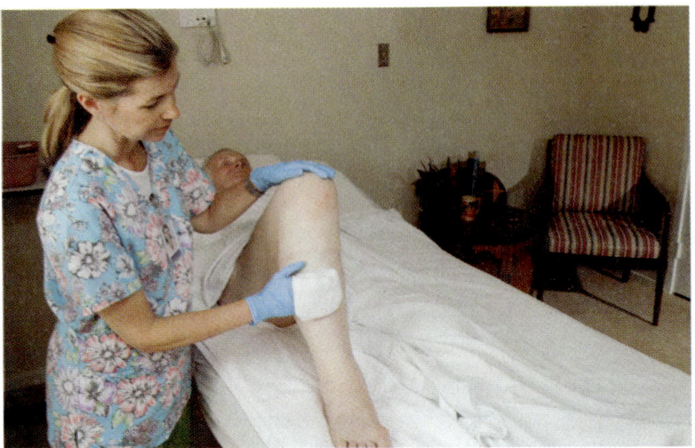

Figure 4

38. Re-cover the leg with the bath blanket. Remove the towel from under the leg.
39. Change the water.

Task 5: Wash the Person's Back and Buttocks

40. Help the person turn onto one side so that his back is facing you.
41. Place the towel on the sheet behind the person's neck, back and buttocks. Adjust the bath blanket so that it covers the person's chest, shoulders, abdomen and legs.
42. Wash, rinse and dry the person's neck, back and buttocks (Figure 5). Inspect the skin as you work.

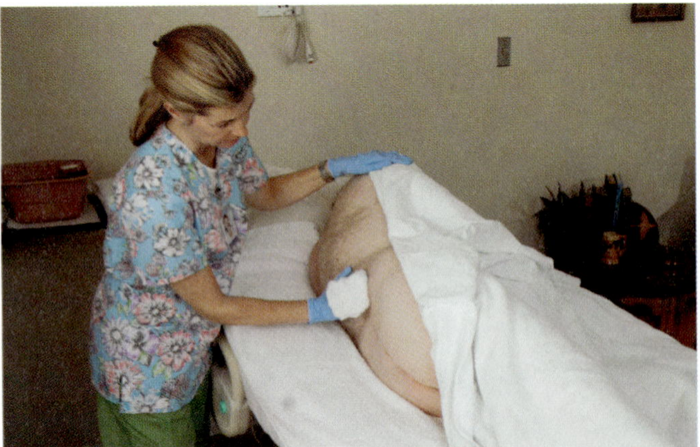

Figure 5

43. If the person would like a back rub, provide a back rub as in Skill 13-14.

Task 6: Wash the Perineal Area

44. Place the towel so that it will be under the person's hips when you help the person back into the supine position. If the person is able to do his own perinal care, provide a fresh washcloth, soap and clean water. Give the person a few minutes alone to complete perineal care. If the person is not able to do his own perineal care, provide perineal care as in Skill 13-11.
45. Remove and dispose of your gloves.

Task 7: Help the Person Dress

46. Help the person back into the supine position.
47. Help the person to apply deodorant or antiperspirant (optional).
48. Help the person to put on clean clothing.
49. If the linens are soiled or wet, change the linens.
50. Pull up the top linens and remove the bath blanket.

COMPLETION

51. Ensure the person's comfort and good body alignment.
52. Adjust equipment for safety: Lower the bed to the level specified in the person's care plan. Make sure the wheels on the bed are locked. Place the person's method of calling for help within reach. Lower or raise the side rails according to the person's care plan.
53. Clean up your work area.
54. Wash your hands.
55. Report and record.

Skill 13-13
Helping a Person with a Shower or Tub Bath

PREPARATION

1. Prepare the shower or tub room. Obtain a shower chair, if one is needed. Cover the seat of the shower chair (or the tub, if the tub has a seat) with a folded towel for comfort. Also place a folded towel on the seat where the person will sit to dry off.
2. Wash your hands.
3. Gather your supplies:
   - Washcloths
   - Towels
   - Bath blanket
   - Bath thermometer
   - Soap
   - Gloves
   - Clean clothing
   - Plastic apron (optional)
   - Shower cap (optional)
   - Shampoo and conditioner (optional)
   - Lotion (optional)
4. Knock, greet the person and ensure privacy.
5. Explain the procedure.
6. Adjust equipment for body mechanics and safety: Lower the bed to the level specified in the person's care plan. Make sure the wheels on the bed are locked.

PROCEDURE

7. Help the person put on a robe and footwear, and assist the person to the shower or tub room. If you are taking the person to the shower or tub room in a wheelchair, have the person hold the supplies in his lap.
8. Run the water:
   - **Shower:** Turn the faucet on, and adjust the temperature of the water so that it is warm to the touch. Use the bath thermometer to verify that the water temperature is between 105° F and 115° F.
   - **Tub:** Turn the faucet on, and allow the tub to fill halfway. Turn the hot water faucet off first to prevent hot water from dripping from the faucet and onto the person. Use the bath thermometer to verify that the water temperature is between 105° F and 115° F.
9. Ask the person if the water feels too warm before the person gets into the tub (sometimes even water at 105° F will feel too warm to the person).
10. Put on the plastic apron, if you are using one.
11. If the person's hair is not going to be washed, offer a shower cap.
12. Help the person undress. If the person seems chilled or concerned about being exposed, offer the person a bath blanket or towel to place over the shoulders. The person can leave the bath blanket or towel in place while he bathes.
13. Using good body mechanics, help the person into the shower or tub. If a shower chair is used, lock the brakes or place the chair against the shower wall.
14. Give the person the soap and a washcloth and encourage the person to complete as much of the bathing as possible independently. Stay in the shower or tub room with the person. If safety allows, you can provide the person with some privacy by staying on the other side of the curtain.
15. Put on the gloves.
16. Ask the person what parts of the body he needs help washing. Wash from the cleanest areas of the body to the dirtiest areas of the body: eyes; face, neck and ears; arms, armpits and hands; chest and abdomen; legs and feet; back and buttocks; perineal area.
17. Assist the person to rinse all of the soap off the skin.
18. Assist the person to wash the hair, if necessary. If washing the hair in the tub, give the person a clean washcloth to hold over his eyes while you rinse the hair with clean water from a pitcher.
19. Help the person to get out of the shower or tub and transfer to the towel-covered chair. Wrap the person in a towel or bath blanket. If the person's hair is wet, wrap the person's hair in another towel.
20. If the person was taking a shower, shut off the water.

Continued on next page

Skill 13-13
Helping a Person with a Shower or Tub Bath *Continued*

21. Help the person to dry off completely. Make sure areas where "skin meets skin" are dry (Figure 1).

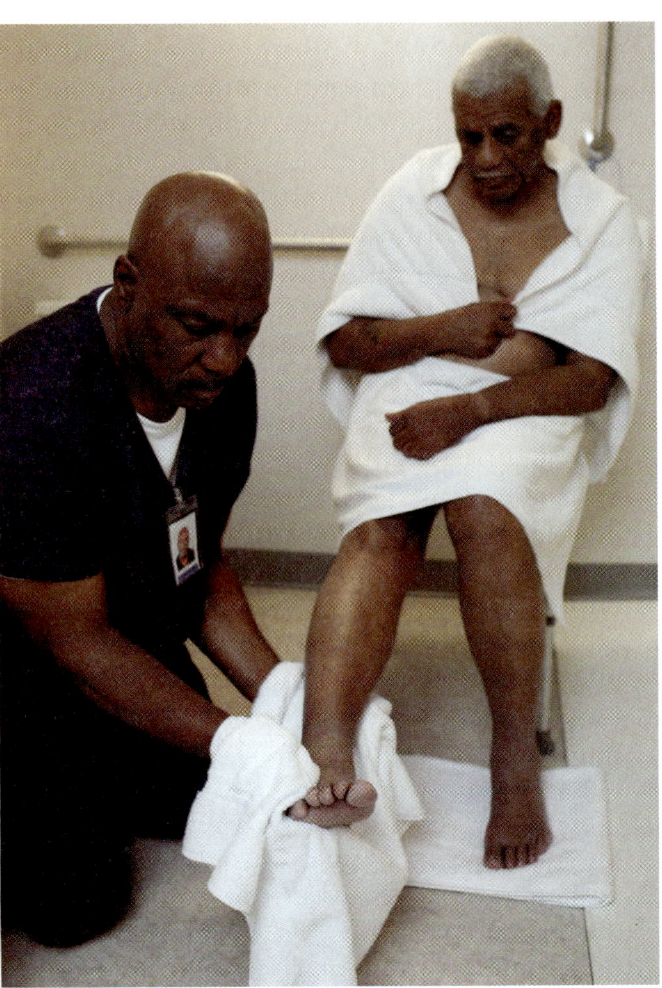

Figure 1

22. Help the person to apply lotion, deodorant or antiperspirant, or other products as the person requests.
23. Help the person to dress.
24. Assist the person back to his room.

COMPLETION

25. Ensure the person's comfort and good body alignment.
26. Adjust equipment for safety: Lower the bed to the level specified in the person's care plan. Make sure the wheels on the bed are locked. Place the person's method of calling for help within reach. Lower or raise the side rails according to the person's care plan.
27. Clean up your work area.
28. Wash your hands.
29. Report and record.

Skill 13-14
Giving a Back Rub

PREPARATION

1. Wash your hands.
2. Gather your supplies:
   - Bath blanket
   - Wash basin
   - Lotion
   - Gloves (optional)
3. Knock, greet the person and ensure privacy.
4. Explain the procedure.
5. Adjust equipment for body mechanics and safety: Raise the bed to a comfortable working height. Make sure the wheels on the bed are locked.

PROCEDURE

6. Cover the over-bed table with the paper towels and arrange your supplies. Fill the wash basin with warm water. Warm the lotion by placing the bottle in the wash basin full of warm water.
7. Lower the head of the bed as low as the person can tolerate.
8. Cover the person and the top sheet with the bath blanket (to provide privacy and warmth). Ask the person to hold the edge of the bath blanket (or tuck the edges under the person's shoulders) while you fold the top linens down to the bottom of the bed.
9. Help the person to remove his top.
10. Help the person turn onto one side so that his back is facing you. Adjust the bath blanket so that only the person's back is exposed.
11. Put on the gloves, if you are using them.
12. Squeeze some lotion onto the palm of your hand and distribute it over your hands by rubbing your palms together.
13. Put your hands at the base of the person's spine. Rub the lotion into the person's back, moving up the spine to the shoulders, and then down the sides of the back (Figure 1). Use big circular motions. Start at the base of the back and move upward toward the shoulders. Continue rubbing the back in this way for 3 to 5 minutes.

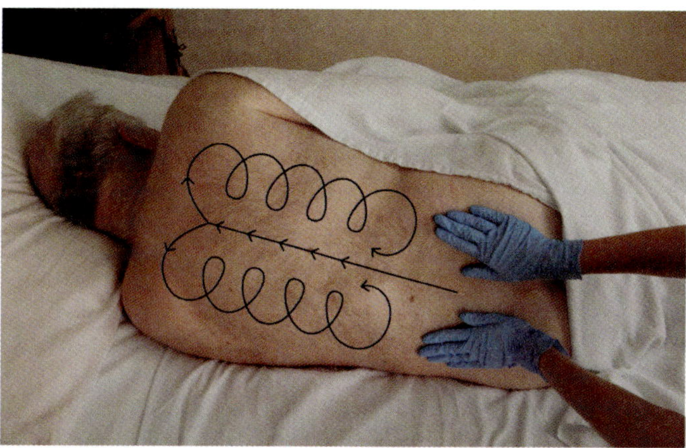

Figure 1

14. Remove and dispose of your gloves, if using.
15. Help the person back into the supine position.
16. Help the person to put his top back on.
17. Pull up the top linens and remove the bath blanket.

COMPLETION

18. Ensure the person's comfort and good body alignment.
19. Adjust equipment for safety: Lower the bed to the level specified in the person's care plan. Make sure the wheels on the bed are locked. Place the person's method of calling for help within reach. Lower or raise the side rails according to the person's care plan.
20. Clean up your work area.
21. Wash your hands.
22. Report and record.

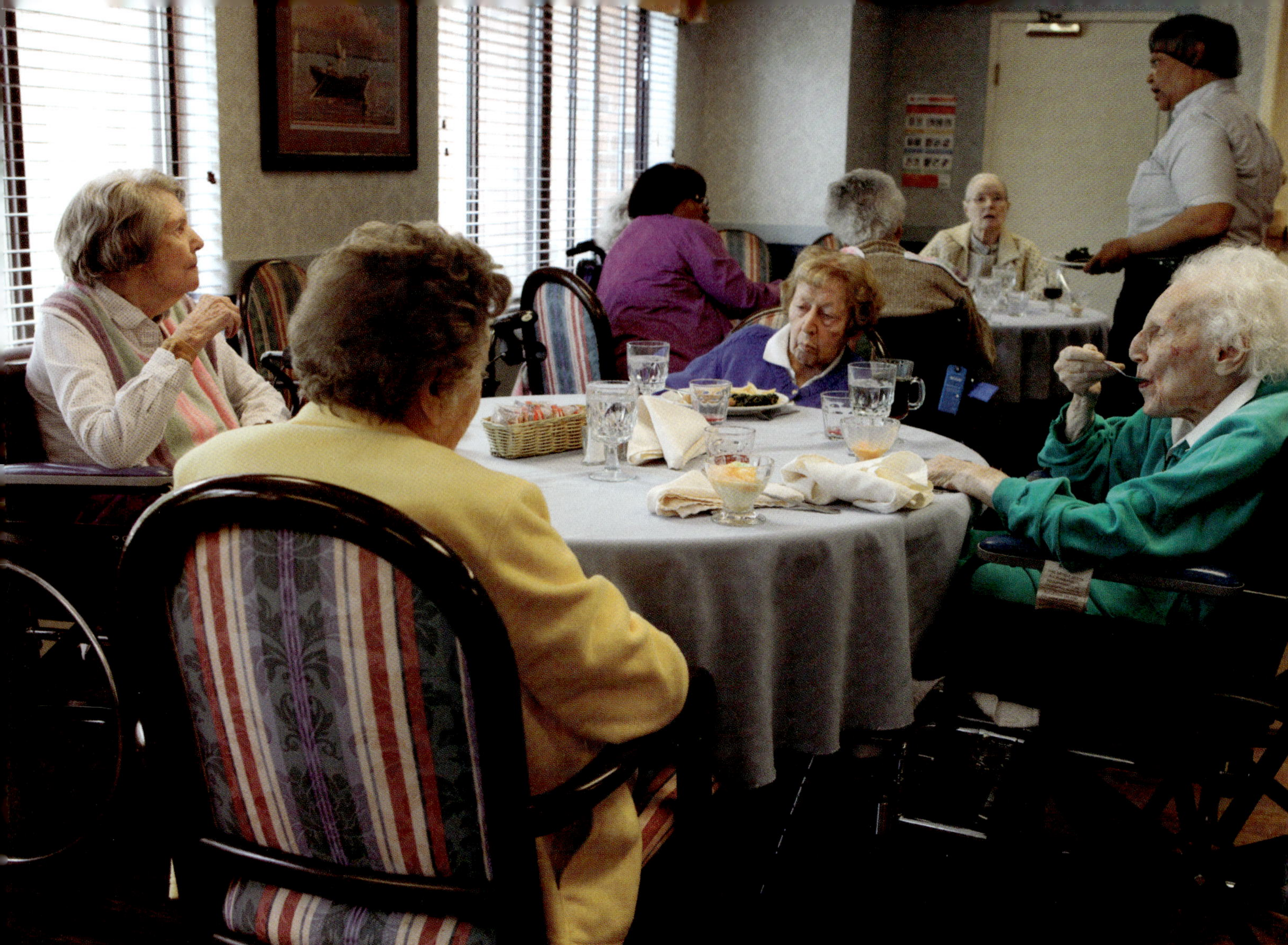

CHAPTER

14 Assisting with Meals and Fluids

Goals

After reading this chapter, you will have the information needed to:

- Describe general types of nutrients that are essential for health.
- Explain general principles of a healthy diet, and describe two tools that can be used to help plan a healthy diet.
- Describe factors that can affect the choices a person makes about food.
- Describe orders that may be in place concerning diet and nutrition.
- Describe common therapeutic diets, and explain the reasons each of these diets may be prescribed.
- List reasons why meal time may be a difficult time for a person who is receiving health care.

Goals

- Describe actions a nurse assistant can take to make meal time as pleasant as possible for the person, and explain why this is important.
- Describe how to prepare a person for a meal, how to serve a meal and how to assist the person with eating.
- Describe how to estimate, report and record a person's food intake.
- Explain the importance of maintaining fluid balance, and describe actions a nurse assistant can take to ensure that a person takes in enough fluids.
- Describe how to measure and record a person's fluid intake.
- Describe the nurse assistant's role in caring for a person who is receiving intravenous (IV) therapy or enteral nutrition (tube feedings).

After practicing the corresponding skill, you will have the information needed to:

- Help a person to eat.

Key Terms:

nutrition	**fiber**	**anorexia**	**fluid balance**
nutrients	**calorie**	**nausea**	**dehydration**
diet	**dietitian**	**malnutrition**	**edema**
glucose	**appetite**	**therapeutic diet**	

Victor Minnetti and his wife, Angela, live by themselves in a large two-bedroom apartment. Mr. Minnetti, who is 79 years old, had a heart attack 2 weeks ago, and has recently come home from the hospital. Mrs. Minnetti, who is 72 years old, has severe arthritis that makes taking care of herself, her husband and their home difficult. You are a home health care aide, and one of your assignments today is to help both Mr. and Mrs. Minnetti with bathing, grooming and meals. The nurse has told you that the doctor has prescribed a low-salt, low-fat diet for Mr. Minnetti. When you mention this to Mrs. Minnetti, she says, "He's going to hate this diet. He just loves his butter and that salt shaker. And meals are really a big part of what we do."

WHAT IS GOOD NUTRITION?

Nutrition is the process of taking in and using **nutrients**, which are substances that the body needs to grow, maintain itself and stay healthy. Nutrients can be obtained through vitamin and mineral supplements, but our main and best source of nutrients is through **diet** (that is, the food we eat and the beverages we drink). Eating a healthy, nutritious diet (that is, one that contains a wide variety of nutrients) helps to maintain good health and can improve poor health.

To get all the necessary nutrients, a person needs to eat a variety of foods. No single food or group of foods supplies all the nutrients the body needs. Different types of nutrients include the following:

- **Carbohydrates** supply the body with **glucose**, the body's most basic source of energy. The most nutritious sources of carbohydrates include whole grains (such as whole wheat bread, brown rice and oatmeal) and fruits and vegetables, because in addition to providing energy, these types of carbohydrates also supply **fiber**, a substance that helps the digestive tract function properly and lowers risk for heart disease and diabetes. Other, less nutritious sources of carbohydrates include table sugar, white bread, white rice and white pasta.
- **Proteins** help the body to build muscle and other body tissue. For this reason, proteins are especially important when a person is healing from an injury or surgery. Proteins are also an important source of energy for the body. Common foods that supply proteins include meat, poultry, fish, beans, eggs and dairy products.
- **Fats** are a concentrated source of energy. Fat in the diet helps us to feel full and makes food taste better. Fat also helps the body use certain vitamins more efficiently, helps to keep us warm and protects our internal organs. For good health, however, only a small amount of fat is needed each day, and healthy fats should be chosen over unhealthy ones. Examples of healthy fats include olive oil, canola oil and peanut

oil. Examples of less healthy fats include butter, margarine, lard and the fat found in red meats.

- **Minerals** and **vitamins** are small molecules that help to regulate body functions and form cells and tissues. Examples of minerals include iron, calcium, sodium, potassium and iodine. Examples of vitamins include vitamins A, B, C, D, E and K. Minerals and vitamins are found in many different types of foods. Good sources include whole grains, fruits and vegetables, lean meats and dairy products.

PLANNING A HEALTHY DIET

A healthy diet helps to ensure that we consume the nutrients we need in the right amounts to stay healthy (or to regain health). It also helps to maintain a healthy body weight (that is, a body weight that is not too high or too low). Being overweight or underweight puts a person at risk for health problems. Two tools that are available to help people plan a healthy diet include MyPlate and nutrition labels.

- **MyPlate** was developed by the United States government to help Americans "build a healthy plate" (Figure 14-1). MyPlate focuses on five food groups that supply important nutrients (fruits, vegetables, grains, protein foods and dairy) and uses a place setting to show how much of each food group should be eaten (relative to the other food groups) at each meal. MyPlate encourages people to choose fruits, vegetables, whole grains, lean meats and low-fat dairy over less nutritious foods, and to cut back on sodium, unhealthy fats and added sugars.
- **Nutrition labels.** All packaged foods are required to have a nutrition label that provides information about serving size, calories, the nutrients supplied by the food and the ingredients in the food (Figure 14-2). Reading these labels can help people make good choices about nutrition. These labels are also an important tool for people who are trying to manage their weight, because they give information about appropriate serving sizes and the number of calories the food contains. A **calorie** is the unit of measure used to describe the amount of energy a food supplies. Taking in more calories than the body uses through daily activity leads to weight gain, because the excess calories are stored in the body as fat.

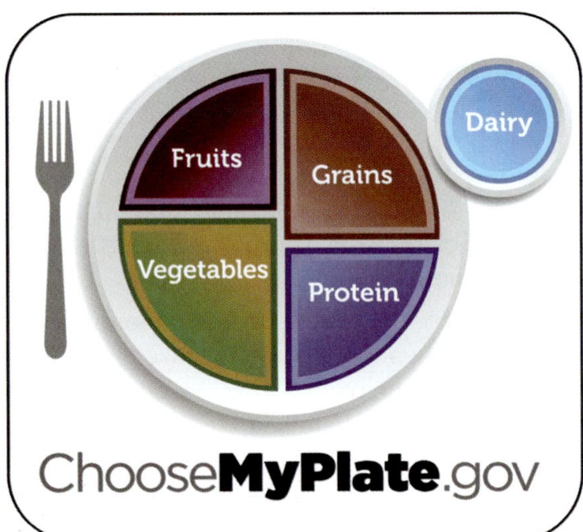

Figure 14-1 MyPlate helps Americans to make healthy food choices.

Although the general principles of following a healthy diet are the same for everyone, the types of nutrients and the number of calories a person needs to take in each day can vary according to the person's gender, age and situation. For example:

- Men tend to need more calories than women do.
- Infants, children and teenagers have increased needs for nutrients and calories because they are growing.
- Pregnant women and women who are breastfeeding require more of certain types of nutrients, such as protein and calcium.
- People who are ill or injured will have different nutritional needs, depending on what type of illness

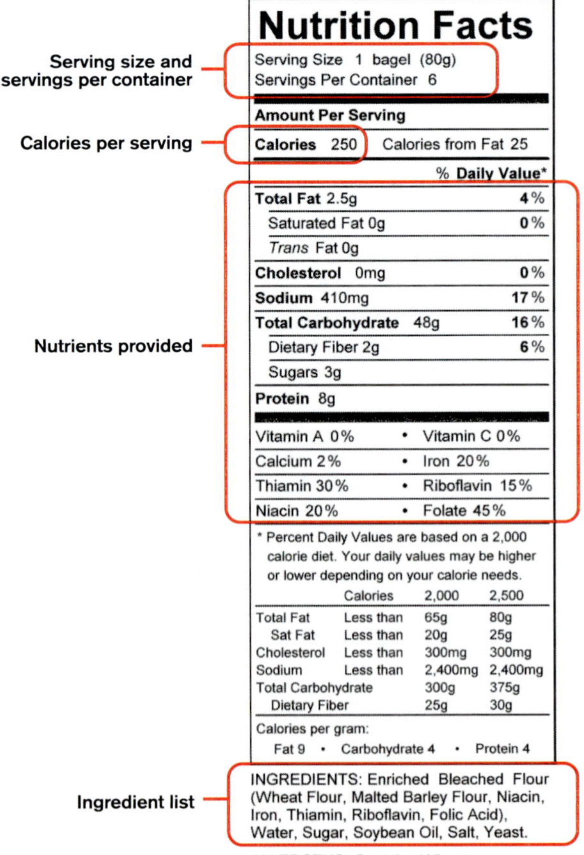

Figure 14-2 Nutrition labels provide information about the ingredients in packaged foods, the nutrients and calories the food provides and the recommended serving size.

or injury they have. For example, a person who is recovering from an injury, burn or surgery usually requires more protein and calories because the body is using a great deal of energy to repair the damaged tissues.

- Older people who are frail usually do not need to take in as many calories, because they are usually less active.

A **dietitian** (a health care professional who has specialized knowledge and training in the field of nutrition) is often consulted when it is necessary to plan a diet for a person with special needs.

FACTORS THAT AFFECT WHAT AND HOW WE EAT

People differ in what they eat, when they eat and how they prepare food. As a nurse assistant, you will play an important role in encouraging those in your care to eat a diet that helps them to maintain or regain health. Knowing about the factors that can affect the choices a person makes about food can help you to respect those choices when you are providing care. This knowledge can also help you identify reasons why a person may not be eating a healthy diet, and take steps to help the person eat more healthfully. Examples of factors that can affect what and how a person eats include:

- **Personal taste.** Each person has certain likes and dislikes when it comes to food. One person may not like green beans, while another may not like chocolate.
- **Allergies and intolerances.** Some people may have reactions that can range from unpleasant to life-threatening if they eat certain foods.
- **Culture and religion.** A person's food choices, likes and dislikes are influenced by social customs, religious practices and the availability of ingredients. Culture and religion can also affect how foods are prepared and when they are served.
- **Budget.** People make choices about food based on what they can afford.
- **Willingness or ability to cook.** Many people rely on prepared convenience foods or restaurant meals because they lack the time, interest, strength or skills needed to cook.
- **Appetite.** A person's desire for food, or **appetite**, influences what and how a person eats. Physical and emotional factors can cause a person's appetite to increase or decrease. **Anorexia**, a loss of appetite, is very common among people who are receiving health care. Factors that can contribute to anorexia include pain, **nausea** (a sick feeling in the stomach often accompanied by the urge to vomit), medication side effects, depression or an impaired sense of taste or smell.

ELDER CARE NOTE. Older people often have several risk factors for malnutrition (failure to take in enough of the right kinds of nutrients to stay healthy). Being on a fixed income may make it difficult for an older person to afford food. Physical disabilities (such as those caused by stroke, vision loss or tooth loss) may make it harder for the person to prepare food, or to chew and swallow it. Emotional difficulties (such as grief, depression and loneliness) can cause the person to lose interest in eating. Conditions that affect the person's memory, such as dementia, can cause the person to forget how to eat. Sensory changes that occur with aging, such as decreased senses of taste and smell, can also negatively affect a person's appetite. When caring for an older person, be alert to signs that the person may not be getting enough to eat (such as weight loss or a lack of interest in food), and report any concerns to the nurse right away. Also, make a special effort to make meal time enjoyable for the person.

As you prepare lunch, Mrs. Minnetti sits at the kitchen table and talks with you. She says, "I'm really grateful you're here. To be honest with you, I've been having more and more trouble managing. My arthritis is so bad I can't lift my cast-iron skillet anymore, and I have trouble chopping vegetables and using the can opener. Before Victor's hospitalization and before you came to help, we were eating a lot of frozen dinners because it was all I could manage on some days."

How did Mrs. Minnetti's increasing difficulty with preparing meals affect the choices Mr. and Mrs. Minnetti made about food?

Mrs. Minnetti said to you, "Meals are a really big part of what we do." What other factors might influence the choices Mr. and Mrs. Minnetti make about food?

Think about the choices you make regarding food. What influences these choices?

SPECIAL ORDERS CONCERNING NUTRITION

When a person is receiving health care, there may be special orders in place. Examples include orders for therapeutic diets, meal supplements, thickened liquids or NPO (nothing by mouth) status.

Therapeutic Diets

A **therapeutic diet** is a special diet that is ordered to help a person regain or maintain her health. The person's primary care provider orders the therapeutic diet, and the dietitian helps to plan meals that meet the requirements of the diet but also suit the person's individual tastes and needs. When you are caring for a person who is receiving a therapeutic diet, you will need to be familiar with the type of therapeutic diet that was ordered, and also the reason why the therapeutic diet was ordered. This knowledge will help you to identify errors (for example, a mix-up with meal trays) and reinforce information the nurse has given the person about the reason for, and benefits of, the therapeutic diet. It is important to help and encourage the person to follow any therapeutic diet that has been ordered, because not following the diet can cause health problems. Commonly ordered therapeutic diets are summarized in Box 14-1.

ELDER CARE NOTE. Although following a therapeutic diet when one has been ordered is important for the person's health, a balance needs to be maintained between meeting nutritional requirements and maintaining the person's quality of life. Particularly with an older person, the health care team may decide to take the person off the therapeutic diet if the special diet seems to be negatively affecting the person's desire to eat and ability to enjoy her food. Often in older people, the risks associated with malnutrition and weight loss (resulting from loss of a desire to eat because the therapeutic diet is unappealing) are greater than the risks associated with not following the therapeutic diet. If an older person in your care is on a therapeutic diet but does not seem to be taking in adequate amounts of food or enjoying his meals, make the nurse aware of this.

Box 14-1 Commonly Ordered Therapeutic Diets

Soft, Mechanical or Pureed Diet. Food can be prepared in special ways to make it easier for a person to chew, swallow and digest. A soft diet includes soft and mashed foods, such as hot breakfast cereal and mashed potatoes. A mechanical diet includes foods that are chopped very small, or ground up (such as ground meat). A pureed diet includes foods that are blended to a very smooth consistency, similar to that of pudding or a milkshake. A pureed diet can look very unappealing, but keeping the individual foods separate from one another and having a positive attitude toward the food can help the person accept it.

Liquid Diet. A liquid diet may be ordered for a person who has digestive problems or has had recent surgery. A clear liquid diet or a full liquid diet may be ordered. A clear liquid diet includes liquids you can see through, such as broth, gelatin, tea, clear carbonated sodas and clear juices (for example, apple, grape, cranberry). A full liquid diet includes fruit juices such as orange and grapefruit juice, strained soups, ice cream, milk and thinned cooked cereal. Because a liquid diet does not provide adequate nutrition, it is usually only used for 1 to 2 days.

Sodium-Restricted Diet. Sodium may be limited for people with high blood pressure or kidney or heart disease. Foods in this diet must be prepared with no added salt, and foods that are naturally high in sodium (such as lunch meat, cured meats, pickles and cheeses) should be avoided. The person is usually not allowed to add salt to foods at the table, but the primary care provider may approve the use of a salt substitute. Often foods are prepared with or accompanied by other spices to increase flavor and make up for the lack of salt.

Carbohydrate-Controlled Diet. This diet is ordered for people with diabetes. The dietician determines the amount of carbohydrates, fat and protein the person can have each day based on the person's activity level and nutritional needs. Meals are planned so that the person's daily budget of carbohydrates, fat and protein is spaced throughout the day to help keep blood glucose levels steady.

Calorie-Restricted Diet. A diet with 1,200, 1,500, 1,800 or 2,000 calories per day may be ordered for a person who needs to control his weight. The primary care provider or dietitian may recommend multivitamin and mineral supplements for a daily diet of 1,200 calories or fewer. For minor calorie restriction, the doctor may order a regular no-concentrated-sweets (NCS) diet that eliminates only sweets, such as candy and cookies.

Heart Healthy Diet. A heart healthy diet is usually ordered for people with heart disease. Foods on this diet are naturally low in unhealthy fats. Lean meats, low-fat or non-fat dairy products, fruits, vegetables and whole grains are encouraged. Cooking techniques that involve the use of additional fats (such as frying) are avoided. Although unhealthy fats like butter should be avoided, spreads and condiments that contain healthy fats can be used in moderation.

High-Protein Diet. A doctor prescribes this diet for people who do not eat enough protein or who need additional protein to rebuild injured tissue.

Meal Supplements

When a person has not been eating well or is losing weight because of an illness, the person's primary care provider may order a meal supplement. These supplements, which are similar in taste and appearance to a milkshake, are usually high in calories, fat and protein. The meal supplement may be given with or between meals, as a snack. If a meal supplement has been ordered for one of the people in your care, be sure to serve the supplement at the specified time. If the person declines the supplement, you should report this to the nurse.

Thickened Liquids

Some medical conditions, such as stroke, may make it difficult for a person to swallow liquids without choking. For these people, the person's primary care provider may order the use of a thickening agent. The thickening agent is added to liquids to thicken them and make them easier for the person to swallow. Liquids can be thickened to different consistencies:

- A nectar consistency is like thin, runny syrup. The liquid pours in a ribbon-like stream.
- A honey consistency is thicker than a nectar consistency. The liquid drizzles slowly when poured.
- A pudding consistency is very thick. The liquid does not pour and must be eaten with a spoon.

The person's primary care provider will specify which consistency should be used. Follow your employer's policies and procedures related to thickening liquids. If you are permitted to use a thickening agent to thicken the person's liquids, follow the directions on the container of thickening agent exactly. These directions will tell you how much product to add to achieve the necessary consistency.

NPO Status

NPO stands for *nil per os*, or "nothing by mouth" in Latin. When a person is placed on NPO status, he is not allowed to have *anything*, not even water, by mouth for the specified amount of time. NPO status is most often ordered for several hours before a person has surgery or other procedures (such as some diagnostic procedures) that involve general anesthesia. This is because the anesthesia may cause the person to vomit, which can lead to aspiration and complications such as pneumonia. It is safer for the person if he goes into the surgery or procedure with an empty stomach.

Being on NPO status can be uncomfortable for the person. Providing frequent mouth care to keep the tissues of the mouth moist can help. Be sensitive to the person's discomfort, and encourage visitors to enjoy their own food or beverages outside of the person's room. To remind everyone that the person may not eat or drink, post a sign on the room door saying "NPO."

You finish preparing lunch and go to help Mr. Minnetti to the table. When he sits down, he looks at his plate with disappointment. "I was really hoping for a ham and cheese sandwich and a dill pickle," he tells you. He picks at his meal and leaves most of it uneaten. He says, "It just has no taste!"After Mr. Minnetti leaves the room, Mrs. Minnetti says to you, "Do you see what I mean? I'm afraid if he can't have what he is used to eating, he might not eat. I don't want mealtimes to become a battleground."

Consider the role that meals and eating play in your life. How would you feel if you couldn't eat certain foods that you enjoy?

How might you approach Mr. Minnetti to ease this transition?

Is there anyone else on the health care team you could ask for help?

MEAL TIME WHEN A PERSON IS RECEIVING HEALTH CARE

Meal time can be difficult for a person who is receiving health care. As you have already learned, many physical and emotional factors can cause a person who is receiving health care to have little or no appetite. For a person who is ill or has a physical disability, the act of eating can require a great deal of physical effort and can be very tiring and frustrating. The person may be embarrassed about needing help with an activity as basic as eating.

There are two major goals for meal times when a person is receiving health care. First, you want to make the meal as positive and pleasurable an experience as possible for the person. Secondly, you want to maintain or improve the person's food intake. Usually, achieving the first goal can help you to achieve the second. To make the meal as positive and pleasurable an experience as possible:

- Involve the person in decisions about when to eat, what to eat and where to eat as much as possible.
- Support rituals and traditions the person may have related to eating and mealtimes, such as giving thanks before a meal.

- Take steps to promote the person's dignity and self-esteem throughout the meal.
- Help the person to enjoy the company of others during the meal (even if the only other person present is you).
- Present the meal attractively (for example, by removing items from the meal tray and placing them on the table to create a more home-like environment if you work in a facility setting, or by planning, preparing and serving visually appealing meals if you work in a home setting).
- Create a pleasant, clean, relaxing environment for eating.

Preparing the Person for the Meal

There is more to assisting a person with meals than simply getting the meal tray and putting it down in front of her. Before the meal is even served, there are several things that must be done to help prepare the person for the meal. Give yourself adequate time to accomplish the following before the meal:

- Ensure the person's physical comfort by assisting her to use the bathroom and wash her hands before the meal.
- Provide mouth care, because a clean mouth makes food taste better. If the person wears dentures, make sure the dentures are clean and in place.
- Assist the person with putting on glasses or inserting a hearing aid, if she uses these devices.
- Create a comfortable, pleasant environment for eating. If the person will be taking the meal in her room, make sure the room is neat, clean and free of odors. Make sure there is adequate lighting.
- Position the person properly for eating. In many long-term care facilities, residents go to the dining room to eat. Even if they must be taken to the dining room in a wheelchair, they are often encouraged to move from the wheelchair to a regular dining chair during the meal. Whether the person is eating in the dining room or in her room, help the person into a comfortable, upright, sitting position, with her head up and her hips at a 90-degree angle. This position makes it easier for the person to chew, swallow, and manage eating utensils. If the person is seated in a chair, make sure her feet are flat on the floor, and have her rest her elbows or forearms on the table if she needs support.
- If the person would like to use a clothing protector to protect her clothing from spills, assist her with putting the clothing protector on. To protect the person's dignity, avoid referring to the clothing protector as a bib.

Serving the Meal

Once these preparations are completed, it is time to get the person's meal tray. Make sure you are delivering the right meal tray to the person by checking the name on the card on the meal tray (Figure 14-3). If the person is on a therapeutic diet, make sure that the diet noted on the card is the same one the person is supposed to be receiving. If you suspect that an error has been made, check with the nurse before serving the meal. It is possible that the person's diet has been changed, but if not, you will need to obtain a replacement meal with the correct diet. Organize your time so that you can help the person to eat shortly after delivering the tray. Foods are much more appealing when they are served at the proper temperature.

Assisting the Person to Eat

Many people will be able to eat on their own, if you help them with tasks such as opening cartons, cutting up meat or identifying the location of items on the table and on the plate. The use of assistive devices for eating (Table 14-1) can further increase the person's ability to eat independently. At each meal, talk with the person about the amount of help he needs, because he may have different needs at different meals. For example, at lunchtime the person may be able to eat a sandwich by himself, but at dinnertime he may need help cutting his meat. Always encourage the people in your care to do as much as they can for themselves. Even when a person is totally dependent on you to feed him, involve him in the process as much as possible (for example, by asking him to hold his napkin). This helps to promote independence and protect the person's dignity and self-esteem. Remember that meals are not just about the food. Being in the company of others and socializing

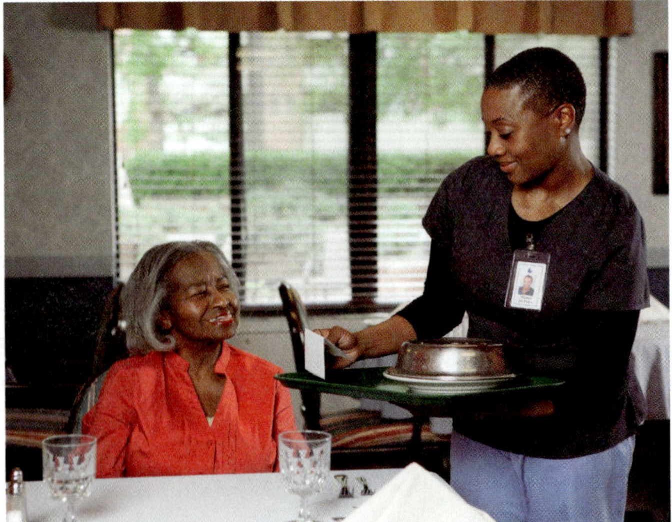

Figure 14-3 Always make sure you are serving the right meal tray to the right person.

Table 14-1 **Assistive Devices for Eating**

Problem	Device	What It Does	How to Improvise
The person has trouble getting food on the utensil	Plate guard 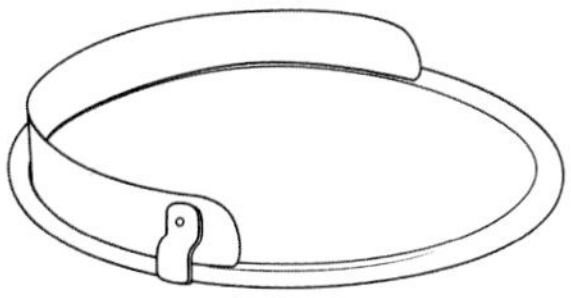	The raised rim gives the person something to push the food against	Have the person hold a piece of bread on the plate to push the food against
	Scoop dish 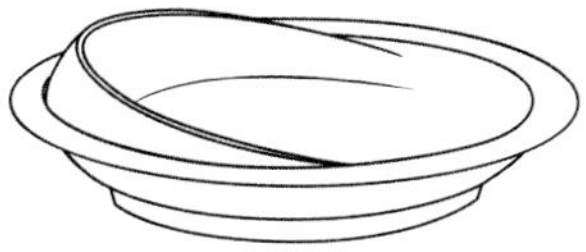	The rounded side gives the person something to push the food against	
	Spork 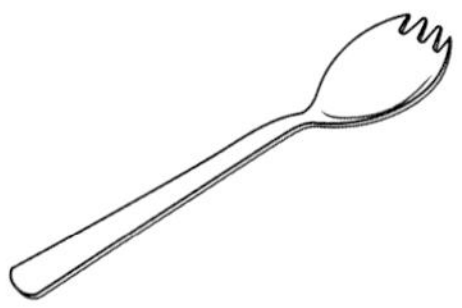	The end of the utensil allows the person to spear or scoop food	
The plate slips or moves	Suction base 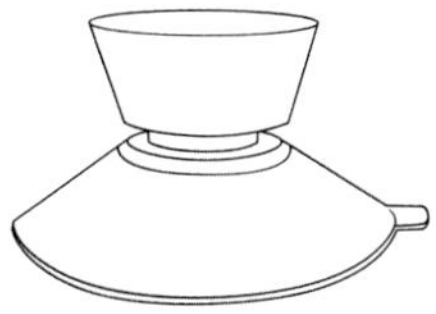	The suction base holds the plate securely to the table	Place a wet washcloth under the plate
The person has trouble grasping the utensil	Built-up handle utensil 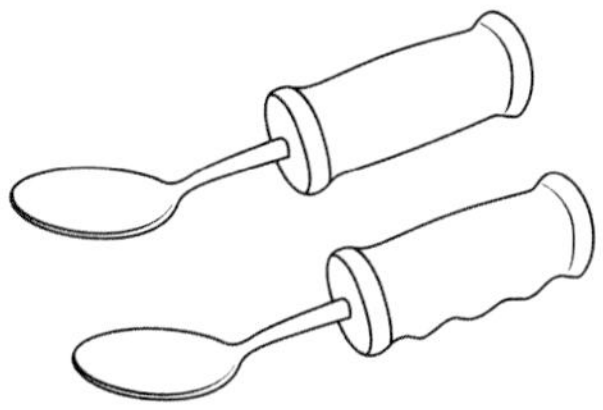	The larger handle is easier to hold	Use foam rubber or leather to build up the handle of a standard utensil, or place the handle of the utensil through a tennis ball 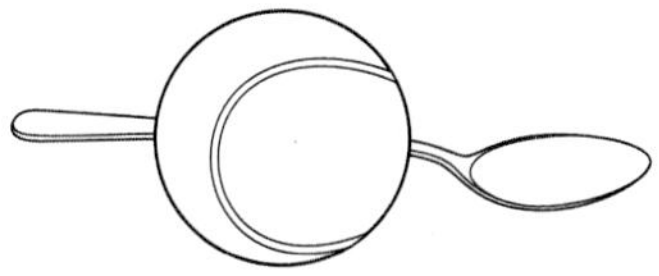
	Vertical or horizontal palm self-handle utensils 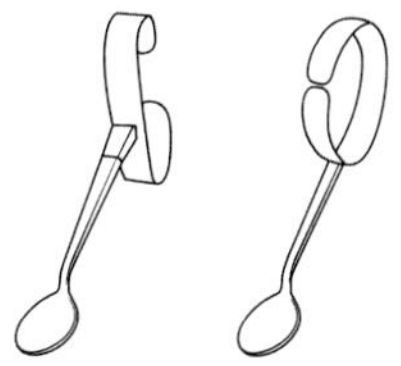	The handle slips over the palm of the hand so the person does not have to grasp it	
	Utensil holder 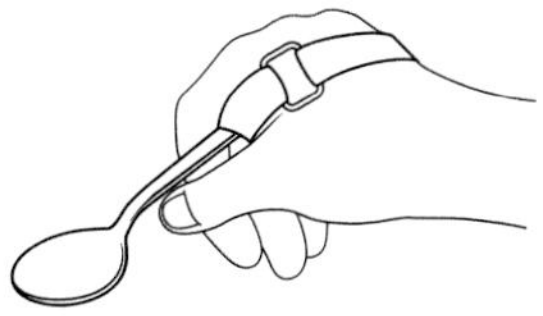	The holder slips over the person's palm and the utensil is placed in the holder, making the utensil easier to grasp	

Continued on next page

Table 14-1 **Assistive Devices for Eating** *continued*

Problem	Device	What It Does	How to Improvise
	Universal cuff	The strap is fastened to the person's hand and the utensil is placed in the strap, making the utensil easier to grasp	
The person has trouble keeping food on the utensil because of a tremor or weakness	Swivel fork or spoon	The end of the fork or spoon remains level even if the person's hand shakes	Rest the person's elbow on a soft, spongy surface (such as a piece of foam or a sponge) to lessen tremors; help to steady the person's hand as needed
The person is only able to use one hand to cut food	Rocker knife	The person rocks the sharp edge of the knife back and forth over the food to cut it	
The person has trouble drinking without spilling the liquid	Modified drinking cup	The handles make it easier for the person to grasp the cup, and the cover and spout keep the liquid from spilling	
	Commercial straw holder	The holder goes across the rim of the cup to keep the straw in place	Secure plastic wrap over the rim of the cup with a rubber band and poke a straw through the plastic wrap
The person has limited arm movement and cannot reach his mouth	Extension utensil	The handle extends to make it easier for the person to bring the food to the mouth	

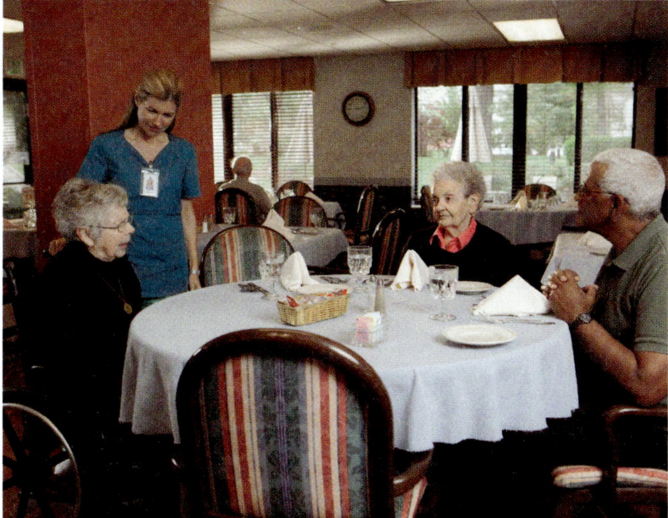

Figure 14-4 Being in the company of others and socializing during meals is important.

are important during the meal as well (Figure 14-4). Sit down and take the time to talk with the person during the meal, even if he cannot answer you.

Avoid rushing the person during the meal. Observe the person to determine whether he needs help eating. If the person does not eat a certain food, ask him why. Sometimes people leave part of a meal uneaten because they get too tired to finish. In this case, the person may eat more if you offer to help. Or the person may just not care for the food. If the person simply did not care for the food, ask if there is something else you can get him to eat that he might find more appetizing. Knowing why a person did not eat part or all of a meal can help the health care team plan future meals that will be more appealing to the person, or address other issues that may be affecting the person's appetite.

When the person has finished eating, remove the dishes and tidy up the table. Assist the person with mouth care and changing any articles of clothing that became soiled during the meal.

Skill 14-1 describes step-by-step how to assist a person during mealtime. Special considerations during mealtime for people with specific conditions are described in the sections that follow.

Helping a person who is visually impaired

A person with visual impairment can usually eat independently if he has no other disabilities. To help the person during meal time, you may only need to do the following:

- Identify the location of foods on the table and on the plate. Describe their locations as if the plate were the face of a clock (Figure 14-5).
- Cut up meats or anything else that needs cutting.
- Open containers.

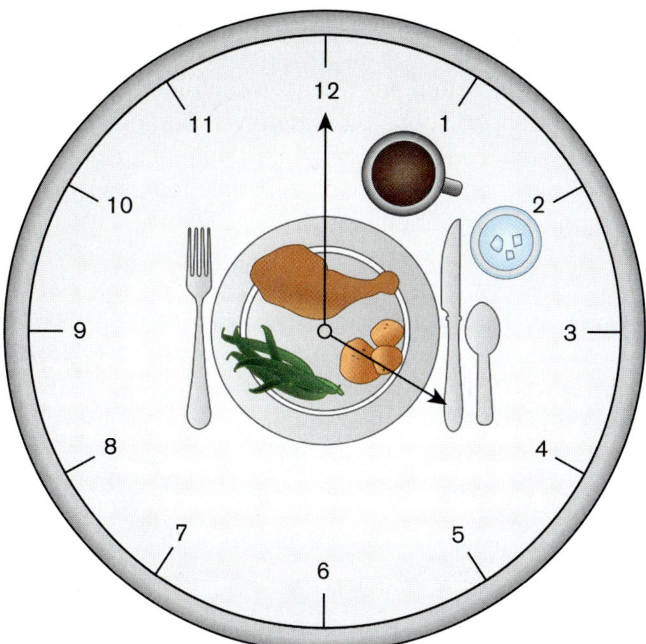

Figure 14-5 Describing the location of items on the table and on the plate in terms of a clock face is useful when assisting a person who is visually impaired to eat. For example, here the chicken is at 12:00, the potatoes are at 4:00, and the green beans are at 7:00. The coffee is at 1:00 and the water is at 2:00.

- Describe the location of the eating utensils.
- During the meal, occasionally check on the person to see whether he has overlooked some of the food, and if so, offer assistance.

Helping a person who has difficulty swallowing

A person who has had a stroke that has resulted in speech difficulties may also have trouble swallowing food. A person who has difficulty swallowing may be on a soft diet, and there may also be orders to use liquid thickeners. When helping a person who has trouble swallowing during meal time:

- Remain with the person while he is eating.
- If the person is working with a speech therapist to relearn safe swallowing techniques, make sure you are aware of these techniques so that you can help the person practice them.
- If liquid thickeners have been ordered, make sure that all of the liquids on the tray, including soup, are thickened before serving them.
- Encourage the person to chew slowly and thoroughly.
- Eliminate distractions, such as television or many visitors, so that the person can concentrate on eating.
- Keep the person's head elevated during eating and for at least 30 minutes after eating.

Helping a person in isolation

Before bringing a meal tray to a person who is in isolation, put on the necessary personal protective equipment (PPE). Because the person's ability to socialize with others is limited, offer the person companionship during the meal. When the person has finished eating, dispose of any leftover food or liquid per your employer's policy. Double-bag reusable and disposable eating utensils, plates and cups for washing or disposal, per your employer's policy.

Monitoring Food Intake

In most facilities, you will be required to estimate, report and record the amount of food the person ate at each meal. You may be asked to estimate how much of the total meal the person ate, and give a rough percentage (Figure 14-6). Usually, you will be required to report a food intake of less than 70% to the nurse.

For some people in your care, you may be required to estimate the percentage eaten of each food that was served. For example, you might say that the person ate 50% of the pork chop, 50% of the mixed vegetables, 100% of the mashed potatoes and 100% of the pudding.

THE IMPORTANCE OF FLUIDS

Earlier you learned about key nutrients that are supplied by food and beverages. In addition to supplying the body with nutrients, foods and beverages supply the body with water. Water is extremely important to life. A person can actually live longer without food than he can without water. Every cell in our bodies contains water, and water forms the basis for many important body fluids, including blood (which circulates oxygen and nutrients throughout the body), sweat (which helps to cool the body) and urine (which helps to remove wastes from the body). We take in the water our bodies need through drinking (water, as well as other beverages) and through eating foods that have high water contents (such as fruits and vegetables, soups, ice cream and gelatin).

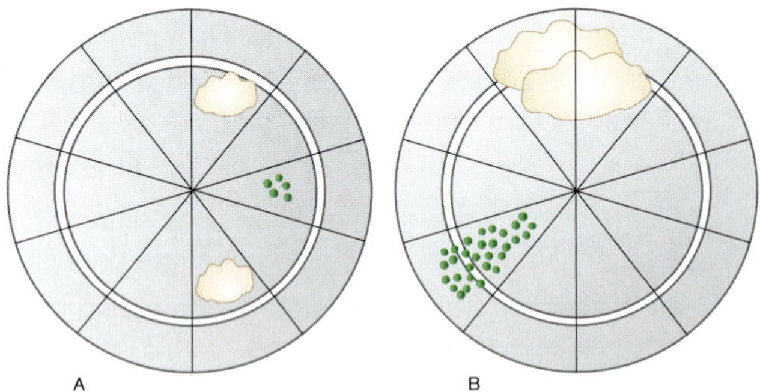

Figure 14-6 Food intake is usually stated as a percentage of the total foods offered. (A) This person ate about 90% of what he was offered. (B) This person ate about 70% of what he was offered. A food intake of less than 70% usually must be reported to the nurse.

Observations Into Action!

When you are assisting a person with eating, be sure to report any of the following observations to the nurse right away:

- **Lack of appetite**
- **Sudden change in appetite**
- **Difficulty chewing or swallowing**
- **Difficulty managing, or extreme frustration with using, assistive devices for eating**
- **Refusal to eat a therapeutic diet, or decreased food intake while on a therapeutic diet**
- **Food intake of less than 70% at a meal**

Fluid Balance

Fluid balance occurs when the amount of fluids a person takes in equals the amount of fluids the person loses. Each day, we lose fluid in the form of urine, sweat, bowel movements and breath vapor. To maintain a state of fluid balance, we must take in enough fluid each day to equal, or balance, these losses. When fluid balance is not maintained, the person develops either **dehydration** (too little fluid in the body) or **edema** (too much fluid in the body).

Dehydration

Dehydration can result from conditions such as vomiting, diarrhea, fever or severe blood loss. A very common cause of dehydration, however, is simply not drinking enough fluids. Many people who are receiving health care have conditions that put them at risk for not drinking enough fluids and becoming dehydrated. For example, a person who has problems with mobility or other disabilities may have a difficult time getting up to get a drink. The person may also cut back on fluids because she is trying to reduce the number of times she needs to get up and go to the bathroom, or she is afraid that she will not be able to make it to the bathroom in time. Some people who are incontinent of urine may also reduce their fluid intake because they think this will lower their risk for having an episode of incontinence. However, it is important to know that decreasing fluid intake does not decrease incontinence, nor does it decrease trips to the bathroom. In fact, the opposite may be true. As the urine becomes more concentrated, it irritates the bladder and may increase the urge to urinate, resulting in the need to urinate more frequently.

As a nurse assistant, you will play an important role in helping to ensure that those in your care take in enough fluids.

- Frequently offer fluids that the person likes at the temperature she prefers (Figure 14-7).
- Encourage the person to drink plenty of fluids with each meal.
- Frequently provide the person with a pitcher of clean, fresh water. Encourage the person to drink each time you enter the room.
- Be sure the person has a clean drinking glass or cup within easy reach. Refill the glass if the person cannot do it. A drinking straw or a plastic water bottle with a screw-on lid and a straw may make it easier for some people to drink independently.
- If the person frequently refuses beverages, check with the nurse to see if you can offer fluid-rich foods instead, such as ice cream, popsicles, gelatin or fruit.

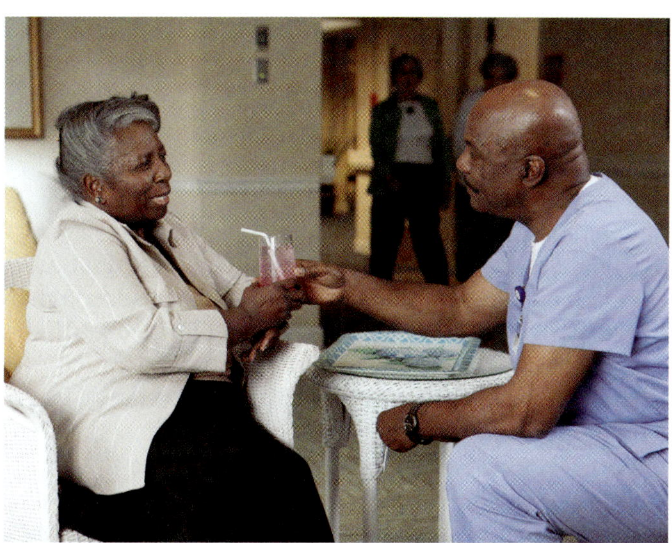

Figure 14-7 A person may hesitate to ask for a drink but will accept one if it is offered.

ELDER CARE NOTE. In an older person, dehydration can occur rapidly and be life-threatening. Many older people often are not as quick to feel thirst as younger people are, so they may not be drinking enough fluids to begin with. This, combined with health concerns that might cause the person to reduce his fluid intake, puts the older person at high risk for dehydration. When you are caring for an older person, offer the person a drink every time you interact with the person, and make sure the person always has fresh water within reach. However, be aware that even when offered water, many older people will say "I'm not thirsty" or "I've already had too much to drink today." You may need to be persistent in encouraging the person to drink.

If a person becomes dehydrated, the person's primary care provider may give an order to "encourage fluids" or "push fluids." This means that the person should be urged to drink as much fluid as possible. Encourage the person to drink each time you enter the room and again on your way out. Keep a record of the amount of fluid the person does drink.

Observations Into Action!

Dehydration is a serious condition. If you suspect that a person in your care is dehydrated, tell the nurse immediately. Signs and symptoms of dehydration include the following:

- **Confusion**
- **Poor skin turgor (the skin does not return to its normal shape when gently squeezed or pinched)**
- **Passing of small amounts of dark-colored urine**
- **Constipation**
- **Drowsiness**
- **Very dry skin or chapped lips**
- **Elevated temperature**

Edema

Edema, or the state of retaining too much water, can result from medical conditions (such as chronic heart failure or kidney disease) that make it hard for the body to rid itself of excess water. The person's primary care provider may place restrictions on the amount of fluid the person is allowed to have each day. When you are caring for a person and fluid restrictions are in place, the nurse will tell you how much fluid the person is allowed to have over the course of your shift. Offer small amounts of fluid at regular intervals. This will help to prevent the person from becoming too thirsty.

Measuring and Recording Fluid Intake

When orders to encourage or restrict fluids are in place, you will need to measure and record the person's fluid intake. A person's fluid intake includes all of the liquids the person drinks, as well as foods that are primarily liquid (such as soups) or that are liquid at body temperature (such as ice cream or popsicles). Although in everyday life fluids are usually measured in ounces (oz), in health care, fluids are measured and recorded in milliliters (mL) or cubic centimeters (cc). A milliliter (mL) is equal to a cubic centimeter (cc). One ounce equals 30 milliliters or 30 cubic centimeters. Follow your employer's policy regarding which abbreviation (mL or cc) to use when documenting fluid intake.

With prepackaged items, printed information on the container indicates how much it holds. For example, a small prepackaged milk container contains 8 ounces, or 240 mL (remember, there are 30 mL in an ounce). In other cases, you will need to determine how much fluid the container holds. Most facilities have a list you can check to determine the amount of fluid the cups, glasses and bowls in use in the facility hold. If you are caring for a person in her home and need to measure fluid intake, you can determine the amount of fluid the person's cups, glasses and bowls hold by filling them with water and then pouring the water into a measuring cup.

To measure and record fluid intake, observe how much fluid the person consumes at each meal and in between meals. For example, if a person had 8 oz (240 mL) of milk, 4 oz (120 mL) of coffee and 12 oz (360 mL) of soup with lunch, you would record the person's fluid intake at lunch time as 720 mL. Then, if the person had another 8 oz (240 mL) of tea in between lunch and dinner, you would record the person's fluid intake as 240 mL. Sometimes the person may not consume all of the fluid in the container. In this case, estimate how much of the total was consumed. For example, if the person only drank about half of his coffee at lunch, you would estimate the amount to be 2 oz (60 mL) instead of the full 4 oz (120 mL).

OTHER WAYS OF PROVIDING NUTRITION AND FLUIDS

Some people will have conditions that make it impossible for them to take food and fluids by mouth. For these people, intravenous (IV) therapy or enteral nutrition (tube feedings) may be ordered.

Intravenous Therapy

Although a person's nutritional needs cannot be met using IV therapy, IV therapy is very useful for administering fluids. A small catheter (tube) is placed in a vein on the back of the person's hand or in the person's arm. Fluid drips slowly from the IV bag, through the IV tubing and into the catheter. Sometimes medications may be administered through the IV tubing as well. Although you will not be responsible for administering IV therapy, you may care for a person who is receiving IV therapy.

Observations Into Action!

When caring for a person who is receiving IV therapy, be sure to report any of the following observations to the nurse right away:

- **Disconnected IV line**
- **Empty fluid bag**
- **Pain, swelling or redness at the IV site**

Enteral Nutrition

Enteral nutrition is often called tube feeding because the person receives nutrition (in the form of a nutrient-rich formula) and fluids through a tube that is placed directly into the stomach or intestines. If the person will only need enteral nutrition for a few days, a nasogastric or nasointestinal tube may be used. These types of tubes are inserted through the person's nose and passed down the person's throat to the stomach or the intestines. If the person is expected to require enteral nutrition for more than a few days, a gastrostomy tube may be used. This type of feeding tube is inserted directly into the stomach through an incision made in the abdomen. The tube is clamped and held in place by sutures (stitches) and covered with a dressing.

You will not be responsible for administering enteral nutrition; however, you may care for a person who is receiving enteral nutrition. Guidelines for caring for a person who is receiving enteral nutrition are given in Box 14-2.

Box 14-2 Nurse Assistant DO's and DON'Ts

Enteral Nutrition

DON'T give the person any food or fluids by mouth.

DO remember that only the nurse may give the person formula or fluids through the tube.

DO keep the head of the person's bed elevated (in low Fowler's position) for at least 30 minutes after the nurse administers a tube feeding. This helps prevent aspiration.

DO position a person with a gastrostomy tube so that he is not lying on the tube.

DO find out from the nurse how to care for the gastrostomy tube insertion site.

DON'T get the dressing covering the gastrostomy tube insertion site wet.

 Observations Into Action!

When caring for a person who is receiving enteral nutrition, be sure to report any of the following observations to the nurse right away:

- **Pain or discomfort in the abdomen**
- **Nausea**
- **Excessive gas**
- **Redness, irritation or drainage around the tube insertion site**
- **The person repeatedly tries to pull out the feeding tube**

CHECK YOUR UNDERSTANDING

Questions for Review

1. Which nutrient helps the body build and repair tissue?

a. Carbohydrates
b. Fat
c. Protein
d. Water

2. A healthy diet is one that:

a. The person will eat.
b. Emphasizes whole grains, fruits and vegetables, lean meats and low-fat dairy.
c. The person's primary care provider prescribes.
d. The person grew up eating.

3. Which nutrient supplies the body with its most basic form of energy?

a. Carbohydrates
b. Vitamins and minerals
c. Protein
d. Fat

4. All of the following can affect the choices a person makes about food EXCEPT:

a. The person's height.
b. The person's culture.
c. The person's religious beliefs.
d. The person's ability to prepare food.

5. Mrs. Powell has had little appetite since her husband of 65 years passed away recently. What action could a nurse assistant take to encourage Mrs. Powell to eat?

a. Remind Mrs. Powell that if she does not eat, she could get sick.
b. Sit with Mrs. Powell while she is eating and make pleasant conversation.
c. Explain to Mrs. Powell the importance of following the MyPlate guidelines.
d. Tell Mrs. Powell that if she does not finish her meal, she cannot have dessert.

6. All of the following can affect a person's appetite EXCEPT:

a. Medications the person is taking.
b. An inability to smell the food.
c. Pain.
d. The person's fluid balance.

7. Which therapeutic diet might be ordered for a person who has trouble chewing or swallowing food?

a. A carbohydrate-controlled diet
b. A liquid diet
c. A soft, mechanical or pureed diet
d. A high-protein diet

8. The doctor has ordered a meal supplement shake for Mrs. Johnson, to be served between lunch and dinner. Today when you tell Mrs. Johnson it is time for her shake, she shakes her head and says she does not want it today. What should you do?

a. Report Mrs. Johnson's refusal of the shake to the nurse.
b. Return the shake to the refrigerator and try offering it to Mrs. Johnson again later.
c. Record Mrs. Johnson's refusal of the shake in her chart, but do not report it to the nurse.
d. Nothing; it is all right if Mrs. Johnson skips the shake because it might spoil her appetite for dinner.

9. Which of the following should you do when assisting with a meal for a person who cannot see?

a. Tell the person loudly what you are feeding him, as you feed it to him.
b. Orient the person to the location of items on the plate and on the table, using the *clock face* method.
c. Insist that the person wear a clothing protector, because he is likely to spill food on himself.
d. Make sure all of the liquids on the tray have been thickened.

10. **Mr. Singer has orders to have his fluid intake measured. At breakfast, Mr. Singer drinks an 8-oz carton of milk, a glass of orange juice and a cup of coffee. The glass holds 180 mL and the coffee cup holds 120 mL. How much fluid, in mL, did Mr. Singer drink?**
    a. 308 mL
    b. 300 mL
    c. 540 mL
    d. 18 mL

11. **Which of the following is a sign of dehydration?**
    a. Swelling in the feet and ankles
    b. Frequent urination
    c. Loss of appetite
    d. Confusion

12. **Mrs. Welker is receiving enteral nutrition through a gastrostomy tube. Which of the following actions should the nurse assistant take?**
    a. Keep Mrs. Welker lying flat for 30 minutes after a tube feeding.
    b. Give Mrs. Welker water by mouth.
    c. Use cotton balls moistened with alcohol to clean around Mrs. Welker's mouth and nose.
    d. Keep the head of the bed elevated for 30 minutes following a tube feeding.

Questions to Ask Yourself

1. *You notice that Mr. Rivera did not eat much of his breakfast or lunch. He says he feels okay and asks you not to worry. What should you do?*

2. *Mrs. Garcia eats very little. She says she is not hungry. You suspect that she may tire easily and find it difficult to feed herself. You offer to help her eat, but she says she is too old to be fed like a baby. What should you do?*

3. *Because of Parkinson's disease, Mr. Linkins has a great deal of difficulty using utensils to eat. His hand shakes, and food falls off the utensil before he can get it to his mouth. What types of assistive devices would you expect the occupational therapist will recommend for Mr. Linkins?*

4. *Mrs. Woods is a new resident at the long-term care facility where you work. When you go to get her ready to go to the dining room for dinner, she tells you that she doesn't want to go and she doesn't feel like eating. She says, "My family just put me here to die anyway." How would you respond to Mrs. Woods? What feelings could be contributing to Mrs. Woods' refusal to go to the dining room and loss of appetite? Is there anything you could do to help Mrs. Woods feel better about her current situation?*

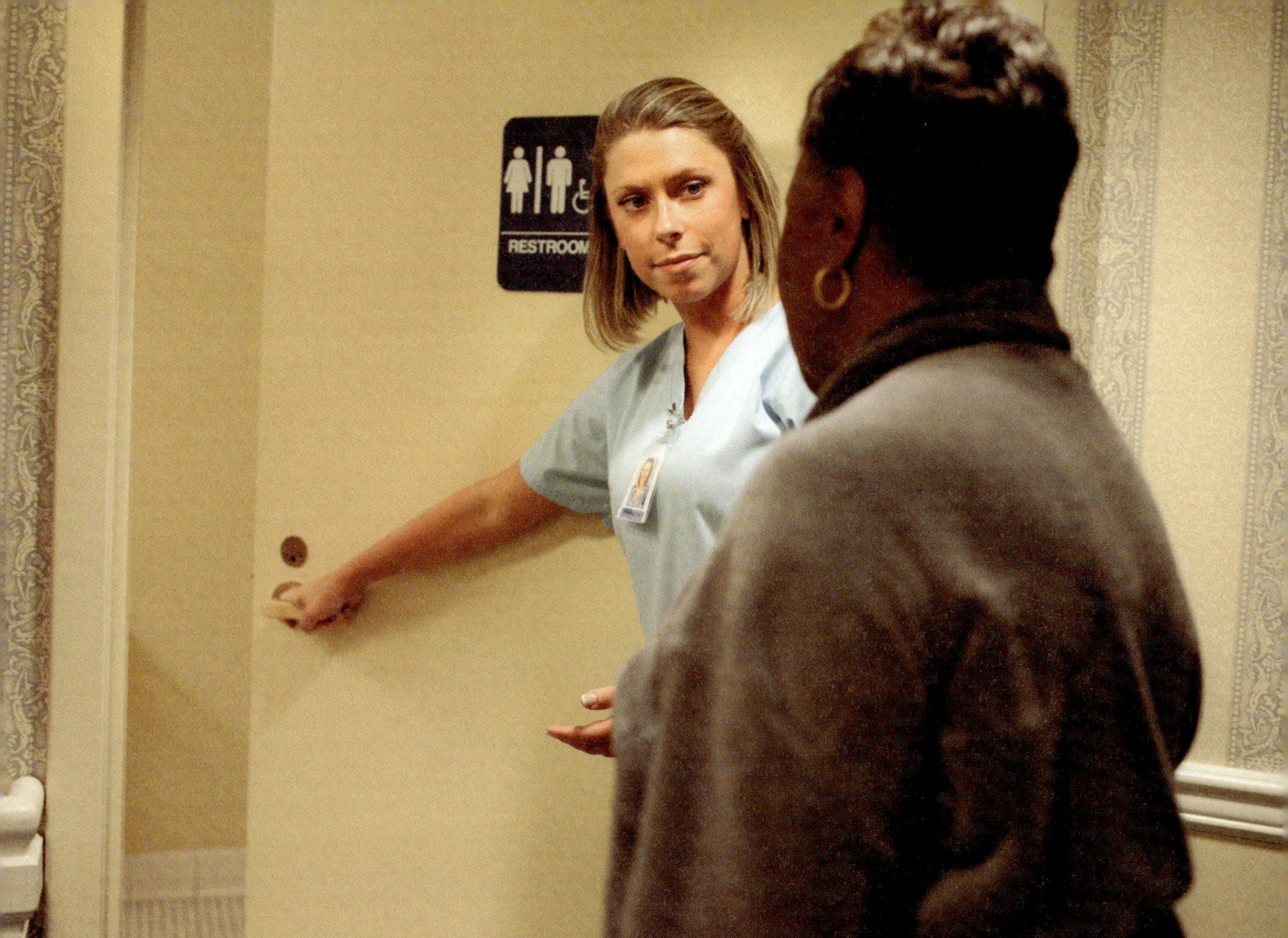

Assisting with Elimination

CHAPTER
15

Goals

After reading this chapter, you will have the information needed to:

- Assist people in your care with elimination in a sensitive, professional way.
- Describe the characteristics of normal urine and feces.
- Explain the importance of knowing a person's regular elimination pattern.
- List actions nurse assistants can take to promote normal elimination.
- Define the word *incontinence* and describe the care needs of a person who is incontinent.
- Describe the signs and symptoms of a urinary tract infection and actions nurse assistants can take to help prevent those in their care from developing urinary tract infections.
- Describe care measures for a person who has diarrhea.

Continued on next page

Goals

Continued from previous page

- Describe actions nurse assistants can take to prevent those in their care from becoming constipated or developing a fecal impaction.
- List observations that a nurse assistant may make while assisting a person with elimination that should be reported to the nurse right away.
- Describe the care needs of a person with an indwelling urinary catheter.
- Explain what an ostomy appliance is and how to care for a person who has an ostomy appliance.
- Describe types of enemas and precautions that should be taken when administering an enema.

After practicing the corresponding skills, you will have the information needed to:

- Help a person use a toilet, portable commode, bedpan or urinal.
- Apply a condom catheter.
- Measure urine output.
- Obtain urine and stool specimens.
- Provide catheter care for a person with a urinary catheter.
- Empty a urine drainage bag.
- Change an ostomy appliance.
- Give a tap water, soap solution or commercially prepared enema.

Key Terms:

urine
feces
urination
defecation
incontinence
condom catheter
diarrhea
constipation
fecal impaction
indwelling urinary catheter
stoma
ostomy appliance
enema

It is almost the end of your shift, but before you leave you decide to check in on Mrs. Doris Wilson one last time. Mrs. Wilson was admitted to Morningside yesterday, and she's been feeling a little homesick. When you knock on Mrs. Wilson's door and ask if you can come in, Mrs. Wilson answers you in a quivering voice and you can tell she has been crying. You enter the room and see a puddle of urine on the floor. Mrs. Wilson is sitting on the chair near the bed in her wet clothes. She looks up and says, "I tried to get to the bathroom by myself and I just couldn't make it in time. I'm so embarrassed." And she starts to cry again. You pat Mrs. Wilson on the shoulder and say, "Don't worry, Mrs. Wilson. It's OK. Here, let me help you."

INTRODUCTION TO ELIMINATION

Waste products such as **urine** (liquid body waste) and **feces** (solid body waste) are formed as the result of normal processes in the body. Urine is formed by the kidneys, which filter the blood to remove dissolved waste products and excess fluid. Feces are formed through the process of digesting food. As food passes through the digestive tract, the usable parts of the food are absorbed into the body, and the unusable parts of the food are eliminated as feces. (Feces are also sometimes referred to as *stool* after they leave the body.) Urine and feces are removed from the body through the processes of urinary and bowel elimination, respectively.

Most people consider elimination to be a personal, private matter. In a health care setting, it may become more difficult for the person to keep elimination personal and private. Some people receiving health care will need to ask for help each time they need to use the bathroom. Others may not be able to get out of bed or walk the distance to the bathroom, and will have to use a bedpan, urinal or portable commode while being separated from others in the room by only a privacy curtain. Members of the health care team may ask the person questions about her elimination habits, or request samples of urine or feces. As you can see, a person who is receiving health care may be required to think and talk about elimination much more than she normally would.

A person who needs help with elimination may feel embarrassed, helpless or angry. Be sensitive to the person's feelings about needing help with a very personal function, and take steps to protect the person's privacy and dignity. Treating elimination as a routine, normal occurrence and maintaining a positive, professional attitude can help to lessen the person's embarrassment and help him to feel better about needing help with elimination. Although it is normal for you to feel embarrassed or uncomfortable while assisting another person with elimination, especially at first, try not to show your feelings. If the person senses that you are embarrassed or uncomfortable, he will likely become more embarrassed and uncomfortable as well.

When discussing elimination, use professional language. Passing urine is referred to as **urination** or voiding. Passing feces is referred to as **defecation**, or having a bowel movement. Always use professional language when you are communicating with other members of the health care team about elimination. When you are communicating with those in your care about elimination, it is always correct to use professional language, but in some situations it is okay to use terms preferred by the person, if doing so helps to ensure clear communication and gain the person's cooperation. For example, when discussing elimination with a person who has dementia, your meaning may be clearer and you may get a better response if you use terms that are familiar to her.

PROMOTING NORMAL ELIMINATION

Normal urine ranges in color from pale to deep yellow and has a slight odor. It is clear, not cloudy. In the morning, the color of urine is darker, and it may have a strong odor. As the day goes on, the urine becomes lighter in color and the odor lessens. This is because decreased fluid intake at night causes urine to become more concentrated (that is, it contains less water). During the day, when the person drinks more fluids, the urine becomes more diluted (that is, it contains more water). The more dilute the urine, the lighter it is in color and the less odor it has. Feces are normally brown in color, soft in texture and formed, with a distinctive odor.

All of us follow fairly predictable patterns for elimination of urine and feces, although elimination patterns vary from person to person. When describing a person's urinary elimination pattern, you note the number of times each day the person typically voids and how much time passes between voiding. When describing a person's bowel elimination pattern, you note what time the person usually has a bowel movement, and how frequently bowel movements occur. Some people have bowel movements every day, others every 2 to 3 days. You must learn the elimination pattern of each person in your care so that you can help maintain the pattern and recognize changes in it. To learn about a person's elimination pattern, ask these questions:

- How often do you urinate?
- Is there anything special about your urination habits that I should know?
- How often do you have a bowel movement?
- What time of day do you usually have a bowel movement?
- Is there anything special about your bowel movement habits that I should know?

If the person cannot provide the information, ask the person's family members or check the person's chart to determine a pattern.

Normal elimination is important for the person's health and comfort. As a nurse assistant, there are many things you can do to help promote normal elimination for the people in your care.

- **Maintain the person's normal elimination pattern.** A change in routine can disrupt a person's elimination pattern, leading to problems such as constipation (difficulty having a bowel movement) or incontinence (the inability to control the release of urine or feces). Take the person's normal elimination pattern into account when planning care, rather than trying to have the person adapt to a schedule that is convenient for you. Also, answer requests for help promptly (Figure 15-1).

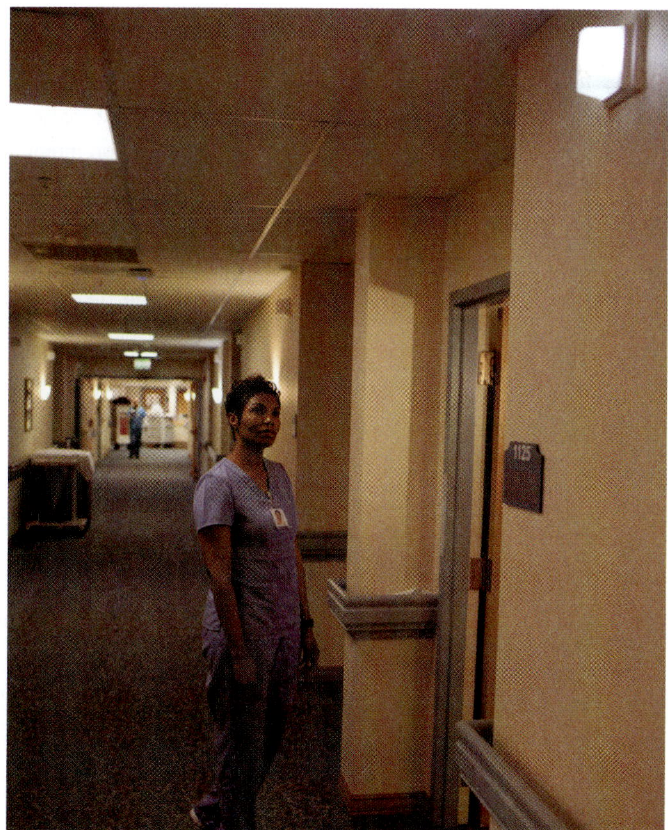

Figure 15-1 Respond to a person's request for help with elimination promptly.

Holding urine or feces is uncomfortable for the person, and can disrupt the person's normal elimination pattern.

- **Encourage adequate fluid intake.** Drinking enough fluid helps to promote regular urination and helps to keep the feces soft (Figure 15-2).

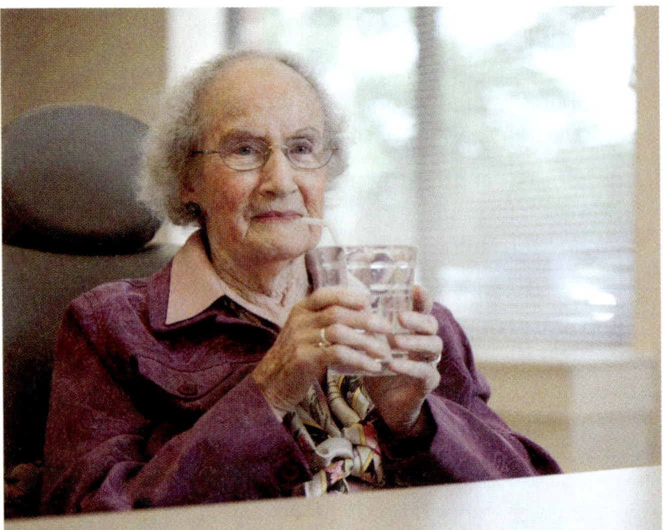

Figure 15-2 Taking in enough fluid helps to prevent problems with elimination.

Regular urination helps to flush bacteria from the urinary tract that can cause infection. Feces that are soft are easier to pass, helping to prevent constipation.

- **Encourage exercise and foods that are high in fiber.** Getting up and moving helps to promote regular bowel movements. The fiber in foods such as whole grains, fruits and vegetables helps to keep the feces moist, making them easier to pass and preventing constipation.
- **Provide privacy.** A sense of privacy makes it easier for the person to urinate or have a bowel movement.
- **Promote comfort.** Being chilled or feeling rushed can make it difficult for a person to urinate or have a bowel movement. Make sure the person is warm enough, and give him plenty of time to meet his elimination needs. If you are aware of routines the person follows related to elimination (for example, some people like to read while using the toilet), help the person maintain those habits.

General guidelines for assisting a person with elimination are given in Box 15-1.

Box 15-1 Nurse Assistant DO's and DON'Ts

Assisting with Elimination

DO maintain a professional attitude when assisting a person with elimination. Treating the person with kindness and respect and treating the task as something normal and routine helps to put the person at ease and lessens feelings of embarrassment.

DO take measures to protect the person's privacy and dignity. Shut doors and pull privacy curtains. If safety considerations allow, leave the room (but check on the person frequently, and make sure the call signal is within the person's reach). Be sensitive to how the person may feel about discussing her elimination needs and habits when other people are present. Approach unpleasant tasks (such as cleaning up a bowel movement) positively, and make sure that your facial expressions and gestures do not show displeasure with the person or the task.

DO learn about the person's normal elimination patterns and habits, and help the person maintain these patterns and habits to the greatest extent possible.

DO promote healthy elimination by encouraging fluids, high-fiber foods (such as fruits, vegetables and whole grains) and regular exercise.

DO answer requests for help promptly. Doing so helps the person maintain her normal elimination pattern and helps to prevent problems such as falls (which could occur if the person cannot wait any longer and tries to get up to go to the bathroom unassisted) and episodes of incontinence (which could happen if the person simply cannot hold the urine or feces any longer).

DO follow the toileting plan as written in the person's care plan.

DO give the person plenty of time to take care of her elimination needs, but check on her regularly so that you do not leave her stranded on the bedpan or alone in the bathroom for too long.

DO offer frequent assistance with elimination. Some people may be reluctant to ask for help, even if they need it. Accepting an offer of help may be easier for them.

DO observe the characteristics and amount of urine and feces before emptying a urinal, bedpan or commode container or flushing the toilet. Changes in urine or feces could be a sign of a health problem and should be reported to the nurse.

DO follow standard precautions when you are assisting a person with elimination.

DON'T place equipment used for elimination, such as bedpans or urinals, on the person's bedside table or over-bed table, even if they are clean.

After you finish getting Mrs. Wilson into clean, dry clothes, you sit beside her on the bed and say, "Now, Mrs. Wilson, I know it can be embarrassing or difficult to have to ask for help, especially with something as personal as needing to use the bathroom. But we're here to help, and we'd much rather you call us when you need us, rather than risk a fall trying to get to the bathroom on your own." Mrs. Wilson nods and says, "I know. It's just so embarrassing to have to ask for help. You've been so kind. I guess my new situation is just going to take a little getting used to."

What could you do or say to make it easier for Mrs. Wilson to ask for help with elimination?

It is always important to answer requests for help promptly. List some reasons why this is especially important when the person is calling for help with elimination.

Mrs. Wilson was obviously very embarrassed and upset by her accident, and she appreciated your kind and caring response. In what other ways could you help to protect Mrs. Wilson's dignity and self-respect?

ASSISTING THE PERSON TO USE A TOILET, A PORTABLE COMMODE, A BEDPAN OR A URINAL

Assisting a Person to Use the Toilet

Many of the people in your care will be able to use the toilet to meet their elimination needs, although they may need your help to get to the bathroom safely, move clothing out of the way, sit down on the toilet or get up from it. Some men may need you to help them stand while they urinate. When assisting a person to use the toilet, help him to put on a robe and slippers before transferring to the bathroom. For safety reasons, you may have to remain in the bathroom with the person. If you need to remain in the bathroom with the person, you may be able to turn your back (to give the person a sense of privacy) while still keeping a hand on the person's arm (so that you can feel if the person starts to stand up unassisted). If it is safe to leave the person alone in the bathroom, make sure the call light and toilet paper are within reach, and reassure the person that you will be nearby if she needs help (Figure 15-3). Stay outside the bathroom door and check on the person every 5 minutes to make sure she is okay and to see whether she needs assistance. When the person is ready, put on gloves and assist the person with wiping, if necessary. Help the person to stand up, if necessary, and adjust clothing as needed. Give the person the opportunity to wash her hands before leaving the bathroom.

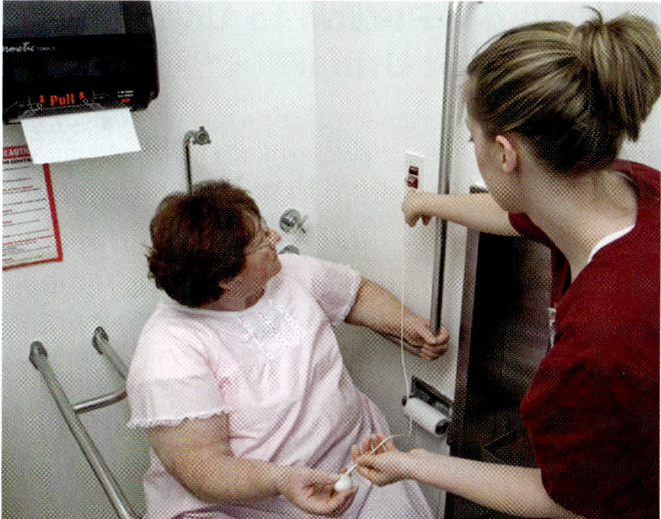

Figure 15-3 Before leaving a person alone in the bathroom, make sure the toilet paper and call signal are within reach. Stay close by and check on the person every 5 minutes.

Assisting a Person to Use a Portable Commode

A portable commode looks like a chair with a toilet seat (Figure 15-4). Under the seat is a collection container that can be removed for emptying and cleaning. A portable commode is used for a person who is able to get out of bed, but is not able to transfer the distance to the bathroom. To use the commode, the person must be able to stand and pivot, and sit up with little assistance. Skill 15-1 describes step-by-step how to help a person to use a portable commode.

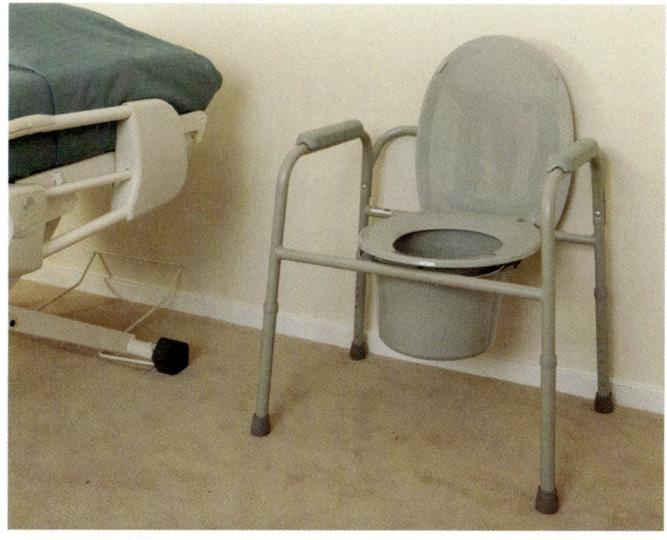

Figure 15-4 A portable commode.

Assisting a Person to Use a Bedpan or Urinal

Bedpans and urinals are used for people who cannot get out of bed to meet their elimination needs. A man may use a urinal to urinate and a bedpan to have a bowel movement. A woman uses a bedpan for both types of elimination. Using a bedpan is not very comfortable. In addition to being uncomfortable, it often feels unnatural to the person to urinate or have a bowel movement while lying in bed. These factors can make elimination more difficult for the person.

The urinal rests between the man's legs. The man places his penis in the opening (or you may need to help him do this). A bedpan is positioned underneath the person's buttocks. There are two different styles of bedpans: a standard bedpan and a fracture pan (Figure 15-5). A fracture pan, which is thinner than a standard bedpan and wedge-shaped, is used when the person has a condition that makes positioning a regular bedpan underneath the person difficult. A regular bedpan is placed with the narrow end pointing toward the person's feet, while a fracture pan is placed with the narrow end pointing toward the person's head.

Check at least every 5 minutes on a person who is using a bedpan or urinal. Help the person off the bedpan or remove the urinal as soon as the person is finished using it. Sitting on a bedpan or having a urinal in place causes pressure that can put the person at risk for developing pressure ulcers, so it is important to remove that pressure source as soon as possible.

ELDER CARE NOTE. Remember that elderly skin is fragile and can tear and bruise easily. Use special care when positioning the bedpan under the person, and remove the bedpan as soon as the person is finished using it.

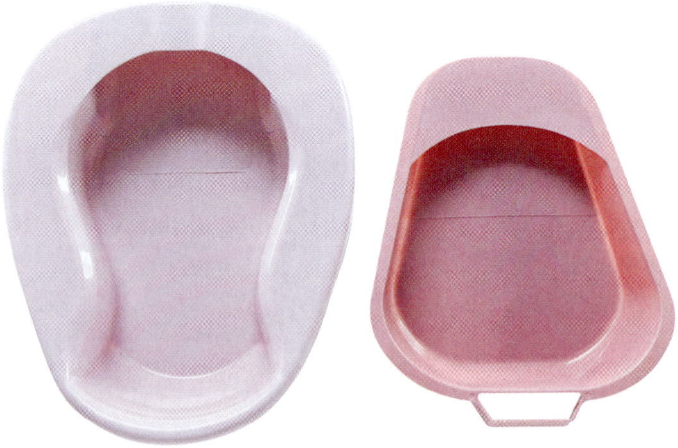

Figure 15-5 A standard bedpan and a fracture pan.

Skill 15-2 describes how to assist a person with using a bedpan, and Skill 15-3 describes how to assist a man with using a urinal.

PROBLEMS WITH ELIMINATION

Common problems with elimination include incontinence, urinary tract infections, diarrhea, constipation and fecal impaction.

Incontinence

Incontinence is the inability to control the release of urine or feces. Incontinence can be temporary or it can be permanent. When it is permanent, incontinence is a leading cause of admission to long-term care facilities. It can be very frustrating to care for a person who is incontinent, but it is important to remember that the person cannot help her condition. In fact, the person may be very embarrassed by her condition. Although many of the people you will care for who are incontinent will be elderly, incontinence is not an expected consequence of aging. Several factors can lead to incontinence:

- Acute conditions, such as a urinary tract infection or diarrhea, that can cause the person to urinate or have a bowel movement almost immediately after recognizing the need to go to the bathroom
- Certain medications, which can also produce an urgent need to use the bathroom
- Conditions such as confusion or dementia that reduce the person's ability to interpret the feeling of having to go to the bathroom and make it hard for the person to remember how to call for help, find the bathroom and remember how to move clothing out of the way
- Conditions such as arthritis that limit a person's mobility, making it difficult for the person to reach the bathroom in time or move clothing out of the way in time
- Brain, spinal cord or nerve damage that prevents the person from feeling the urge to urinate or have a bowel movement
- Weakness of the muscles that normally prevent the involuntary release of urine or feces

Bladder or bowel training programs and scheduled toileting programs

A bladder or bowel training program is usually developed for a person who is incontinent of urine or feces and has the ability to recognize the urge to eliminate and to retrain the muscles used to control elimination. The bladder or bowel training program helps the person to regain control over elimination by promoting urination or defecation at predictable times. For example, as part of a bladder training program, you may be required to give the person the opportunity to urinate at regular intervals according to the schedule specified in the person's care plan. You would assist the person to the bathroom (or offer a bedpan, urinal or portable commode) and allow the person sufficient time to urinate each time. Supporting a bladder training program means following the schedule during the night as well (if the person typically gets up during the night to urinate), although the intervals between using the toilet may be longer during the night. A bowel training program works in much the same way as a bladder training program, except the person is only assisted to use the toilet (or bedpan or bedside commode) during the time when a bowel movement is expected, based on the person's usual bowel elimination pattern.

A person with dementia may become incontinent because she cannot recognize the urge to eliminate or remember how to control the muscles used for elimination. In this situation, a training program will not work. Instead, a scheduled toileting program is set up for the person. The scheduled toileting program, which also involves giving the person the opportunity to eliminate at regular intervals based on the person's past elimination patterns, helps to maintain the person's dignity by reducing the likelihood that an episode of incontinence will occur.

Both training programs and scheduled toileting programs are based on accurate assessment of the person's elimination patterns. As a nurse assistant, you will be involved in gathering data about when the person normally eliminates in preparation for placing the person on either type of program, and you will play a very important role in helping the person adhere to the plan by assisting the person with elimination at the scheduled times. Following a bladder or bowel training or scheduled toileting program when a person is incontinent is an important part of providing restorative care.

Products used for managing incontinence

Even when a bowel or bladder training or scheduled toileting program is in place, the person may still have episodes of incontinence. Different products are available to help manage incontinence, including incontinence pads, incontinence briefs and condom catheters.

- **Incontinence pads** are absorbent pads that are placed inside the person's underpants to absorb urine and pull it away from the person's skin. **Incontinence briefs** are worn instead of underpants, and like incontinence pads, they absorb urine and help to keep the person's skin dry. To protect the person's self-esteem, always refer to adult briefs as briefs, not diapers. Incontinence pads and briefs should be used according to the person's care plan, and never for staff convenience. Change soiled pads or briefs promptly and provide good perineal care to prevent skin breakdown.
- A **condom catheter** may be used for a man who is incontinent of urine. The condom catheter consists of a condom-like device, tubing and a drainage bag (Figure 15-6). The condom fits over the man's penis and is attached to the tubing, which is connected to a urine drainage bag. A large urine drainage bag (the same type that is used with an indwelling urinary catheter) may be attached to the system, or a leg bag may be used. A leg bag is strapped to the man's thigh, so it can be worn underneath pants. Because the leg bag is small, it must be emptied frequently (for example, every few hours, depending on the person's urine output). Remove the condom once daily to clean the skin, and then apply a new condom. When applying the condom, make sure the skin is dry so that the adhesive will stick during application. Unroll the condom completely, so that it does not interfere with the person's circulation. Check the person frequently to make sure the condom is not too tight and that circulation is good. If you notice any swelling or color change in the man's penis, remove the condom and report your observations to the nurse. Skill 15-4 describes step-by-step how to apply a condom catheter.

Caring for a person with incontinence

When caring for a person who is incontinent, change soiled clothing promptly and provide good perineal care to prevent embarrassing odors and protect the person's self-esteem. Dry clothing and good skin care are also important to prevent skin breakdown, which can put the person at risk for pressure ulcers.

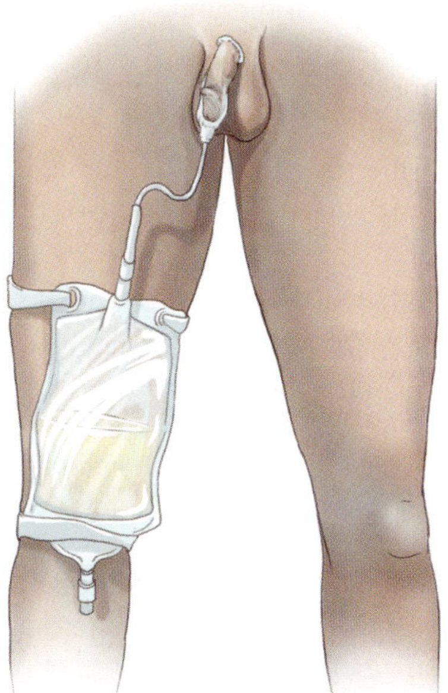

Figure 15-6 A condom catheter may be used for a man who is incontinent of urine.

Be aware that incontinence is a condition that the person cannot correct easily or sometimes at all. When the person experiences an episode of incontinence, never scold the person. Avoid saying things like, "I was just down the hall; I wish you would have waited." If the person could have waited, he would have! Soiling garments and leaving puddles are not normal behaviors for adults. People who are aware of their episodes of incontinence are often very embarrassed and feel very bad about themselves and their condition.

You leave Mrs. Wilson's room and stop by the nurse's station on your way to clock out to report Mrs. Wilson's episode of incontinence to the nurse. The nurse says, "You know, episodes like this are pretty common with new residents. Sometimes just being in a new, unfamiliar place is enough to cause a resident to develop temporary incontinence. I know Mrs. Wilson has been having a hard time settling in. Thank you for taking the time to reassure her. We'll keep an eye on her and rule out any physical causes for the incontinence, but I'm pretty sure this is a one-time occurrence. Now you go and enjoy your daughter's concert tonight!"

What else could potentially be a cause for Mrs. Wilson's incontinence?

Urinary Tract Infections

A urinary tract infection occurs when bacteria gain access to the urinary system. A urinary tract infection can occur in any part of the urinary system—the kidneys (which filter the blood to produce urine), the ureters (the tubes that carry the urine from the kidneys to the bladder), the bladder (where the urine is stored) or the urethra (the tube that carries urine out of the body). Figure B-8 in Appendix B shows the urinary system.

Urinary tract infections are often caused by bacteria in feces. When the person has a bowel movement, the area around the anus becomes contaminated with bacteria. It is very easy, especially in women, for the bacteria on the skin to then enter the urethra. Once inside the urethra, the bacteria can travel to any part of the urinary system and cause a urinary tract infection. To help prevent urinary tract infections, always encourage the people in your care to wipe from front to back after having a bowel movement. And when you are assisting a person with perineal care, remember to always clean from the urethra outward, and to use a clean part of the washcloth for each pass.

People who have indwelling urinary catheters are at high risk for developing urinary tract infections, because the catheter tubing provides a direct pathway into the urinary system for bacteria. Later in this chapter, you will learn more about indwelling urinary catheters and how to provide care for a person who has one. Many of the care principles you will learn have to do with preventing urinary tract infections.

Incomplete emptying of the bladder can also put a person at risk for developing a urinary tract infection. For example, in men, an enlarged prostate gland can squeeze against the urethra, making it difficult for the man to empty his bladder completely each time he urinates. When you are assisting a person with elimination, always give the person enough time to empty the bladder as completely as possible. Making sure the person takes in enough fluids can also help to prevent urinary tract infections, because frequent urination helps to flush out any bacteria that may gain access to the urinary tract.

You may be the first to become aware that a person in your care has developed a urinary tract infection. Signs and symptoms of a urinary tract infection include:

- Pain or a burning sensation when urinating.
- A frequent and often urgent need to urinate.
- The ability to pass only a small amount of urine, despite feeling the need to urinate.
- Cloudy, dark yellow and possibly foul-smelling urine.
- Mucus (which gives the urine a milky appearance) or blood in the urine.
- Fever.
- New unusual behaviors in a person with dementia, such as leaning to one side (this occurs because the person cannot accurately identify the source of her discomfort and her only way of expressing this discomfort is through behavior).
- Changes in mental status (especially in older people).

ELDER CARE NOTE. Urinary tract infections are very common in older people. However, an older person with a urinary tract infection may not have these common signs and symptoms. The only sign of a urinary tract infection in an older person may be a change in the person's mental status (such as confusion in a person who is not normally confused).

If a person develops any signs or symptoms of a urinary tract infection, be sure to report them to the nurse right away so that steps can be taken to diagnose and treat the infection.

Diarrhea

Diarrhea is the frequent passage of loose, watery feces that are often foul-smelling and accompanied by cramping. Common causes of diarrhea include infections (such as *Clostridium difficile,* or "C diff"), food poisoning (which is caused by eating or drinking contaminated food or water) and medical conditions (such as irritable bowel syndrome). Some medications and treatments (such as cancer treatments) may also cause diarrhea.

Sometimes no medical treatment is prescribed for diarrhea, and the diarrhea is simply allowed to run its course. The person may be put on a clear liquid diet to rest the bowel and replace fluids. However, ongoing diarrhea that is not relieved can cause the person to become dehydrated, especially if the person is young, elderly or frail. In this case, a medication may be prescribed for the person to stop the diarrhea.

You can help a person who has diarrhea by understanding the discomfort associated with it. Respond promptly to the person's requests for help with elimination. After the person has a bowel movement, provide good perineal care. Be gentle, because the skin around the anus may be irritated and sore.

When assisting a person who has diarrhea with elimination, always take standard precautions because the diarrhea may be caused by viruses or bacteria that can be transmitted to others. For example, *C. difficile*, a type of bacteria, is a common cause of diarrhea in people who are receiving health care. "C. diff" is highly contagious and hard to kill. When you are caring for a person who is known to have "C. diff," remember to wash your hands with soap and water (instead of using an alcohol-based hand rub) and use a disinfectant containing bleach to clean hard surfaces.

Constipation

The difficult elimination of hard, dry feces is called **constipation**. It occurs when feces move too slowly through the intestine. The longer the feces remain in the intestine, the harder and drier they become, making them very difficult to pass. The following factors contribute to constipation:

- Immobility
- Inadequate fluid intake
- Inadequate intake of high-fiber foods, such as fruits, vegetables and whole grains
- Disruptions in the person's normal bowel elimination pattern (for example, not being able to access a toilet shortly after feeling the need to have a bowel movement)
- Changes in diet
- Aging
- Certain medications

A person who is constipated feels uncomfortable and may be irritable. He may complain that his abdomen feels hard. When he tries to move his bowels, he may feel pain, which is caused by straining to eliminate the hard, dry feces. A laxative or an enema may be prescribed to relieve the constipation. A laxative is a medication that is taken orally to produce a bowel movement. An enema is a solution that is placed into the rectum to cause a bowel movement.

Fecal Impaction

Fecal impaction is a more serious form of constipation that occurs when constipation is not relieved. The feces continue to build up in the bowel until the bowel is almost completely blocked. A person with fecal impaction has pain, discomfort and abdominal swelling. The person may pass small amounts of watery, diarrhea-like feces around the impacted mass, but this diarrhea-like discharge should not be confused for a bowel movement. To treat fecal impaction, a special type of enema may be ordered to soften the feces. Often, an enema alone is not enough to clear the bowel. The nurse or doctor may need to insert a finger into the person's anus and scoop the feces out piece by piece. This procedure is called *disimpaction* and it can be very uncomfortable for the person. As a nurse assistant, you will play a very important role in helping to prevent fecal impaction from occurring by reporting changes in the person's normal bowel elimination pattern to the nurse promptly. This will allow constipation to be treated before it develops into a fecal impaction.

! Observations Into Action!

Whenever you assist a person with elimination, observe for changes that could be a sign of a problem. Report any of the following:

- **Urine that is cloudy, or that has an unusual color or odor**
- **Urinary frequency (the need to urinate more frequently)**
- **Urinary urgency (the need to urinate immediately)**
- **Pain or difficulty urinating or having a bowel movement**
- **Feces that are loose or very dry**
- **Feces that are foul-smelling or an unusual color**
- **Changes in the person's usual bowel elimination pattern**
- **Episodes of incontinence, if the person is not usually incontinent**

SPECIAL TASKS RELATED TO ASSISTING WITH ELIMINATION

In addition to assisting those in your care with meeting their elimination needs, you may be asked to perform other tasks related to elimination.

Measuring Urine Output

In Chapter 14, you learned about fluid balance in the body. To maintain fluid balance, the amount of fluid lost through urine, feces, sweat and breath vapor must be equal to the amount of fluid taken in through beverages and food. Because urine accounts for the most fluid loss from the body, measuring urine output and comparing it to the person's fluid intake can provide valuable information about the person's fluid balance. People who take medications or have conditions that affect their ability to maintain fluid balance usually have orders to have their fluid intake and urine output (intake and output, or I & O) measured and recorded.

You learned about measuring fluid intake in Chapter 14. There are many different ways to measure urine output. If the person uses a portable commode, bedpan or urinal, simply pour the urine into a graduate (a pitcher-like measuring device). Look at the fluid level to determine the amount of urine in the graduate, using the measurement markings on the side (Figure 15-7). If the person uses a toilet for elimination, a collection device called a *commode hat* can be fitted over the toilet seat (Figure 15-8). After the person urinates, the contents of the commode hat can be measured using the markings on the side. Some people will have indwelling urinary catheters. For these people, urine output is measured by emptying the urine drainage bag into a graduate.

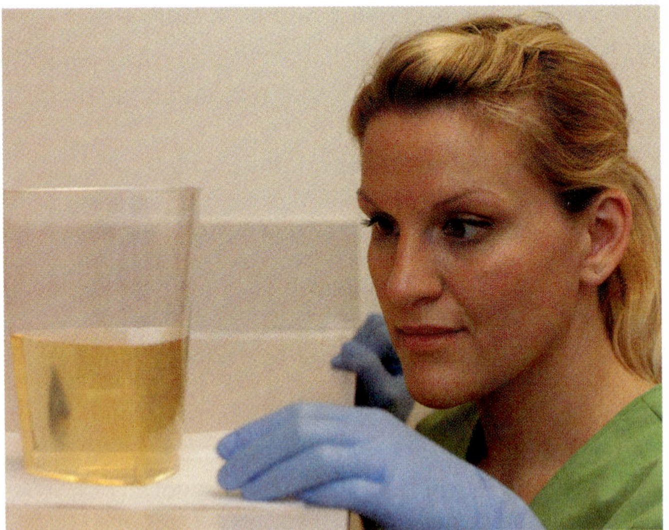

Figure 15-7 A graduate is used to measure urine output.

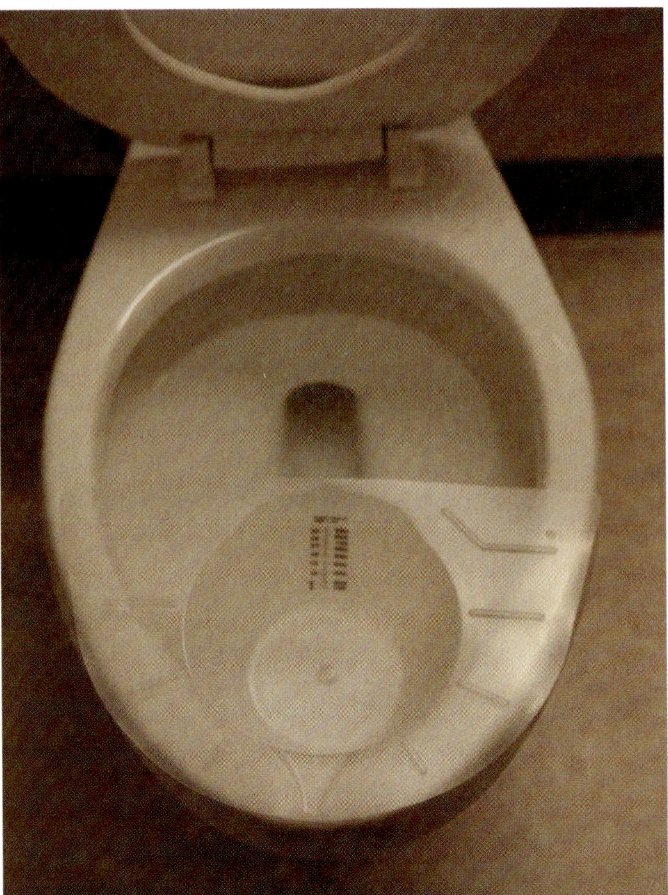

Figure 15-8 A commode hat fits in place over the rim of the toilet seat and may be used when a person uses the toilet for elimination and it is necessary to collect urine for measuring, or to obtain a urine or stool sample.

Obtaining Specimens

You may be asked to obtain samples of the person's urine or feces for laboratory testing. The person's primary care provider (a doctor or advanced practice nurse) uses the information obtained from laboratory tests on the urine or feces to evaluate the person's health status, to diagnose medical conditions and to determine proper treatment. Guidelines for obtaining specimens of any type are given in Box 15-2. Following these guidelines helps to ensure that the person's test results are accurate and that the test will not need to be repeated.

Urine specimens

Collecting urine

Three methods of collecting urine specimens are routine urine collection, clean catch (midstream) urine collection and 24-hour urine collection. Each method is ordered for a particular purpose, so use only the method ordered.

- **Routine urine specimen.** A routine urine specimen is collected by having the person void directly into the specimen container, or by pouring

Box 15-2 Nurse Assistant DO's and DON'Ts

Collecting Specimens

DO check with the nurse to ensure that you know the method to be used for collecting the specimen.

DO know what to do with the specimen after you have obtained it. Some specimens will need to be delivered to the laboratory right away, while others may be placed in a designated area for pick-up.

DO make sure the specimen container is labeled properly, per your employer's policy.

DO remind the person not to place toilet paper in the collection device (if using a bedpan, urinal, portable commode or commode hat) because this can affect test results. Provide an alternative place for the person to dispose of the toilet paper.

DO remind the person not to have a bowel movement in the collection device if a urine sample is being collected, and not to urinate in the collection device if a stool sample is being collected. This can also affect test results.

DO follow standard precautions when handling any specimen.

urine from a urinal, bedpan, portable commode collection container or urine drainage bag into a specimen container. Skill 15-5 describes how to obtain a routine urine specimen.

- **Clean catch (midstream) urine specimen.** A clean catch (midstream) urine specimen is collected when the person is thought to have an infection (such as a urinary tract infection). A clean catch specimen can be collected while the person is using the toilet, portable commode, bedpan or urinal. Before the person starts to void, the opening of the urethra is cleaned to remove any microbes in the area. The person then starts to void (*not* in the container), then stops, then voids into the container. The initial flow of urine washes away microbes that might be around the urethral opening. These steps help to avoid contamination of the urine sample with microbes other than the ones causing the infection, giving more accurate test results. For the same reason, you should avoid touching the inside of the specimen container or lid when obtaining a clean catch (midstream) urine specimen, because doing so could contaminate the sample. Skill 15-6 describes how to obtain a clean catch (midstream) urine specimen.
- **24-hour urine specimen.** A 24-hour urine specimen is collected over 24 consecutive hours. To collect a 24-hour urine specimen, have the person empty his bladder. Discard the urine, and note the time. For the next 24 hours, each time the person voids, collect the urine and transfer it to the specimen container. At the end of the 24-hour period, have the person void one last time and add this urine to the specimen container. During the 24-hour urine collection, be sure to label and store the specimen container according to your employer's policy.

Straining urine

When a person has kidney stones, you may be asked to strain the urine to collect the stones for laboratory analysis. To strain the urine, have the person urinate in a commode hat, portable commode, bedpan or urinal. Place a disposable strainer or a 4 x 4–inch gauze square over the rim of a graduate and pour the urine into the graduate. Any stones or fragments of stones will be left behind in the strainer or gauze. Place the strainer or gauze in a labeled specimen container and dispose of the urine.

Testing urine

For some of the people in your care, you may be asked to test the urine for certain substances by dipping a chemically treated strip of paper into a urine sample. The squares on the strip of paper change color as the chemicals they contain react with different substances that may be found in the urine. To read the test results, compare the color of the square on the strip of paper to the chart that comes with the strips. If you are required to do this type of urine testing, the nurse will show you how.

Stool specimens

A stool specimen can be collected using a commode hat, portable commode or bedpan. Be sure to give the person advance notice when a stool sample is required, since bowel movements occur much less frequently than voiding. Remind the person not to urinate or dispose of toilet paper in the commode hat, portable commode or bedpan, because this can affect the sample. Skill 15-5 describes how to collect a stool specimen.

Caring for a Person with an Indwelling Urinary Catheter

An **indwelling urinary catheter** (also called a Foley catheter) is a small tube that is inserted through the urethra and into the bladder to allow urine to drain out of the body. A small balloon at the end of the catheter is inflated to hold the catheter in place within the bladder. The urine drains from the bladder through the catheter and is collected in a urine drainage bag, which is connected to the catheter by a length of tubing (Figure 15-9).

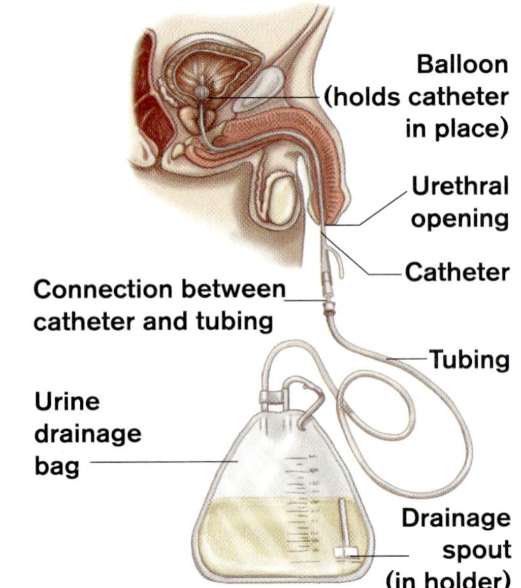

Figure 15-9 An indwelling urinary catheter is inserted through the urethra and into the bladder. It is held in place in the bladder by a small inflated balloon. A length of tubing connects the catheter to the urine drainage bag.

There are many different reasons why an indwelling urinary catheter may be needed, such as:

- When a person has a medical condition or injury that prevents him from being able to empty his bladder when he needs to.
- Before, during and after certain types of surgeries.
- When a person is incontinent of urine and has a pressure ulcer that would become worse if the skin came in contact with urine.
- When a person has lower-body paralysis or nerve damage and cannot sense the need to urinate.

Because having an indwelling urinary catheter greatly increases the person's risk for developing a urinary tract infection, indwelling urinary catheters are only used when there is a medical reason for their use, and an effort is made to remove the indwelling urinary catheter as soon as the person is able to void normally or the medical reason for the catheter has been resolved. Instead of having an indwelling urinary catheter that is left in place, some people will use a straight catheter to empty the bladder at regular intervals. This is called *intermittent catheterization*. In intermittent catheterization, the catheter is inserted, the bladder is drained and then the catheter is removed. Intermittent catheterization is useful when a person has a condition such as paralysis below the waist that causes her to be unable to sense the urge to void. In this case, the person inserts the catheter and drains the bladder at regular intervals to avoid having episodes of incontinence.

As a nurse assistant, inserting and removing urinary catheters is outside of your scope of practice unless you have received advanced training. However, you will be required to provide care for people who have indwelling urinary catheters. General guidelines for caring for a person with an indwelling urinary catheter are given in Box 15-3.

Box 15-3 Nurse Assistant DO's and DON'Ts

Indwelling Urinary Catheters

DO secure the catheter tubing to the person's thigh to prevent pulling.

DO make sure the catheter tubing is lower than the person's bladder, and the urine drainage bag is lower than the catheter tubing.

DO make sure the tubing is free of kinks, bends or creases.

DO secure the urine drainage bag to a stationary object that is lower than the person's bladder (for example, the bed frame or the back of the wheelchair).

DO use extra care when assisting the person to reposition or transfer, to avoid pulling on the catheter tubing.

DO protect the person's modesty by placing the urine drainage bag in a cloth cover.

DO offer fluids frequently to help promote urination and flush bacteria from the urinary tract.

DO provide catheter care on a regular schedule per your employer's policy and whenever the perineal area is soiled.

DO follow standard precautions when providing catheter care or emptying the urine drainage bag.

DON'T allow the catheter tubing or the urine drainage bag to touch the floor.

DON'T allow the end of the drainage tube (used to empty the urine drainage bag) to come in contact with anything except its holder.

DON'T disconnect the catheter tubing from the urine drainage bag.

Handling the catheter tubing and urine drainage bag

The urine drainage bag is connected to the catheter by a long length of tubing. It is important to handle this tubing properly to prevent the tubing from pulling at the entrance to the urethra, maintain the free flow of urine into the drainage bag and lower the person's risk for infection.

Pulling on the catheter tubing is uncomfortable for the person and could cause the catheter to come out of the person's body. To prevent pulling, secure the tubing with tape or a catheter strap to the top of the person's thigh. If the person is in bed, gently make a loop in the remaining length of tubing and secure it to the bed linens (Figure 15-10). Attach the urine drainage bag to the bed frame (which does not move), rather than the side rail. If the person is in a wheelchair, attach the urine drainage bag to the back of the chair at a level lower than the person's bladder. Be sure the tubing and bag are secure and cannot get tangled in the moving parts of the wheelchair. When helping the person with repositioning or transferring, unclip tubing that is secured to the bed linens and move the urine drainage bag before moving the person. Otherwise, the movement will cause pulling on the catheter.

To maintain the free flow of urine, make sure the tubing is free of kinks or bends, and that the person is not lying or sitting on it. Keep the tubing lower than the person's bladder and the urine drainage bag lower than the tubing, because urine flows downward by the force of gravity. Kinking of the tubing or raising the tubing or bag higher than the person's bladder can cause urine to back up into the bladder, possibly causing an infection or serious bladder damage.

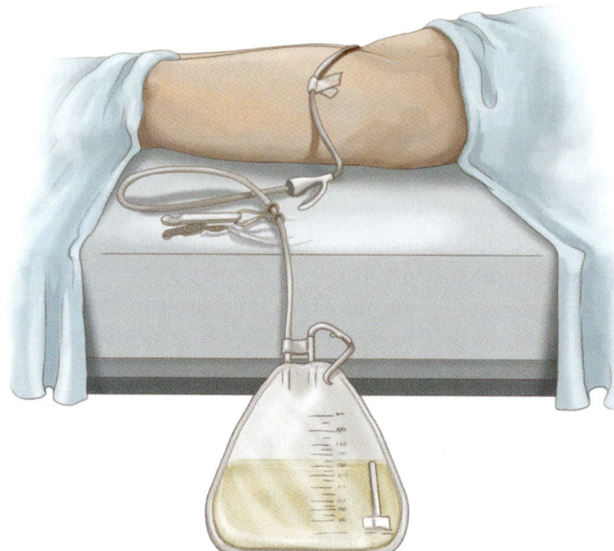

Figure 15-10 Securing the catheter tubing to the person's upper thigh helps to prevent the tubing from pulling on the opening of the urethra. Gently looping the tubing and clipping it to the bed linens helps to prevent kinking.

Remember that the catheter provides a direct pathway for microbes to enter the person's body. To help reduce the person's risk for infection, never disconnect the tubing from the urine drainage bag. Keep the tubing and urine drainage bag from touching the floor, because the floor is dirty.

The urine drainage bag is clear to make it easier for the health care staff to observe the amount and characteristics of the urine. However, for the person, it may be embarrassing to have a bag of her own urine in view. Placing the urine drainage bag in a cloth cover made to conceal the bag helps to protect the person's dignity and self-esteem.

Providing catheter care

Catheter care is cleansing of the perineal area and the length of catheter tubing that extends from the body. Catheter care is provided at least once daily (or per your employer's policy) and whenever the perineal area becomes soiled (for example, with feces). Careful, regular catheter care helps to lower the person's risk for developing a urinary tract infection. Skill 15-7 describes how to provide catheter care.

Emptying the urine drainage bag

In many facilities, the urine drainage bag is routinely emptied at the end of each shift. The urine drainage bag also needs to be emptied whenever it becomes full. The urine drainage bag has a drainage tube that is opened to empty the bag. Never touch the end of the drainage tube with your fingers, or allow the end of the drainage tube to touch the floor or other surface. This could cause the end of the drainage tube to become contaminated with microbes, which could then travel through the catheter system and into the person's body, causing an infection. Skill 15-8 describes how to empty a urine drainage bag.

Observations Into Action!

When providing care for a person with a catheter, be alert to problems that should be reported to the nurse:

- **Cloudy or foul-smelling urine**
- **A change in the amount of urine**
- **A change in the color of the urine**
- **Pain or discomfort as a result of the catheter**
- **Blood, redness, swelling or a discharge near the urethral opening**
- **Urine that does not flow freely through the tubing and into the urine drainage bag**
- **The catheter has come out**

Caring for a Person with an Ostomy Appliance

Sometimes, because of disease or injury, all or part of the bowel must be surgically removed. If the bowel is no longer complete, the person is no longer able to pass feces through the anus. To allow the person to eliminate feces, the surgeon creates an opening in the abdominal wall (called a **stoma**) and sutures the end of the healthy bowel to it (Figure 15-11). Feces pass through the stoma and are collected in a pouch the person wears on the outside of the body called an **ostomy appliance** (Figure 15-12). A person who has had her bladder removed due to disease or injury will also wear an ostomy appliance to allow for elimination of urine from the body.

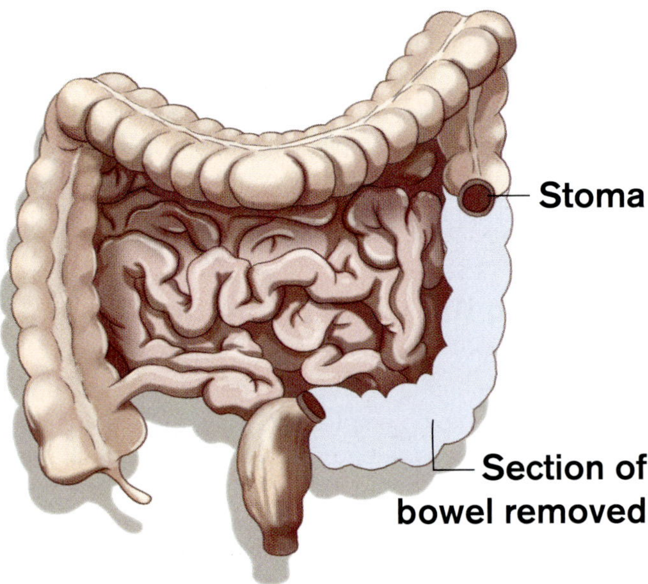

Figure 15-11 A stoma is created and the healthy end of the bowel is sutured to it to create a way for the person to eliminate feces following surgical removal of part of the intestine.

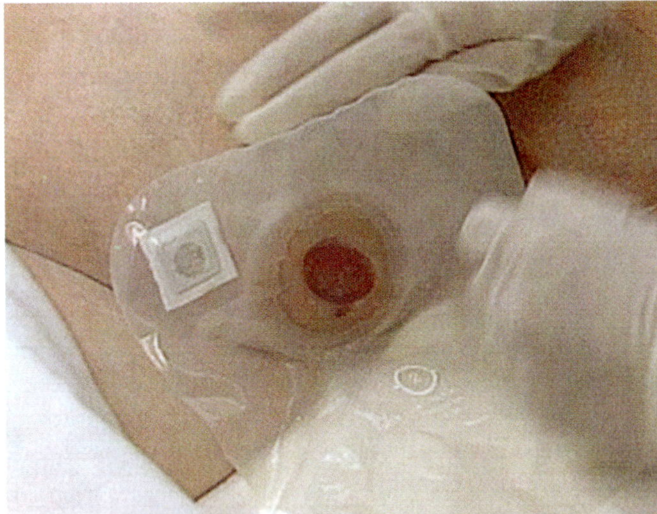

Figure 15-12 A person who has had all or part of the bowel removed wears an ostomy appliance to collect feces. A person who has had the bladder removed wears a similar appliance to collect urine.

You may care for people who need assistance changing their ostomy appliances and caring for the skin around the stoma. Because the skin around the stoma comes into contact with feces or urine, it must be kept clean and dry to prevent irritation and breakdown. Skill 15-9 describes the general procedure for changing an ostomy appliance. There are many different types and styles of ostomy appliances. Although the general principles of care are the same, the ostomy appliance may attach in different ways or have slightly different parts. Check with the nurse or the person to make sure you know specifically how to change the type of appliance the person is using.

Assisting with Enemas

An **enema** is the introduction of fluid into the bowel through the anus to remove feces from the bowel. Nurses are usually responsible for administering enemas, although nurse assistants who have received the proper training may be allowed to give enemas in some facilities. Always act within your scope of practice. If you are responsible for giving an enema, follow the written orders exactly. Know what type of enema was ordered, and how many times the person is allowed to receive an enema within a given period of time. If the person complains of pain when you are giving an enema, stop the procedure and wait until the pain goes away. Reassure the person and have him take some deep breaths. If the pain continues, stop and report the situation to the nurse.

There are different types of enemas. Commercially prepared enemas come in pre-filled plastic bottles with a tip that is designed to be placed into the anus. Alternatively, an enema can be administered using an enema bag and tubing. An enema bag and tubing are often used to administer tap water or soap solution enemas. The bag is filled with warm tap water (for a tap water enema) or tap water and a small amount of a mild soap called castile soap (for a soap solution enema). Always follow the written orders exactly regarding the amount of water (and, if applicable, soap) to be used when preparing the enema solution. Also, make sure that the enema solution is the proper temperature (105° F). If the solution is too cold, the person could experience cramping and pain. A solution that is too hot can cause more serious injury.

Skill 15-10 describes how to give an enema.

CHECK YOUR UNDERSTANDING

Questions for Review

1. **The nurse asks you to obtain a midstream (clean catch) urine specimen. What should you do?**
   a. Collect and store all of the urine the person voids in a 24-hour period.
   b. Empty urine from the bedpan into a specimen container.
   c. Remind the person to start the stream of urine, then stop, then collect the urine sample from the restarted stream of urine.
   d. Provide catheter care before obtaining the urine sample.

2. **Mrs. Klein uses the toilet to void. The nurse asks you to obtain a urine specimen. Which piece of equipment would be best to use to obtain a urine specimen from Mrs. Klein?**
   a. A bottle
   b. A urinal
   c. A commode hat
   d. A bedpan

3. **What is the purpose of a scheduled toileting program for a person with dementia who is incontinent?**
   a. To punish the person for episodes of incontinence
   b. To teach the person how to use the toilet again
   c. To give the person the opportunity to void or have a bowel movement just before the person would normally void or have a bowel movement (as indicated by the person's normal elimination patterns), to reduce the likelihood that the person will have an episode of incontinence
   d. To reduce the number of times the nurse assistant needs to help the person with elimination

4. **How often should a person's incontinence pad or briefs be changed?**
   a. When you detect an odor
   b. Whenever they become soiled
   c. At the end of every shift
   d. Every hour

5. **Mrs. Summers can get out of bed but she can only walk a few feet before becoming very weak. She is able to sit up without assistance. Which piece of equipment would be best to use when assisting Mrs. Summers with elimination?**
   a. Bedpan
   b. Toilet
   c. Portable commode
   d. Indwelling urinary catheter

6. **Which of the following could increase a person's risk for developing a urinary tract infection?**
   a. Not drinking enough water
   b. Not emptying the bladder completely
   c. Having an indwelling urinary catheter
   d. All of the above

7. **Mr. Reynolds has not had a bowel movement in 3 days. Usually he has a bowel movement every other day, after breakfast. What should you do?**
   a. Give Mr. Reynolds an enema.
   b. Encourage Mr. Reynolds to rest.
   c. Nothing, since Mr. Reynolds does not seem to be complaining.
   d. Report the change in Mr. Reynolds' bowel elimination pattern to the nurse.

8. **Mrs. Cummings has an indwelling urinary catheter. When caring for Mrs. Cummings you should:**
   a. Remove the catheter to provide perineal care.
   b. Secure the tubing and urine drainage bag to the side rail of the bed.
   c. Make sure the tubing and urine drainage bag are lower than Mrs. Cummings' bladder.
   d. Disconnect the urine drainage bag from the tubing to empty it.

9. **When is an ostomy appliance used?**
   a. When a person is incontinent of urine or feces
   b. When a stool sample is required of the person
   c. When a person has had the bladder or a portion of the bowel surgically removed
   d. Before, during or after surgery

10. **Mrs. Ito can use the toilet to meet her elimination needs, but she needs help transferring to the bathroom, sitting down on the toilet and getting up from it. When assisting Mrs. Ito with elimination, you should:**
    a. Make sure the toilet paper and call signal are within her reach, and then leave her alone (but stay nearby and check on her every 5 minutes).
    b. Stay with Mrs. Ito in the bathroom.

c. Encourage Mrs. Ito to use a bedpan instead, because it is safer.
d. Encourage Mrs. Ito to use a portable commode instead, because it is less work to assist her to transfer to the commode.

Questions to Ask Yourself

1. *When assisting a person onto the toilet or portable commode, how would you use good body mechanics?*
2. *What can you do to help a person become more independent in managing his elimination needs?*
3. *Mrs. Simmons is incontinent of urine. According to Mrs. Simmons' care plan, she is to wear incontinence briefs in the afternoon, when she participates in activities at the facility. Today, while you are helping Mrs. Simmons get ready for bingo at 2:00, you tell her that it is time to "put on her briefs." Mrs. Simmons becomes angry with you and says, "I hate wearing those things! I'm not going to go to bingo today." What should you do?*
4. *You have helped Mrs. McWilliams onto the portable commode. While you are waiting outside the curtain for her to signal that she is finished, her roommate asks you to help her get back into bed. What should you do?*
5. *Mr. Smith has an indwelling urinary catheter and is expecting company. He tells you that he would like to meet with his visitors in the common area, but he is embarrassed by the urine collection bag. What can you do to enhance his self-esteem and protect his dignity and privacy?*
6. *Mr. Spatola is incontinent of feces. You are changing his briefs when your supervisor calls for you from the hall. What should you do?*

Skill 15-1
Helping a Person to Use a Portable Commode

PREPARATION

1. Wash your hands.
2. Gather your supplies:
   - Portable commode with collection container
   - Collection container cover
   - Toilet paper
   - Gloves
   - Wash basin
   - Soap
   - Washcloth
   - Towel
3. Knock, greet the person and ensure privacy.
4. Explain the procedure.
5. Adjust equipment for body mechanics and safety: Lower the bed to the level specified in the person's care plan. Make sure the wheels on the bed are locked.

PROCEDURE

6. Position the portable commode near the side of the bed on the person's stronger side so that it faces the foot of the bed. If the commode has wheels, make sure they are locked.
7. Lift the lid of the commode. Make sure the collection container is under the seat. If the collection container has a cover, remove it.
8. Transfer the person to the commode as you would transfer him to a chair. Before helping the person to sit down on the commode, help him to move clothing out of the way as needed.
9. Make sure the toilet paper and the person's method of calling for help are within reach. If you do not need to stay with the person to ensure his safety, ask the person to call you when he is finished and leave the room. Remember to shut the door on your way out, and to check on the person every 5 minutes.
10. When the person is finished using the portable commode, put on gloves. Help the person to stand and assist the person with wiping and adjusting his clothing as needed.
11. Remove your gloves and wash your hands. Put on a clean pair of gloves.
12. Fill the wash basin with warm water and help the person to wash and dry his hands.
13. Put on a clean pair of gloves. Remove the collection container from the commode and replace the cover. Take the collection container to the bathroom. Observe and (if ordered) measure the contents of the collection container before emptying it and cleaning it.
14. Remove your gloves and wash your hands.

COMPLETION

15. Ensure the person's comfort and good body alignment.
16. Adjust equipment for safety: Lower the bed to the level specified in the person's care plan. Make sure the wheels on the bed are locked. Place the person's method of calling for help within reach. Lower or raise the side rails according to the person's care plan.
17. Clean up your work area.
18. Wash your hands.
19. Report and record.

Skill 15-2
Helping a Person to Use a Bedpan

PREPARATION

1. Wash your hands.
2. Gather your supplies:
   - Bedpan
     - Bedpan cover
     - Bed protector
     - Toilet paper
     - Gloves
     - Wash basin
     - Soap
     - Washcloth
     - Towel
3. Knock, greet the person and ensure privacy.
4. Explain the procedure.
5. Adjust equipment for body mechanics and safety: Raise the bed to a comfortable working height. Make sure the wheels on the bed are locked.

PROCEDURE

6. Lower the head of the bed as low as the person can tolerate.
7. Fold the top linens out of the way, keeping the person's legs covered. Adjust the person's clothing as needed to expose the buttocks.
8. Put on gloves.
9. Position the bedpan underneath the person's buttocks.
   - **Option A:** Ask the person to bend her knees, place her feet firmly on the bed and raise her buttocks. Assist as necessary by slipping your hand under the person's lower back and lifting slightly. Position the bed protector under the person's buttocks, and place the bedpan on the bed protector. Help the person to lower herself onto the bedpan.
   - **Option B:** Assist the person to turn onto her side so that she is facing away from you. Position the bed protector under the person's buttocks. Hold the bedpan firmly against the person's buttocks and then gently turn the person back onto the bedpan (Figure 1).

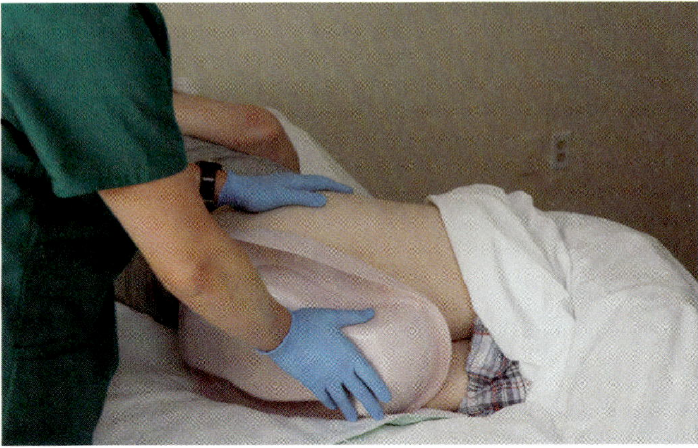

Figure 1

10. Arrange the top linens back over the person. Raise the head of the bed as tolerated so that the person is in a comfortable sitting position.
11. Make sure the toilet paper and the person's method of calling for help are within reach.
12. If you do not need to stay with the person to ensure her safety, remove your gloves and wash your hands. Ask the person to call you when she is finished and leave the room. Remember to shut the door on your way out, and to check on the person every 5 minutes.
13. When the person is finished using the bedpan, lower the head of the bed as low as the person can tolerate. Fold the top linens out of the way.
14. Put on gloves and assist the person with wiping, as needed.
15. Remove the bedpan.
    - **Option A:** Ask the person to bend her knees, place her feet firmly on the bed and raise her buttocks. Remove the bedpan and bed protector.
    - **Option B:** Assist the person to turn onto her side (facing away from you) while you hold the bedpan against the mattress to prevent the contents from spilling. Remove the bedpan and bed protector, and then help the person to roll back.
16. Cover the bedpan with the cover and set it aside on the bed protector, in a place where it will not spill. Remove your gloves.

17. Help the person to adjust her clothing, as needed. Arrange the top linens back over the person. Raise the head of the bed as the person requests.
18. Put on a clean pair of gloves. Fill the wash basin with warm water and help the person to wash and dry her hands.
19. Take the bedpan to the bathroom. Observe and (if ordered) measure the contents of the bedpan before emptying it and cleaning it.
20. Remove your gloves and wash your hands.

COMPLETION

21. Ensure the person's comfort and good body alignment.
22. Adjust equipment for safety: Lower the bed to the level specified in the person's care plan. Make sure the wheels on the bed are locked. Place the person's method of calling for help within reach. Lower or raise the side rails according to the person's care plan.
23. Clean up your work area.
24. Wash your hands.
25. Report and record.

Skill 15-3
Helping a Man to Use a Urinal

PREPARATION

1. Wash your hands.
2. Gather your supplies:
   - Urinal
   - Toilet paper
   - Gloves
   - Wash basin
   - Soap
   - Washcloth
   - Towel
3. Knock, greet the person and ensure privacy.
4. Explain the procedure.
5. Adjust equipment for body mechanics and safety: Make sure the wheels on the bed are locked.

PROCEDURE

6. Position the man to use the urinal. The man may sit up in bed, sit on the side of the bed or stand by the bed to use the urinal.
7. Put on gloves. Assist the man with positioning the urinal, as needed.
8. Make sure the toilet paper and the person's method of calling for help are within reach.
9. If you do not need to stay with the man to ensure his safety, remove your gloves and wash your hands. Ask the man to call you when he is finished and leave the room. Remember to shut the door on your way out, and to check on the man every 5 minutes.
10. When the man is finished using the urinal, put on a clean pair of gloves. Ask the man to hand you the urinal, or help him to remove it. Close the lid on the urinal and hang the urinal on the side rail in a place where it will not spill. Assist the man with wiping, as needed.
11. Remove your gloves and wash your hands.
12. Help the man adjust his clothing, as needed. Help him back into a comfortable position in bed.
13. Put on a clean pair of gloves. Fill the wash basin with warm water and help the man to wash and dry his hands.
14. Take the urinal to the bathroom. Observe and (if ordered) measure the contents of the urinal before emptying it and cleaning it.
15. Remove your gloves and wash your hands.

COMPLETION

16. Ensure the person's comfort and good body alignment.
17. Adjust equipment for safety: Lower the bed to the level specified in the person's care plan. Make sure the wheels on the bed are locked. Place the person's method of calling for help within reach. Lower or raise the side rails according to the person's care plan.
18. Clean up your work area.
19. Wash your hands.
20. Report and record.

Skill 15-4
Applying a Condom Catheter

PREPARATION

1. Wash your hands.
2. Gather your supplies:
   - Condom catheter kit (includes the condom catheter, catheter tubing and a method of securing the condom, such as adhesive or a strap)
   - Leg bag or large urine drainage bag
   - Leg strap (if a leg bag is used)
   - Catheter strap, or bandage scissors and tape (to secure the catheter tubing if a large urine drainage bag is used)
   - Gloves
   - Perineal care supplies
3. Knock, greet the person and ensure privacy.
4. Explain the procedure.
5. Adjust equipment for body mechanics and safety: Raise the bed to a comfortable working height. Make sure the wheels on the bed are locked.

PROCEDURE

6. Put on gloves.
7. Provide perineal care and thoroughly dry the skin.
8. Put the head of the man's penis in the condom. Unroll the condom over the penis. Allow room at the tip of the penis.
9. Secure the condom.
   - **Option A:** If the condom is self-adhesive, gently press the condom to the penis to cause it to adhere.
   - **Option B:** If the condom is secured using a strap, wrap the strap around the condom according to the manufacturer's instructions. Do not wrap the strap too tightly.
10. Attach the condom to the leg bag or large urine drainage bag.
11. Secure the catheter tubing and drainage bag:

    Option A: If using a leg bag, leave some slack in the catheter tubing and secure the leg bag to the man's thigh using the leg strap.

    Option B: If using a large urine drainage bag, secure the catheter tubing to the man's thigh using the catheter strap or tape, and hang the urine drainage bag from the bed frame. Make sure the urine drainage bag is lower than the man's bladder.

COMPLETION

12. Ensure the person's comfort and good body alignment.
13. Adjust equipment for safety: Lower the bed to the level specified in the person's care plan. Make sure the wheels on the bed are locked. Place the person's method of calling for help within reach. Lower or raise the side rails according to the person's care plan.
14. Clean up your work area.
15. Wash your hands.
16. Report and record.

Skill 15-5
Collecting a Routine Urine Specimen or Stool Specimen

PREPARATION

1. Wash your hands.
2. Gather your supplies:
   - Gloves
   - Paper towels
   - Specimen container and label
   - Commode hat (if person uses toilet)
   - Two tongue depressors (if collecting a stool sample)
   - Toilet paper
   - Plastic bag
3. Knock, greet the person and ensure privacy.
4. Explain the procedure.
5. Adjust equipment for body mechanics and safety: Make sure the wheels on the bed are locked.

PROCEDURE

6. Complete the label per your employer's policy. Take the specimen container to the bathroom. Remove the lid from the specimen container and place it face-up on a paper towel on the counter, being careful not to touch the inside of the lid.
7. If the person will be using the toilet, place the commode hat over the rim of the toilet seat.
8. Assist the person to use the toilet, a portable commode, a bedpan or a urinal as needed. Provide the person with the plastic bag for disposing of the toilet paper. Remind the person not to have a bowel movement (if a urine sample is being collected) or urinate (if a stool sample is being collected).
9. When the person is finished, help the person to wash the hands, as needed. Help the person back to bed if necessary.
10. Put on gloves. Take the portable commode collection container, bedpan or urinal to the bathroom, or remove the commode hat from the toilet seat.
11. Transfer the specimen to the specimen container.
    - **Urine.** Holding the specimen container over the toilet, pour the urine into the labeled specimen container, filling the container about halfway.
    - **Stool.** Use the tongue depressors to remove 1 to 2 tablespoons of the stool and place it in the labeled specimen container.
12. Place the lid tightly on the specimen container and place it on a paper towel on the counter. Apply the completed label to the specimen container.
13. Remove your gloves and wash your hands.

COMPLETION

14. Ensure the person's comfort and good body alignment.
15. Adjust equipment for safety: Lower the bed to the level specified in the person's care plan. Make sure the wheels on the bed are locked. Place the person's method of calling for help within reach. Lower or raise the side rails according to the person's care plan.
16. Clean up your work area.
17. Take the specimen container to the designated area for pick-up.
18. Wash your hands.
19. Report and record.

Skill 15-6

Collecting a Clean Catch (Midstream) Urine Specimen

PREPARATION

1. Wash your hands.
2. Gather your supplies:
   - Gloves
   - Paper towels
   - Clean catch kit
   - Toilet paper
   - Plastic bag
3. Knock, greet the person and ensure privacy.
4. Explain the procedure.
5. Adjust equipment for body mechanics and safety: Make sure the wheels on the bed are locked.

PROCEDURE

6. Complete the label per your employer's policy.
7. Cover the over-bed table or bathroom counter with paper towels. Open the clean catch kit and arrange the contents on the paper towels. Remove the lid from the specimen container and place it face-up on the paper towels, being careful not to touch the inside of the lid.
8. Put on gloves.
9. Assist the person as needed to cleanse the area around the urethral opening using the wipes in the clean catch kit.
   - **Female:** While separating the labia with the thumb and forefinger of one hand, wipe down the middle, then one side, and then the other side, using a clean wipe for each pass. Always wipe from front to back.
   - **Male:** Clean the tip of the penis by wiping three times in a circular pattern, moving from the urethral opening outward and using a clean wipe for each pass. If the man is uncircumcised, retract the foreskin and keep it retracted while cleansing the tip of the penis.
10. To obtain the specimen, the person must start the flow of urine, then stop it. The specimen is collected from the restarted flow, by having the person urinate directly into the specimen container. Remind the person not to touch the inside of the specimen container, and to keep the labia separated (if the person is a woman) or the foreskin retracted (if the man is an uncircumcised man). Provide the person with the plastic bag for disposing of the toilet paper.
11. When the person is finished urinating, place the lid tightly on the specimen container, being careful not to touch the inside of the lid. Apply the completed label to the specimen container. Place the specimen container on a paper towel on the counter.
12. Help the person to wash the hands, as needed. Help the person back to bed if necessary.
13. Remove your gloves and wash your hands.

COMPLETION

14. Ensure the person's comfort and good body alignment.
15. Adjust equipment for safety: Lower the bed to the level specified in the person's care plan. Make sure the wheels on the bed are locked. Place the person's method of calling for help within reach. Lower or raise the side rails according to the person's care plan.
16. Clean up your work area.
17. Take the specimen container to the designated area for pick-up.
18. Wash your hands.
19. Report and record.

Skill 15-7
Providing Catheter Care

PREPARATION

1. Wash your hands.
2. Gather your supplies:
    - Washcloths
    - Towels
    - Bath blanket
    - Bed protector
    - Wash basin
    - Bath thermometer
    - Soap or other cleansing agent, per your employer's policy
    - Paper towels
    - Gloves
3. Knock, greet the person and ensure privacy.
4. Explain the procedure.
5. Adjust equipment for body mechanics and safety: Raise the bed to a comfortable working height. Make sure the wheels on the bed are locked.

PROCEDURE

6. Cover the over-bed table with the paper towels and arrange your supplies. Fill the wash basin with warm water. Use the bath thermometer to verify that the water temperature is between 105° F and 115° F. Place the wash basin on the over-bed table.
7. Lower the head of the bed as low as the person can tolerate.
8. Cover the person and the top linens with the bath blanket (to provide privacy and warmth). Ask the person to hold the edge of the bath blanket (or tuck the edges under the person's shoulders) while you fold the top linens down to the bottom of the bed.
9. Put on the gloves.
10. Help the person to remove soiled clothing.
11. Have the person bend her knees and spread her legs as much as possible.
12. Have the person raise her buttocks off the bed, and place a bed protector under the person's hips. If providing catheter care for a woman, elevate the woman's pelvis by placing a bedpan or a folded towel or bath blanket under her buttocks.
13. Adjust the bath blanket as needed so that only the perineal area is exposed.
14. Wet the washcloth and make a mitt. Apply soap or other cleansing agent to the mitt, per your employer's policy.
15. Cleanse the perineal area.
    - **Female:** Separate the labia with one hand. Place the washcloth mitt at the top of the vulva and stroke downward, toward the anus. Clean the middle, then one side, then the other side, using a clean part of the mitt for each stroke. Rinse and dry the area.
    - **Male:** Hold the man's penis in one hand. If the man is uncircumcised, retract the foreskin. Moving from the urethral opening outward, wash the penis using a circular motion, starting with the tip and moving down to the base. Rinse and dry the area. If the man is uncircumcised, return the foreskin to its natural position.
16. Wet another washcloth and make a mitt. Apply soap or other cleansing agent to the mitt, per your employer's policy.
17. Hold the catheter near the urethral opening and clean about 4 inches of the catheter tubing, starting where the tubing leaves the body and moving outward (Figure 1). Rinse and dry the catheter tubing.

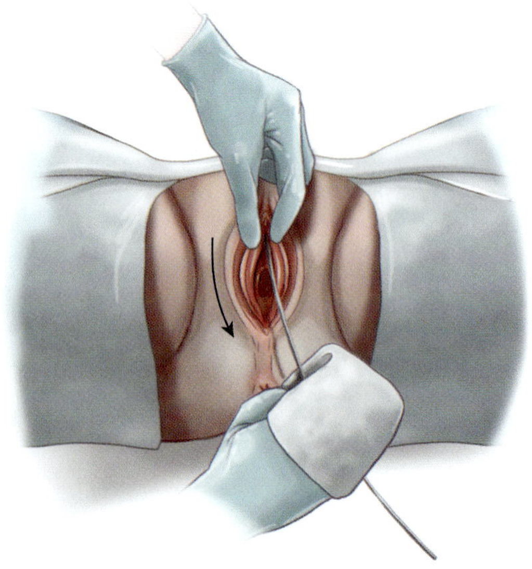

Figure 1

18. Make sure the catheter tubing is secured by tape or a catheter strap to the person's inner thigh.
19. Remove the bed protector.
20. Remove and dispose of your gloves.
21. Help the person back into the supine position.
22. Help the person to put on clean clothing as necessary.
23. If the linens are soiled or wet, change the linens.
24. Pull up the top linens and remove the bath blanket.

COMPLETION

25. Ensure the person's comfort and good body alignment.
26. Adjust equipment for safety: Lower the bed to the level specified in the person's care plan. Make sure the wheels on the bed are locked. Place the person's method of calling for help within reach. Lower or raise the side rails according to the person's care plan.
27. Clean up your work area.
28. Wash your hands.
29. Report and record.

Skill 15-8
Emptying a Urine Drainage Bag

PREPARATION

1. Wash your hands.
2. Gather your supplies:
   - Gloves
   - Graduate
   - Alcohol wipe
   - Paper towels
3. Knock, greet the person and ensure privacy.
4. Explain the procedure.
5. Adjust equipment for body mechanics and safety: Make sure the wheels on the bed are locked.

PROCEDURE

6. Put on gloves.
7. Place a paper towel on the floor underneath the drainage spout on the urine drainage bag. Place the graduate on the paper towel.
8. Remove the drainage spout from its holder on the side of the drainage bag and open the clamp. Allow the urine to flow into the graduate container (Figure 1). Do not touch the end of the drainage spout or allow it to come into contact with the graduate or any other surface except its holder.

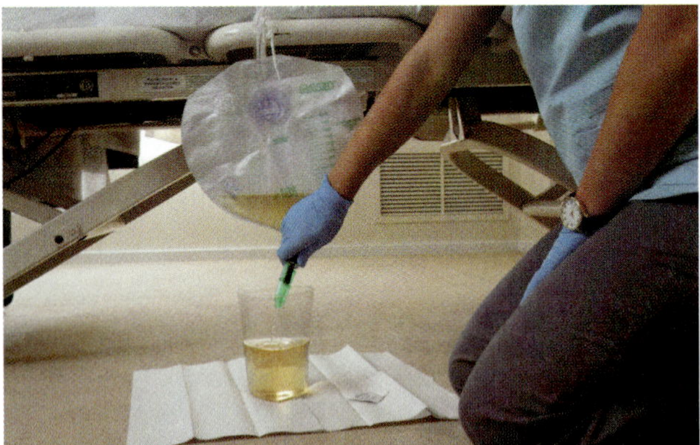

Figure 1

9. Close the clamp. Wipe the end of the drainage tube with an alcohol wipe. Return the drainage spout to its holder.
10. Take the graduate to the bathroom. Observe and (if ordered) measure the contents of the graduate before emptying it and cleaning it.
11. Remove your gloves and wash your hands.

COMPLETION

12. Ensure the person's comfort and good body alignment.
13. Adjust equipment for safety: Lower the bed to the level specified in the person's care plan. Make sure the wheels on the bed are locked. Place the person's method of calling for help within reach. Lower or raise the side rails according to the person's care plan.
14. Clean up your work area.
15. Wash your hands.
16. Report and record.

Skill 15-9
Changing an Ostomy Appliance

PREPARATION

1. Wash your hands.
2. Gather your supplies:
   - Gloves
   - Bed protector
   - Toilet paper
   - Washcloth
   - Towel
   - Clean ostomy appliance
   - Ostomy appliance deodorant (if used)
   - Skin adhesive (if used)
   - Scissors
   - Bedpan
   - Bedpan cover
   - Paper towels
   - Soap or other cleansing agent, per your employer's policy
3. Knock, greet the person and ensure privacy.
4. Explain the procedure.
5. Adjust equipment for body mechanics and safety: Raise the bed to a comfortable working height. Make sure the wheels on the bed are locked.

PROCEDURE

6. Cover the over-bed table with the paper towels and arrange your supplies. Fill the wash basin with warm water. Use the bath thermometer to verify that the water temperature is between 105° F and 115° F. Place the wash basin on the over-bed table.
7. Lower the head of the bed as low as the person can tolerate.
8. Fold the top linens out of the way, keeping the person's legs covered. Adjust the person's clothing as needed to expose the stoma. Position the bed protector alongside the person.
9. Put on gloves.
10. Remove the soiled ostomy appliance by holding the skin and gently peeling the appliance off, starting at the top. Place the soiled ostomy appliance in the bedpan.
11. Wipe around the stoma with toilet paper and place the toilet paper in the bedpan. Cover the bedpan with the cover.
12. Wet the washcloth and make a mitt. Apply soap or other cleansing agent, if ordered. Wash, rinse and dry the area around the stoma.
13. If the person uses as ostomy appliance deodorant, place the deodorant in the new ostomy appliance. Apply skin adhesive, if used. Apply the new appliance over the stoma, making sure there are no wrinkles.
14. Remove your gloves and wash your hands.
15. Help the person to adjust her clothing, as needed. Arrange the top linens back over the person. Raise the head of the bed as the person requests.
16. Put on a clean pair of gloves. Take the bedpan to the bathroom and dispose of the ostomy appliance by placing it in a labeled biohazard bag.
17. Remove your gloves and wash your hands.

COMPLETION

18. Ensure the person's comfort and good body alignment.
19. Adjust equipment for safety: Lower the bed to the level specified in the person's care plan. Make sure the wheels on the bed are locked. Place the person's method of calling for help within reach. Lower or raise the side rails according to the person's care plan.
20. Clean up your work area.
21. Wash your hands.
22. Report and record.

Skill 15-10
Giving a Person an Enema

PREPARATION

1. Wash your hands.
2. Gather your supplies:

   Tap water or soap solution enema:

   - Enema unit (bag, tubing and clamp)
   - Lubricating jelly
   - Packet of castile soap (if giving a soap solution enema)
   - Bath thermometer
   - Gloves
   - Bedpan or portable commode (if the person is not able to use the toilet)
   - Bedpan or collection container cover
   - Bed protector
   - Bath blanket
   - Washcloth
   - Towel

   Commercially prepared enema:

   - Commercially prepared enema
   - Bath thermometer
   - Gloves
   - Bedpan or portable commode (if the person is not able to use the toilet)
   - Bedpan or portable commode cover
   - Bed protector
   - Bath blanket
   - Washcloth
   - Towel
3. Knock, greet the person and ensure privacy.
4. Explain the procedure.
5. Adjust equipment for body mechanics and safety: Raise the bed to a comfortable working height. Make sure the wheels are locked.

PROCEDURE

6. Prepare the enema.
   - **Tap water enema:** Clamp the tubing and fill the enema bag with the amount of warm water (usually 500 to 1000 mL, 105° F on the bath thermometer), per the written orders.
   - **Soap solution enema:** Clamp the tubing and fill the enema bag with the amount of warm water (500 to 1000 mL, 105° F on the bath thermometer), per the written orders. Add the packet of soap and gently rotate the enema bag to mix the solution. Avoid shaking the enema bag to mix.
   - **Commercially prepared enema:** Open the enema package and take off the protective cover.
7. Lower the head of the bed as low as the person can tolerate.
8. Cover the person and the top linens with the bath blanket. Ask the person to hold the edge of the bath blanket (or tuck the edges under the person's shoulders) while you fold the top linens down to the bottom of the bed.
9. Assist the person to turn onto her left side with her back toward you and the right knee flexed (Sims' position).
10. Adjust the bath blanket and the person's clothing as necessary to expose the buttocks. Position the bed protector alongside the person.
11. If giving a tap water or soap solution enema, lubricate the tip of the tubing (2 to 4 inches) by placing a small amount of lubricating jelly on a tissue and dipping the tip of the tubing into it. Commercially prepared enemas usually have a pre-lubricated tip.
12. Put on gloves.
13. Lift the person's upper buttock and insert the tubing or the tip of the commercially prepared enema into the anus no more than 2 to 4 inches. If you have difficulty inserting the tubing or the tip of the commercially prepared enema bottle at least 2 inches into the person's rectum, stop the procedure and tell the nurse.
14. Administer the enema solution.
    - **Tap water or soap solution enema:** Open the clamp and, holding the bag no higher than 12 inches above the anus, allow the solution to flow slowly into the person's rectum. Hold the tubing in place so that it does not slip out of the rectum.
    - **Commercially prepared enema:** Squeeze the plastic bottle.

15. When all of the enema solution has been administered, remove the tubing or the tip of the commercially prepared enema from the person's rectum and encourage her to hold the solution in a side-lying position for as long as possible.
16. Help the person to eliminate the enema solution, using a bedpan, portable commode or the toilet.
17. Fill the wash basin with warm water and help the person to wash and dry her hands. Assist the person with perineal care as needed.
18. Remove the bed protector. Adjust the person's clothing to cover the buttocks and help her into a comfortable position.
19. If the person used a bedpan or portable commode, cover the bedpan or collection container and take it to the bathroom. Observe the contents of the bedpan or collection container before emptying it and cleaning it.
20. Remove your gloves and wash your hands.

COMPLETION

21. Ensure the person's comfort and good body alignment.
22. Adjust equipment for safety: Lower the bed to the level specified in the person's care plan. Make sure the wheels on the bed are locked. Place the person's method of calling for help within reach. Lower or raise the side rails according to the person's care plan.
23. Clean up your work area.
24. Wash your hands.
25. Report and record.

▼ Box 16-1 Common Conditions Associated with Chronic Pain

Arthritis

- Inflammation of a joint is characterized by pain, swelling and stiffness.

Osteoarthritis

- In this form of arthritis, loss of the cartilage that covers the ends of the bones causes bones to rub together during movement, which produces pain.

Osteoporosis

- The bones become weak and brittle, which often results in fractures that produce pain.

Peripheral artery disease

- Blocked blood flow to the legs decreases the delivery of oxygen and nutrients to the tissues, which results in pain, skin ulcers and possibly gangrene (tissue death).

Amputation

- Amputation (surgical removal of all or part of a limb) results in *phantom pain*, or the sensation of pain that originates in the part of the body that was removed.

Peripheral neuropathy

- Damage to the nerves causes pain and numbness in the hands and feet; this kind of pain is often a result of diabetes.

Cancer

- Pain can be caused by the disease or by the treatment.
- A growing tumor or the excessive build-up of fluid can push against other organs or tissues, which causes pain.
- Medical tests and treatments (for example, biopsies, chemotherapy) can be painful because they frequently involve injections with large needles, chemicals that can irritate the veins or both.

Gastroesophageal reflux disease (GERD)

- Backflow of gastric acid from the stomach into the esophagus (the passageway that food travels through to get from the mouth to the stomach) irritates the esophageal lining, which produces a burning sensation that extends from the stomach into the chest and throat.

- **The person's previous experiences with pain.** A person who has had a great deal of experience with pain in the past may be better able to tolerate similar experiences in the future. Or, the person may be so worn down by past experiences with pain that each new episode of pain becomes more difficult for the person to handle.
- **The person's emotional state.** Anxiety, worry or emotional upset can make it more difficult for the person to handle physical discomfort and pain.

Think back to Mr. Murphy. What type of pain do you think Mr. Murphy is experiencing now? What type of pain do you think Mr. Murphy experienced in the past? How could Mr. Murphy's past experiences with chronic hip pain affect his response to the pain that he is currently experiencing after his surgery?

Individual differences in pain responses often influence the actions of health care providers. For example, a person who does not complain of pain, even when enduring a treatment that is known to be painful, may not be offered pain relief because the health care provider may assume that the person is not experiencing pain. However, a person who demonstrates a very emotional reaction to pain may be thought of as being overly dramatic. In this case, the health care provider may view that person's response as beyond what is necessary for the expected level of pain, and the person's report of pain may be minimized or sometimes even ignored! It is important to recognize that people experience and react to pain in different ways and we must be respectful of each person's response.

Pain is a personal experience. In health care, we routinely use objective measurements to determine what is happening in a person's body. For example, we count pulses and respirations and measure blood pressure, weights and urinary output. However, with pain, there is nothing that we can measure. The only information that we have about a person's pain is the description of the pain that the person gives us. All people who are receiving health care have the right to have relief from pain. To meet this goal, we must listen to what the person says about pain, accept it as truth, and respond with appropriate actions to promote comfort and relieve suffering.

Recognizing Pain

The very first step toward relieving pain is recognizing that it exists. Failure of health care providers to recognize the existence of pain is a major factor that interferes with pain relief. Some health care providers assume that if a person has pain, he will tell someone in order to get relief. However, some people may not be able to report pain (for example, because of language problems related to a stroke or dementia). Others may simply be unwilling to report pain. Reasons why a person may choose not to report pain include the following:

- Not wanting to be thought of as a bother
- Being fearful of what the pain means
- Not wanting to worry loved ones
- Cultural or social pressure to be strong and stoic
- Concern about uncomfortable or unpleasant side effects (such as constipation) from pain medications
- Fear of developing a dependency on, or an addiction to, pain medications (Box 16-2)

ELDER CARE NOTE. Many people believe that pain is just a natural part of old age and has to be tolerated. However, pain is not a normal or expected consequence of aging! Still, because of this false belief, an older person may be less likely to report pain. Also, even if the person does complain of pain, family members may be less likely to follow up on the complaint because they may also believe that the pain is normal and that nothing can be done about it.

Sometimes, simply asking about the presence of pain is all that is needed to get the person to tell you about pain that he is having. However, you must also be alert to nonverbal expressions of pain (Figure 16-1, Box 16-3). No member of the health care team spends more time

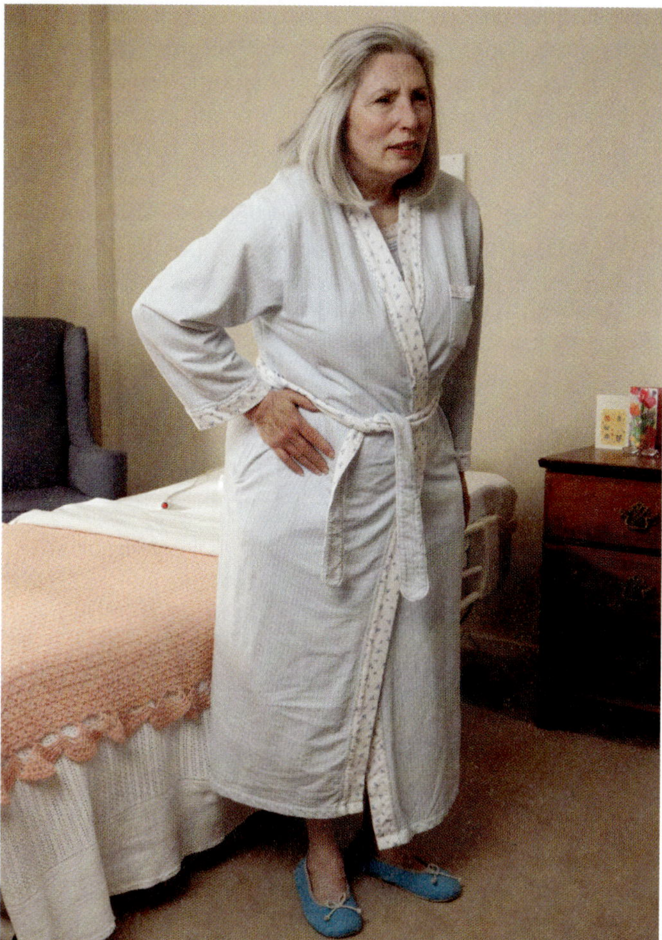

Figure 16-1 Many people will not tell you about pain that they are having, but their facial expressions or behaviors will give you clues to their discomfort.

Box 16-2 Pain Medications, Dependence and Addiction

Some types of pain are effectively treated with medications called *opioids*. Opioids work on the central nervous system to block the perception of pain. In most cases, people who have pain function better with use of these medications. When opioids are used for a long time, the body becomes physically dependent on the medication, and higher doses are required to achieve the same effect. This is called *dependence*, and it is expected when a person takes a medication for a long period. In drug dependence, the drug improves the person's ability to function. Dependence is different from *addiction*. Addiction has a mental basis as well as a physical one. The person is driven to seek the drug at all costs, and obtaining the drug becomes the focus of his efforts. With drug addiction, the person's ability to function is decreased. If a person expresses concerns about taking pain medications because of a fear of becoming addicted to them, be sure to report these concerns to the nurse, so that the nurse can follow up accordingly.

Box 16-3 Nonverbal Expressions of Pain

- Wincing or grimacing
- Frowning or showing a worried facial expression
- Rocking
- Pacing
- Restlessness
- Rubbing the painful body part
- Guarding (protecting) the painful body part
- Moaning or crying
- Resisting care
- Behaving aggressively (especially in response to attempts to give care)
- Wakefulness
- Having less appetite

providing hands-on care than the nurse assistant does. This puts you in an ideal position to recognize a person's pain. The pain associated with many of the conditions that affect older people is triggered by movement. For this reason, it is particularly important to look for nonverbal expressions of pain when you are giving care. For example, a person who cannot verbally express how she is feeling may resist care or react with aggression when something that you are doing causes pain. If you observe any signs that may indicate that a person is experiencing pain, you should report your observations to the nurse immediately so that a thorough assessment can be done and treatment for pain, if found, can be started.

Reporting Pain

Prompt reporting of pain to the nurse is very important (Figure 16-2). However, *what* you report is just as important. What you report helps the other members of the health care team to identify the source of the pain and determine what treatment would work best to achieve relief. Important facts to report are:

- **The location of the pain.** Be as specific as possible. For example, rather than reporting that a person complains of pain in her leg, try to find out exactly where it hurts. If the person cannot tell you exactly what hurts, then watch for behavioral clues that might indicate the specific location of the pain. For example, you noticed that Mrs. Bateman is limping on the right side when she walks, but on further observation, you notice that when she is sitting, she constantly rubs her right knee. This information will be very helpful to the nurse because it identifies the knee as the most likely source of Mrs. Bateman's discomfort.
- **The characteristics of the pain.** Different kinds of problems in the body result in different kinds of pain. For example, pain associated with nerve damage is often described as *burning* or *tingling*, whereas pain from arthritis is described as *dull* or *achy*. Box 16-4 provides a list of words commonly used to describe pain. If the person has difficulty finding a word to describe his pain, it may be helpful to offer suggestions from this list to help him identify the type of pain he is experiencing. The most effective treatment for the pain may depend on the characteristics of the pain. For example, medicines effective in treating arthritis pain are usually not as effective for treating nerve pain.
- **The intensity of the pain.** *Intensity* refers to the level of pain. Words such as mild, moderate and severe can be used to indicate the level of a person's pain. A pain scale can also be used to help the person communicate the level of pain that she is experiencing. There are many different types of pain scales. Some scales are based on a number system. The person indicates her level of pain on a scale of 1 to 10, with 1 being no pain and 10 being the worst pain possible. Other pain scales work in a similar way but use diagrams of faces or colors of increasing intensity. Although a person's pain cannot truly be measured, having the person rate the intensity of her pain on a pain scale gives a baseline for evaluating the person's pain in the future. For example, a person rates her pain as a 9 on the pain scale before taking medication, but after taking medication she rates her pain as a 6. Using the pain scale makes it easier to judge the amount of relief the medication is providing.

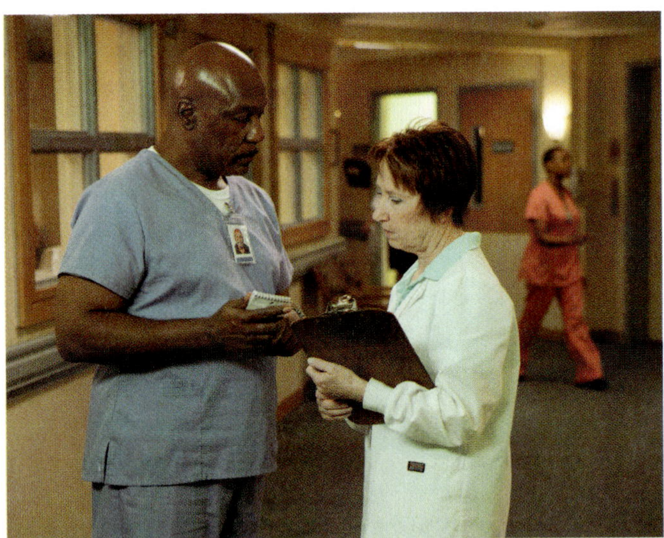

Figure 16-2 Reporting a person's pain to the nurse promptly is one of the most effective things that you can do to help provide the person with relief.

Box 16-4 **Words Used to Describe Pain**

- Dull
- Sharp, piercing, stabbing or shooting
- Achy or sore
- Nagging
- Throbbing, pulsating or pounding
- Burning, tingling, or a pins and needles sensation
- Gnawing
- Spasm
- Crampy
- Squeezing, crushing or feeling of pressure
- Radiating or spreading

Box 16-5 **Consequences of Untreated Pain**

- Decreased mobility
- Decreased ability or desire to perform usual activities
- Decreased ability or desire to attend social functions and interact with others
- Sleep disturbances
- Changes in appetite and weight
- Emotional effects, such as depression or anxiety
- Slowed healing

- **The frequency of the pain.** If the pain is there all the time, it is described as *constant.* When pain comes and goes, it is called *intermittent.* Other words that describe frequency include *occasional, seldom* and *daily.* When pain is not present all of the time, it is important to try to identify exactly when the pain occurs. This can provide clues about the cause of the pain. For example, ask the person what he was doing when the pain started. It is also helpful to find out what makes the pain better, and what makes it worse.

Think back to your interaction with Mr. Murphy this morning.

What questions would you ask Mr. Murphy to find out more about the pain he is having? What observations would you report to the nurse?

Relieving Pain

Pain contributes to suffering that impacts every part of a person's life (Box 16-5). A person who is in pain may not be able to do things he likes to do (such as engage in hobbies) and he may not feel like socializing with others. In addition, a person who is in pain may have reduced mobility and may not be able to participate in self-care activities, and as a result may experience a decrease in independence and abilities. A decreased ability to do things independently and to engage in enjoyable activities can lead to emotional problems, such as depression and loneliness. Unrelieved pain also negatively impacts the person's physical health by causing physical and emotional stress, interfering with sleep and appetite and slowing healing. Therefore, providing relief from pain is very important to the person's overall health and well-being.

A person's pain can be managed in many ways. Effective pain management often involves the use of medication in addition to other comfort measures, such as the application of heat or cold. Although nurse assistants are not responsible for prescribing or administering medications, you will play an important role in observing and reporting the person's response to them. The observations that you make to report pain are the same observations that you make to help determine the effectiveness of treatment. For example, you notice that since Mrs. Bateman has been taking medication for pain, she no longer limps when she walks. This is important for the nurse to know, because it suggests that the medication is working to relieve Mrs. Bateman's pain. It is also important to report any observations that may be signs of an unwanted side effect from the medication. For example, you noticed that since Mr. Evans has been taking his new pain medication, he has not had a bowel movement. This is important to report, because many pain medications cause constipation. Or perhaps you noticed that Mr. Evans has had periods of confusion and disorientation that did not occur before he started taking his new pain medication. Again, the nurse needs to know this so that the medications can be properly adjusted.

As a nurse assistant, you may be involved in administering treatments for pain that do not involve medication. For example, heat or cold applications may be ordered for the person to relieve muscle aches and joint pains. It is important to check with the nurse prior to performing these procedures to review precautions that should be taken and to find out specifics, such as the temperature and the length of time for the treatment. Box 16-6 describes general guidelines for the safe use of heat and cold applications. Skills 16-1 through 16-4 describe step by step how to apply a warm or cold compress, assist with a warm soak, apply an aquathermia pad and apply a warm water bottle or ice bag.

There are also many simple comfort measures you can use every day to help decrease pain:

- Distraction is literally helping the person take her mind off of her pain. The brain can only pay attention to so many signals at a time. When the brain becomes occupied by other things, it tends to pay less attention to the pain signals. Listening to music, watching a favorite television program, reading a book or playing a game are all ways to divert attention away from pain. Using distraction techniques can be particularly useful at night. At night, the person has little to think about except the pain she is experiencing. If you find that a person is awake at night, engaging in a quiet activity with the person may help the person get back to sleep.

Skill 16-2
Assisting with a Warm Soak

PREPARATION

1. Wash your hands.
2. Gather your supplies:
   - Towel
   - Bed protector
   - Wash basin
   - Watch
   - Bath thermometer
3. Knock, greet the person and ensure privacy.
4. Explain the procedure.
5. Adjust equipment for body mechanics and safety: Raise the bed to a comfortable working height. Make sure that the wheels on the bed are locked.

PROCEDURE

6. Fill the wash basin with warm water and use the bath thermometer to verify that the water temperature is between 100° F and 105° F.
7. Help the person into a comfortable position and expose the part of the body that is to receive the treatment.
8. Place the bed protector under the part of the body that is to receive the treatment, and then place the wash basin on the bed protector. Position the part of the body that is to receive the treatment in the wash basin.
9. Note the time on your watch and calculate the time that the treatment should end (usually after 20 minutes). If you intend to leave the room, place the person's method of calling for help within reach.
10. Check the skin every 5 minutes. If the skin is bright red, pale or blue, or if the person reports pain, tingling or burning, stop the treatment and report to the nurse.
11. When the treatment is finished, remove the part of the body that received the treatment from the wash basin and dry the skin with a clean towel.

COMPLETION

12. Ensure the person's comfort and good body alignment.
13. Adjust equipment for safety: Lower the bed to the level specified in the person's care plan. Make sure that the wheels on the bed are locked. Place the person's method of calling for help within reach. Lower or raise the side rails according to the person's care plan.
14. Clean up your work area.
15. Wash your hands.
16. Report and record.

Skill 16-3
Applying an Aquathermia Pad

PREPARATION

1. Wash your hands.
2. Gather your supplies:
   - Aquathermia pad and heating unit
   - Distilled water
   - Flannel cover or towel
   - Tape or roller gauze
   - Watch
3. Knock, greet the person and ensure privacy.
4. Explain the procedure.
5. Adjust equipment for body mechanics and safety: Raise the bed to a comfortable working height. Make sure that the wheels on the bed are locked.

PROCEDURE

6. Fill the heating unit to the fill line with distilled water.
7. Place the pad and tubing below the heating unit and tilt the heating unit from side to side to remove bubbles from the tubing.
8. Place the heating unit so that the unit will be level with the aquathermia pad and connecting hoses. Plug in the unit and turn it on.
9. Set the temperature as directed by the nurse (usually 105° F). Remove the key.
10. Place the aquathermia pad in the flannel cover or wrap it in a dry towel.
11. Let the water warm to the set temperature.
12. Help the person into a comfortable position and expose the part of the body that is to receive the treatment.
13. Apply the pad to the part of the body that is to receive the treatment. If necessary, secure the pad in place with tape or roller gauze. Do not use pins.
14. Note the time on your watch and calculate the time that the treatment should end (usually after 20 minutes). If you intend to leave the room, place the person's method of calling for help within reach.
15. Check the skin every 5 minutes. If the skin is bright red, pale or blue, or if the person reports pain, tingling or burning, stop the treatment and report to the nurse.
16. When the treatment is finished, remove the pad.

COMPLETION

17. Ensure the person's comfort and good body alignment.
18. Adjust equipment for safety: Lower the bed to the level specified in the person's care plan. Make sure that the wheels on the bed are locked. Place the person's method of calling for help within reach. Lower or raise the side rails according to the person's care plan.
19. Clean up your work area.
20. Wash your hands.
21. Report and record.

Skill 16-4
Applying a Warm Water Bottle or Ice Bag

PREPARATION

1. Wash your hands.
2. Gather your supplies:
   - Warm water bottle or ice bag
   - Flannel cover or towel
   - Towel
   - Bath thermometer
   - Watch
3. Knock, greet the person and ensure privacy.
4. Explain the procedure.
5. Adjust equipment for body mechanics and safety: Raise the bed to a comfortable working height. Make sure that the wheels on the bed are locked.

PROCEDURE

6. If you are using a warm water bottle, use the bath thermometer to verify that the water temperature is between 100° F and 105° F and then fill the bottle one-half to two-thirds full. If you are using an ice bag, fill the bag two-thirds full with ice (Figure 1).

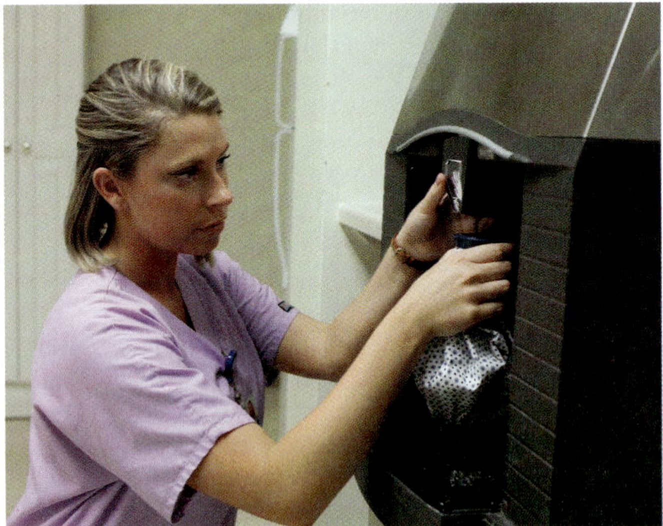

Figure 1

7. Check for leaks by putting on the cap and turning the water bottle or ice bag upside down. Use a towel to dry the outside of the water bottle or ice bag.
8. Place the water bottle or ice bag in the cover or wrap it in a dry towel.
9. Help the person into a comfortable position and expose the part of the body that is to receive the treatment.
10. Apply the water bottle or ice bag to the part of the body that is to receive the treatment. Hold the water bottle or ice bag in place, or ask the person to assist by holding the water bottle or ice bag in place.
11. Note the time on your watch and calculate the time that the treatment should end (usually after 20 minutes).
12. Check the skin under the water bottle or ice bag every 5 minutes. If the skin is bright red, pale or blue, or if the person reports pain, tingling or burning, stop the treatment and report to the nurse.
13. When the treatment is finished, remove the water bottle or ice bag.

COMPLETION

14. Ensure the person's comfort and good body alignment.
15. Adjust equipment for safety: Lower the bed to the level specified in the person's care plan. Make sure that the wheels on the bed are locked. Place the person's method of calling for help within reach. Lower or raise the side rails according to the person's care plan.
16. Clean up your work area.
17. Wash your hands.
18. Report and record.

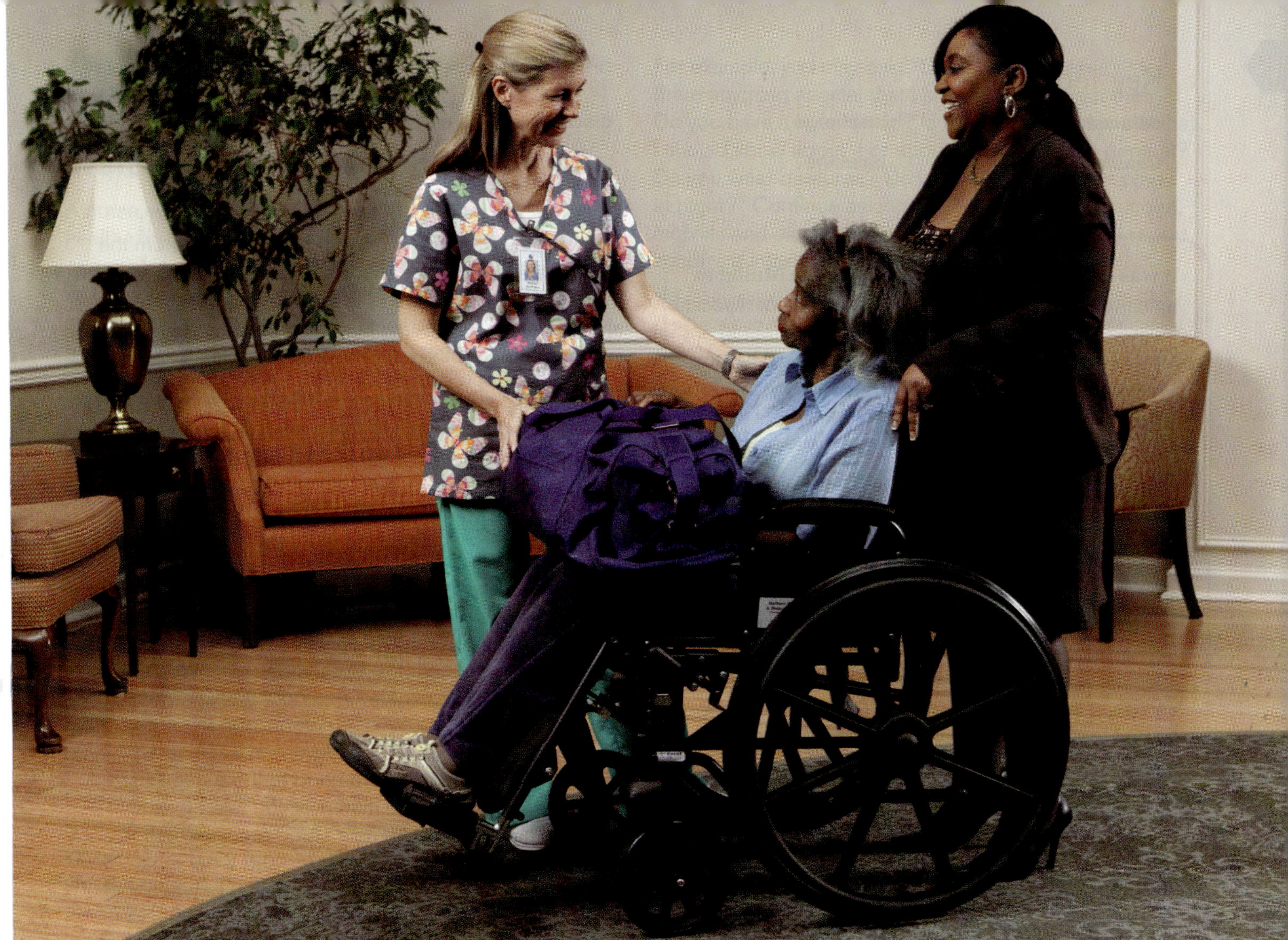

Assisting with Admissions, Transfers and Discharges

CHAPTER 17

Goals

After reading this chapter, you will have the information needed to:

- Assist with admissions to a health care facility.
- Make a person feel welcome and comfortable during his or her stay at a health care facility.
- Assist with transfers within a health care facility.
- Assist with discharges from a health care facility.

example, a person may be discharged from a hospital to a sub-acute care facility, a nursing home or his own home as his condition improves and he no longer requires hospital care.

To ensure that the person's health care needs continue to be met after the person leaves the facility where he is receiving care, the health care team follows a process called **discharge planning**. Discharge planning involves identifying the person's ongoing care needs and making arrangements to have those needs met after the person leaves the facility (Figure 17-6). Discharge planning begins as soon as the person is admitted to the health care setting and continues throughout the person's stay. The nurse and, in many facilities, the discharge planner, are primarily responsible for discharge planning, although you will help with discharge planning by communicating information about the person's needs to the other members of the health care team.

On the day that a person is ready to be discharged from the facility, help her gather all her belongings and pack her suitcase. Check items against the personal belongings inventory list to make sure that she has everything she brought with her. Check with the nurse to make sure that the proper forms are filled out and ready to go with the person. If the person is being discharged to another facility, it is often helpful to send a detailed description of the person's physical needs and personal habits, as well as medications and usual vital signs, to the receiving facility. Stay with the person and comfort her until she is discharged because she may be very frightened.

Help the person into a wheelchair or onto a stretcher and transport her to the exit. Tell the person how much you have enjoyed helping her, and wish her well in her recovery. If the person is being transported by ambulance, introduce the person to the ambulance crew. If necessary, help the ambulance attendants move the person into the ambulance. Make sure that the person's belongings and forms are placed in the vehicle with the person.

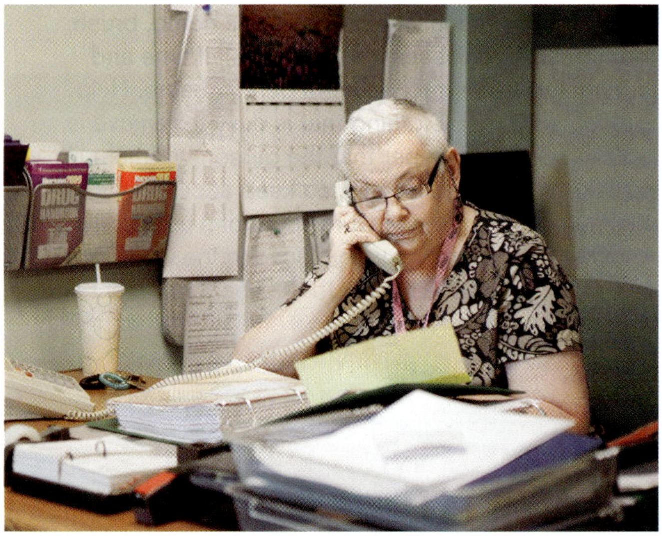

Report to the nurse that the person's discharge has been completed. Provide important information, such as the time of the discharge, mode of transportation, how the person responded and any important observations.

Figure 17-6 A discharge planner helps make arrangements so that the person's care needs can be met after the person leaves the facility.

For several months, you and other nurse assistants have helped Mrs. Mulligan with bathing, dressing and walking and have assisted her with special exercises that she learned from the physical therapist. The nursing care and physical therapy have strengthened Mrs. Mulligan's hip and enabled her to walk with a walker. After a few more months, Mrs. Mulligan is stronger and more confident and is able to walk without assistance. She now bathes and dresses herself. She has recovered well enough to be discharged from the nursing home to her own home.

What will your responsibilities be in assisting with Mrs. Mulligan's discharge?

How do you think Mrs. Mulligan may feel about leaving Morningside Nursing Home and returning home? What about her daughter?

CHECK YOUR UNDERSTANDING

Questions for Review

1. **When a person moves into and out of health care situations, the nurse assistant looks after the person and the person's:**
   a. Finances.
   b. Pets.
   c. Doctor.
   d. Belongings.

2. **When you admit a new resident to a nursing home, one of your tasks may be to label:**
   a. The person's bed.
   b. The person's clothing.
   c. The back of the person's hand.
   d. The bed linens.

3. **The nurse assistant takes and records a new person's vital signs, height and weight when he arrives at a health care facility. Why are these measurements important?**
   a. Because the person may not know his current height and weight.
   b. Because other health care workers use them as a baseline reference point when the same measurements are taken at other times.
   c. Because the nurse assistant needs to assess the person's nutrition requirements.
   d. Because the billing department requires this information to submit to health insurance companies.

4. **What sort of information is the nursing assistant most interested in when she asks a new person in her care questions?**
   a. Information that will help make the person's stay more comfortable.
   b. Signs that the person needs psychological help.
   c. Clues about any underlying health problems such as diabetes.
   d. Information about the person's ability to pay for care.

5. **How should a nurse assistant address a person in her care?**
   a. Use the person's ID number instead of her name.
   b. Refer to a person by his medical condition.
   c. Use the person's first name.
   d. Ask the person how she would like to be addressed and use that name.

6. **Which of the following is one of the ways that a nurse assistant helps transfer a person in her care?**
   a. Pack up the person's belongings.
   b. Write up a transfer plan.
   c. Give the person a bath so that he is relaxed.
   d. Nothing. The nurse assistant is not involved in transfers.

7. **When a person's transfer or discharge is complete, you should report all of the following to the nurse EXCEPT:**
   a. Time of the discharge.
   b. Mode of transportation.
   c. The person's emotional status.
   d. The person's method of payment.

8. **When a person is being discharged, how can the nurse assistant be sure that she packed all the belongings that a person brought with her?**
   a. Ask the person. She will remember her belongings.
   b. Consult family members.
   c. Refer to the personal belongings inventory sheet.
   d. Check the safe for items with the person's name.

9. **What is the purpose of discharge planning?**
   a. It gives the staff an end date for the care that they are giving.
   b. It ensures ongoing care for a person even after the person leaves the health care facility.
   c. It helps the nursing staff prepare the room for the next person.
   d. It serves as proof of the care that was given.

Questions to Ask Yourself

1. *Mrs. Wilson insists that she was wearing a ruby ring when she was transferred from the nursing home to the hospital. She is adamant that it was stolen, and she is beginning to despair because it was a family heirloom that was passed on to her from her mother. How would you respond to Mrs. Wilson? What would you do?*
2. *Mr. Garcia is a new patient at the hospital, and he is going into surgery tomorrow. You overhear him speaking to his wife, and it is clear that he is confused about the upcoming surgery and his medical condition. What would you do?*
3. *You are introducing yourself to Mrs. Woods, a new resident in the nursing home. She tells you that she dislikes the plainness of the room and is worried that she will be lonely here. She also tells you that she really wanted to live with one of her sons' families. What can you do to alleviate her concerns? How can you help her to feel welcome and at home in her new environment? How would you respond to her comments about her sons?*
4. *Mr. Mendez is being transferred out of your unit to the intensive care unit (ICU) because his condition has worsened. He confides in you that he is very frightened about his health and worried about the change in the nursing staff. How would you respond to Mr. Mendez? What can you to do to help?*

Key Terms:

acute condition

chronic condition

arthritis

osteoporosis

angina

chronic heart failure

hypertension

influenza

pneumonia

aspiration pneumonia

chronic obstructive pulmonary disease (COPD)

pulse oximetry

asthma

Parkinson's disease

multiple sclerosis (MS)

hemiplegia

hemiparesis

paralysis

paraplegia

quadriplegia

diabetes

insulin

hypoglycemia

hyperglycemia

kidney (renal) failure

dialysis

cancer

tumor

benign

malignant

metastasize

chemotherapy

radiation

depression

suicide

anxiety

The first time you went to Craig and Karen Trainer's home to provide care for 63-year-old Mr. Trainer, he had received a diagnosis of lung cancer 2 months earlier. He had surgery to remove part of his left lung and is receiving chemotherapy. You are there to help with personal care and to observe how he tolerates chemotherapy treatment.

When you arrive, Mrs. Trainer greets you at the door and you can see that her eyes are puffy and red and her eye makeup is smudged. After you hang up your coat in the hall closet, you ask Mrs. Trainer what you can do to help her. "Nobody can help me!" she says in a loud, high-pitched voice. Then she sits down in a chair and bursts into tears. You put your hands on her shoulders to try to comfort her. When she calms down, she says, "I'm sorry. It's just that the cancer has made everything so difficult. We can't go out together because I can't handle his wheelchair and oxygen tank, and I'm afraid to leave him alone. I feel like a prisoner. I never get out of this house. All I do is take care of Craig. I don't mind taking care of him, because I love him. But I'm so tired. I don't see how we can continue to live like this."

Think about the last time you were sick. Did the illness occur suddenly? Perhaps one day you felt fine, and the next day you were ill with a cold or an infection. Or perhaps someone you know had surgery to remove an infected appendix (appendicitis). In both of these cases, the illness is considered an **acute condition**. That is, the illness happened fairly suddenly and lasted a short time.

Some illnesses, such as diabetes and arthritis, do not resolve with time. These conditions are **chronic conditions**. In many cases, a person who has a chronic condition lives the rest of his life with an illness or condition that never really goes away, and the person requires ongoing treatment to manage it. Sometimes a person can have a chronic condition that continues for years without many serious symptoms, and then suddenly it flares up. When it flares up, the chronic condition is in an acute phase. The person feels ill and may need medical attention. After treatment, the acute phase resolves, but the person continues to live with the chronic condition.

Many people in your care will have chronic conditions, especially if you work in a nursing home. Living with a chronic condition can be very difficult for a person. Often, the condition affects the person's ability to manage activities of daily living (ADLs) independently. The person may have good days, when she is able to do quite a lot, and bad days, when pain or disability prevents her from doing much at all. A chronic condition also impacts a person's emotional health. The person may become depressed or angry because the condition affects her ability to do the things she likes to do. It can be very difficult for the person to cope day to day with a condition that may prevent her from ever feeling really well. As a nurse assistant, you must try to help the person live the fullest life possible. Show empathy, and recognize that the person's abilities may change from day to day. Therefore, your care and the amount of assistance you provide may need to change from day to day as well.

Family members and friends are also affected by the person's chronic condition. If a person's diet changes, his family may have to eat differently, too. If the person cannot move without help, he may need assistance with a variety of tasks. Family members and friends may also be sad, angry or depressed about the change in the person's health.

MUSCULOSKELETAL CONDITIONS

Common conditions that affect the musculoskeletal system include arthritis, osteoporosis and hip fractures.

Arthritis

Arthritis is a condition that causes joints to become inflamed, swollen, stiff and painful (Figure 18-1). A few or many joints may be affected. The smooth tissue that covers the ends of bones becomes rough or wears away, causing painful friction between bones when the person moves. The remaining tissues around the joints swell, which leads to stiffness. This stiffness makes normal movement difficult. Even an activity like unscrewing the lid of a jar or walking up stairs can be difficult and cause pain.

Imagine what it might be like being in constant pain or not being able to move without pain. When you provide care for a person with arthritis, focus on relieving pain, assisting with mobility and promoting independence.

- Let the person know that you understand that movement is painful and that you are there to help. Ask the person about ways to make movement easier and less painful.
- If the person takes pain medication, plan her morning care so that it is scheduled to occur after she takes her morning dose of pain medication. When the person has less pain, she may be able to participate more in her own care.
- Because warm water and heat soothe joints and help reduce stiffness and pain, assist the person with tub baths, warm soaks or heat therapy, according to the person's care plan.
- To reduce stiffness and pain, encourage the person to wear warm clothing that covers the affected joints.
- Encourage the person to exercise the affected joints, or assist her with range-of-motion exercises according to the care plan. Activity promotes independence and keeps the joints more flexible. However, never move a joint that is painful, red or swollen.
- Encourage the person to use assistive devices as needed. For example, toothbrushes, hair brushes and combs with built-up handles may be easier for a person with arthritis in the hands to hold, allowing more independence.

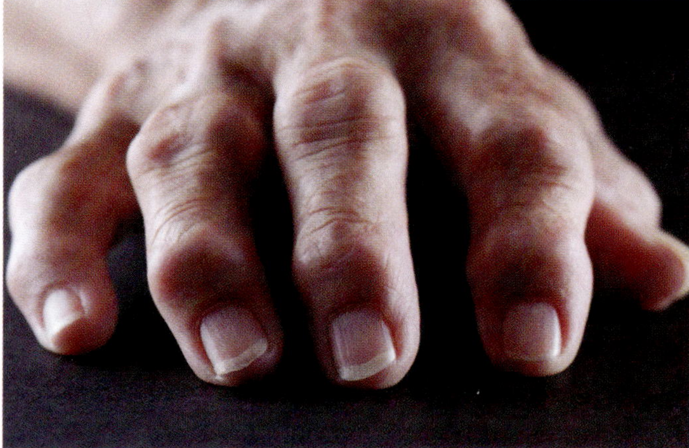

Figure 18-1 Arthritis affects the joints and makes movement difficult and painful. © *iStockphoto.com/Richard Rudisill*

Osteoporosis

Osteoporosis (a disease in which loss of bone tissue causes the bones to become very fragile and prone to breaking) occurs mainly in older women but may also occur in men. The disease is caused by a gradual loss of minerals, especially calcium, in the bones. Calcium helps make bones hard and strong. When calcium is lacking, bones become soft and weak, and they break more easily. Fractures in the spine can cause the person to develop a stooped posture and a rounded upper back (Figure 18-2). This posture is very painful for the person. As the disease progresses, the person may have severe pain in the parts of the body that support her weight. The person often tires easily and may be fearful of falling while walking. If a person with osteoporosis breaks a bone, it can take a very long time for the bone to heal.

When you provide care for a person who has osteoporosis, it is important to focus on safety. In addition, do the following things:

- Help the person exercise as much as he can do comfortably. Gentle exercise may help slow down bone loss.

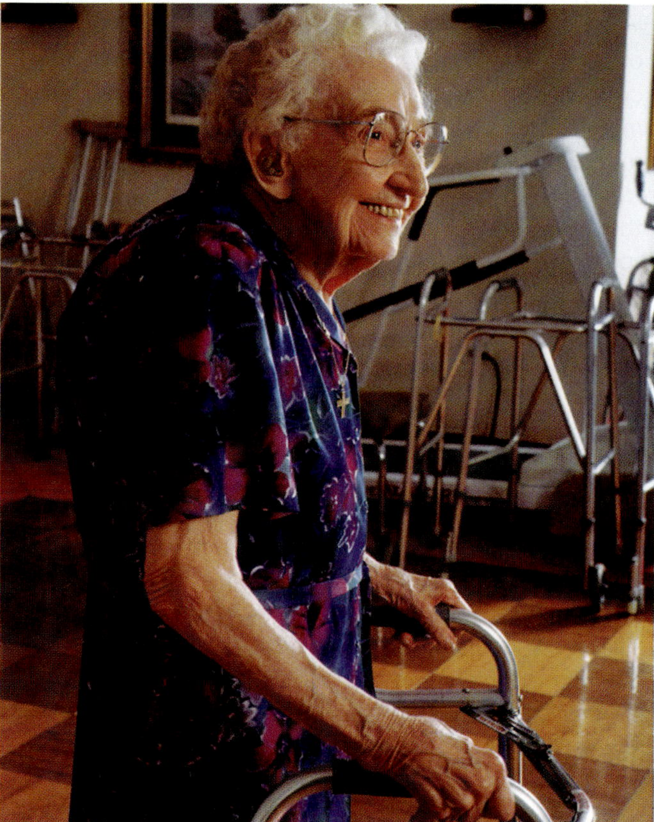

Figure 18-2 A person with osteoporosis may develop a rounded upper back. This happens when the bones of the spine weaken and collapse. © *2012 Custom Medical Stock Photo, Inc.*

- Use a transfer belt when assisting the person to walk or move, according to the person's care plan. Use the belt very carefully. Remember, the person's bones are very fragile.
- Keep areas where the person walks clear and free of tripping hazards, such as throw rugs. Make sure that chairs are the proper height and that grab bars are fastened in appropriate places. These precautions help reduce the risk of injury.
- Follow care measures that may be necessary because of medications the person is taking to treat the osteoporosis. For example, the person may have to remain upright and may not be allowed to have food or fluids for a period of time after the medication is administered. These measures, if applicable, will be detailed on the person's care plan.
- Be aware that the person's visual range may be limited due to postural changes, which cause her to lean forward and down and make it difficult for her to look up. Place objects the person needs where she can see them easily, and ensure the person's safety while walking.
- Report any new pain, loss of function or swelling. These could be signs of a broken bone.

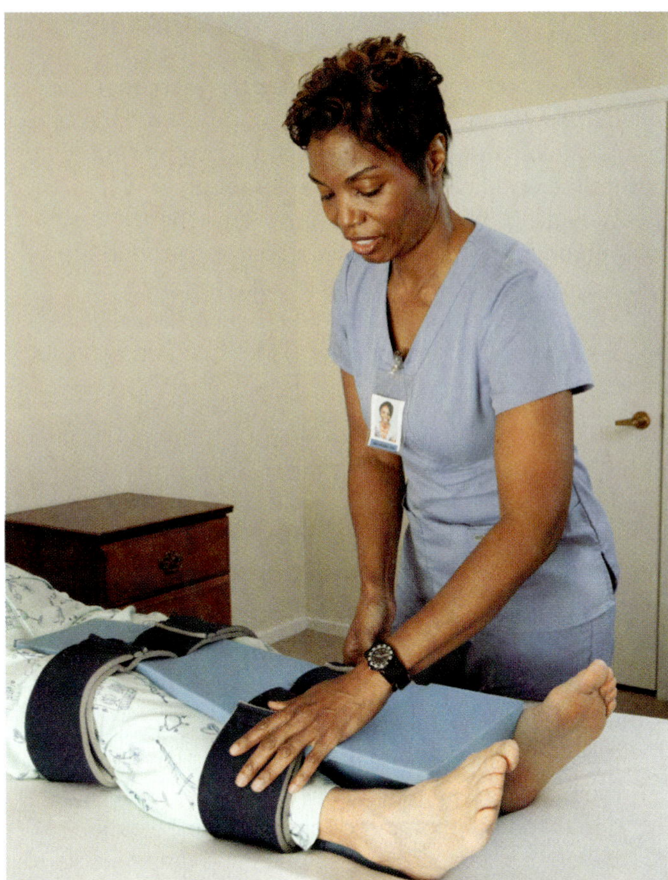

Figure 18-3 A person who is recovering from hip joint replacement surgery may use an abduction pillow to keep the hips properly aligned until the joint heals fully.

Hip Fracture

A hip fracture is a break in the bone of the upper thigh, just below the hip joint. Hip fractures are very common in older people who experience a fall and can have serious consequences. Hip fractures are usually treated with surgery. Sometimes the bone can be repaired, but other times it is necessary to replace the entire hip joint with an artificial joint. Following the surgery, the person will require weeks to months of physical therapy. Sometimes, other conditions that the person has will make surgical repair impossible. In this case, the person will be put on non-weight-bearing status and physical therapy may possibly not be permitted.

While the person recovers from a hip fracture, he will have difficulty changing position on his own. You will need to assist the person with repositioning according to the person's care plan, to lower the person's risk for pressure ulcers. Encourage the person to help as much as he can by using assistive devices such as a trapeze suspended above the bed. Use positioning aids, such an abduction pillow as ordered, to keep the hip joint aligned properly (Figure 18-3). It is also important to make sure that the person maintains good alignment when seated. The person's feet should be flat on the floor, and his hips should be flexed no more than 90 degrees.

The person may also have weight-bearing restrictions. During this period, the person will need assistance with transfers by using a mechanical lift, or assistance with pivoting to the chair using only the unaffected leg. As the person continues to heal, these weight-bearing restrictions may be changed. For example, at first the person may not be allowed to bear any weight on the affected leg, but as healing progresses, the person may be allowed to increase weight bearing to 25%, then 50%, and so on. The physical therapist will teach the person how to use appropriate assistive devices for walking. You should encourage the person to practice the skills she has learned in physical therapy, and you should monitor her technique to make sure that she uses assistive devices properly. Always follow the person's care plan exactly, regarding how much, if any, weight the person is allowed to bear. Bearing too much weight too soon could result in increased pain, swelling and possible re-fracture of the hip, which would delay the person's recovery.

A person recovering from a hip fracture may require a great deal of emotional support. The person may be frustrated by needing so much assistance and by the length of the recovery period. In addition, the person may be very worried about whether she will fully recover from the fracture, and what this could mean for the future. Listen to the person's concerns, practice empathy and provide encouragement by acknowledging the person's progress toward recovery.

CARDIOVASCULAR CONDITIONS

The cardiovascular system transports nutrients and oxygen to all the tissues of the body and then carries away the wastes from these same tissues. Common conditions that affect the cardiovascular system include angina, chronic heart failure and hypertension.

Angina

Angina is chest pain that occurs because the heart is not getting enough oxygen. An angina attack can be caused by activity, exercise or stress. A person who has angina may take nitroglycerin to relieve the chest pain. The nitroglycerin may be in the form of a pill that is placed under the tongue or in the form of a patch that is applied to the skin.

When caring for a person with angina, be aware that the person may try to limit activity out of fear of bringing on an angina attack. Encourage the person to be as independent as possible by allowing him to move at his own pace. If he does feel any chest discomfort with activity, encourage him to rest and breathe deeply to help relieve the pain, and then report the episode of angina to the nurse.

Chronic Heart Failure

In people with **chronic heart failure**, the heart muscle is weak and cannot pump effectively. Heart failure may cause fluids to build up in the body, resulting in swelling of the feet, legs, hands, and face and difficulty breathing. Shortness of breath can cause the person to feel anxious and restless. The shortness of breath and anxiety may be worse when the person lies down. If you notice that a person in your care becomes anxious and short of breath only when lying down, report this to the nurse. This could be an early sign of heart failure.

When you provide care for a person who has chronic heart failure, do the following things:

- Provide frequent rest periods when helping the person with daily care activities. People with chronic heart failure often become tired after only a little exertion. Help the person see that by pacing her activities during the day, she accomplishes more.
- Help the person maintain a position that lets her breathe more comfortably. Many people find a sitting position supported by pillows to be best. Keep the person's legs elevated to reduce swelling of the legs and feet.
- Provide regular mouth care. A person with chronic heart failure may breathe through the mouth or receive oxygen, which makes the mouth dry.
- Provide frequent opportunities for the person to use the toilet. The medications used to manage chronic heart failure can increase both urinary output and frequency of urination. As always, answer requests for help promptly.
- Measure and record the person's intake, output and weight every day, or according to the person's care plan. These measurements are used to determine how well the person is eliminating excess fluid.
- Be aware that a person with chronic heart failure may also have fluid restrictions in place.
- Provide diversion (such as enjoyable activities) to calm the person and reduce strain on the heart.

Hypertension

Hypertension is chronically high blood pressure. Blood pressure that remains elevated over time places a great deal of stress on the heart and blood vessels. Hypertension often does not cause symptoms but can cause serious health problems. Many people who have been diagnosed with hypertension take medications to lower blood pressure. It is important that the person take these medications as ordered. If a person tells you that he has stopped taking blood pressure medication (for example, because he is not having any symptoms, or because the medication causes unwanted side effects), report this to the nurse right away. The nurse can help explain to the person the importance of taking the medication. If the person has stopped taking the medication because of unpleasant side effects, the nurse can work with the person's primary care provider to adjust the person's medication regimen to eliminate or reduce the side effects.

As you talk with Mrs. Trainer, she mentions that she has hypertension for which she takes medication. She says, "But honestly, I'm under so much stress right now, and so focused on Craig, my own health is the least of my worries. Half the time I don't even remember to take my medication."

How would you respond to Mrs. Trainer's comment?

RESPIRATORY CONDITIONS

The respiratory system supplies the body with oxygen and rids the body of carbon dioxide. Disorders of the respiratory system include influenza (flu), pneumonia, chronic obstructive pulmonary disease (COPD) and asthma.

Influenza

Influenza is a highly contagious viral infection that affects the respiratory tract. Symptoms of influenza include a sore throat, stuffy nose, dry cough, headache and body aches, fatigue and fever.

ELDER CARE NOTE. An older adult may not have typical signs and symptoms of the flu. In an older adult, a change in behavior, body temperature that is below normal, decreased blood pressure, rapid pulse, fatigue and decreased appetite may be signs and symptoms of the flu.

Influenza is highly contagious. Flu season is from November until April, with peak activity between late December and early March. In young adults and middle-aged people, influenza is usually a mild disease, but in older adults, people with chronic illnesses and people with compromised immune systems, influenza can be life-threatening. The best protection against influenza is prevention. To lower your risk of getting the flu (and possibly passing it to those in your care), you should receive an annual flu shot in the fall, before the peak flu season. You should also encourage those in your care to do the same. If a person in your care does become ill with the flu, be sure to practice strict infection control measures to help prevent others from getting sick.

ELDER CARE NOTE. Receiving an annual flu shot can reduce an older person's risk of being hospitalized because of influenza by 50 to 60 percent, and the risk of death by 80 percent (U.S. Department of Health and Human Services, Centers for Disease Control and Prevention, www.cdc.gov/flu).

Pneumonia

Pneumonia is inflammation of the lungs. Because of the inflammation, the air sacs in the lungs begin to fill with fluid. Oxygen has trouble reaching the bloodstream. Pneumonia may be caused by infection with bacteria, viruses or fungi and is often a complication of the flu. A person may also develop **aspiration pneumonia**, which occurs when foreign material (such as food, fluid or vomit) is inhaled into the lungs. The foreign material can damage the lung tissue or introduce bacteria that can cause an infection. People who are in a coma or who are receiving nutrition through a feeding tube are especially at risk for developing aspiration pneumonia.

ELDER CARE NOTE. Several factors, including reduced immune function that occurs with age, immobility and a reduced ability to cough forcefully (because of muscle weakness), can put an older person at increased risk for developing pneumonia. Pneumonia can be a very serious, even fatal, illness in older adults.

When you care for a person with pneumonia, be aware that droplet precautions may be in effect. Follow the person's care plan carefully regarding turning and positioning schedules, and encourage the person to drink fluids, rest and cough. You may be required to obtain a sputum specimen for testing. Have the person take one or two breaths, cough deeply and expel sputum directly into the specimen container. Having the person cough deeply helps to ensure that the sample contains thick mucus (sputum) from deep within the lungs, rather than saliva. As when you are collecting any type of specimen, observe standard precautions and make sure the container is labeled and stored properly.

Mr. Trainer is receiving chemotherapy that places him at risk for infection. In addition, he has had a portion of his left lung removed. Together, these put him at risk for developing pneumonia.

What areas would you need to focus on when giving him care?

Chronic Obstructive Pulmonary Disease

Chronic obstructive pulmonary disease (COPD) is a term used to describe lung disorders that make it difficult for air to enter or leave the lungs. There are different forms of COPD. One form occurs when alveoli (tiny air sacs where gas exchange takes place in the lungs) are damaged. The alveoli break and lose their ability to expand with air. As a result, air gets trapped in the lungs. Another form occurs when the airways are constantly inflamed and irritated (for example, by cigarette smoke). The irritation and inflammation cause the airways to produce excessive mucus, which clogs them and makes it difficult for air to pass through.

A person with COPD often has a great deal of trouble breathing, which can be very frightening. Because the person is not getting enough oxygen, she tires easily. She may carry herself with bent posture, with her shoulders elevated and her lips pursed, because these measures make breathing easier. The person's chest may be enlarged and rounded, like a barrel, because over several years, the air trapped in the lungs causes the chest cavity to enlarge. The person may have a poor appetite. As her condition worsens, the person will require supplemental oxygen.

When you provide care for a person who has COPD:

- Encourage the person to relax and breathe slowly but as deeply as possible. Relaxation and slow, deep breathing increase the flow of oxygen to the lungs and help maintain flexibility in the chest wall. The person may have special exercises to do to improve her ability to relax and breathe slowly. If so, encourage the person to do these exercises as prescribed.

- Provide good mouth care. Breathing through the mouth and supplemental oxygen therapy can make mouth tissues dry and uncomfortable.
- Follow the guidelines in Box 18-1 for caring for a person who is receiving oxygen therapy.
- Obtain **pulse oximetry** readings as requested or specified in the person's care plan. (Pulse oximetry readings are often taken along with the person's vital sign measurements.) A pulse oximeter is a device that is clipped to the fingertip to measure the oxygen level of the blood (Figure 18-4).
- Provide a portable commode when the person needs it. Sometimes using the commode is easier than getting to the bathroom when the person needs to conserve energy or has shortness of breath. A commode is also more comfortable than a bedpan.
- Offer small, frequent meals to reduce fatigue associated with eating and help ensure that the person receives adequate nutrition.
- Encourage the person to cough to help clear air passages of excess mucus. To promote infection control and maintain the person's dignity, keep tissues and trash containers within the person's reach.
- Raise the head of the bed for comfort.

Asthma

Asthma is an illness in which certain substances or conditions, called triggers, cause inflammation and constriction of the airways, making breathing difficult. Common triggers include exercise, temperature extremes, allergies, irritants (such as dust, smoke or pollution), perfume or cologne, and stress or anxiety. People who have asthma usually know what can trigger an attack and take measures to avoid these triggers. Many people who have been diagnosed with asthma also take medication on a regular basis to prevent asthma attacks. However, when an asthma attack does occur, it can be very frightening for the person. Signs of an asthma attack include wheezing; rapid, shallow breathing (or difficulty breathing); sweating; and an inability to talk.

A person who has been diagnosed with asthma may take two forms of medication. Long-term control medications are taken every day, whether the person has symptoms or not. These medications help prevent asthma attacks. A person who is experiencing an acute asthma attack may also need to take a quick-relief (or rescue) medication to open the airways right away. Both long-term control medications and quick-relief medications may be given through an inhaler or orally.

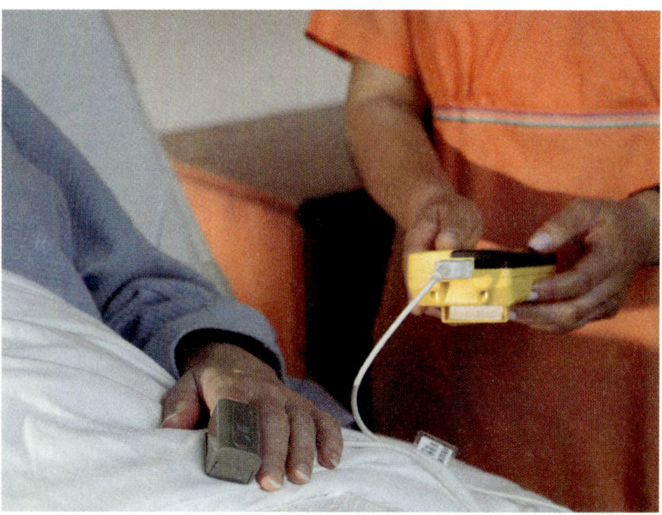

Figure 18-4 A pulse oximeter is placed on the person's fingertip to measure the oxygen level in the person's blood.

Box 18-1 Nurse Assistant DO's and DON'Ts

Caring for a Person Who Is Receiving Oxygen Therapy

DO check regularly to see that tubes are in place and not kinked.

DO provide good skin care around the nose, cheeks and ears if the person is receiving oxygen through a nasal cannula (a device with two prongs that is inserted into the nostrils). The cannula and tubing can put pressure on the skin in these areas and cause skin breakdown.

DON'T adjust the flow rate. Oxygen is considered a medication, and the amount of oxygen that the person is supposed to receive (the flow rate) is specified by the person's primary care provider.

DO tell the nurse if the flow rate on the flowmeter does not match the ordered flow rate.

DON'T remove the person's cannula to provide care, unless you are instructed to by the nurse.

DO take precautions to prevent fire and make sure that others do the same. Oxygen therapy raises the amount of oxygen in the surrounding air, which increases the risk for a fire.

DO ensure that Oxygen in Use signs are prominently displayed according to your employer's policy.

NEUROLOGICAL CONDITIONS

Chronic conditions of the nervous system include Parkinson's disease, multiple sclerosis (MS), stroke and spinal cord injury.

Parkinson's Disease

Parkinson's disease is one of the most common nervous system disorders affecting older adults. In **Parkinson's disease**, a brain chemical called dopamine is not produced in adequate amounts. Dopamine is needed for proper functioning of the nerves that control movement. As a result, communication between the brain and the nerves that control muscle movement is disrupted. A person with Parkinson's disease has muscle tremors (shaking or repetitive motions of the muscles), especially in the hands. The tremors are worse when the person is resting and decrease when the person attempts movement. As the disorder gets worse over time, muscles become weak and stiff. The person may shuffle and lean forward during walking, and it can be difficult for the person to stop suddenly once he is walking. These factors put the person at risk for falling. As the muscles of the face are affected, the person may have trouble chewing and swallowing, and he may drool. Speech may also be affected; the person may speak in a low tone without much variation. The person may lose the ability to smile, frown or show other facial expressions.

When you provide care for a person who has Parkinson's disease, focus your care on promoting safety, independence, good nutrition and mobility. Care strategies for a person with Parkinson's disease include the following:

- Avoid rushing the person. Muscle tremors increase when the person becomes anxious.
- Encourage the person to use assistive devices as needed. Be patient and allow the person to take the time that she needs.
- Encourage the person to exercise within his capabilities and according to his care plan. Activity can help prevent worsening of stiffness and balance problems. Frequent rest periods can help the person avoid becoming too tired or frustrated.
- When the person is walking, remind her to take big steps. A person with Parkinson's disease has to make a conscious effort to do what comes naturally to people who can control their movements.
- Use a high toilet or elevated toilet seat set on top of a regular toilet seat. This can make it easier for the person to sit down on, and get up from, the toilet.
- Many people with Parkinson's disease work with a speech therapist to learn safe techniques for eating and swallowing. Remind the person to use these techniques and check to make sure that he uses them properly.
- Offer small, frequent meals and snacks. People with Parkinson's disease usually lose weight because they become tired before they finish a meal. They may also be embarrassed by spilling food or by how slowly they eat, and they may lose interest in eating.
- Be aware that Parkinson's disease can affect the muscles used for speech, which makes it difficult for the person to express herself. Be patient and give the person time to respond to a question or request. When appropriate, asking questions that can be answered with a simple "yes" or "no" may make it easier for the person to express herself.
- Provide emotional support.

Multiple Sclerosis

Multiple sclerosis (MS) is a chronic disease that gradually destroys the protective coating on the nerves in the brain and spinal cord. This condition creates a situation similar to a short circuit or crossed wire. Nerves cannot communicate with each other or with the brain. A person with MS may have difficulty walking; loss of balance; muscle tremors and muscle weakness; feelings of numbness, tingling and burning; vision problems; speech problems (such as slurred speech); bowel and bladder problems; pain; and overwhelming fatigue. Late in the disease, the person may become paralyzed. The person may experience periods of remission, with no symptoms, but then the symptoms return and are much worse. There is no cure for MS.

When you care for a person with MS, encourage the person to do as much for herself as possible to maintain independence. As always, focus on what the person can do rather than what she cannot do. Encourage the person to do active range-of-motion exercises when possible, or help her with range-of-motion exercises according to her care plan, to prevent contractures and maintain joint mobility.

Stroke

A stroke (cerebrovascular accident [CVA]) occurs when blood flow to a part of the brain is interrupted, which results in death of brain cells. A stroke can also be caused by bleeding into brain tissue. A stroke can cause **hemiplegia** (paralysis on one side) or **hemiparesis** (weakness on one side). The person may have a decreased sense of pain, touch and temperature on the affected side. In addition, the person may have difficulty swallowing (Figure 18-5). Other effects of stroke may include aphasia (difficulty speaking, reading or writing), vision impairments, and bowel or bladder incontinence (or both).

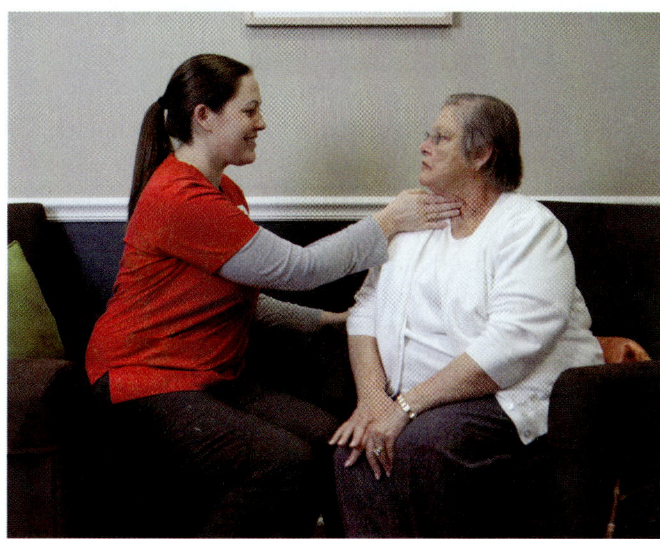

Figure 18-5 A person who has had a stroke may work with a speech-language therapist to learn techniques that will help her to swallow without choking.

Depending on the area of the brain damaged by the stroke, the person may have trouble forming words or understanding the meaning of words. If the person has trouble forming words, allow the person extra time to express her thoughts. The person may rely heavily on nonverbal forms of expression (such as body language or gestures) or pointing to pictures to communicate with others. As appropriate, ask "yes" or "no" questions to make it easier for the person to respond. If the person has trouble understanding the meaning of words, speak slowly and clearly in a normal tone of voice. Choose simple words rather than complex ones, and speak in simple, direct sentences (for example, "Mr. Lewis, please sit here" instead of "Mr. Lewis, could you please sit down?"). Use hand gestures (such as patting the seat of the chair), pictures or written messages to help the person understand your meaning.

When you provide care for a person who has had a stroke, encourage her to do as much as possible for herself. If the dominant side of her body is affected, she may have to relearn how to do activities using her other side. Encourage the person to use assistive devices for eating, mouth care and other activities to maintain her independence. In addition:

- Encourage the person to do active-assistive range-of-motion exercises or assist the person with passive range-of-motion exercises, according to the person's care plan.
- Be aware that the person's sense of touch may be affected. He may be unable to recognize pain and temperature and will be unaware of how his affected body parts are positioned. Take measures to keep the person safe.
- Follow measures on the person's care plan designed to prevent pressure ulcers, such as following a repositioning schedule and using positioning aids to support weak or paralyzed limbs and ensure good body alignment.
- Supervise the person while she eats. If the person cannot eat independently, always put food on the side of the mouth that is not affected by paralysis. Make sure that no food is left in the person's mouth after the meal is finished to lower the person's risk of choking. Make sure that the person sits up to eat so that she can swallow food more easily. As when assisting a person with Parkinson's disease to eat, be aware of the techniques the person has learned from the speech therapist, and help the person practice these techniques while eating.
- Because the person may drool on the paralyzed side and her skin may become irritated, keep her face clean and dry. If ordered, apply a protective skin cream.
- Supervise the person while he shaves. The person may miss spots that he cannot feel, or he may cut himself and not feel it.
- Help the person walk, according to the physical therapist's directions. The person may need a walker or cane to steady herself.
- Put articles that the person needs, such as the person's method for calling for help, eyeglasses, hearing aid, telephone and a glass of water, within reach on his unaffected side.

Spinal Cord Injury

Messages to and from the brain travel through the spinal cord. Spinal cord injuries often occur suddenly, as a result of trauma (for example, a motor vehicle crash or diving accident). Spinal cord injuries can cause **paralysis** (the loss of movement and sensation) below the level of the injury. **Paraplegia** is paralysis that affects both legs and the lower trunk and can result from injury to the lower spinal cord (for example, at waist level or below). **Quadriplegia** is paralysis that affects both arms, the trunk and both legs. An injury in the neck or upper spinal cord can result in quadriplegia. Depending on the location of the damage to the spinal cord, as well as the severity of the injury, the person may experience:

- Loss of sensation in the affected body parts.
- Loss of movement in the affected body parts.
- Loss of bladder control, bowel control or both.
- Loss of the ability to breathe without mechanical assistance.

Loss of sensation puts the person at risk for injuring the affected body parts, and loss of movement can affect the person's ability to manage some tasks. When you provide care for someone with a spinal cord injury, focus on promoting safety and independence. Follow the person's care plan concerning care measures such as schedules for repositioning and toileting. Remember the principles that you learned about providing restorative care. Physical rehabilitation from a spinal cord injury can be long and difficult, so providing emotional support and encouragement is important.

DIABETES

Diabetes, sometimes called diabetes mellitus, is a disorder characterized by the body's inability to process glucose (sugar) in the bloodstream. Normally, an organ called the pancreas secretes **insulin**, a hormone that causes glucose to be moved from the bloodstream into the cells, where it is used for energy. In a person with diabetes, either the pancreas fails to make insulin or the body's cells are unable to respond to insulin. Either situation causes glucose levels in the bloodstream to increase. As a result of the high levels of glucose in the bloodstream, the person may develop symptoms such as excessive thirst, increased urination, chronic fatigue, blurred vision, and slow healing of wounds or infections.

ELDER CARE NOTE. In an older person, falling and dehydration could be early signs of undiagnosed diabetes and high blood glucose levels.

If the glucose levels are not controlled, the person can develop severe complications, including heart disease, blindness, kidney failure and nerve damage. The person is also at higher risk for increased blood pressure and stroke. Circulatory problems and nerve damage associated with high blood glucose levels may delay healing of injuries to the lower legs and feet, which can necessitate amputation (surgical removal) of a toe, the foot or the lower leg.

A person with diabetes may manage the condition with insulin injections or oral medications. Diet and exercise play an important role as well. To keep blood glucose levels within an acceptable range, food intake, exercise and medication must be balanced. A person with diabetes must follow a well-balanced diet, with limited sweets and fats. The timing of meals, relative to exercise and medication, is important as well.

If food intake, exercise and medication are not in balance, the person may develop **hypoglycemia** (excessively low blood glucose levels) or **hyperglycemia** (excessively high blood glucose levels).

- Hypoglycemia can result if a person misses a meal or snack, eats too little food, exercises more than usual, vomits or takes too much medication. A person who is experiencing hypoglycemia may experience symptoms such as dizziness; shakiness; sudden changes in behavior (for example, combativeness, argumentativeness, aggression or anger); cool, clammy skin; and headache.
- Hyperglycemia can result from eating too much food, taking too little medication, exercising less than usual, or from physical or emotional stress. The signs and symptoms of hyperglycemia are similar to those of undiagnosed diabetes (for example, excessive thirst and urination). The person's pulse may be rapid and weak, the person may have a headache, and the person's breath may have a fruity or sweet odor.

Severe hypoglycemia or hyperglycemia can result in seizures and loss of consciousness and is life-threatening.

A person with diabetes needs to monitor her blood glucose levels regularly. The person may use a glucometer, which tests a drop of blood drawn from the person's finger, or the person may test the urine for glucose using a chemically treated strip of paper. If you are expected to perform blood or urine glucose monitoring for a person in your care, the nurse will show you how. When assisting with blood glucose monitoring, take standard precautions and dispose of the lancet (the small device used to prick the skin) in a sharps container.

General care measures for a person with diabetes include the following:

- Serve meals and snacks on time, and report to the nurse if the person does not finish the meal or snack (Figure 18-6).
- Provide good foot care. Examine the person's feet each day for small cuts or breaks in the skin (Figure 18-7). In people who have diabetes, cuts do not heal well because of decreased circulation, and even the smallest cut can become badly infected. The sensation of touch may also be impaired, and a person with diabetes may not

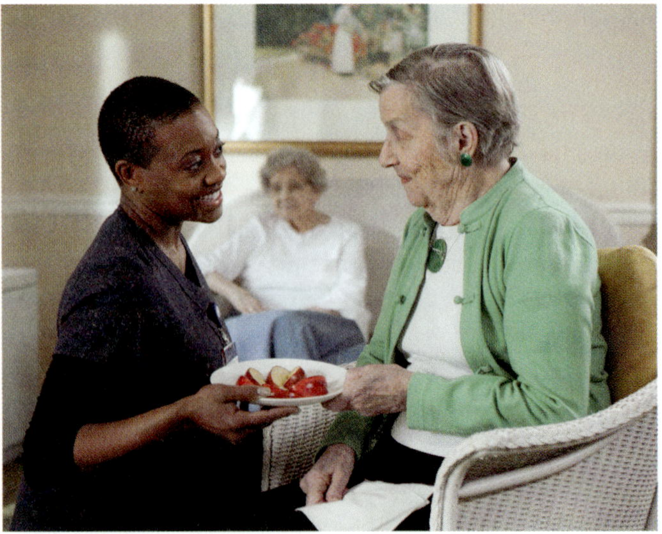

Figure 18-6 The timing of meals and snacks is important for a person with diabetes.

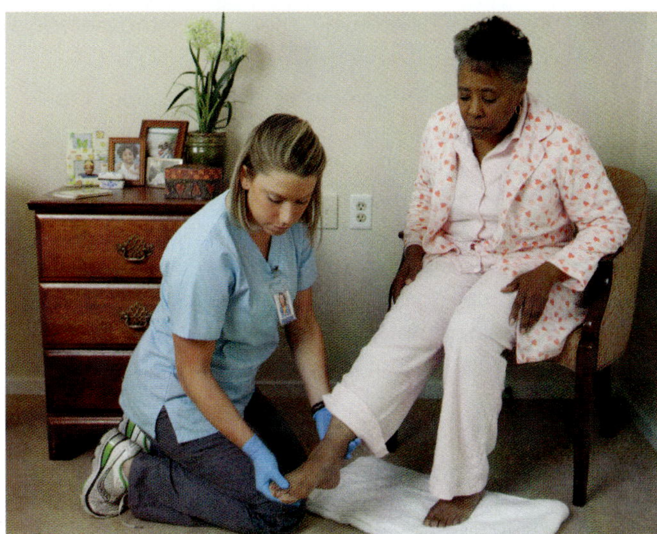

Figure 18-7 A person with diabetes often has poor circulation and may not realize that her shoes do not fit properly until a sore develops. To detect early signs of trouble, regularly inspect the tops and bottoms of her feet for red or sore areas.

feel an injury. Inform the nurse when the person's toenails need to be cut.

- Assist the person with exercise as needed. Exercise improves circulation and helps the person maintain a healthy body weight, both of which are key for people with diabetes.

Observations Into Action!

When you care for a person with diabetes, be sure to report the following to the nurse right away:

- **Any change in the usual amount of exercise, activity or stress in the person's life**
- **The person does not eat all or part of a meal or snack**
- **The person vomits**
- **The person has signs of hypoglycemia (for example, dizziness, shakiness, behavioral changes, clammy skin, headache)**
- **The person has signs of hyperglycemia (for example, excessive thirst and urination, sweet-smelling breath, rapid pulse)**
- **The person's blood glucose monitoring test results are high or low**
- **The person has a cut or wound on the foot, or the person's toenails need trimming**

KIDNEY FAILURE

Kidney (renal) failure is the inability of the kidneys to filter waste products from the blood. Kidney failure can be the result of an acute disease (such as poisoning or a severe infection) or a complication of a chronic condition, such as diabetes. Acute kidney failure may be reversible, but chronic kidney failure is not.

When waste products accumulate in the body, they produce symptoms such as:

- Fatigue, weakness and confusion.
- Puffiness around the eyes and swelling in the hands and feet.
- Muscle twitching or cramping.
- Nausea, vomiting and an unpleasant taste in the mouth, which often lead to decreased food intake.
- Itching skin that is often severe.
- High blood pressure.

A person with kidney failure often needs **dialysis**, a treatment that replaces the function of the kidneys by removing waste products and excess fluid from the body. There are different types of dialysis. *Peritoneal dialysis* involves injecting a solution through the abdominal wall and then withdrawing it after a period of time. *Hemodialysis* uses a machine to clean the blood of waste products. Dialysis treatments take several hours and may be done a few times a week.

When you provide care for a person with kidney failure, focus on the following things:

- Carefully monitor and report the person's food and fluid intake.
- Plan care to conserve the person's energy and to provide periods of rest. Be aware that after dialysis, it is common for the person to feel very tired, and the person may need more assistance than on nondialysis days.
- Take increased care to prevent infections. If the person is on dialysis, pay special attention to keeping the access site (for either peritoneal dialysis or hemodialysis) clean and dry.
- Provide good skin care.
- Obtain vital sign and weight measurements according to the person's care plan. If the person receives hemodialysis, avoid measuring blood pressure in the arm where the access site for the hemodialysis is located.

CANCER

Cancer is the abnormal growth of new cells that crowd out or destroy other body tissues. A **tumor** (a solid mass of tissue) can be noncancerous (**benign**) or cancerous (**malignant**). Benign tumors usually grow slowly and do not spread to other areas of the body. Malignant tumors can spread, or **metastasize**, to other parts of the body.

Cancer can affect almost any organ in the body. The outcome of the disease depends on the type of cancer, how early the cancer was detected and many other factors. Although signs and symptoms differ according to the type of cancer, the American Cancer Society has identified seven general signs and symptoms that may be early signs of cancer:

- A change in bowel or bladder habits
- A sore that does not heal
- Unusual bleeding or discharge
- Unusual lumps
- Indigestion or difficulty swallowing
- A change in a mole or wart
- A persistent cough or hoarseness

Any of these signs warrants further medical investigation.

Cancer is treated in different ways, depending on the kind of cancer, the location and whether the cancer has spread. Some cancers are treated with surgery. **Chemotherapy** (the use of drugs to stop or slow the growth of cancer cells), **radiation** (the use of high-energy X-rays to destroy cancer cells) or both may be used instead of or in addition to surgery. A person undergoing chemotherapy or radiation therapy may experience unpleasant side effects. The drugs used for chemotherapy are powerful and affect all of the systems in a person's body. As a result, the person may experience nausea, diarrhea, loss of appetite, hair loss and extremely dry skin. Radiation therapy can also have unpleasant side effects, including skin burns, fatigue and possibly nausea, vomiting and hair loss.

When you provide care for a person who is being treated for cancer:

- Provide emotional support. If the cancer is newly diagnosed, the person may be very worried about the effects of treatment, whether the treatment will be successful and what the future holds. Although many cancers are treatable and many people with cancer recover fully, some people in your care with cancer may be coming to terms with the fact that their cancer is terminal. The emotional support that you provide during these times will be a great help and comfort to the person.
- Remember that infection control is extremely important. Chemotherapy and radiation affect a person's immune system and put the person at higher risk for infections. If you have a contagious illness such as a cold or the flu, ask to be temporarily reassigned to limit your exposure to the person until you recover fully.
- Provide good mouth care to promote comfort and prevent infection. Treatments such as radiation and chemotherapy can make the mouth dry and may cause painful sores in the mouth. Use special rinses or sprays according to the person's care plan.
- The drugs used for chemotherapy can affect the person's sense of smell and taste so that nothing seems appetizing. A person being treated with chemotherapy or radiation may also experience nausea, vomiting, diarrhea and painful mouth sores that can make eating difficult. Still, it is important for the person to receive adequate nutrition. Offer small snacks of nutritious, appealing foods (such as milkshakes or fruit smoothies) frequently. If the person requests a special food, try to accommodate the request.
- Chemotherapy can cause people to become very sensitive to certain smells. Even scents that would normally be considered pleasant can become offensive, so take steps to eliminate odors that the person finds offensive.
- The drugs used for chemotherapy are excreted in the person's urine, feces and vomit for 48 to 72 hours after treatment. To protect yourself from exposure to these drugs when contact with body fluids is likely, put on two pairs of gloves.
- Help the person with grooming routines to promote self-esteem. Some people who experience hair loss as a result of treatment may wish to wear a scarf, wig or hat until the hair grows back.
- Exercise is beneficial for the person and should be encouraged when the person feels up to it. Be aware that the person may experience extreme fatigue after chemotherapy or radiation treatment, however. Plan care to allow for periods of rest, and encourage the person to take naps as needed.
- Pain is common, as a result of either the cancer or the treatment. Frequently ask the person about pain and report any complaints of pain or discomfort to the nurse.
- Provide good skin care.

What precautions will you take while providing care for Mr. Trainer, who is undergoing chemotherapy treatments? What special care needs will you anticipate that Mr. Trainer might have?

HIV/AIDS

Acquired immunodeficiency syndrome (AIDS) is a condition that results from human immunodeficiency virus (HIV) infection. HIV infection is passed from one person to another primarily through unprotected sexual contact and blood-to-blood contact through needles and syringes. In addition, infected pregnant women can pass HIV to their babies during pregnancy or delivery, as well as through breast-feeding.

When a person is exposed to HIV, the virus enters the body, multiplies in the blood and other organs and damages the immune system. The person can be infected with HIV for many years without showing any signs or symptoms of AIDS. As a person's HIV infection worsens and the immune system weakens, the person may begin to experience signs and symptoms, including:

- Yeast infections (candidiasis) in the mouth (called thrush) or in other areas of the body, such as the vagina.
- Repeated episodes of diarrhea.
- Dry cough or shortness of breath.
- Swelling in the glands that does not go away.
- Fatigue.
- Fevers that occur again and again.
- Night sweats.
- Weight loss.
- Memory loss or confusion.
- Pain and difficulty when moving.

By the time a person with HIV develops AIDS, his immune system is very damaged and the person is no longer able to fight off other infections. This makes the person vulnerable to opportunistic infections (infections that healthy people can resist or control), such as pneumocystis pneumonia (PCP). The person may also develop cancers rarely found among people with healthy body defenses, such as Kaposi's sarcoma (which causes red or purplish spots on the skin) and invasive cervical cancer.

You may be afraid to care for a person with HIV/AIDS. Knowing the facts about how HIV/AIDS is transmitted can help to relieve some of those fears (Table 18-1). Practice standard precautions when you provide care for someone who has HIV/AIDS, just as you practice standard precautions when you provide care for anyone. You do not have to do anything differently when caring for a person with HIV/AIDS. You can safely touch, help and hug the person, as well as laugh and talk with her.

Table 18-1 **Myths About HIV/AIDS**

Myth	Fact
You can get HIV through casual contact (shaking hands, hugging, using a toilet, drinking from the same glass).	HIV is not transmitted through casual contact. The virus does not live long outside of the body.
You can get HIV by breathing the air after an infected person coughs or sneezes, or by sharing food with the person.	HIV is not an airborne or food-borne virus.
Only homosexuals are at risk for HIV infection.	Any person, regardless of sexual orientation, can get HIV as a result of unprotected sexual activity.
Men cannot get HIV from women.	Any person, regardless of gender, can get HIV as a result of unprotected sexual activity.
You can get HIV through receiving donated blood or organs.	Stringent policies for HIV screening and testing of blood transfusion products and donated organs have been in place in the United States since 1985, making the U.S. supply of donated blood and organs among the safest in the world.
You can get HIV through donating blood.	Donating blood does not put a person at risk for becoming infected with HIV. Sterile procedures and disposable equipment are used when collecting blood. Each needle is used only once.
There are medications that can cure HIV/AIDS.	There are medications that can delay the progression of the disease, but currently, there is no cure for HIV/AIDS.

Adapted from the Centers for Disease Control and Prevention: *HIV Transmission.* http://www.cdc.gov/hiv/resources/qa/transmission.htm

Care measures for the person with HIV/AIDS include taking steps to relieve uncomfortable symptoms and protecting the person from opportunistic infections. A person who has AIDS is particularly susceptible to infection caused by contact with people who have contagious illnesses, foods that have not been handled safely and pets. Prevent the person from being exposed to people who are ill with contagious illnesses, such as a cold or the flu. Practice good infection control measures, including the safe handling of food. Finally, be aware that the person should not perform pet care activities that involve possible contact with animal stool (for example, cleaning litter boxes or bird cages, or changing the water in fish tanks).

The person may also require a great deal of emotional support and compassion. People who used to be close to the person may stop coming to visit when they learn of the person's diagnosis (for example, because they do not understand how the virus is transmitted and are afraid of getting the disease themselves, or because they do not approve of behaviors that may have led to the person getting the infection). Because HIV/AIDS is a terminal condition, the person may have many worries about what the future holds. As with each person in your care, be a good listener and practice the five principles of caregiving.

MENTAL HEALTH CONDITIONS

Mental health conditions affect a person's emotions and thoughts. There are many different types of mental health disorders. Two common types of mental health disorders are depression and anxiety disorders.

Depression

Depression is a persistent feeling of sadness. A person who is experiencing depression loses interest in activities that used to give him pleasure. He may say that he feels sad, empty, helpless or hopeless, and he may complain of feeling very tired all the time. He may have crying spells. A person who is depressed may eat or sleep too much or too little. The person may be irritable or angry. Sometimes depression will cause physical complaints, such as headaches, stomaches or backaches. An extremely depressed person may talk about or try to commit **suicide** (the act of deliberately taking one's own life).

Depression can be triggered by an event (such as the death of a spouse or having to give up one's home to move to a nursing home) but often is not related to a single event. Signs of depression may be similar to those of a physical illness, and often the person is treated for the physical illness while the depression goes untreated.

ELDER CARE NOTE. Depression is a common problem in older adults. Older adults experience many life changes that can trigger a bout of depression, such as the deaths of friends and family members and the loss of independence as a result of a decline in physical abilities. As a result, people often assume that depression is just part of getting old and that the depression must be accepted. However, this is not true! If you think that an older person in your care is showing signs of depression, report your concerns to the nurse so that the person can be assessed and treatment, if needed, can be initiated.

When you provide care for a person with depression, focus on maintaining her safety and increasing her self-esteem. To accomplish this:

- Encourage independence to promote feelings of self-worth.
- Give the person appropriate positive feedback and reinforce her accomplishments.
- Work with the person to set simple, attainable goals. Be sure to praise her when she meets the goals.
- Listen when the person expresses sadness, and allow the person to cry (Figure 18-8).
- Because the person's energy level is low, schedule rest periods throughout the day.
- Monitor the person's food intake to make sure that nutrition is adequate.
- Provide fluids frequently, because the person may not drink enough fluids on her own.
- Report all complaints of pain so that her symptoms do not get overlooked.

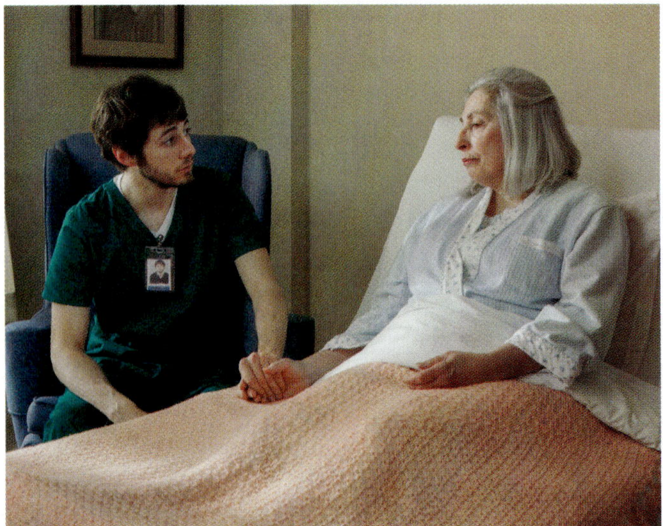

Figure 18-8 Listening is an important skill when caring for a person who is depressed.

- Encourage the person to use a prescribed hearing aid or eyeglasses so that she is more in touch with the world around her.
- Encourage the person to participate in activities, especially those that involve contact with other people and those that are physical (as much as she can). Avoid overly stressful or tiring activities.
- Take all comments about suicidal thoughts seriously and report them to the nurse right away.

! Observations Into Action!

A person with untreated depression may try to commit suicide or talk about committing suicide or wanting to die. Take all such actions and comments seriously and report them to the nurse right away. Do not conclude that a suicide threat or attempt is just a way to get attention. Also report any of the following observations to the nurse:

- **The person shows a dramatic change in mood or behavior, such as increased withdrawal or a very excited, elevated mood.**
- **The person hoards medication or purchases a gun or other weapon.**
- **The person gives away belongings.**
- **The person increases her use of alcohol.**
- **The person becomes preoccupied with inner thoughts.**
- **The person becomes secretive.**

ELDER CARE NOTE. Older men, especially those who are without a partner (because of death or divorce), have a higher rate of suicide than any other group.

Anxiety Disorders

Anxiety is a feeling of unease, dread or worry. At times, we all experience periods of anxiety, but usually this anxiety is only temporary. A person with an anxiety disorder experiences anxiety that continues to build and will not go away, until the person can no longer function. Examples of specific types of anxiety disorders include:

- **Panic disorder.** The person experiences episodes of intense anxiety and fear, commonly called panic attacks. The emotional symptoms are often accompanied by physical symptoms such as chest or abdominal pain, dizziness, shortness of breath or racing heartbeat.
- **Obsessive-compulsive disorder.** A person with obsessive-compulsive disorder has recurrent unwanted thoughts (called obsessions). To calm the obsessions, the person feels that he must engage in certain rituals (called compulsions). Performing these rituals helps reduce the person's anxiety. However, performing these rituals may interfere with the person's ability to function and live a normal life.
- **Post-traumatic stress disorder.** Post-traumatic stress disorder is a type of anxiety disorder that is brought on by experiencing a life-threatening event. For example, veterans returning from war, people who survive natural disasters or terrorist attacks, and people who have been victims of rape or abuse are at risk for developing post-traumatic stress disorder. The person may not be able to stop thinking about the event and may have flashbacks and recurrent nightmares.

When caring for a person with an anxiety disorder, learn what causes the person's anxiety to increase, and try to avoid those situations. For example, making basic decisions can be difficult for a person with an anxiety disorder. Offering two or three choices, instead of multiple choices, can help limit the person's anxiety. When caring for a person with an anxiety disorder, continuity of care is important. Communicate to the nurse what strategies work well for minimizing the person's anxiety, so that these strategies can be included in the person's care plan for all members of the health care team to use when caring for the person.

CHECK YOUR UNDERSTANDING

Questions for Review

1. **A person with arthritis should be encouraged to:**
   a. Avoid the pain by not moving.
   b. Take cold showers to reduce swelling of joints.
   c. Exercise strenuously to keep joints flexible.
   d. Do active or passive range-of-motion exercises regularly.
2. **A person with chronic heart failure generally is most comfortable when:**
   a. Lying flat.
   b. Sitting up.
   c. Lying on the left side.
   d. Lying on the right side.
3. **A person with diabetes:**
   a. Needs to eat extra sugar and protein to maintain her strength.
   b. May have reduced sensation in his feet.
   c. Needs to eliminate exercise completely.
   d. Needs to have the nurse assistant cut his toenails daily so that they do not become too long.

4. **A person with chronic obstructive pulmonary disease (COPD) should be encouraged to:**
   a. Eat one large meal per day instead of several smaller meals.
   b. Lie flat after eating.
   c. Breathe deeply often during the day.
   d. Smoke to relieve tension.

5. **When you provide care for someone who has had a stroke, you must:**
   a. Place the person's method of calling for help within reach on the person's unaffected side.
   b. Position the person so that he lies flat when he eats, because he may be paralyzed and may drool.
   c. Place food in the person's mouth on the affected side.
   d. Keep the paralyzed arm or leg lower than the rest of the body to keep blood flowing into it.

6. **A person can get human immunodeficiency virus (HIV) by:**
   a. Sharing eating utensils with an infected person.
   b. Getting bitten by an infected dog.
   c. Sharing needles with an infected drug user.
   d. Coming into contact with someone's sweat during a basketball game.

7. **Which of the following statements about depression is true?**
   a. Depression is a normal consequence of aging.
   b. There is no treatment for depression.
   c. A person who is severely depressed may try to commit suicide.
   d. A person who is depressed just wants extra attention.

8. **All of the following statements about chemotherapy are true EXCEPT:**
   a. Chemotherapy makes the person less susceptible to infection.
   b. Chemotherapy can affect the person's senses of taste and smell.
   c. Chemotherapy can cause the person to feel very tired.
   d. Chemotherapy can be combined with radiation therapy.

9. **Mrs. Knight is recovering from a broken hip. Which of the following most accurately describes Mrs. Knight's care needs?**
   a. Mrs. Knight may have weight-bearing restrictions and will need help with repositioning.
   b. Mrs. Knight will need warm tub baths to promote healing of the bone.
   c. When Mrs. Knight is sitting down, her hips should be flexed more than 90 degrees.
   d. All of the above

Questions to Ask Yourself

1. *Today, while you are providing care for Mrs. Roth, who has diabetes, her hands start shaking. You ask her whether she is okay. "I'm fine!" she snaps, "Leave me alone!" What do you think might be happening? What should you do?*
2. *Mrs. Reilly, who has chronic obstructive pulmonary disease (COPD), is very short of breath. She has difficulty with any amount of exertion and needs to rest frequently. Today Mrs. Reilly's daughter is bringing her 6-month-old son to visit at 10:30 a.m. Mrs. Reilly wants to look especially nice, but she also does not want to be too tired to enjoy the visit. How would you help her plan her morning care so that she can accomplish both goals?*
3. *Mrs. Lindquist is one of your home health clients. Mrs. Lindquist has diabetes but is not very conscientious about managing her condition. She has a real sweet tooth and always has a box of chocolates on the sideboard. You can tell from the number of wrappers lying around that Mrs. Lindquist is treating herself to a piece of chocolate frequently. You also know that she is not very strict about monitoring her blood glucose levels. One of the reasons Mrs. Lindquist is receiving home care is because she recently had to have her foot amputated due to complications from her diabetes. What measures could you take to help Mrs. Lindquist better understand the need for keeping her blood glucose levels under control?*

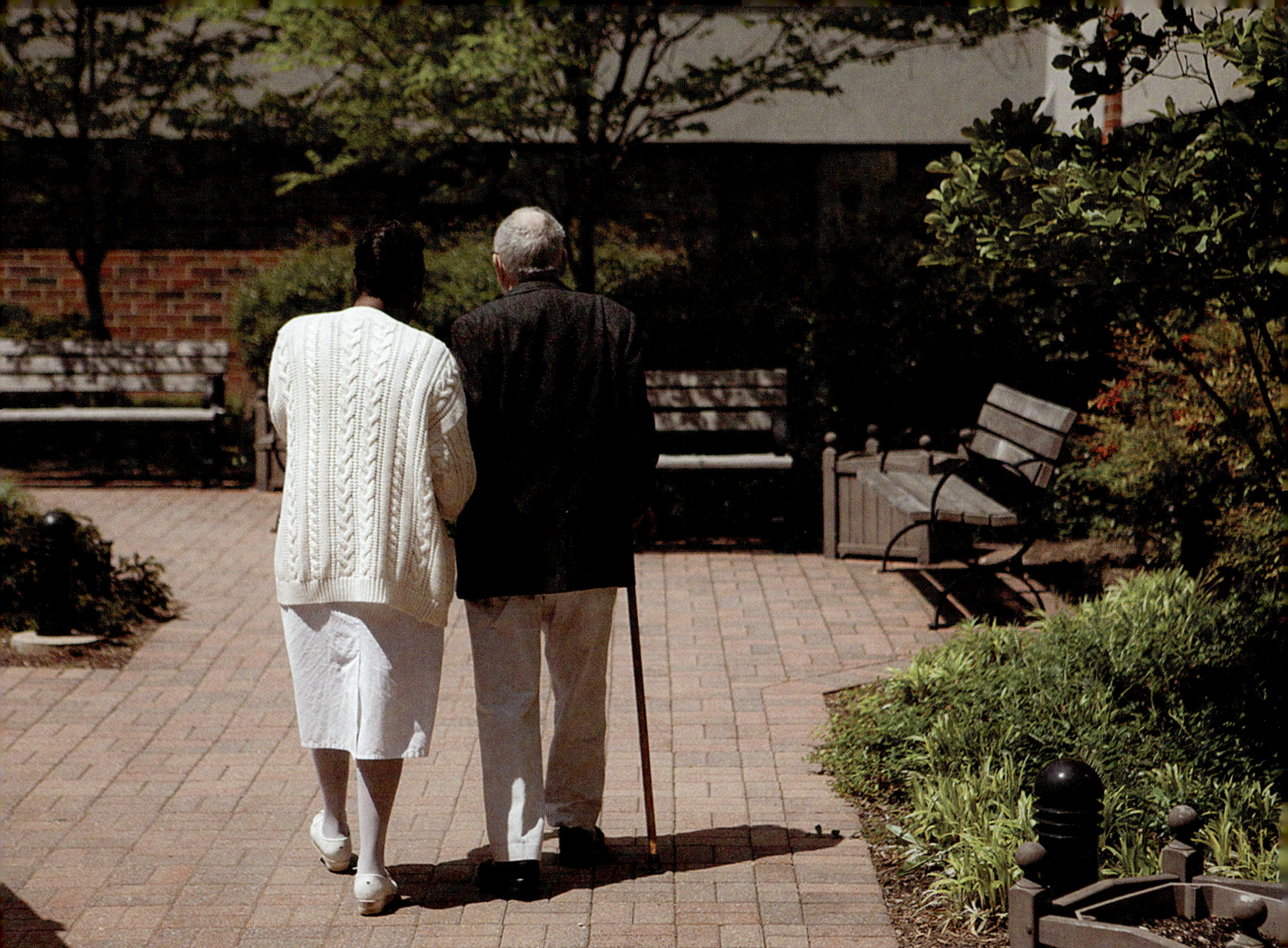

Providing Care for People with Cognitive Changes and Dementia

CHAPTER 19

Goals

After reading this chapter, you will have the information needed to:

- Describe different types of cognitive changes, including age-related memory impairment, mild cognitive impairment, dementia and delirium.
- Describe the course of illness for people with dementia and list common symptoms that occur in each stage.
- Identify common mental health symptoms often experienced by those with dementia.
- Describe appropriate care measures to meet the needs of people with dementia over the course of the illness.
- Identify the issues specific to caring for those with dementia, including the display of challenging behaviors.

Continued on next page

Continued from previous page

Goals

- Discuss effective communication techniques to use when caring for people with dementia.
- Discuss the needs of those who provide care for those with dementia, including family members and nurse assistants.

Key Terms:

cognition
age-related memory impairment
mild cognitive impairment
dementia
delirium
amnesia
short-term memory
long-term memory
validation therapy
aphasia
expressive aphasia
receptive aphasia
agnosia
apraxia
hallucinations
delusions
paranoia
catastrophic reaction

Today you meet Mrs. Elizabeth Davis for the first time, as she is on her way home after spending the day with her husband, Will, who was just admitted to Morningside Nursing Home because of dementia. Tearfully, Mrs. Davis shares with you that her husband is nothing like he used to be. "He was such a charming, fun-loving, thoughtful husband and family man," she says. "He worked hard to make a good life for us. We were so looking forward to his retirement, so that we could travel and spend time with our grandchildren." But, she continues, "We didn't get much of a chance. A few months after Will retired, I started noticing increasing problems. He became very forgetful and increasingly confused. I started finding odd things like mail in the freezer and gardening tools in the pantry! And, I found that he was making lots of mistakes handling our money. This was really concerning to me, because Will was an accountant for 40 years." You give Mrs. Davis a tissue and she dabs at her eyes. She says, "I feel so guilty for placing him here, but I am so tired and I just don't know what else to do. As things got worse, Will was picked up by the police twice because he got so lost while driving. I took his car keys away, but twice I found him wandering through the neighborhood on foot. It got to the point where I felt I had to watch him every minute to make sure he didn't get himself in trouble." You hand Mrs. Davis another tissue and tell her that she can be sure her husband will be well cared for at Morningside.

TYPES OF COGNITIVE CHANGES

Cognition is the term used to describe thinking processes, which include memory, reasoning, judgment and language.

Normal Age-Related Changes

As we age, changes occur that affect how the body functions. These changes affect all organs and processes in the body, including the brain and thinking processes. Many older people complain about the forgetfulness that occurs with aging. Forgetfulness happens because of the gradual loss of brain cells and a decrease in the chemicals that help the brain to work. As a result, it becomes harder to remember or recall things. For example, a person may remember a piece of news but cannot recall when or how she heard it. Or perhaps the person remembers who told her the news but cannot immediately recall that person's name—even if it is a close friend! Frequently that forgotten information just pops into mind a few hours later. Other examples of normal forgetfulness are misplacing commonly used items, such as keys or eyeglasses, or having a word on the tip of the tongue and being unable to say it. Although it may take a little longer for older people to learn something new (such as the features of a new cell phone), they are capable of learning. Such experiences may be annoying, but they do not interfere with the ability to carry out normal activities of life. These types of changes are known as **age-related memory impairments**.

Mild Cognitive Impairment

Cognitive impairment refers to changes in thinking processes (such as memory, reasoning, judgment and language) that are caused by disease or injury. People with **mild cognitive impairment** demonstrate problems with memory and thinking that are noticeable to others but are not severe enough to interfere with daily life. Problems are worse than those associated with age-related memory impairment, but are not severe enough to indicate dementia. Some people with mild cognitive impairment remain stable without experiencing further decline; however all people with this condition are at increased risk for developing dementia.

Dementia

Dementia is a term that is used to describe the group of symptoms that occur with a progressive decline in memory and thinking. Dementia is not a specific disease. Rather, there are many different types of dementia. The most common types are summarized in Table 19-1. Although variations exist among the types of dementia, they are similar enough that the only way to tell what type of dementia a person has is by examining the person's brain after the person dies, during an autopsy. Often, autopsy shows that a person had more than one type of dementia. A person's specific symptoms depend

Table 19-1 Types of Dementia

Type of Dementia	Cause	Characteristics	General Information
Alzheimer's disease	Plaques (abnormal sticky clumps of amyloid, a protein) and tangles (twisted protein fibers within nerve cells) build up in the brain. Together, they cause cell death and ultimately destroy the brain tissue.	■ Progressive memory loss; difficulties thinking, problem solving and performing familiar tasks ■ Problems recognizing people and objects ■ Loss of language skills ■ Personality changes	■ Accounts for more than 50% of all dementias ■ Lasts on average 8 to 12 years ■ Usually occurs after age 60, with risk increasing with advanced age; however, a rare form (early-onset Alzheimer's disease) can occur between the ages of 30 and 60 years
Lewy body dementia	Abnormal protein deposits, called *Lewy bodies*, occur in the brain, and throughout the gray matter covering of the brain.	■ Has features of both Parkinson's disease and Alzheimer's disease: problems with motor movement, memory, language and thought processes ■ Possible alternating periods of confusion and periods of alertness and orientation ■ Vivid visual hallucinations common; also possible delusions (fixed, false beliefs), or acting out of dreams	■ Second-most-common cause of dementia ■ Affects men slightly more than women ■ Generally occurs between the ages of 50 and 85 years, but can occur earlier
Vascular dementia	Blood supply to the brain is impaired because of damaged blood vessels, which deprive the brain tissue of nutrients and oxygen. Can occur suddenly with a total blockage of a blood vessel (as in a stroke), or over time because of gradual closing off of a vessel.	■ Type and severity of symptoms depend on the area of the brain that has been damaged ■ Problems with memory, confusion, thinking processes and problem solving ■ Unsteady gait ■ Restlessness ■ Urge to urinate or difficulty passing urine ■ Depression	■ About as common as Lewy body dementia ■ Rarely occurs before age 65; increasing likelihood with advanced age ■ Has the same risk factors as heart attack and stroke (history of heart problems, strokes, mini-strokes, high cholesterol, high blood pressure, diabetes, smoking)

Continued on next page

Table 19-1 **Types of Dementia** *Continued*

Type of Dementia	Cause	Characteristics	General Information
Frontotemporal dementia	Damage to the front part of the brain occurs.	■ Language difficulties: trouble naming things and misuse of words ■ Impulsive, inappropriate behavior and lack of concern for others ■ Increased irritability, decreased judgment ■ Possible apathy (loss of interest and motivation) ■ Memory generally spared until later in the disease	■ Accounts for 10 to 20 percent of all dementias ■ Lasts from 2 to 20 years, with people living 8 years, on average, after symptoms start ■ Generally affects people in their 50s and 60s

on what areas of the brain are damaged and how much damage there is (Figure 19-1).

Most forms of dementia affect older people. The diseases that cause dementia last for years and ultimately lead to death. As brain cells become damaged, the person gradually loses the ability to remember, to think and to use language. Physical abilities are lost, and the person becomes totally dependent on others for care. Despite widespread research, there is still no cure for dementia. Some medications have helped slow the progression of symptoms, but they do not work for everyone, they are not useful in all forms of dementia and they do not prevent decline from occurring. Dementia ultimately robs the person of all memories, personality and abilities—the things that make up the very essence of an individual.

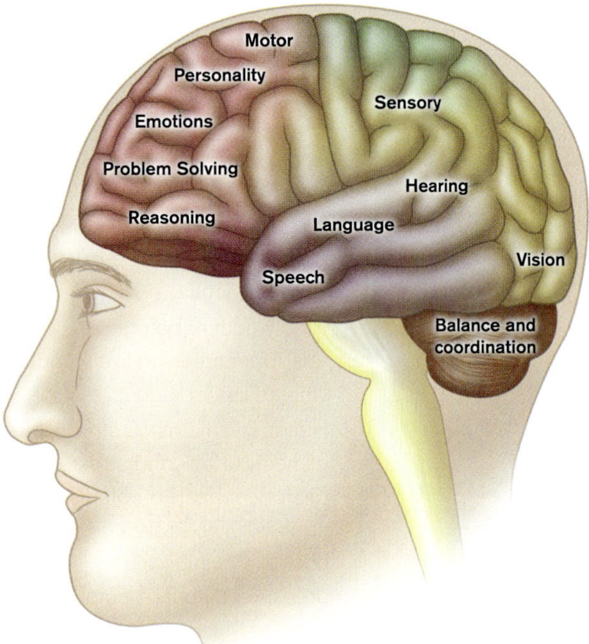

Figure 19-1 Not everyone with dementia may show exactly the same symptoms. The symptoms depend on what area of the brain is damaged and how much damage there is. The function that is controlled by the damaged area of the brain will be the function that is impaired.

Most people with dementia whom you will care for will have Alzheimer's disease, the most common type of dementia. Table 19-2 provides an overview of the changes that occur over the years as Alzheimer's disease runs its course.

- **Early stage.** In the early stages of Alzheimer's disease, changes occur very gradually and may not be immediately noticeable to others. When they do become noticeable, many people misinterpret them as normal changes of aging. Often those in the early stages of Alzheimer's disease are able to cover up their symptoms by using their social skills. For example, in answer to the question "How many grandchildren do you have?" a person in the early stages of Alzheimer's disease might reply, "Oh, so many, so many! We are blessed! We love them all!" The person did not really answer the question, but her answer is socially acceptable because she acknowledges that she has grandchildren and that she loves them very much. However, social interactions become more challenging for the person over time, as the person experiences an increasing loss of ability to follow the thread of a conversation and a decreased ability to recognize or remember people.
- **Middle stage.** As the person's symptoms worsen, it becomes apparent that something is very wrong. The person's perceptions and understanding of the world change significantly at this time. The person's personality may change. For example, a person who was always sweet-natured may become more argumentative. The person requires a great deal of attention to ensure his safety. Often, caring for the person at home becomes too much for family members, and it becomes necessary to consider admission to a long-term care facility or other options for care.

Table 19-2 **Characteristics of the Stages of Alzheimer's Disease**

Early	Middle	Late
■ Memory problems (amnesia) ■ Some difficulties finding and using the right words (aphasia) ■ Misplacing things in odd places ■ Difficulties with usual routines such as shopping or handling money ■ Getting lost in familiar places ■ Changes in mood or personality ■ Loss of initiative or motivation	■ Increasing loss of memory (amnesia) ■ Increasing difficulties with language (aphasia) ■ Problems with recognition (agnosia) ■ Difficulties performing tasks (apraxia) ■ Incontinence	■ Loss of language ■ Swallowing difficulties and weight loss ■ Dependent for all care; confined to bed or chair ■ At increased risk for serious infection ■ Death

- **Late stage.** In the final stages of the disease, the person shows significant decline. The person becomes physically dependent on others for all aspects of care. In addition, the person is at high risk for complications related to pressure ulcers, contractures and infections. Problems with nutrition and fluid balance commonly develop as the person forgets how to swallow. Although tube feeding may be an option, it is not necessarily beneficial and often increases the risk of complications related to aspiration (inhalation of food or fluid into the airway during breathing) and pneumonia. Language skills are also lost, and the person becomes mute. The person's physical condition progressively declines and eventually the person dies, often as a result of an infection. Care during the final stage of dementia is directed toward promoting comfort at the end of life and supporting a peaceful death (Box 19-1; see also Chapter 20).

Delirium

Delirium is a change in cognition that has a rapid onset and is related to chemical changes in the body. These changes can occur within a few days or even hours. Delirium is usually reversible, although the person may experience changes in cognition that are permanent even after the delirium is treated. Quick identification and treatment of the underlying cause of the delirium is necessary to reduce the person's risk for experiencing long-term effects.

Common causes of delirium include medications and their side effects, lack of fluids (dehydration), lack of sleep, pain and infections. Signs and symptoms of delirium include:

- Seeing, feeling or hearing something that is not there (hallucinations)
- Not being able to recognize a familiar person
- Being extremely restless, especially at night
- Failing to remember things that happened quite recently
- Wandering, even though person knows her way around
- Not being able to concentrate or follow instructions
- Becoming lethargic and displaying little movement or activity

Box 19-1 **Care Measures for the Final Stage of Dementia**

- Routine pain medication for comfort
- Laxatives as needed to prevent constipation
- Oxygen support to ease breathing
- Good skin care to prevent pressure ulcers
- Food and fluids mechanically altered for ease and safety of intake (pureed food, thickened liquids)
- Discontinuation of weight measurements (weight loss is expected)
- Respect of advance directives

ELDER CARE NOTE. Delirium in older people is sometimes mistaken for dementia because some people assume that all confusion in older people is caused by dementia. Similarly, the presence of delirium in someone who has dementia is sometimes missed because the person with dementia already has a change in mental processes. It is important to recognize and report sudden changes in mental status (regardless of the person's baseline level of confusion) because delirium is often a red flag for a pending medical emergency—especially among older people.

DEMENTIA

The 4 A's of Dementia

Four words beginning with the letter *A* are often used to describe common symptoms in dementia. These words are:

- Amnesia, from the Greek words meaning *without memory.*
- Aphasia, from the Greek words meaning *without speech.*
- Agnosia, from the Greek words meaning *without knowing.*
- Apraxia, from the Greek words meaning *without doing.*

Understanding these symptoms and how they change the person's interpretation of the world will give you a foundation for meeting the challenges that arise when you provide care.

Amnesia

Amnesia is the term used to describe memory loss. In most forms of dementia, memory loss occurs early in the disease and is often the first symptom noticed. Usually, **short-term memory** (memory of recent events) is affected. For example, a person in the early stage of dementia commonly remembers details of events that occurred in childhood (**long-term memory**, or memory of the past) but cannot recall what happened earlier in the day. Damage to the hippocampus, a small structure in the brain that stores and retrieves memory, is responsible for the short-term memory loss associated with dementia. The hippocampus acts very much like the *save* button on your computer. When you save a computer file, you give it a name and press *save*. The computer then stores your file so that you can use it again another time. Sometimes, however, something goes wrong, and when you try to open your file you get a *file not found* message. Now imagine your hippocampus as the save button for your brain. If that button becomes damaged, new events cannot be properly saved by the brain. So, the next time you need to recall your memory of an event, it is not there. However, all of your previous memories are still there, having been stored when your hippocampus was working. As the disease progresses and more and more of the brain becomes damaged, even the earlier memories will disappear.

Can you imagine how strange the world would seem if you could not recall the events in your life? How would you feel if you could not remember where you were and how you got there? The loss of memory causes a great deal of confusion as the person with dementia tries to make sense out of the present circumstances. Table 19-3 highlights some of the more common behaviors that result from the memory loss associated with dementia, as well as strategies for managing them.

When you care for a person with memory loss as a result of dementia, focus on what the person feels to be true rather than what is really true. Trying to argue or reason with the person to accept the truth will most likely cause the person a great deal of distress. It is important to remember that the brain is diseased, which makes the person incapable of understanding facts. Accepting and responding to what the person feels to be true is consistent with a technique called **validation therapy**. Validation therapy shows respect for the person's thoughts and feelings and validates (acknowledges) what the person feels, regardless of the actual truth. When you use validation therapy techniques, you do not tell the person that what she believes is incorrect, but you do acknowledge whatever emotions correspond to that belief. For example, Mrs. Wesley tells you that her husband is coming for a visit. You know that Mrs. Wesley's husband died more than 20 years ago. In this situation, you would not acknowledge Mr. Wesley's visit as a fact, but you would acknowledge that Mrs. Wesley is feeling excited and happy about the prospect of a visit from her husband. To validate, or acknowledge, Mrs. Wesley's feelings, you could ask her questions about her husband (but not about the visit that will not occur). Talking about her husband may provide some distraction for Mrs. Wesley and will let her recall pleasant memories from the past and connect with the good feelings that she had about her husband. By using validation therapy techniques, the caregiver helps preserve the person's dignity and sense of self.

Aphasia

Aphasia refers to problems with communication resulting from damage to the brain from injury or disease. The problem is one of communication. The person's intelligence is not affected. For example, in the early stage of dementia, the person first shows problems with communication by having difficulties finding words. Language difficulties increase throughout the middle stage of illness with expressive aphasia, receptive aphasia or both. **Expressive aphasia** refers to the inability to use language to express oneself, verbally or in writing (or both). **Receptive aphasia** refers to the inability to understand communication (spoken and written) from others. To imagine what this is like, picture yourself in a foreign country where you do not speak or understand the language. What if you got lost and had to ask for directions back to your hotel, but you did not know the right words to use? How would you feel if someone became impatient with you because you could not express what you needed or understand what the person was trying to explain to you? Would you feel anxious or frightened?

Expressive aphasia is easy to detect from the person's verbal expression. You may notice the person struggles to find the right word, uses the wrong words or sometimes jumbles words together that do not make sense. The

Table 19-3 **Helping Someone with Amnesia (Memory Loss)**

Behavior	What to Do	What Not to Do
Asks the same questions over and over	■ Be patient. The person is not trying to be difficult or get on your nerves. ■ Write down the requested information where the person can easily find it or see it. ■ Provide reassurance.	■ Do not scold the person or keep reminding her that you already answered that question multiple times. ■ Do not ignore, or refuse to answer, the person.
Rummages, or searches for lost items and accuses others of stealing (sometimes items were truly misplaced, and other times the person may never have had that item or has not had that item in a very long time)	■ Show concern for what is missing, without regard to whether the person really had the item in the first place. If the person believed that he had something and is upset about it, then react to his belief. Offer to help the person look for the missing item or to report the loss. ■ Label all personal belongings so that they can be returned when the misplaced item is found. ■ Label the fronts of closets or dresser drawers with the contents to help the person locate frequently searched-for items. ■ Have the family provide a substitute for a precious item with something similar of lesser value to avoid significant emotional or financial loss if the item truly becomes lost.	■ Do not argue with the person about what he did or did not have. ■ Do not disregard the person's concern about the lost item.
Cannot remember the names of familiar people or how she knows them	■ Use words that help the person correctly identify other people, or explain who they are. For example, "Your sister Gladys and her husband Tom are here to visit."	■ Do not assume that the person will remember people when she sees them. ■ Do not use statements that will increase confusion, such as, "Oh, look who came see you! Do you know who that is?"
Constantly tries to find a way back home or searches for deceased loved ones, not remembering that they died	■ Create reasonable explanations for the inability to go home at that time, or for why the deceased person is not there. ■ Use distraction to divert the person's attention from her searches. For example: "They are calling for bad weather so you can stay here tonight and we will see that you get home tomorrow." Or "Your husband called and said that he had an emergency at work and will be late. He wants you to eat without him and he will see you later."	■ Do not tell the person the truth, because the truth may only bring about sadness, anger or distrust. Because the person does not remember ever moving from her home or losing a loved one, the truth would be new and very confusing information that the person will be unable to understand or accept.

person, however, may not seem to recognize that anything is wrong. At some point, the person may not be able to use words at all and will use only sounds for verbalization. However, the rhythm of those sounds may mimic normal speech. Again, the person may not realize that anything is wrong with her speech. When a person has expressive aphasia, watch for the person's nonverbal cues to understand what she is trying to say. For instance, if she is pulling at her clothes and looking worried, she may need to use the toilet. If she strikes out at you whenever you try to put on or take off her blouse, perhaps she is trying to tell you that it hurts when you are moving her arms and shoulders. A person often becomes angry or frustrated with caregivers because caregivers may not understand what she is trying to communicate.

Receptive aphasia is more difficult to detect because you cannot know how the person is interpreting what you say. You may notice that the person cannot follow directions that you give him and that he gets more and more upset the more you talk. In this instance, try using fewer words and more gestures to show the person what you need him to do (Figure 19-2). If he can follow gestures, he likely has receptive aphasia and cannot understand your spoken words. Although the person may not understand your words, he will understand your tone of voice and respond to it. Therefore, approach the person in a calm, nonthreatening manner and use a calm tone of voice to ensure that you do not convey annoyance, impatience or anger. If the person detects those emotions in your voice, you can expect him to react accordingly. As a result, the interaction will be difficult for both of you.

Agnosia

Agnosia is the inability to use the five senses to recognize familiar things or people. For example, a person would be able to hold and feel a key in her hand but would not be able to identify it simply by touch. Likewise, a person may hear a truck drive by and become alarmed by the noise because she does not know what it is. Or a person may see a hair brush but cannot identify it. Agnosia can cause a person to be unable to recognize family members or familiar caregivers, or even her own face when looking in a mirror. Imagine how frightening it would be to always see someone looking back at you and not know who that person is!

Since the person with dementia is not able to recognize familiar things, safety in the environment becomes a huge concern. Leaving cleaning chemicals or medications where they are easily accessible to people with dementia could have disastrous results. These items could be sprayed into the eyes, swallowed or otherwise used in a harmful way. Although it is important to treat adults with dementia with dignity and respect, it is also important to recognize that they share many similarities with young children such as toddlers. Toddlers have not learned enough about the world to recognize what is unsafe. Adults with dementia have forgotten, or lack insight, about safety. All safety measures that you would use when caring for a small child should also be used when caring for someone with dementia.

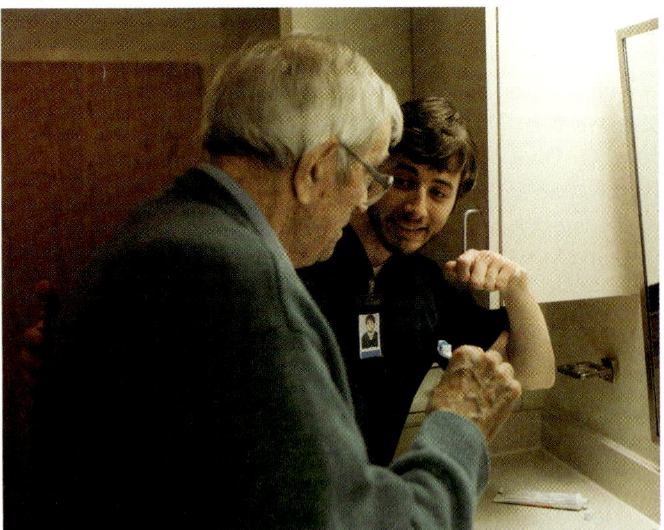

Figure 19-2 Sometimes showing a person what to do is more effective than telling the person what to do.

Apraxia

Apraxia is the inability to perform the steps necessary to complete a task despite having the ability and desire to perform the task. Apraxia causes simple and familiar tasks, such as getting dressed, brushing teeth or eating with utensils, to become overwhelmingly complex. Although it may be easier to take over and perform the task for the person, doing so robs the person of pride and self-esteem and affects the person's dignity and independence. It is important to carefully observe what the person can do, and step in to help only when it becomes clear that the person has done as much as he can on his own.

It helps to break tasks down into a series of steps and give the person simple directions to complete each step. Wait until one step is completed before giving instructions for the next step. Giving instructions one step at a time is necessary because memory loss prevents the person from remembering multiple directions.

Think about ways that tasks can be simplified. For example, dressing is difficult because the person has to figure out the order for putting on each article of clothing. Laying out articles of clothing in the order in which each article is to be put on will help the person dress appropriately (Figure 19-3). Sometimes the person will have trouble dressing and undressing because she cannot remember how to use buttons, snaps, buckles or other fasteners. If this is the case, see if the family can provide clothing that is easier to manage, such as pants with elastic waistbands or shoes with Velcro fasteners. Several companies make adaptive clothing. For example, a man's shirt may look like a regular button-down shirt, but it is fastened with a strip of Velcro behind the buttons. Adaptive clothing can help the person maintain independence with dressing and toileting for a longer time.

Eating also presents challenges. Apraxia makes it difficult for the person to figure out the steps used to get food from the plate to the mouth, and agnosia makes it difficult for the person to recognize utensils or even which items on the table are food and which are not. Offering one food at a time can help minimize this confusion. Hand-over-hand cueing can help the

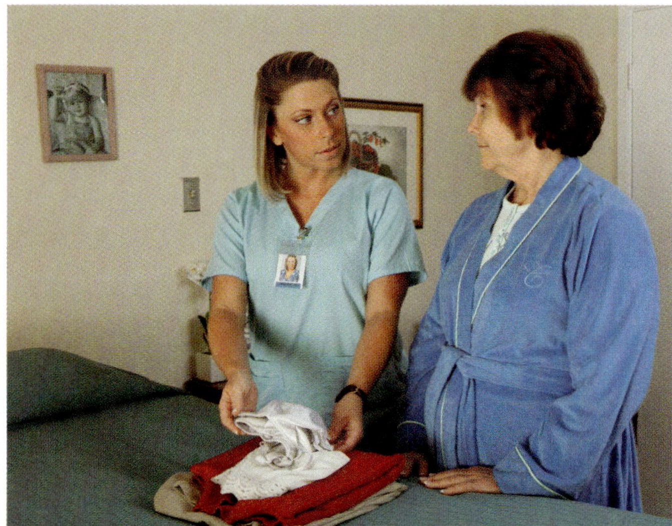

Figure 19-3 Laying out the person's articles of clothing in the order in which each article is to be put on can help a person with dementia dress herself and remain independent longer.

person perform the steps necessary for eating. Place food on the utensil and put the utensil in the person's hand. Put your hand over the person's hand and guide it to the mouth. The person often recognizes the familiar movement and will be able to continue feeding himself, at least for a short time. If trouble using utensils persists, offer finger foods such as sandwiches, chicken nuggets or cheese sticks, or put soup in a cup for the person to sip (Figure 19-4). Hand-over-hand cueing can be effective for involving the person in his own care with other tasks as well, such as brushing the hair or teeth.

Mental Health Symptoms in Dementia

People with dementia can experience problems with mental health as a result of the damage that occurs in the brain or because of the stress of trying to cope with a world that is no longer understood. Just imagine yourself in a world where your only active memories are those of years past. You no longer know the people and places of your more recent life, and you constantly search for people and places that no longer exist except in your long-term memory. You do not recognize where you are or the people you meet. You have difficulty making your wants and needs known. You cannot perform your own care, yet you do not understand caregivers' attempts to help. It is not only frustrating, but frightening, intrusive and very embarrassing.

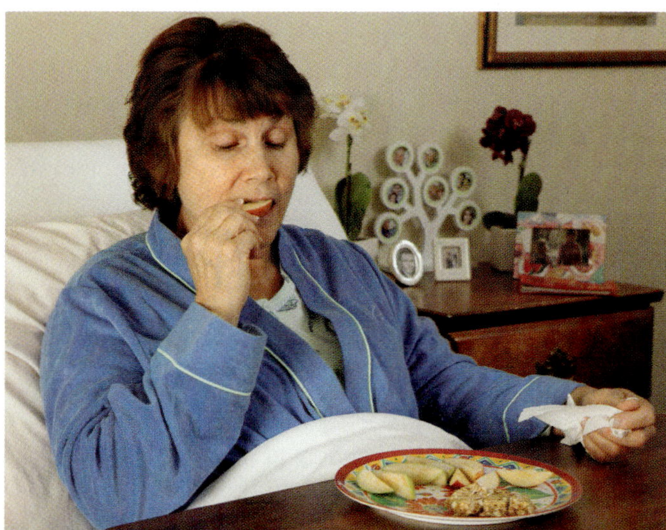

Figure 19-4 Finger foods may be easier for a person with dementia to manage, which promotes independence with eating.

Common mental health symptoms include depression, anxiety, hallucinations, delusions and paranoia:

- **Depression** (characterized by a low or sad mood, loss of interest, and loss of energy and motivation) can easily result as the person struggles to come to terms with the loss of memory and abilities, experiences confusion about surroundings and loses self-esteem. A person who is depressed may be sad or tearful, may lose interest in usual activities, may experience changes in eating and sleeping patterns, and may show increased irritability or anger.
- **Anxiety.** Anxiety is intense, exaggerated and persistent worry about everyday things. A person who is anxious may have difficulty concentrating and find it hard to make decisions. The person may be restless or irritable and may have physical symptoms, such as digestive problems, headaches and fatigue.
- **Hallucinations and delusions. Hallucinations** occur when the person sees, hears, tastes, smells or feels something that does not exist. For example, a person who is having hallucinations may tell you that spiders are crawling over the bed linens. Hallucinations can be caused by the disease in the brain or may result from the presence of delirium. **Delusions** (fixed false beliefs) can also result from changes in the brain or from the person trying to make sense of the confusion around him. For example, a person who is having delusions may view family members, caregivers or other residents as dangerous intruders or may say that people are stealing from her or are going to harm her. If the person cannot understand where she is or what is happening, she may create a story in her mind that helps her make sense of her situation. Despite the fact that there is no reality base for hallucinations and delusions, they are very real to the person experiencing them. Telling the person that what she is experiencing or believes is not real will only cause frustration and additional confusion.

- **Paranoia.** Common delusions often involve the person feeling threatened with some kind of harm or wrongdoing by others, which can lead to **paranoia** (excessive suspicion without cause). A person who is experiencing paranoia may express fear of caregivers who are attempting to provide personal care. The person may refuse to eat because he is afraid that the food has been poisoned. Arguing or trying to reason with the person to convince him that the threat is not real is not productive. Instead, acknowledge any threats that the person *perceives*, and try to be helpful in that situation. For example, if the person believes that another person is out to harm him, provide reassurance that you are watching out for his safety and will provide protection.

Sometimes, the distress caused by mental health symptoms is so severe that it causes the person to act out in aggressive ways. When this occurs, medications may help manage these symptoms and reduce aggression, but because of side effects these medications must be used with caution and only as a last resort. Ideally, the person's symptoms can be successfully managed using creative care approaches that address the underlying cause of the person's mental health symptoms.

CHALLENGING BEHAVIORS

Challenging behaviors are often associated with the middle stage of dementia. These behaviors are called *challenging* because they pose difficulties for caregivers in providing care and in maintaining the safety and well-being of the person and others around her. Sometimes these behaviors are associated with damage to the brain. More often, they are expressions of the fear and frustration that the person feels. Common behaviors in people with dementia include wandering and pacing, hoarding, resisting care, inappropriate sexual behaviors and sundowning (Table 19-4). Sometimes the person has an intense emotional and behavioral outburst over a seemingly small event. This is referred to as a **catastrophic reaction**.

As the person's language skills decline, behaviors become the way the person expresses his wants, needs or feelings. As a nurse assistant, you must carefully observe the person's behavior and the circumstances to figure out what the person is trying to tell you. First, you will try to identify the trigger (what sparks the behavior), and then you will take a systematic approach to figure out what the behavior means. Once you know what causes or triggers the behavior, you can take steps to eliminate or minimize the behavior. All team members involved in the person's care play a role in this fact-finding and problem-solving process.

Identifying Triggers and Minimizing Challenging Behaviors

The first step in identifying behavioral triggers is to gather facts. Focus on the facts you observe rather than jumping to conclusions about what you think may be happening. Note exactly what you saw, what you heard, where it occurred, when it occurred, who else was with the person and what activity was happening at the time of the incident. By collecting and reviewing this information each time the behavior occurs, you may be able to detect a pattern that reveals what sparks the behavior. For example, the person demonstrates behavioral problems only at bath time. This timing would be a clue that something about the bathing process is causing distress. Perhaps the behavior occurs only in the dining room. It could be the noise in the room, confusion about how and what to eat or even mouth pain related to ill-fitting dentures. Regardless of the reason, gathering the facts provides a foundation and focus for problem solving. The questions in Box 19-2 may help you identify the triggers for challenging behaviors.

Pay special attention to pain as a possible trigger for behavior. Most older people experience pain because of physical changes of aging or the presence of medical conditions, such as arthritis. Therefore, if most older people have pain, and most people with dementia are older, it is logical to conclude that most people with dementia will experience pain. However, a person with dementia may not be able to report pain. As a result, the person may express the pain she is feeling through behavior. Keep in mind that assisting with personal care often involves a fair amount of physical movement. For example, the person may have to raise her arms over her head to put on a sweater or comb her hair. Or the person may need to bend at the waist to put on socks or tie shoes. She may have to use her hands to button a shirt or jacket. Any of these activities could increase the person's pain. Because you are the staff member most often involved in assisting with personal care, you may be a common target for behavioral outbursts during these activities. If you observe that the person demonstrates behavior problems during personal care, report this to the nurse so that a proper pain assessment can be completed and an appropriate pain management plan can be developed.

Once a suspected trigger is identified, care approaches should be planned to eliminate or minimize that trigger. By eliminating or minimizing the trigger, challenging behaviors may also be eliminated or minimized. Everyone who cares for the person should know what the trigger is, what approaches to

Table 19-4 **Challenging Behaviors**

Behavior	Common Causes	Suggestions for Management
Wandering Walking around aimlessly, or searching	■ Need for movement or exercise ■ Boredom ■ Searching for someone or someplace	■ Incorporate exercise into the person's day. ■ Provide a safe, contained place for walking; create barriers to unsafe places. ■ Use pictures or other familiar items to help the person identify the door to her room. ■ Take the person to the bathroom; to help the person locate the bathroom independently, place a picture of a toilet on the bathroom door. ■ Listen to what the person says for hints as to what the person is searching for, and respond with validation therapy techniques.
Pacing Walking back and forth	■ Physical need, such as hunger or elimination, not being met ■ Overstimulation from the environment ■ Fear of being lost	■ Assist the person in getting to bathroom; offer something to eat. ■ Walk with the person until the behavior stops. ■ Guide the person to a quiet, less stimulating environment. ■ Gently remind the person where he is and that you are there to help.
Hoarding Stashing food, linens or other items in purses, dresser drawers or closets; trying to take items away causes great distress	■ Fear that items may be wanted or needed later, and the person will not be able to obtain them	■ Do not try to remove the items while the person is present. ■ Arrange for room cleaning when the person is distracted with an activity taking place outside of the room. ■ Provide reassurance that the person's needs will be met.
Resisting care Verbally and physically aggressive behaviors (examples: screaming, yelling, or grabbing, hitting or pushing caregiver)	■ Embarrassment or feeling of exposure because of nakedness ■ An uncomfortable environment (for example, the room is too bright, too noisy, too cluttered or too cold) ■ Distressing caregiver approach (rushing, being too loud, giving confusing directions)	■ Slow down; focus on the person, not on the task. ■ Use good communication techniques and be mindful of your own body language and tone of voice. ■ Identify and address triggers (for example, if the person feels exposed during a shower, drape a bath blanket over the person's shoulders; if the person dislikes the shower spray, try a bath; if the person wants to wear one outfit all time, have the family supply multiples of the same outfit). ■ Ensure the person's physical comfort (for example, make sure that the room is warm enough and that the person has had the chance to use the toilet).
Inappropriate sexual behaviors Removing clothing or masturbating in public; making sexually suggestive comments or advances; pinching, grabbing or touching personal body parts of others	■ Lack of impulse control	■ Approach the person calmly and redirect person away from the behavior; use distraction techniques.
Sundowning Increased confusion, agitation, restlessness and irritability in the late afternoon or early evening	■ Change in the person's routine ■ Overstimulation ■ Fatigue ■ Disrupted sleep ■ Reduced vision because of reduced lighting	■ Keep to the person's routine as much as possible. ■ Keep the person's environment well lit and turn on inside lights as it gets darker outside. ■ Make sure that the person gets enough sleep at night and does not get over-tired during the day.

Box 19-2 **Identifying Triggers for Challenging Behaviors**

Cognitive losses

- Are problems with memory, communication, recognition of people or objects, or difficulties performing tasks involved with the behaviors?

Mental health symptoms

- Does the person show signs of depression or anxiety (anger, irritability, withdrawal, tearfulness, constant worry)?
- Does the person show evidence of hallucinations (seeing, hearing, tasting, smelling or feeling something that is not there) or delusions (false beliefs or suspicions about others) that are upsetting?

Physical conditions

- Is the person hungry or thirsty or does she need to use the toilet?
- Does the person show any verbal or nonverbal signs of pain?
- Are there symptoms of an underlying medical condition (for example, fever, swelling)?

Past personal history

- Does the person try to act out past life roles or usual habits?

Environment

- Is the person too hot or too cold or wearing ill-fitting or otherwise uncomfortable clothes?
- Is the setting too bright, too dark, too noisy or too quiet for the person's comfort?
- Is there too much going on around the person or is the person bored?

Other people

- Does the person react negatively to your tone of voice? Manner of touch? Close physical presence?
- Does the person react negatively in the presence of only one person?

use to eliminate the trigger and how to use the approaches. Be sure to report to the nurse which care measures work and which do not so that the person's care plan can be updated with that important information.

Responding to Aggressive Behaviors

Dementia can cause a person to act in an aggressive or combative manner. The person may assault you physically (for example, hitting, spitting, kicking, slapping or throwing an object at you) or verbally (for example, shouting, threatening you with harm or making offensive statements). This behavior may be the person's way of communicating fear, frustration, pain or an unmet physical need, such as hunger, thirst or the need to use the toilet. If a person becomes aggressive while you are trying to provide care, stop what you are doing and step back from the person to maintain your own safety. Then, refocus on the person and alter your approach to restore calm. Because the person is upset, respond with concern and comfort. Distract the person with another activity or change the topic and tone of the conversation to something pleasant. This distraction helps re-establish a connection with the person and may reduce the aggressive behavior, allowing you to continue to provide care. If your efforts to calm the person are unsuccessful and you still feel threatened after taking a step back, ensure the person's safety and then leave the area.

It is never acceptable for you to respond in kind to aggressive behavior (for example, by hitting a person who hits you). However, you can take steps to keep yourself safe and minimize this type of behavior. If you know that a person is likely to display aggressive behavior with certain care activities, it often helps to use the buddy system and arrange for help from a co-worker when you provide that type of care to the person. It is also important to always report any incident of violence or aggression and complete an incident report according to your employer's policy. This report will allow other members of the health care team to perform assessments and follow up as necessary to help minimize this type of behavior in the future.

COMMUNICATING WITH A PERSON WITH DEMENTIA

Successful care results from making a connection with the person for whom you are providing care. Good communication is the starting point. Keep in mind the effects of dementia on the person's abilities and maintain an awareness of the person's mood and her individual qualities. Sometimes when giving care, the task, rather than the person, becomes the focus of care, and the person's emotions and personal preferences are forgotten or ignored. Try being social first, then clinical. This approach allows the person to feel comfortable with you before you start touching or handling her in a personal way.

Communicating with a person with dementia can be difficult because the person is easily distracted and can easily become overwhelmed. The person has difficulty determining what he should or should not be paying attention to, especially when the setting is a busy one. Minimize distractions by turning off the TV or radio, or take the person to a quieter area. Adjust the lighting so that it is not too bright or too dim. Keep in mind that communication may also be complicated by changes in hearing resulting from aging. Be sure to announce yourself before touching the person to avoid startling the person and triggering a challenging behavior. Face the person directly so that she can see your face (Figure 19-5). Speak slowly and clearly and use simple words. When you phrase requests, use simple, direct, positively worded sentences (for example, "Please put that down here" rather than "Don't put that there!"). Also, use gestures to help to convey your message.

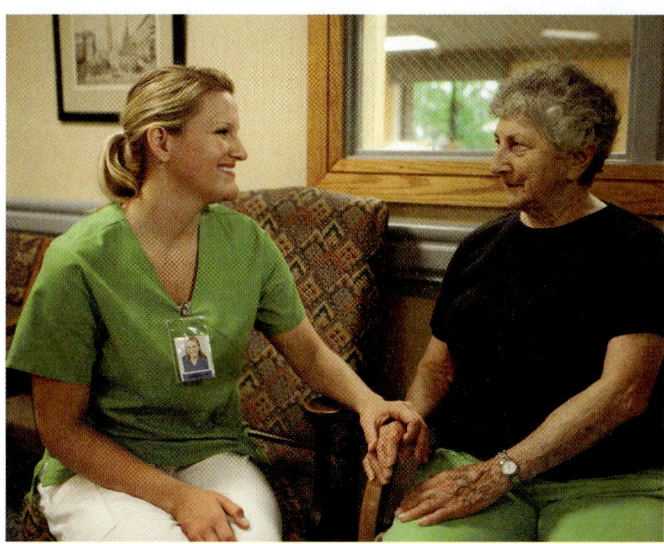

Figure 19-5 Use good eye contact, gentle touch and a calm tone of voice when communicating with a person with dementia.

Table 19-5 summarizes helpful tips to use when communicating with someone with dementia.

Julie is your new co-worker. Today, Julie approaches you for help. She is assigned to Mr. Davis and she reports that she is having a lot of difficulty trying to care for him, and, quite frankly, she is a little scared of him. She states that he does not seem to understand why he is here. He repeatedly talks about his home in Deer Park and his need to return there. Julie constantly finds him wandering the halls trying to find the way out. When she explains that he lives here now, he yells and screams, calling her a liar. He gets angry very quickly and is constantly accusing her, as well as others, of stealing from him. He believes that someone has taken his car keys and all of his money.

Mr. Davis needs help with bathing, dressing and toileting. Julie tells you that she tries as best as she can, but Mr. Davis often strikes out when she is trying to provide this care. He disregards her explanations and yells that he does not need help. Because he is much bigger than she is, Julie feels nervous whenever she approaches him for care. Julie asks you for your advice.

How would you explain some of Mr. Davis's behaviors to Julie? What approach would you advise her to take with regard to finding the cause of the behaviors?

What advice would you give Julie about how to protect Mr. Davis's dignity and self-esteem, and keep him safe?

What advice would you give Julie about how to respond to Mr. Davis's aggressive behaviors and keep herself safe?

THE NEEDS OF THE CAREGIVER

Providing care for a person with dementia is very difficult. As the illness progresses over time, the person becomes increasingly dependent on others. It becomes more difficult for the person to communicate needs and wants. In addition, the caregiver must come up with creative approaches to encourage the person to cooperate with care and to keep the person safe. This need puts a tremendous amount of stress on the caregiver and requires enormous amounts of physical and emotional energy. The constant stress of caregiving can negatively affect the caregiver's ability to cope with the difficult behaviors characteristic of dementia. As a result, the caregiver may react with anger or impatience. These reactions trigger additional problems. Abuse is possible if the caregiver loses control out of frustration and fatigue.

Family Caregivers

Most people who have dementia are initially cared for at home, which requires the support of family members 24 hours a day, 7 days a week. This situation places a great deal of responsibility on the family members and can disrupt family routines and relationships. Family caregivers tend to focus on the needs of the person with dementia, at the cost of attending to their own needs and those of other family members. To care for their own physical and emotional needs, caregivers need periodic breaks (respite) from their caregiving responsibilities. Other family members, friends and neighbors can often assist by watching the person for a short time to give the primary caregiver a break. Home health care agencies and adult day care centers can also provide respite care.

Table 19-5 **Communicating with a Person with Dementia**

Action	Reason
Always approach from the front.	Approaching from the back or side can startle the person and trigger a challenging behavior.
Make eye contact, preferably at eye level.	Making eye contact helps the person connect with you. Standing over a person conveys power or authority and is overwhelming.
Respect the person's personal space.	Standing too close is threatening.
Eliminate distractions.	Distractions interfere with the person's ability to focus.
Be social first, then clinical.	Establishing a personal connection and comfort level first is important before providing personal care.
Observe the person's body language.	Body language provides information about the person's mood and needs.
Match your tone and responses to the person's mood. For example, if the person is sad, respond with concern.	Responding in a way that agrees with the person's mood shows the person that you recognize her feelings and helps foster trust.
Be aware of your own tone of voice and body language.	Displays of impatience, frustration or anger will upset the person and could trigger a challenging behavior or aggressive response.
Explain what you are doing with simple words, gestures or both. Allow time for the person to process the information.	Explanation increases the person's ability to understand what you are doing, or what you want him to do.
Give only one instruction at a time.	The person cannot remember or successfully follow multiple instructions. Multiple instructions may overwhelm the person and add to her frustration and anxiety level.
Never rush the person.	Rushing causes increased anxiety because the person cannot process information or act on instructions quickly.
Maintain the same familiar routines.	The person has limited mental abilities to cope with change. A change in structure or routine overwhelms the person and can increase the person's level of frustration and agitation.

Even after a person with dementia is admitted to a nursing home for care, family members carry a tremendous burden. Dementia is a progressive disease, which means that it only gets worse, not better. As the disease robs the person of memories, abilities and personality, family members must cope with the gradual disappearance of the person they have known and loved. This involves grieving for each loss as it occurs, grief that can last for years. As a nurse assistant, you can do many things to help the person's family members:

- Encourage family members to have at least one thing each day that they can look forward to for themselves and to arrange for a break from their caregiving responsibilities at least once per week.
- Reassure family members that the person's needs will be met, even when they are not there.
- Put family members in touch with members of the health care team (such as a social worker or chaplain) who are knowledgeable about resources to help the family, such as support groups. Being able to talk about feelings and problems with other people who are going through the same thing can help family members feel less alone with their burdens.
- Provide family members, as appropriate, with information about their loved one's daily life. Because of language difficulties, the person with dementia cannot share with family members the events of the day or week.
- Suggest activities that family members can do together, such as taking a walk, looking at pictures in a book or singing songs (Figure 19-6). Often family members do not know how to have a meaningful visit, especially if the person does not really remember them or cannot meaningfully share information. These activities do not rely on

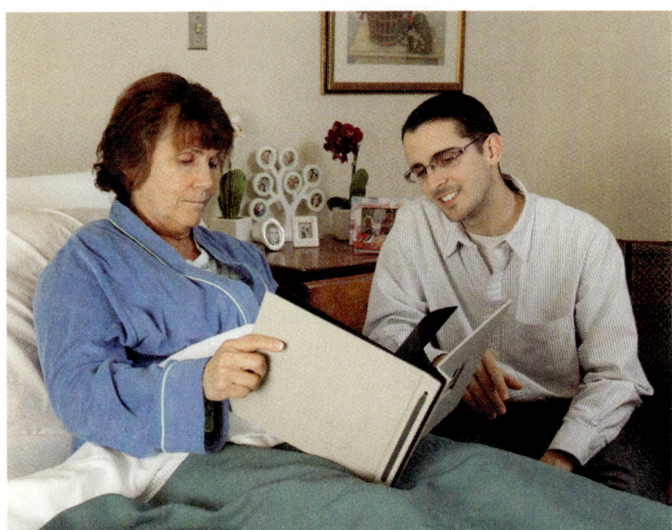

Figure 19-6 Activities that do not rely on knowledge of relationships and past memories can help promote a feeling of togetherness and shared enjoyment for family members and the person with dementia.

knowledge of relationships and past memories and yet can still promote a feeling of togetherness and shared enjoyment. Even if the person cannot remember the family member, she will have positive feelings from the encounter.

Mrs. Davis visits her husband every day. One day, you see Mrs. Davis in the hall and ask her how she is doing. She tells you that she thought life would be easier once she had her husband admitted here, but she still worries about him all the time and just feels so sad. She doesn't really do anything with her days other than to come and see him. You tell Mrs. Davis that you are worried about her and would like to help.

What things could you say or do that might help Mrs. Davis?

What losses has Mrs. Davis has experienced as a result of her husband's disease?

Nurse Assistants

Statistics show that at least half of the people who live in nursing homes have dementia. Sometimes they may live on a special unit for dementia care, and other times they live among the general facility population. In either case, the nurse assistants who work in those facilities are faced with caring for multiple people with dementia at the same time. People with dementia need constant supervision and frequent redirection. Meeting physical care needs is often difficult because of challenging behaviors. In addition, nurse assistants often feel burdened by their workload, feeling as if there is never enough help to get the job done. Many nurse assistants are not only caregivers at work but are caregivers for children or other family members when off duty. Like family caregivers, nurse assistants fall victim to the physical and emotional toll of care.

Be sure to know your limits. Stay alert and recognize when to ask for help so that you do not find yourself in a situation where you are overwhelmed. Also, be alert for possible signs of stress in your co-workers. You can help relieve some of that stress by stepping in to assist.

It is also important for you to find ways of coping successfully with your own stress. Activities such as exercising, listening to music, getting together with friends or engaging in hobbies can help you relieve stress. Activities do not need to be expensive or time-consuming. It is always possible to find something enjoyable that fits your lifestyle. The important thing is to find what works and commit to it so you can function at your best whether you are caring for people at work or caring for your family at home.

CHECK YOUR UNDERSTANDING

Questions for Review

1. **Forgetting where you put your wristwatch is an example the memory loss that occurs with:**
   a. Delirium.
   b. Dementia.
   c. Illness.
   d. Normal aging.
2. **Dementia is defined as:**
   a. Another word for Alzheimer's disease.
   b. A group of symptoms involving loss of memory and thinking abilities.
   c. A specific disease that affects memory.
   d. Personality change related to aging.
3. **Of the people diagnosed with dementia, most have which type?**
   a. Alzheimer's disease
   b. Lewy body dementia
   c. Vascular dementia
   d. Frontotemporal dementia
4. **You have repeatedly asked a resident with dementia to sit in the chair, but he continues to stand looking at you with a confused look. You then point to the chair and bend your knees as**

you demonstrate a sitting motion, and he sits in the chair. The resident is showing:

a. Amnesia.
b. Expressive aphasia.
c. Receptive aphasia.
d. Apraxia.

5. You are giving care to a woman who becomes frightened of her reflection in the mirror because she does not recognize herself. This is an example of:

a. Agnosia.
b. Amnesia.
c. Delusions.
d. Hallucinations.

6. A resident has been walking the halls looking into rooms and behind doors. He is looking worried and keeps pulling at his clothes. This behavior suggests:

a. A catastrophic reaction.
b. A delusion.
c. Hoarding.
d. Possible need for toileting.

7. You have taken care of Mr. Edwards, a resident with dementia, for a long time now. He can no longer walk or talk and is beginning to have difficulty swallowing. Mr. Edwards is showing signs of:

a. Advanced Alzheimer's disease.
b. Middle stage Alzheimer's disease.
c. Vascular dementia.
d. Depression.

8. Every time you try to wash a resident's hair in the shower, she starts screaming and tries to hit you. You now realize that wetting her hair:

a. Causes her pain.
b. Makes her feel like a child.
c. Must be done quickly to complete the task.
d. Is the trigger for her behavior.

9. The best way to calm a resident who is experiencing a catastrophic reaction is to:

a. Smile at him.
b. Look into his eyes to show concern.
c. Leave the room.
d. Ignore the behavior so that he will stop, and continue with your task.

10. Mrs. McDay confronts Mrs. Morgan in the hall and accuses her of wearing her clothes. Your co-worker raises her voice to Mrs. McDay, saying, "I have already told you several times that Mrs. Morgan's outfit doesn't belong to you. You need to stop bothering her because I don't have time for this nonsense." Your best response would be to:

a. Report this abuse to your supervisor.
b. Stay out of it because neither Mrs. McDay nor Mrs. Morgan is assigned to you.
c. Offer to provide assistance to give your co-worker a break from Mrs. McDay.
d. Remind your co-worker that Mrs. McDay has dementia.

11. Mr. Knight has dementia. This morning when you tried to help Mr. Knight get dressed, he hit you with his cane. What is the best way of responding to this behavior?

a. Ignore it. Mr. Knight cannot help his actions.
b. Take Mr. Knight's cane away from him.
c. Stop what you are doing, speak to Mr. Knight in a calm, comforting tone of voice, and try distracting him with another activity before attempting to help him with dressing again.
d. Report Mr. Knight's behavior to the nurse and request that he be given medication to calm him.

12. Mrs. McBride, who is normally alert and oriented, is acting very strangely today. When you answer her call light, she tells you that mice are running up the walls. This could be a sign of:

a. Alzheimer's disease.
b. Delirium.
c. Age-related memory impairment.
d. Mental illness.

Questions to Ask Yourself

1. *Describe how you might feel if you were providing care for someone who paces and wanders for most of the day and then becomes very agitated when you try to help.*
2. *Imagine that you are providing care for a client at home who has dementia. The client lives with his elderly wife. What safety issues might you encounter?*
3. *What could you do to promote the dignity and self-esteem of a person who has dementia?*

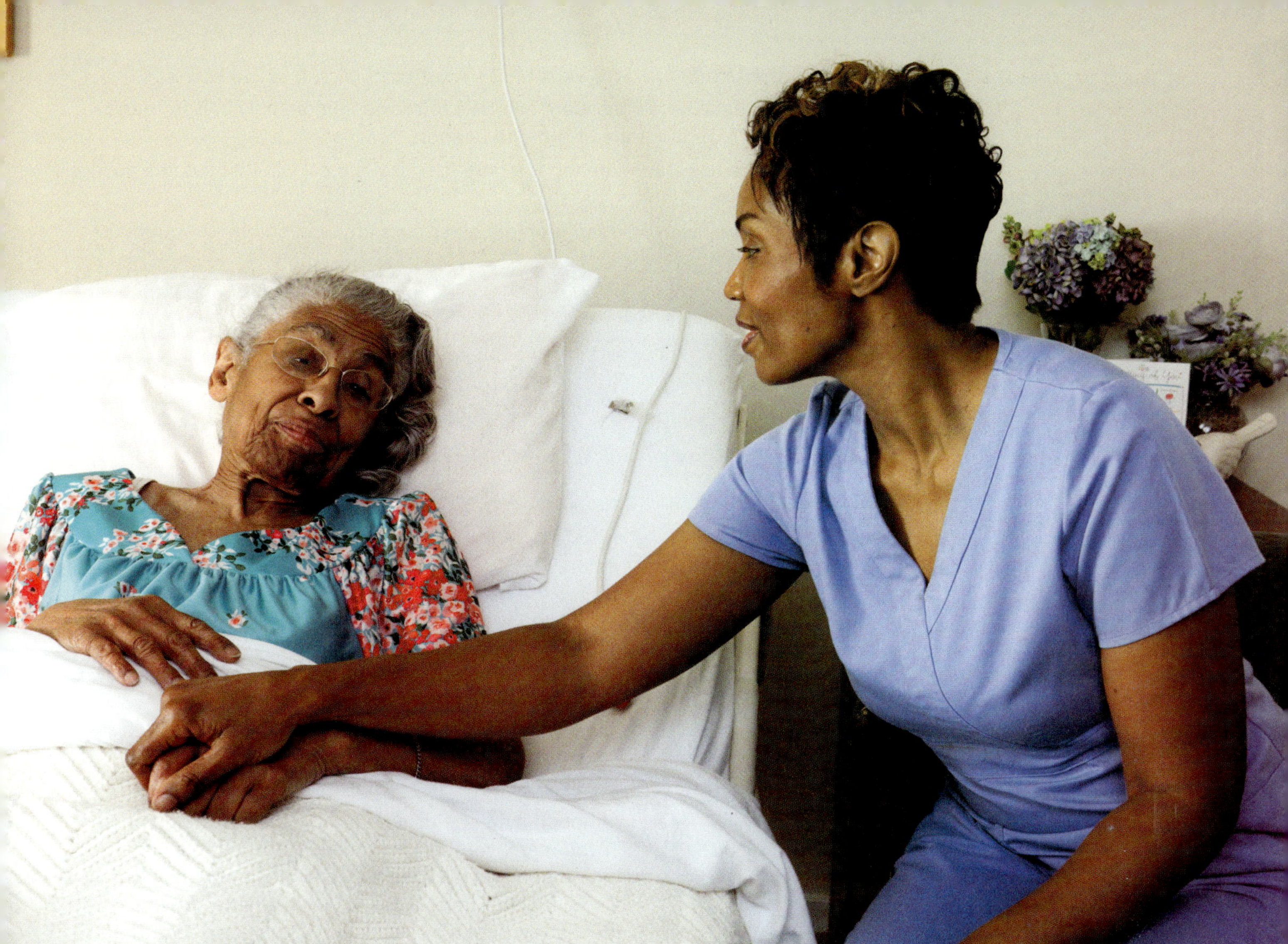

Providing Care for People at the End of Life

CHAPTER 20

Goals

After reading this chapter, you will have the information needed to:

- Discuss measures that may be taken to ensure that a person's death is as peaceful and comfortable as possible.
- Discuss how a nurse assistant can prepare to provide end-of-life care, and why this preparation is important.
- Describe basic needs that a person who is dying may have.
- List factors that may influence a person's feelings about death and dying.
- Describe common emotions that a person who is dying, and those close to the person, may experience throughout the end-of-life period.

Continued on next page

Continued from previous page

Goals

- Describe actions that a nurse assistant can take to provide emotional support to the person and family throughout the end-of-life period.
- Explain how a nurse assistant can honor a person's religious or cultural customs during the end-of-life period.
- Describe how a nurse assistant can promote a person's physical comfort throughout the end-of-life period.
- Describe ways in which the nurse assistant can support the family throughout the end-of-life period.
- Describe the care that is provided in the hours leading up to and following a person's death.
- Discuss the bereavement process for family, friends and staff.

After practicing the corresponding skill, you will have the information needed to:

- Provide postmortem care.

Key Terms:

terminal illness	**comfort (supportive) care**	**grief**	**rigor mortis**
life-sustaining treatments	**palliative treatments**	**postmortem care**	**bereavement care**
do-not-resuscitate (DNR) order	**hospice**	**shroud**	

Ellen Miller has been a resident at Morningside Nursing Home for the past 2 years. She has advanced heart and lung disease that limits her ability to care for herself. She can no longer walk in her room because of shortness of breath and severe arthritis. During the past 6 months, Mrs. Miller has been hospitalized for pneumonia and exacerbations of her chronic heart failure three times. After the last time, Mrs. Miller told her family that she does not want to go back to the hospital again. She signed an advance directive saying that she wants to be kept comfortable but does not want any special measures taken to prolong her life.

As a health care worker, you will most likely have the opportunity to care for people during the last phase of their lives (the end-of-life period). Sometimes death occurs suddenly, and the end-of-life period is short or nonexistent. Often, a period of time leads up to a person's death when the person and the family anticipate the likelihood of the person's death and prepare for it. Some people in your care will have **terminal illnesses** (illnesses for which there is no treatment and that are expected to lead to the person's death). Other people will develop acute illnesses (illnesses of sudden onset) that lead to their death. Many others will simply die as a result of one or more long-term, chronic conditions.

Although it can be difficult to face the death of a person in your care, you will play a very important role in helping the person and family through this time of transition. Dr. Elisabeth Kübler-Ross, a psychiatrist who wrote the classic book *On Death and Dying*, said that dying people teach us how to live, how to look at our own lives and how to see every day as a precious gift. This is the gift that we receive when we provide end-of-life care.

A PEACEFUL AND COMFORTABLE DEATH

All people have the right to a peaceful and comfortable death. For many people, this means choosing to forego **life-sustaining treatments** (treatments that will prolong life, such as cardiopulmonary resuscitation [CPR] or mechanical ventilation) at the end of life, if having these treatments will prolong their suffering. When a person chooses to forego life-sustaining treatments at the end of life, the person's primary care provider will write a **do-not-resuscitate (DNR) order**. This order means that the health care team should not start CPR if the person's heart stops or breathing stops. When a person has a DNR order, all members of the health care team should be aware of this, so that the person's wishes can be honored.

A desire to forego life-sustaining treatments at the end of life does not mean that the person wishes to forego *all* care at the end of life. Instead, many people choose to receive only **comfort (supportive) care** (care that will make the person more comfortable but will not prolong the person's life, such as oxygen therapy, administration of pain medications and personal care). In some states, these wishes are communicated through a do-not-resuscitate/comfort care (DNR-CC) order. As part of comfort care, **palliative treatments** may be offered. Palliative treatments are provided to relieve uncomfortable symptoms without actually curing the disease that is causing the symptoms. For example, if a person has a cancerous tumor that is pressing on another organ and causing pain, surgery may be done to reduce the size of the tumor to relieve the pain. In this case, the surgery is palliative because it was done to provide pain relief, not to cure the person's cancer. Sometimes comfort care also involves eliminating routine procedures or treatments that are no longer of benefit to the person, such as routine weight measurements, providing a therapeutic diet or routine blood glucose testing. The goal of comfort care is to help the person have the best quality of life up until the time of death.

Hospice is a model of care that focuses on providing comfort care to people who are dying, and on supporting their families, during the end-of-life period. The hospice model of care is based on several core beliefs:

- Dying is a normal and expected part of the life cycle.
- The dying person should not be separated from family and other support systems.
- Care for the dying person and family must address the person's and family's physical, emotional, social and spiritual needs.
- Care for the dying person seeks to relieve pain and other distressing symptoms that a person may experience during the end-of-life period.
- Care seeks to help the person die with dignity, by honoring the person's preferences for end-of-life care.

Some people receive hospice care through formal hospice programs, which may be provided in a person's home, in a hospice facility or in a special unit of a nursing home or hospital. A person may be enrolled in a formal hospice program when the person's primary care provider documents that the person has a terminal condition and is not expected to live for more than 6 months. However, the principles of hospice are important to practice with all people who are dying, even those who are not enrolled in a formal hospice program.

When a person is enrolled in a hospice program, the coordination of care is extremely important. The hospice personnel will create a schedule specifying the days and times of their visits. Usually the hospice program provides necessary equipment and supplies for those receiving their services, so it is important to communicate any needs that the person may have to the hospice staff when they are in the facility. The hospice program provides visits from both hospice aides and hospice nurses. The hospice aide assists the person with meeting hygiene and mobility needs. When you plan your day, take the hospice aide's schedule into account. When the hospice nurse is scheduled, he or she will visit and assess the status of the person and the family, so that the care plan can be adjusted accordingly. The hospice nurse will then meet with the facility nurse to review and coordinate the person's care. Because changes in the person's condition may necessitate changes in the person's care plan, it is important to check the care plan daily for any changes. When the person's death is expected to occur within a short period, the hospice nurse will be with the person around the clock to offer support to the dying person, family and staff, as needed. During this time, you will also play an important role in assisting the hospice personnel meet the person's and family's needs.

For the past few weeks, Mrs. Miller's condition has gotten worse. She has trouble eating and is losing weight. She does not want to get out of bed because of pain and feels that she is too weak to sit in her chair. The health care team recognizes that Mrs. Miller most likely is starting the next phase of her life, the end-of-life period. Mrs. Miller's primary care provider meets with Mrs. Miller and her children and reassures them that while Mrs. Miller's condition is terminal, much can be done to ensure her comfort in the coming months.

What type of care might be put in place for Mrs. Miller going forward?

Why is honoring Mrs. Miller's wishes regarding end-of-life care important?

PROVIDING END-OF-LIFE CARE

Many caregivers, especially those who have not had much previous experience with death and dying, worry about their ability to provide end-of-life care. Examples of common concerns include:

- What if the person or family wants to talk about the person's death? What should I say?
- How will I feel if a person dies right in front of me?
- Will I be able to handle the emotional stress of losing people in my care?
- What will it be like to provide care for a deceased person's body?

Preparing to provide end-of-life care can also make caregivers uncomfortable because it requires them to think about their own mortality. For many people, this can be very frightening. To effectively help others through the end-of-life period, you must first address your own feelings about death and dying and the concerns that you may have about providing end-of-life care. Your cultural and religious or spiritual beliefs and your past experiences with death and dying can influence how you feel about death and dying. Talking with someone you trust, such as a clergy member or more experienced co-worker, can help you sort through your feelings about death and dying and about providing end-of-life care (Figure 20-1).

Providing end-of-life care can be emotionally difficult, but it can also be very rewarding. You will help all the people in your care meet their physical, emotional, social and spiritual needs. These needs do not go away during the end-of-life period; in fact, they may increase (Box 20-1). By helping the person to meet these needs and showing empathy and compassion, you can make a significant difference in the end-of-life period for the person and his or her family members.

Providing Emotional Support

The end-of-life period is a time of emotional preparation, for both the person and those close to the person.

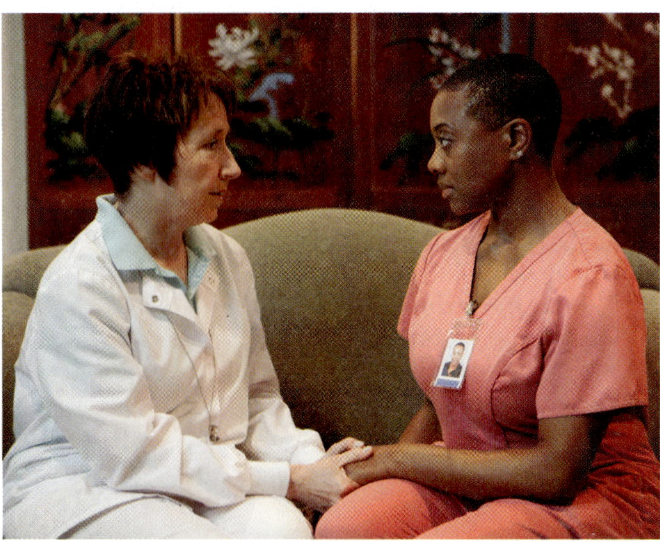

Figure 20-1 Talking with an experienced co-worker, clergy member or other trusted person can help you sort out your feelings about death.

A person's feelings about death can be influenced by many different factors, including:

- The person's culture.
- The person's spiritual or religious beliefs.
- The person's past experiences with death (for example, deaths of family members or friends).
- The person's sense of having lived a full and complete life.
- The person's current quality of life (for example, if the person has had a long and difficult struggle with an illness, death may be viewed as a release from a state of suffering).

Each person prepares for death in her own personal way and at her own emotional speed. The person (as well as those who are close to the person) may experience a wide range of emotions throughout the end-of-life period. No matter what emotion the person experiences at any given point throughout the end-of-life period, she will need your understanding and support. You may be the only one whom the person can talk to, because family members may not be available or may be reluctant to discuss the person's death. Common emotions that a person, and those close to the person, may experience during the end-of-life period include:

- **Grief. Grief** is intense sadness that occurs as a result of loss. Any type of significant loss, not just death, can cause a person to experience grief. For example, the loss of health or the end of a marriage can also cause a person to feel grief. A dying person and those close to the person may experience grief when they learn that death is imminent. After the person's death, those left behind will continue to grieve their loss, sometimes for months or years afterward.
- **Sadness.** Throughout the end-of-life period, the person and those close to him may experience periods of sadness. These feelings can arise from both awareness of future losses and regrets about the past. Some people will want to talk about their feelings of sadness, whereas others will become withdrawn and quiet. Do not try to cheer

Box 20-1 Needs of a Dying Person

- To maintain my dignity
- To feel comfortable with the people who are caring for me
- To be told the truth
- To have someone listen to me
- To have people touch me
- To not feel alone
- To feel prepared to die
- To be free of physical discomfort and pain
- To be kept clean

Adapted from Steinhauser KE, Christakis NA, Clipp EC, McNeilly M, McIntyre L, Tulsky JA: Factors considered important at the end of life by patients, family, physicians, and other care providers, *Journal of the American Medical Association* 284:2476–2482, 2000.

the person up, distract him from his sadness or convince him that he has much to be grateful for in his life. Instead, acknowledge the person's feelings and allow him to talk openly and honestly about them.

- **Fear.** People may have many fears related to death and dying, including fear of the unknown, fear of dying alone and fear of experiencing pain. You can do much to reassure the person and help to relieve some of the fears that the person may have about dying by simply being there for the person. Check on the person frequently, and reassure the person that you will be there with her until the end. Some people will want to talk about their fears. When this is the case, the best thing you can do is listen. Others will not want to talk, and that is okay too. Often, just sitting quietly with the person is all the person needs.
- **Anger.** Many people experience feelings of anger during the end-of-life period. The person may be angry because he feels that the situation is unfair or because he feels that maybe there was something that could have been done to prevent the situation. Sometimes that anger is directed inward, and other times it is directed at others. The person may even direct his anger at a higher being and experience a loss of faith. People show anger in different ways. Some people may become withdrawn and moody, whereas others may criticize others unfairly. If a person's anger is directed unfairly toward you, it is important to try and remember where that anger may be coming from and to avoid taking it personally.
- **Denial.** Denial is a way of dealing with information that is difficult to accept. Denial allows the person to put information aside until she is emotionally ready to deal with it. In this way, denial helps to protect the person from overwhelming sadness. A person who is experiencing denial may insist that members of the health care team are wrong about a diagnosis or may delay following up with recommended tests, treatments or care. The best way to respond to a person who is experiencing denial is in a supportive, yet honest way. For example, if a person says to you, "The doctors must be wrong. My father was fine last week, and now they are telling me he might not live another 6 months?" you could respond, "I'm sorry, this must be very hard for you." Eventually, the person will be able to process the information that she has been given and will begin to accept the reality of the situation, but right now she cannot. It is important to allow her to process the information at her own pace. It is also important to recognize that throughout the end-of-life period, a person may move back and forth between periods of denial and reality.
- **Hope.** Hope is the belief in a better future. Hope gives the person the strength to keep going when a situation is difficult. Throughout the end-of-life period, what a person hopes for may change, but there is always hope. The person may hope for a cure or a new treatment; to live long enough to experience an important event, such as the birth of a child, a marriage or a graduation; or simply to die a peaceful and pain-free death. It is important to support and nurture the person's feelings of hope. For example, a person may say, "If I just make it to my daughter's wedding, I'll be ready to go. I won't ask for anything else." You may not believe that the person's health will allow her to attend her daughter's wedding, but a response such as "I want to see you at your daughter's wedding, too" is supportive and honest and nurtures the person's hope.
- **Acceptance.** Acceptance is a time of peaceful resignation. The person feels at peace with the future and what the future holds. The person may experience a sense of calm and of being able to let go and move on. Acceptance does not mean that the person has given up hope. It simply means that the person has reached a place emotionally that allows him to be at peace with the reality of the situation.

One of the most important skills that you will use as a nurse assistant when caring for people and their families throughout the end-of-life period is your ability to be a good listener (Figure 20-2). The person and the family members may want to talk about the emotions that they feel. Be willing to talk about what the person wants to talk about, even if the subject is sad or frightening. You may worry that you will not know how to respond to a person. Often, simply listening and

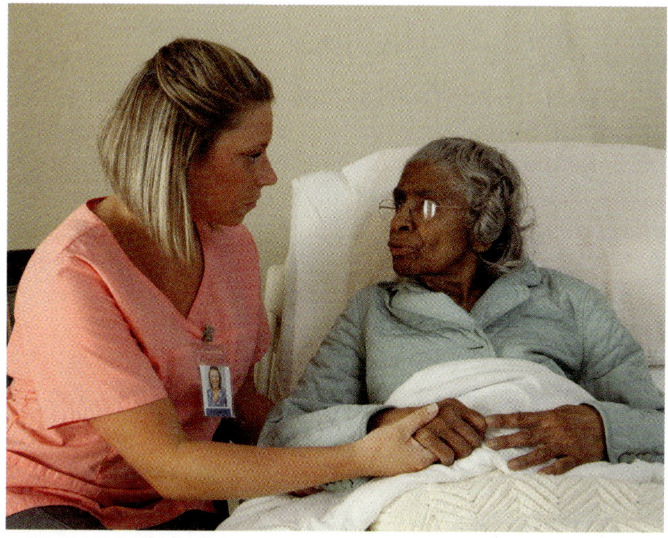

Figure 20-2 Being available to listen is a very important part of providing end-of-life care.

holding the person's hand is enough. Some people who are dying will want to look back on their lives and share important memories with you. Family members may also find it comforting to share memories about the dying person's life. You might encourage them to share family photos so that everyone can see the photos and talk about them. This activity helps the dying person and the family to review the accomplishments and happy times of the person's life. Sometimes, people will want to talk about what they believe the future holds. For example, the person may talk about what she thinks the afterlife will be like or may express a belief in reincarnation (the idea that a person's soul can come back to earth in another body). Be accepting of beliefs and ideas that may be different from your own. In all cases, your ability to listen is key to providing emotional support throughout the end-of-life period.

After the family conference, Mrs. Miller's son, William, runs into you in the hall. He recognizes you as one of the nurse assistants who has been caring for his mother for the last 2 years. He says, "I just don't understand why Mom has given up so easily. She has so much to live for—my sister and me, and her grandchildren." His voice cracks, and his eyes start to fill with tears.

What emotions might William be experiencing now?

How would you respond to William?

What other emotions could William, his sister and Mrs. Miller experience over the next few months?

Respecting Cultural and Religious Customs

Many religions and cultures have their own customs and rituals relating to death. Specific rituals may have to be performed before or at the time of death, or as part of the care that is provided after death. Ahead of time, make sure you are aware if something special needs to be done. This information should be recorded in the person's care plan. If the religious or cultural practices are not followed, the family members may experience additional unnecessary grief. Not only will they have to deal with the loss of a loved one, but they may also feel guilt or anger associated with not performing an important ritual.

Some people may request and receive visits from clergy members throughout the end-of-life period. Report a person's request to see a clergy member to the nurse immediately, so that the necessary arrangements can be made. See to the clergy member's comfort and provide privacy during the visit.

Providing Physical Support

Throughout the end-of-life period, ensuring the person's physical comfort is important. Conditions that a dying person might experience in the months leading up to death may include pain, shortness of breath and digestive problems. These conditions can be uncomfortable for the person and distressing to the family. As a nurse assistant, it is important that you become familiar with these conditions, recognize when they occur and report them promptly so that steps can be taken to relieve them.

- **Pain.** Pain is the most common and most feared symptom that occurs when someone is dying. Many people think that uncontrolled pain must always be part of the dying process. However, even severe pain can be managed. Letting the person and family know this helps to decrease their anxiety. Observe for nonverbal signs of pain (see Chapter 16), and ask the person frequently whether he has pain. If you suspect or know that the person is experiencing pain, report your concerns to the nurse immediately. Some of the daily care tasks you must perform may be associated with pain or discomfort. Alerting the nurse to this is important so that pain medication may be given before the painful activity takes place.
- **Shortness of breath.** Another common condition during the end-of-life period is shortness of breath. Proper positioning can help provide relief for mild shortness of breath. Sometimes, increasing air circulation with a fan in the room provides comfort for those who feel breathless. The person may also learn relaxation and special breathing techniques that can help. Severe shortness of breath may require medication, such as morphine and oxygen.
- **Digestive problems.** Digestive problems, such as nausea, vomiting and constipation, are very uncomfortable. Medications may be given to prevent or relieve these conditions, so be sure to report these conditions to the nurse.

As a nurse assistant, you can do many things to promote the person's physical comfort, including the following:

- **Provide assistance with repositioning according to the person's care plan.** Many people will lose the ability to reposition themselves as their condition worsens. Assisting with repositioning according to the person's care plan reduces the person's risk for pressure ulcers and promotes comfort by ensuring good body alignment. If equipment is available to assist with repositioning, be sure to use it because the person will have a limited ability to help you.

- **Provide frequent skin care.** Wipe away secretions that may form around the person's eyes, nose and mouth with a warm, damp washcloth. If the person is incontinent of urine, feces or both, check the person frequently and provide perineal care as needed.
- **Provide frequent mouth care.** The mouth may become dry, especially if the person is not taking any food or water by mouth. Mouth care helps to keep the tissues of the mouth moist and promotes comfort.
- **Report the need for other comfort measures as appropriate.** Report conditions such as pain, difficulty breathing, constipation, nausea, vomiting or anxiety to the nurse so that measures can be taken to relieve these sources of discomfort.
- **Create a comfortable environment.** Keep the room well-ventilated, clean and neat.

As always, ensure privacy when you provide care. Ask family members who are present to step outside, and draw the privacy curtain. Work quickly and efficiently to minimize the time that family members must be away from the bedside. Some family members may find it comforting to participate in the person's physical care. If this is the case, teach the family member how to do simple tasks that promote the dying person's comfort, such as using a warm washcloth to keep the eyes, nose and corners of the mouth clean, or offering ice chips from a cup (Figure 20-3). Some family members may not want to participate in care activities, but they can still be a source of comfort to the person by sitting with the person, holding her hand and talking to her. Although the person may slip in and out of consciousness as death nears, the person can still hear and feel and may find it very comforting if family members hold her hand and talk about happy times they shared with her.

Remember to take measures to meet the family's physical needs as well as the person's. Many times, family members will spend long hours at the person's bedside. Make sure that they know the location of restrooms, places to get a meal or snack, or places where they can go to rest. Sometimes, family members may be reluctant to leave the bedside to take care of their own needs. Try to arrange your schedule so that you can stay with the person while the family members are gone. That way, the family members can take a break to attend to their own needs without worrying that the person will be left alone. Simple measures, such as making sure everyone in the room has a place to sit and bringing a tray with coffee or tea and snacks to the person's room, are thoughtful gestures that can help the family through this difficult time (Figure 20-4).

Mrs. Miller now cannot get out of bed.
She is very weak and has no appetite. Her daughter, Sheila, has come from out of town to be with her mother during this time. William, who lives locally, visits frequently as well and often brings his wife and children with him.

What care will you provide to Mrs. Miller to ensure her physical comfort during these last few days or weeks of her life?

How can you help William and Sheila as they prepare for their mother's death?

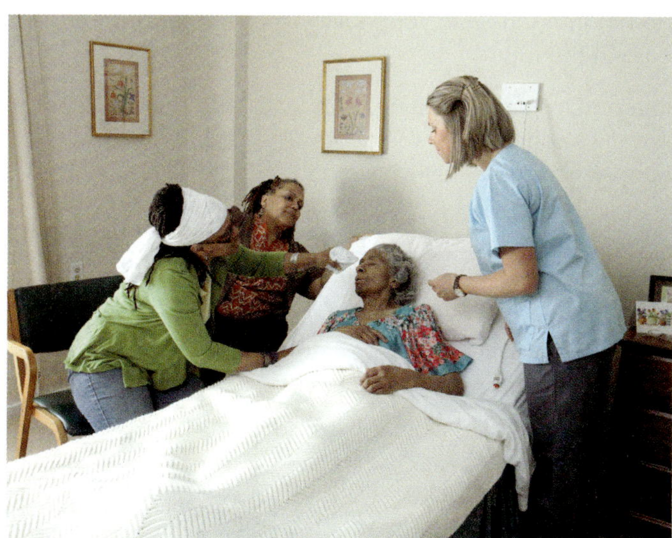

Figure 20-3 Some family members may take comfort from being involved in providing care to a loved one at the end of life.

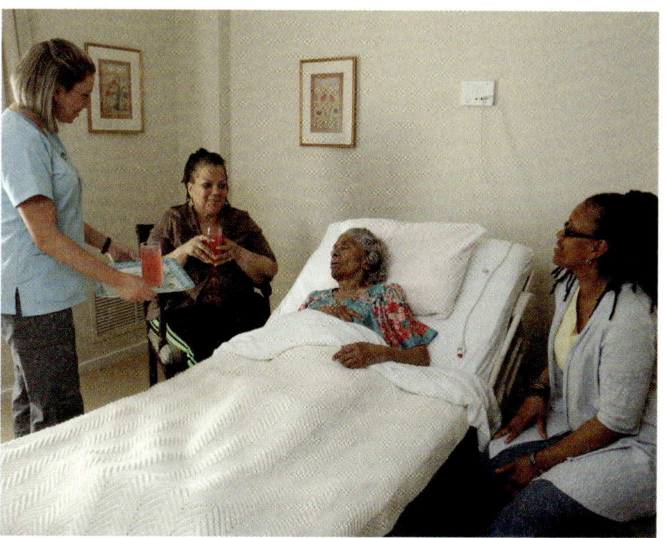

Figure 20-4 Simple gestures, such as ensuring the physical comfort of family members, can help to make a difficult time a little easier.

PROVIDING CARE IN THE HOURS IMMEDIATELY BEFORE AND AFTER DEATH

As death approaches and the person's body systems start to shut down, you may begin to see signs that indicate death is near. The signs do not necessarily occur in the order listed in Box 20-2, and not all the signs may occur in everyone. The onset of these signs may be gradual or rapid.

After death occurs, there is no pulse, respiration or blood pressure. The person's breathing may stop first, and then the heart may stop beating. The pupils of the person's eyes become fixed (no movement) and dilated (widened). If you are with a person when the person dies, notify the nurse immediately. The doctor or someone the doctor delegates (usually the nurse) must examine the person, legally pronounce the person dead and document the time of death. If family members are present when the person dies, they may want time to be alone with the person's body. This need should be respected, and family members should not be rushed.

Postmortem Care

Depending on your employer's policy, you may be responsible for providing or assisting with **postmortem care**. The word postmortem means *after death*. Postmortem care involves cleaning, positioning and identifying the body. After death, the bladder and bowels may empty, so the skin needs to be cleaned and the clothing and linens changed. The body may be wrapped in a cloth covering called a **shroud**. **Rigor mortis** (stiffening of the muscles of the body) starts to develop about 6 to 8 hours after death. It can be very difficult to reposition the body after rigor mortis occurs. Discoloration of the person's skin as a result of pooling of the blood also occurs. Postmortem care is done to ensure that the body is positioned naturally and to preserve the appearance of the body in preparation for subsequent arrangements that the family may wish to make.

Skill 20-1 describes step-by-step how to provide postmortem care. Always follow your employer's policies and procedures and specific instructions that you may be given by the nurse when you perform postmortem care. Certain rituals may need to be followed according to the person's religious or cultural beliefs. Make sure that you are aware of these rituals and that the necessary arrangements have been made to allow the rituals to be carried out according to the family's wishes. When you provide postmortem care, ensure privacy and handle the person's body with care and respect. Always follow standard precautions, because body fluids may still contain pathogens after death. If someone is helping you provide care, your conversation should be respectful and appropriate.

Bereavement Care

Bereavement care is care that is provided for people who are grieving after a person dies. Counselors, social workers, clergy members or trained volunteers may be involved in providing bereavement care for family members and friends after a person's death.

Staff members may also have many feelings to deal with after the death of a person in their care. For example, as a nurse assistant, you may have formed a close relationship with the dying person and her family. Depending on the circumstances surrounding the person's death, you may feel anger about the person's extended suffering, relief that her suffering has ended, sadness over the loss of the relationship or a combination of these. If you cannot work through these or other feelings, or if old memories of your own have been triggered, talk about them with someone you trust, such as a more experienced co-worker or clergy member. Many employers also offer resources to help employees deal with difficult emotional issues. Coming to terms with your own feelings is important so that they do not interfere with your ability to provide end-of-life care in the future.

In a nursing home setting, the death of a resident can greatly sadden other residents. The residents know each other and usually have had time to develop

Box 20-2 Signs of Approaching Death

- Rapid, weak or irregular pulse
- Decreased blood pressure
- Cool, moist and pale skin
- Coolness and mottling (patchy discoloring) of the hands and feet
- Incontinence
- Periods of increased, shallow respiration followed by periods of decreased respiration
- A gargling sound with breathing (caused by mucus in the airway)
- Loss of, or a drifting in and out of, consciousness
- Loss of movement
- Loss of the ability to communicate

friendships. You may tell other residents that the person has died so that they do not wonder and worry. When you give information about the person's death to other residents, be sure the information meets HIPAA privacy requirements. For example, you may tell them that the person died peacefully, where he died and who was with him. Encourage residents to talk about their memories of the person who died and help them remember the good things. Also, encourage them to talk about their own fears about death or their sadness about losing a friend, and encourage them to attend religious or memorial services, if they desire. Residents who were especially close to the person may go through a grieving period and will need extra attention from you during this time.

Mrs. Miller died early this morning from complications of her heart and lung disease. Mrs. Miller's daughter, Sheila, asks if you can help her select a dress for her mother's burial. You say that you will and that you know how much choosing a pretty dress would please her mother, because she was always so particular about her appearance. Sheila says, "You've been so great with us and Mom. This has been a really difficult time for our entire family. I can't tell you how much it has meant to me these last few weeks to know that Mom was receiving such good care."

How have Sheila's memories of her mother's death been affected by the care you provided for her mother throughout the end-of-life period? How would these memories be different if she felt that her mother did not receive excellent care during the end of her life?

CHECK YOUR UNDERSTANDING

Questions for Review

1. **Family members of a person who is dying should be:**
    a. Encouraged to talk about their feelings and their needs.
    b. Discouraged from participating in the care of the person, because it is too upsetting.
    c. Encouraged to visit with the person who is dying for only a few minutes to avoid tiring the person.
    d. Discouraged from expressing how they feel.

2. **CPR is an example of:**
    a. A supportive treatment.
    b. A palliative treatment.
    c. A life-sustaining treatment.
    d. A hospice treatment.

3. **The hospice philosophy is based on all of the following EXCEPT:**
    a. The dying person should not be separated from family and other support systems.
    b. Care for the dying person and family should address the person's and family's emotional needs.
    c. Pain is a normal and expected part of dying.
    d. The person's preferences for end-of-life care should be honored.

4. **Mr. Troyer has a DNR order in place. What does this mean?**
    a. The health care team should withdraw supportive care at the end of life and just allow Mr. Troyer to pass away peacefully.
    b. In the event that Mr. Troyer's heart stops beating or his breathing stops, the health care team should not start CPR.
    c. Mr. Troyer's death will occur soon, and end-of-life care should be provided.
    d. Mr. Troyer has died and requires postmortem care.

5. **All of the following are needs of the dying person EXCEPT:**
    a. The need to be isolated from other people
    b. The need to be kept clean
    c. The need to receive emotional support
    d. The need to be touched

6. **Mrs. Skorgard is in the last stages of a terminal illness. She tells you that she believes science is on the brink of discovering a cure for her condition. Mrs. Skorgard is expressing:**
    a. Denial.
    b. Anger.
    c. Hope.
    d. Grief.

7. **Mrs. Skinner is dying and is experiencing difficulty breathing. What can you do to help Mrs. Skinner?**
    a. Reassure Mrs. Skinner that difficulty breathing is a normal part of dying, and tell her that you will stay with her and see her through it.
    b. Report Mrs. Skinner's difficulty breathing to the nurse immediately.

c. Talk to the nurse about Mrs. Skinner's eligibility for hospice care.
d. Provide mouth care for Mrs. Skinner.

8. Mr. Reynolds is 98 years old. He tells you that he has lived a good life and he's "ready to go when the good Lord takes me." Mr. Reynolds is expressing feelings of:

a. Hope.
b. Acceptance.
c. Denial.
d. Giving up.

9. A new nurse assistant on the unit tells you that she is really upset about the idea of providing postmortem care, because she has never seen a dead body before. What advice would you give her?

a. To tell the nurse that she cannot provide postmortem care
b. To talk about her feelings regarding death and providing end-of-life care with someone she trusts
c. To consider changing jobs
d. To review the skill for providing postmortem care in her textbook

10. When you provide end-of-life care, it is important to:

a. Be prepared to respond to anything a dying person might tell you in a reassuring way.
b. Be a good listener.
c. Leave the person alone as much as possible.
d. Conceal your feelings about the person's death from the person.

Questions to Ask Yourself

1. *Mr. Williams, one of the residents in the nursing home where you work, died suddenly yesterday. Mrs. Casey was a close friend of Mr. Williams and is very upset to learn of his passing. What should you do for Mrs. Casey?*
2. *Mr. Calloway, a 90-year-old nursing home resident, is dying after a long illness. He is a widower whose three children visit him at various times. Two of the children visit regularly to talk with him and comfort him. The third child, a son named Mike, seldom visits, seems quiet and withdrawn and stays for only a short time. One day when you are bathing Mr. Calloway, he says that he is concerned about Mike. He says that Mike does not seem to care that he is dying but that he often seems to be hurt, angry or upset. How would you respond to Mr. Calloway? What, if anything, would you report to the nurse about your conversation with Mr. Calloway? Why do you think Mike is behaving the way he is?*
3. *Mrs. Lukens is one of your home health clients. She is terminally ill. One day when you are helping her, she says, "I don't want to die alone, and I don't have anybody. My husband died years ago, and we never had any children." And she starts to cry. What can you do for Mrs. Lukens?*

Skill 20-1
Providing Postmortem Care

PREPARATION

1. Wash your hands.
2. Gather your supplies:
   - Gloves
   - Bed protector
   - Bath blanket
   - Clean gown
   - Wash cloth
   - Towel
   - Wash basin
   - Soap
   - Identification tags (one or two, depending on whether a shroud is used)
   - Envelope or plastic bag for small personal items and an inventory sheet
   - Shroud (if used)
   - Clean linens (if needed)
3. Knock, greet family members and ensure privacy.
4. Explain the procedure if family members are present.
5. Adjust equipment for body mechanics and safety: Raise the bed to a comfortable working height. Make sure the wheels on the bed are locked.

PROCEDURE

6. Cover the over-bed table with the paper towels and arrange your supplies. Fill the wash basin with warm water. Place the wash basin on the over-bed table. Complete the identification tags with the required information.
7. Put on the gloves.
8. Lower the head of the bed and place the body in the supine position.
9. Close the person's eyes.
10. With approval from the nurse, remove any medical equipment.
11. Remove jewelry. (Follow your employer's policy regarding wedding or engagement rings. Often, these are left in place.) Place any jewelry that you remove in the envelope or plastic bag designated for the person's belongings. Record each item on the inventory sheet as you remove it.
12. If the person wears dentures and they were not in the person's mouth at the time of death, replace the dentures in the person's mouth (or follow the nurse's instructions). Close the person's mouth.
13. Place the bath blanket over the body, and remove the person's clothing. Wash and dry the body, and then dress the body in the clean gown.
14. Put an identification tag around the person's ankle.
15. Replace the linens, if necessary. Place the bed protector under the person's buttocks. Draw the top sheet over the person's legs and torso and make a cuff. Do not cover the person's face.
16. If the family would like to view the body, clean up your work area and dim the lights before inviting the family back in. Provide for privacy and leave the room.
17. After the family leaves, return to the room and complete the postmortem care procedure.
18. If a shroud is to be used:
    a. Unfold the shroud on the bed and place the person's body on it.
    b. Fold the top of the shroud down over the person's head.
    c. Fold the bottom of the shroud up over the person's feet.
    d. Fold the sides of the shroud over the person's body and tape the ends together.
    e. Attach an identification tag to the shroud.

COMPLETION

19. Adjust equipment for safety: Make sure that the wheels on the bed are locked.
20. Clean up your work area.
21. Wash your hands.
22. Report and record.

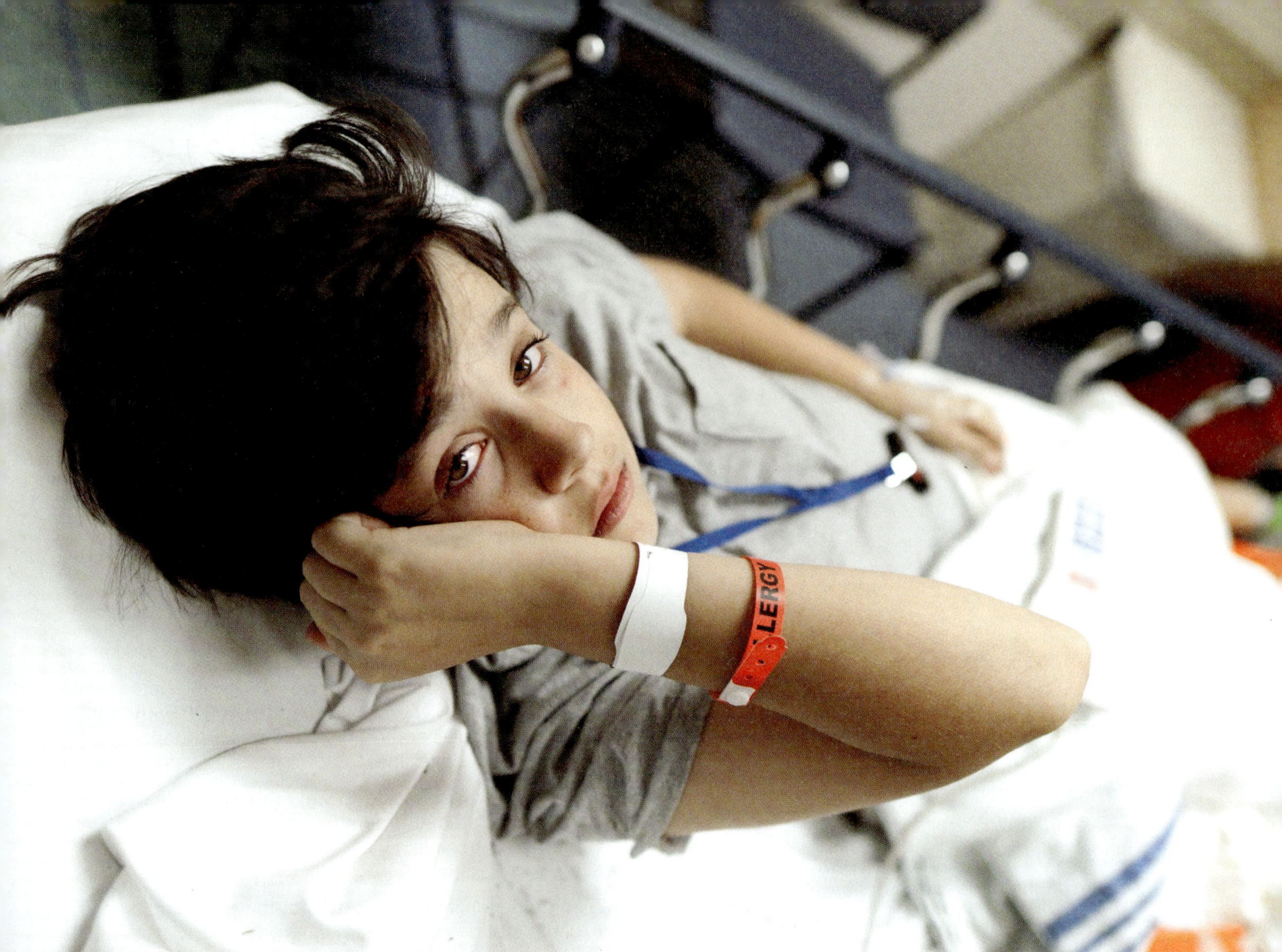

CHAPTER

21 Providing Care to Infants and Children

Goals

After reading this chapter, you will have the information needed to:

- List three common responses to illness, injury or hospitalization that children may show.
- Explain the factors that can affect how a child responds to illness, injury or hospitalization.
- Identify characteristic responses to illness, injury or hospitalization according to developmental level.
- Describe the effect of chronic illness on children and families.
- Discuss the concepts of family-centered care and atraumatic care.
- Discuss the ways a nurse assistant can address the responses of infants and children who are ill, injured or hospitalized.

Goals

- Explain the ways a nurse assistant can maintain a child's safety when ill, injured or hospitalized.
- Discuss the use of play with infants and children.
- List the ways a nurse assistant can help family members deal with an ill, injured or hospitalized infant or child.
- Identify the modifications needed when monitoring the vital signs of infants and children.
- Describe how a nurse assistant meets a child's hygiene needs.
- List the ways a nurse assistant can foster nutrition in infants and children.

Key Terms:

Separation anxiety **Regression** **Family-centered care** **Atraumatic care**

You are assigned to care for Javier Green, a 3½-year-old boy who was admitted to the hospital with an acute asthma attack and pneumonia. Javier is receiving oxygen to help him breathe a little easier, and he is receiving medication to open his airways. The nurse reviews his care plan with you and tells you that this is the fourth time Javier has been admitted in the past 4 months for the same problem. The nurse also tells you that Javier tires easily and needs to drink more fluids because he is a little dehydrated. You enter Javier's room and find his mother, Isabella, at his bedside with tears in her eyes. You introduce yourself to Javier and his mother.

Imagine that you became ill or injured or needed to go to the urgent care center, emergency department or hospital. How would you respond? Now imagine that you were a child in the same situation. How do you think you might react? Typically, when you think about infants and children, you think about cute little babies cooing, giggling and crawling about, and boys and girls running around, playing on the playground and enjoying themselves. Rarely do you think about them becoming ill or injured. Unfortunately they do, and their responses, although similar in some respects to those of adults, are unique. In addition, infants and children continually grow and develop. They are not "mini-adults." So you will need to adapt how you care for infants and children, both physically and emotionally, based on the child's stage of growth and development.

GENERAL CHILDHOOD RESPONSES TO ILLNESS, INJURY AND HOSPITALIZATION

Infants and children are growing emotionally as they experience the outside world. However, their experience is limited. As a result, they have limited means for coping with the changes and stresses associated with being ill or injured. Common emotional responses to illness, injury and hospitalization include fear and anxiety, separation anxiety and a feeling of loss of control.

Fear and Anxiety

Infants and children, like adults, commonly experience fear and anxiety when affected by illness, injury or hospitalization. For most children, the sights and sounds of a care center, emergency department or hospital unit are strange and unfamiliar. There are bright lights, odd smells, large pieces of equipment and people dressed in unusual clothing. The comfort and quiet of the home and a familiar routine are gone. They do not know what is happening to them. For example, the child may have a strange pain in his tummy or be awakened during the night to have his vital signs taken. The child may not be allowed to eat or drink because of a planned procedure. Or the child may undergo a procedure that causes pain. All of these situations can cause the child to experience fear and anxiety related to the unknown.

Separation Anxiety

Separation anxiety is anxiety that is experienced when a child is away from her parents or guardians. It is a normal stage of development that occurs during infancy and toddlerhood as the child becomes familiar with her surroundings and develops trust as she is being cared for by the parents or guardians. The infant learns to recognize that her parents are safe and familiar. Separation anxiety peaks between the ages of 8 and 18 months, when the child becomes frightened in new situations or with new people. However, over time, the child learns that the parent keeps coming back, allowing the anxiety and fear to subside. As a result, the child begins to develop self-confidence. Separation anxiety usually disappears by the end of the toddler's second year.

Children can re-experience separation anxiety when they are faced with unfamiliar situations that cause stress. These situations lead the child to seek the safety, comfort, protection and familiarity of the parent or guardian. However, if the parent or guardian is not present, the child experiences upset and distress and may go through the three stages of separation anxiety (Table 21-1).

Loss of Control

Consider a child's usual routine. He usually follows a similar routine each day, such as getting up and getting dressed, eating meals, participating in activities and going to school or day care. As the child grows, his level of independence in the routine increases, for example, bathing and dressing himself. The child also begins to make decisions, such as what he wants to eat and wear or what activities to do. The child is developing a sense of control over himself and his surroundings. Unfortunately, illness, injury or hospitalization can disrupt the child's routine and sense of control. The child often feels threatened by the loss, which leads to further anxiety and fear.

Because of the effects of the illness or injury and the routines of the facility, an ill, injured or hospitalized child often cannot decide what he wants to do and when. For example, a child who was injured may be required to remain in bed to allow the injury to heal. As a result, the child can no longer use the bathroom. Instead, the child must use a bedpan for elimination and get washed at the bedside. Additionally, he may be unable to perform the care independently and will need to rely on others for help.

Loss of control is also reflected in decisions involving the body. Treatments and procedures often are necessary. In most cases, the child's parents or guardians, not the child, are involved in the decision making along with the health care team. As a result, the child has little input. Additionally, many of these procedures or treatments are invasive, causing trauma to the child.

When children feel a loss of control, they often demonstrate **regression**, or a return to a previous stage of development. Regression is one of the ways that a child copes. For example, a toddler who has achieved toilet training may regress or go back to using diapers. A preschooler who is able to feed himself may need to be fed his meals.

FACTORS AFFECTING A CHILD'S RESPONSE TO ILLNESS, INJURY AND HOSPITALIZATION

Each child responds to illness, injury or hospitalization differently based on a variety of factors. These factors include the child's developmental level; previous experiences with injury, illness or hospitalization; recent stresses and changes; and the family's response to the situation. In addition, a child's response can be affected by whether the condition is acute or chronic.

Developmental Level

A child responds to situations such as illness or hospitalization based on his developmental level (Table 21-2). The child's ability to think and understand what is happening around him influences how he perceives the actual situation. This perception, in turn, affects how the child responds. For example,

Table 21-1 Stages of Separation Anxiety

Stage	Description
Protest	■ Occurs when the child is initially separated from the parent or guardian. ■ The child may respond by crying or becoming very agitated, upset or angry. The child may be inconsolable and reject the attempts of those who try to console the child. ■ Lasts for several hours to several days.
Despair	■ Results from parents' or guardians' failure to return within a short time. ■ The child feels hopeless and withdraws from others. The child may be quiet without crying and loses interest in activities such as playing or eating.
Denial (Detachment)	■ Most commonly occurs with long-term separation. ■ The child begins to develop coping mechanisms to prevent further emotional pain. The child begins to show interest in activities and the environment, and begins to interact and form relationships with others. The child may ignore parents or guardians if they return.

Table 21-2 **Common Fears and Responses to Illness, Injury or Hospitalization by Developmental Stage**

Stage	Characteristics	Common Fears and Responses to Illness, Injury or Hospitalization
Infancy (birth to age 1 year)	■ Awareness of parent's or guardian's presence and absence	■ Separation anxiety related to the absence of parent or guardian
Toddlerhood (age 1 to 3 years)	■ Exploration, curiosity and independence	■ Loss of control, insecurity, separation anxiety ○ Regression (return to a previous comfortable stage) to cope with stress ○ Inability to talk about fears or understand what is happening ○ Pleading, temper tantrums ■ Fear of strangers
Preschoolers (age 3 to 5 years)	■ Egocentric thinking (belief that he or she did something to cause the problem) ■ Magical thinking (fantasies, imagination, creativity) ■ Literal interpretation of words	■ Fear of body mutilation (for example, "cutting off" a body part), or fear of invasive procedures ■ Loss of control leading to fantasy thinking ■ Fear of the dark and nighttime ■ Fear of being alone
School-Age (age 5 to 12 years)	■ Confidence through development of skills and abilities ■ Increased ability to understand reasons and explanations	■ Fear of disability and death ■ Fear of injury and pain ■ Loss of control
Adolescence (age 12 to 20 years)	■ Egocentric with feelings of invincibility ■ Questioning of authority ■ Emphasis on body image and perceptions ■ Independence ■ Self-assertion ■ Desire for privacy and confidentiality	■ Fear of injury ■ Fear of pain ■ Fear of disability, change in body appearance ■ Loss of control ■ Separation anxiety (from peers)

a preschooler is egocentric (that is, the child is centered on himself). In addition, preschoolers often engage in "magical thinking." The stress associated with illness or hospitalization often leads the preschooler to imagine that he did something to cause the problem. The preschooler also has limited understanding of words and is unable to tell the difference between sound-alike words or words with double meanings. For example, the words "dye" and "die" sound alike but mean totally different things. The preschooler may hear the word "dye" but interpret it as "die." Consider the word "dressing." As an adult and a nurse assistant, you know that "dressing" could refer to clothing or to bandaging. However, a preschooler does not have this ability. The child may wonder why he or she is going to be naked or without clothes, when in fact, the child's bandage is being changed. This misinterpretation adds to the stress that the child is already experiencing.

Previous Experiences

A previous experience with illness, injury or hospitalization can go a long way in helping a child deal with a current similar situation. This is true if the experience was a positive one. For example, a child's previous experience with a hospital may have been for the birth of a little brother or sister, which would be viewed as a positive experience. Thus the child may think back on that time and experience less stress when faced with her own current situation.

However, a previous negative experience, such as one involving a serious illness or the death of a loved one, would most likely be viewed as negative, leading the child to perceive the current situation negatively as well. The child may respond by kicking, screaming, crying loudly, clinging to her parents or having a temper tantrum. Or the child may push others away and withdraw into herself.

You need to measure Javier's vital signs. As you approach him, you explain that you are going to take his temperature. Javier puts out his arms and shouts, "Go away!" His mother says, "He's been through so much lately. Between all the questions, exams and tests, I think he's about had it."

What could you do to address Javier's response while completing your task for measuring his vital signs?

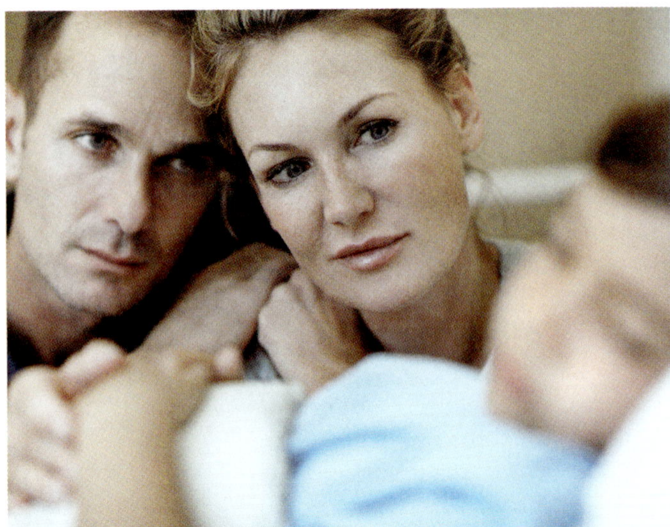

Figure 21-1 Illness in a child creates a crisis for the family.
© iStockPhoto.com/Abel Mitja Varela

Recent Stresses and Changes

A child who is ill or injured already may be experiencing numerous changes and stresses that further affect his ability to cope with the situation. Children are vulnerable because they lack physical and emotional maturity. This vulnerability increases as stresses and changes increase. For example, a child with a serious illness may have to be hospitalized in an intensive care unit. In addition to coping with the stress of the illness, the child also must cope with environmental stresses, such as bright lights, loud sounds and strange smells. The child's senses may become overloaded. As a result, the child might become irritable, agitated or visibly angry. Or the child might become indifferent or uninterested, and withdraw because he is not able to cope.

Family's Response

Children do not exist in isolation. Rather, caring for children *always* involves caring for the family, which includes parents or other primary caregivers, siblings (brothers and sisters) and members of the extended family. Illness, injury or hospitalization of a child can create a crisis situation for the family (Figure 21-1). All members of the family are affected, as are their roles and routines. Children often look to their parents for clues about what is happening and how to respond. The reactions of parents may range from disbelief, fear, irritability, agitation and anger to guilt, uncertainty, confusion, denial, helplessness and hopelessness. These reactions can be heightened by other stresses, such as financial problems, separation from the rest of the family or just the physical and emotional stress that accompanies any illness.

The responses of siblings, like those of the ill or injured child, vary based on the child's developmental stage. Consider a hospitalized school-aged child with a sister who is a preschooler. The sister may have wished for the older child to "go away." With the older child's hospitalization, the preschooler's wish came true. Subsequently, the preschooler may actually believe that she caused the situation and feel guilty for doing so.

Additionally, the sibling may feel neglected because of the focus placed on the ill child. A child's illness can result in separation of family members from one another (for example, if one parent travels with the ill child to a distant hospital to receive specialized treatment, while the other parent stays home with the other children). Even if travel is not involved, the situation of having an ill or injured child will naturally lead to more attention being given to that child. The child's siblings may misinterpret the parents' concern for the ill child, thinking that the ill child is better than or more important than they are. The siblings may be left to feel that they are not loved as much as the ill child. The siblings may become jealous, clingy, demanding or withdrawn.

Moreover, with changes in family routines and roles, siblings may be required to take on additional family responsibilities, such as household chores. Siblings may become angry and possibly come to resent the ill child because of the increased workload or restrictions placed on them. For example, an adolescent sibling might be needed to stay home with an ill brother or sister on a Friday night because both parents are tied up with work. The adolescent is missing a party that all of his friends are attending. As a result, the adolescent is upset at missing the party and blames his ill sibling.

Acute Versus Chronic Illness

Children often face illnesses or injuries that are acute, such as a broken arm. For most children, that means the condition arises suddenly, requires some type of treatment, and then resolves and disappears. However, many children are faced with chronic illness. Chronic illness is commonly defined as any health problem that lasts over 3 months. Examples of common chronic illnesses in children include asthma, diabetes, cerebral palsy, sickle cell anemia, epilepsy and congenital heart conditions. In addition, acute conditions, such as a traumatic injury to the brain or spinal cord, may lead to problems that require long-term follow up and treatment.

A child with a chronic illness typically has times when he feels well and times when he feels ill. However, even during the periods when the child feels well, he is living and dealing with the illness. He must cope with the understanding that the condition is lifelong, permanent, possibly incurable in some cases, and may get worse over time.

Chronic illness affects the child in numerous ways. Children with chronic illnesses often need frequent visits to physicians or other primary care providers for follow-up to evaluate their condition. They also may require more frequent testing, which may be painful or frightening. The need for frequent testing and follow-up can impact the child's school attendance, leading to missed time at school and at school activities. Strict schedules such as for medications or procedures may take priority over routine childhood activities. In addition, certain restrictions may lead to the child's being unable to participate in certain activities, such as sports or school field trips. As a result, the child may feel different and begin to withdraw from others. This adds to further isolation and loneliness.

Chronic illness also places a tremendous amount of stress on parents and families. Parents and families must learn about the illness and come to terms with it. This may be especially difficult if the illness is inherited. Parents may be overwhelmed with guilt, as they are the "cause" of the illness. To compensate for the guilt, they may respond by overprotecting the child.

Family routines are disrupted because the focus is on the ill child. Parents may inadvertently neglect one another as they care for the ill child, becoming overly fatigued and overstressed. Parents also may inadvertently neglect other children in the home or they may have unrealistic expectations for them. Siblings often "blend into the woodwork" unless they demand attention. At times, siblings may act out to get attention.

CARING FOR INFANTS AND CHILDREN

Two major concepts provide the foundation for the care of infants and children: family-centered care and atraumatic care. **Family-centered care** emphasizes an open, working relationship among health care providers, the child and family members. Important components of family-centered care include open 24-hour visitation to the hospital unit, sibling involvement, family conferences, family presence during procedures and family participation in care and decision making. Although decision making involves input from the health care team, the family is ultimately in control of the decisions that are made on behalf of the child.

Atraumatic care is care that focuses on reducing the negative effects associated with illness and injury by minimizing the physical and emotional stress the child and family members experience. Atraumatic care focuses on three areas:

- Identifying stresses for the child and family
- Minimizing the separation of the child from parents or guardians
- Minimizing or preventing pain

As a nurse assistant working with children, you will be involved in promoting family-centered, atraumatic care.

Addressing Overall Childhood Reactions

Children, regardless of their age, become frightened and anxious in new situations. For many children, experiencing illness, injury or hospitalization is a new experience. You can help reduce these feelings by being attentive to the child and family and by promoting a sense of control in the child and family. Table 21-3 summarizes some actions that you can take to address the child's fear, anxiety and loss of control.

Addressing Responses Developmentally

Each child is unique in his or her responses. Those responses are, in part, determined by the child's developmental level. When you are providing care to an ill, injured or hospitalized child, you need to adapt your care based on the stage of the child's development and his or her primary fears.

Table 21-3 **Managing Common Childhood Reactions to Illness, Injury or Hospitalization**

Stage	Fear and Anxiety	Separation Anxiety	Loss of Control
Infants	■ Hold and snuggle the infant closely, rock gently, cuddle. ■ Talk soothingly and gently to the infant, use music. ■ Ask to be consistently assigned to the infant.	■ Encourage parents to room-in if possible. ■ Play peek-a-boo to help infant understand separation.	■ Offer pacifier. ■ Snuggle, cuddle or hold infant close. ■ Change environment periodically—take infant to playroom or nurse's station.
Toddlers/ Preschoolers	■ Ask parents to bring in a familiar item from home that the child likes. ■ Allow the child to express feelings through play such as drawing, hammering on a workbench or throwing a ball.	■ Urge parents to room-in. ■ Use time frames the child understands to explain the absence of parents or guardians, such as "your parents will return when *Sponge Bob* is over." ■ Use play to act out parents leaving and returning.	■ Allow child choices when possible (for example, orange juice or apple juice, or whether to go to the playroom before or after lunch). ■ Try to stick to usual home routines as much as possible, such as bedtime rituals.
School-Age Children	■ Encourage the child to talk about how she is feeling. ■ Listen to the child and be supportive.	■ Encourage parents to allow friends and siblings to visit. ■ Encourage the child to call, chat or text with friends and siblings.	■ Reinforce explanations by other health care staff about condition; if possible allow child to handle equipment being used. ■ Encourage the child to participate in tasks, such as counting the number of cups of water she drinks.
Adolescents	■ Encourage the adolescent to talk about how he is feeling. ■ Be honest when talking with the adolescent. ■ Arrange for the adolescent to interact with others of the same age.	■ Encourage the adolescent to talk and interact with peers.	■ Encourage parent visitation. ■ Include the adolescent in decisions about care and activities; offer choices if possible. ■ Ensure privacy.

Infants

Typically infants experience fear, anxiety, loss of control and separation anxiety. When providing care to infants, be consistent. Learn to recognize the infant's cues and respond accordingly. For example, change the infant's diaper or offer the infant a bottle when she cries. Doing so allows the infant to develop trust that someone is there to meet her needs. As a result, the infant may experience less stress and thus less trauma.

An infant experiences satisfaction through sucking. However, the infant may not be allowed anything by mouth. In these situations, offer a pacifier to satisfy her needs. A pacifier can help to calm and soothe the infant as well as meet her need for sucking.

Separation anxiety is an issue during infancy, regardless of whether the infant is ill or well. It can become more significant if illness, injury or hospitalization causes the infant to be away from his parents or guardians for any period of time. For example, the parents may be unable to stay with the infant during hospitalization because they have to care for other children at home. Or the facility may be a long distance from home. To minimize distress for the infant, encourage the parents or guardians to room-in with the infant if at all possible. If not, encourage the parents or guardians to visit frequently and participate in the infant's care as much as possible. As you provide care to the infant, allow the infant to keep the parents in view. Talk with the parent so that you can learn what the infant's cues are so that you can respond accordingly. Also, ask the nurse to assign you to care for the infant so that she receives consistent care and is exposed to the fewest number of caregivers as possible.

Toddlers

Caring for a toddler can be challenging because the toddler needs structure and routine. However, toddlers also need to be able to explore their surroundings to satisfy their curiosity. Toddlers are attempting to establish their independence as they explore the world around them. Thus, a loss of control is a major issue for this age group. In addition, toddlers have a fear of strangers.

Always introduce yourself to the child and explain your role in terms that the child can understand. Use simple, concrete terms and speak to the child at his eye level. However, do not be surprised if the toddler does not respond immediately to you. Remember, he views you as a stranger. In addition, try to follow the child's normal routines. Perhaps the child has a snack of milk and cookies before going to bed. Or his parents read him a bedtime story. Regardless of what the routine is, try to follow it, if possible, because you will be helping to restore the toddler's feeling of control.

Toddlers, although able to talk, have difficulty putting their feelings into words. In addition, their ability to understand what is happening to them is limited. As a result, they may act out, have temper tantrums or regress to a previous level of functioning to cope. You can help the toddler cope with the situation by spending time with the toddler and helping him understand what is happening. Use the child's natural sense of curiosity at this stage as an aid (Figure 21-2). For example, allow the child to handle or touch the stethoscope before taking vital signs. The child can pretend to listen to his own heart or the heart of a doll. Or let the child put a bandage on the arm of a stuffed toy or doll before or after an invasive procedure. Additionally, you can encourage the child to play with things that he routinely plays with when well. For example, if the child enjoys miniature cars or has a favorite doll, have the parents bring the toy to the hospital with the child. Not only does this bring the child pleasure, it also helps to promote some consistency, which helps the child to feel as if he has some control over the situation.

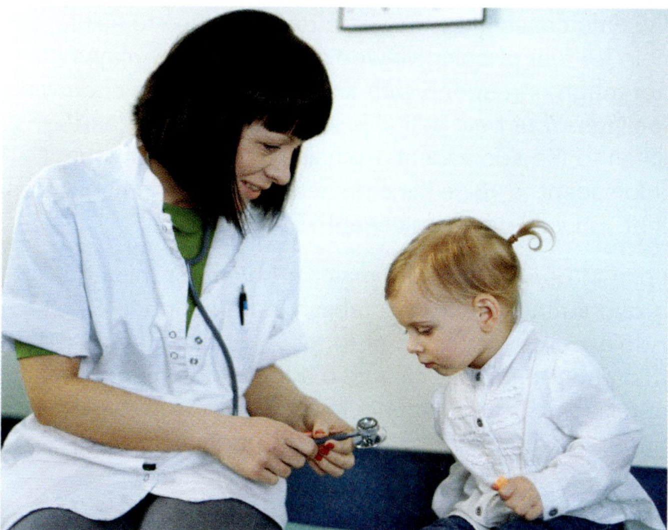

Figure 21-2 Letting a toddler handle equipment satisfies the toddler's natural curiosity and fosters a sense of control. © *iStockPhoto.com/ Anna Zielinska*

You talk with Javier and his mother about the need to drink more fluids. His mother says, "Usually he loves apple juice and iced tea, but today, he's been really fussy."

Based on Javier's age, how could you get him to participate in drinking more fluids? Would your actions promote Javier's dignity and independence? Why or why not?

Preschoolers

Preschoolers are engaged in fantasy and creativity and have a view of the world as revolving around them. Their level of understanding is better than that of a toddler. As a result, they can probably understand that they are sick. However, they are usually unable to understand the cause of the illness or injury or the issues involved. They take information literally. So, when talking with the child, use words that the child will understand and avoid words that sound alike, such as "die" and "dye," or that have double meanings. Think about the word "stool." To you, it would probably imply a bowel movement. However, a preschooler would interpret "stool" to mean a small chair. In this case, use words that would be familiar to the child, such as "poop." Find out from the child's parents what words the child typically uses for routine activities such as going to the bathroom, eating lunch or going to bed.

Preschoolers have a fear of body mutilation. When caring for a child who will need invasive procedures, assist with preparing the child beforehand. Keep the information simple, direct and honest, remembering that this age group interprets things literally. Do not tell the child that the test or procedure will not hurt if it will. Instead, let the child know what she might feel (for example, some pressure, a short pinch or tightness). Work with the nurse on how to minimize the child's risk for pain. As with toddlers, encourage the preschooler to "play" with any materials or equipment that may be used. When appropriate, allow the child to make simple decisions about her care, such as picking out an adhesive bandage to place over the site or choosing a special snack. Doing so promotes feelings of control.

Children in this age group enjoy pretending. Encourage the child to express her feelings through play with dolls, stuffed toys or puppets. Preschoolers will often talk through puppets or dolls as a safe way to express their feelings. Drawing or coloring is also helpful in encouraging the child to express her feelings.

Fear of the dark and nighttime are common fears in this age group. Adhere to the child's typical bedtime routine as much as possible. Reading the child a story or offering the child a small snack may be helpful. Keep a small nightlight on or dim the lights for sleep. If the child is hospitalized, keep the room door slightly ajar to allow light from the hallway to enter, but close blinds or curtains on windows to prevent any strange reflections or sights.

School-age children

School-age children are developing increased self-confidence as they participate in the school environment and expand their skills and abilities. In addition, their ability to understand information, reasons and explanations is growing. They are expanding socially, both with friends and interests. Illness, injury or hospitalization can limit this expansion.

When caring for school-age children, remember that they are gaining confidence in their abilities and like to be involved. They have the mental ability to understand what is happening and are able to follow directions. Talk with the child, using terms that he will understand. Answer the child's questions honestly. Never make promises or statements that you cannot support. If a child asks you a question for which you do not know the answer, be honest and tell the child that you do not know but that you will talk with the nurse and find out. Doing so will help to develop trust with the child and reduce fears of injury, pain and disability.

Encourage the child to participate in his care. Break down tasks into simple steps that the child can accomplish to promote feelings of confidence and control. In addition, allow the child to make decisions about his care. For example, encourage the school-age child to choose what foods he wants to eat based on his specific diet. Let the child decide if he wants to get washed before or after breakfast.

School-age children like to demonstrate their independence but may have difficulty if they need help with something that they previously were able to do by themselves. In these situations, allow the child to do as much as he can for himself. Focus on the child's ability to perform the task, rather than on the fact that he needed assistance. For example, you can tell the child, "You really did well getting dressed this morning. We couldn't have gotten your arm through the pajama sleeve without your help." Offer praise and rewards for activities and tasks well done.

Friends and peers are important to the school-age child. Encourage the child to talk with his friends as often as possible and to have his friends visit. If access to the Internet is available, encourage social networking or visual websites, such as Skype, to maintain contact. If the child is hospitalized, arrange for the child to meet other children of the same age. The facility's activity room (often called a playroom) may be the optimal place for socializing with other children.

As the school-age child nears the teenage years, privacy becomes an important issue. Respect the child's privacy. Closing the curtain around his bed, closing the door and knocking before entering the bathroom are some common examples.

Adolescents

Adolescents are striving for identity, questioning authority and feeling invincible. They are struggling between wanting to be treated as adults while still having some fears about being completely independent. Body image and how they are perceived by others are very important to them. As a result, adolescents can become very distressed by injury or disability, especially if the illness or injury causes a change in body image. Additionally, they may feel embarrassed and self-conscious about their changing bodies, so make every effort to ensure their privacy. These feelings also may arise when adolescents need assistance with tasks such as bathing. In some cases, they may be afraid or refuse to ask for help for fear of being viewed as a child. They may try to act tough or respond with anger to hide these underlying feelings. Your best action is to provide support and listen to the adolescent. Remain impartial. Allow the adolescent to voice his opinions. Doing so demonstrates that you value the adolescent as an individual.

Loss of control is also a major problem for this age group as they work to establish independence. Adolescents may attempt to test limits as they assert their independence. Maintain a firm yet nonjudgmental approach. As adolescents mature, their level of understanding about abstract concepts improves. Therefore, explain the rules with the adolescent and reinforce those that are absolute. Discuss behavioral issues with the nurse, and together with the adolescent, work together on finding a way to meet the adolescent's needs while following necessary rules. The adolescent age group places a high value on peer relationships (Figure 21-3). Illness, injury or hospitalization can isolate the adolescent from friends.

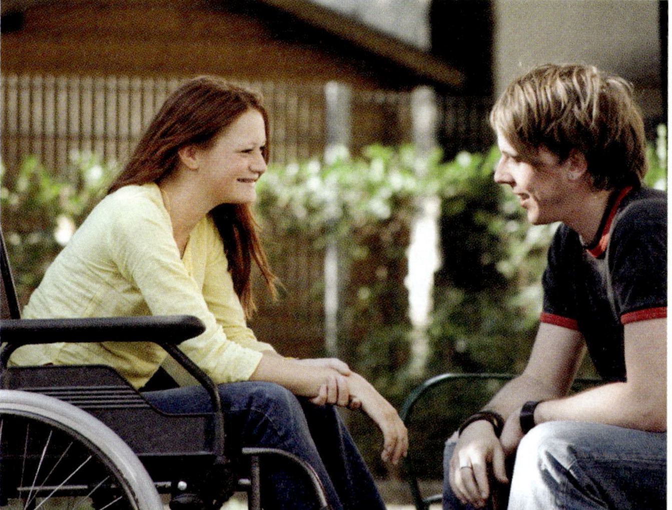

Figure 21-3 Peer relationships are extremely important to an adolescent. © *iStockPhoto.com/franz pfluegl*

Use similar techniques as you would for a school-age child to promote social interaction and contact with peers.

Maintaining Safety

Children are constantly growing and, as they become more mobile and agile, they become more vulnerable to injury. Therefore safety of the child is extremely important. Each age group faces different risks to safety. Box 21-1 summarizes some of these risks and what you can do to ensure the child's safety.

Promoting Play

Play is often referred to as a "child's work." It provides the child with a mechanism for coping, learning and trying out new skills. Unstructured play includes activities that the child routinely engages in to have fun, such as playing with blocks, stuffed animals, coloring books, videos, and board or video games. With this type of play, the child is in control and the

Box 21-1 **Tips for Ensuring Safety**

Each stage of growth and development poses different characteristic safety challenges.

Infants

- Never leave an infant unattended on a surface, even for a second. Always keep the infant in your sight, with at least one hand on the infant at all times. Infants can easily roll and fall.
- Always double-check the safety straps when placing an infant in an infant carrier, swing or high chair. Make sure the straps are securely fastened over the infant's shoulders and around her legs to prevent the infant from sliding down or falling out.
- Be sure to lock the wheels of a stroller.
- Keep the rails of the crib up at all times, and keep the crib free of any pillows. Use only a tight-fitting bottom sheet in the crib.
- Make sure that a protective covering is over the crib (when hospitalized) for an infant over the age of 6 months.
- Remove any mobiles from the crib if the child is 5 months of age or older or if the child can sit up and reach the mobile.
- Use only age-appropriate toys with an infant. Remember that infants like to put everything in their mouths. Be sure that toys have no small parts that can be removed (even inadvertently).

Toddlers and Preschoolers

- Keep sharp objects; small, hard objects; and balloons out of the child's reach. Toddlers and preschoolers still have a tendency to put things in their mouths.
- Maintain a close eye on toddlers and preschoolers. Keep in mind that toddlers are extremely curious and like to go anywhere their legs will take them as they explore their environment.
- Briefly explain the rules in terms that the child will understand. Preschoolers are beginning to learn the difference between right and wrong.
- If the child is in a bed, use side rails to prevent falls.
- Always secure the child in a wheelchair, stroller or other device.
- Never leave the child unattended in the bathtub.
- Make sure that the foods being served to the child are appropriate for the child's age and chewing ability.

School-Age Children

- Review the safety rules for the child, including any issues that may affect his mobility and getting around from place to place.
- Supervise play activities to prevent injury.
- Review safety related to strangers.
- Keep head-of-the-bed side rails up when the child is in bed.

Adolescents

- Remind adolescents of safety rules.

play acts as a diversion. Remember to make sure that the play is appropriate for the child's age and level of development.

Therapeutic play is goal-directed by another person, such as the nurse, to assist the child in coping with her illness, injury or hospitalization. It also provides the child with information to reduce the stress of the unknown. For example, a child is scheduled to undergo an invasive procedure. The nurse uses a doll to explain the procedure to the child. The child then is encouraged to act out the procedure on the doll while the nurse watches (Figure 21-4). As a nurse assistant, you can continue to reinforce what the child learned through the play experience and also encourage the child to continue to play out the procedure (with supervision).

You can also incorporate play into tasks and activities you perform with the child. For example, you may ask a child who needs to improve his lung function to participate in a game of blowing cotton balls across a table. You can set a goal distance that you want the child to reach. Each time the child blows, he can attempt to reach the spot. When he does, you can offer the child a reward. A child with a broken leg can maintain upper body strength by tossing a soft sponge ball back and forth with you. Without realizing it, the child is exercising his arm muscles. In addition, such activity helps to divert the child's attention away from his condition.

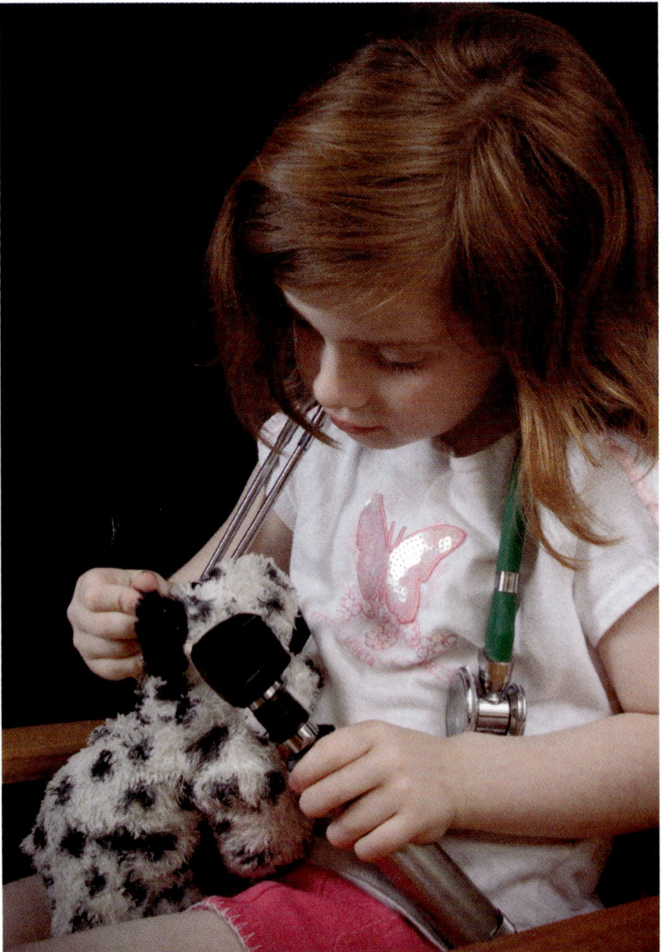

Figure 21-4 Therapeutic play can help a young child work out anxiety and concerns related to a treatment or procedure. © *iStockPhoto.com/ Lisa Eastman*

Assisting Family Members

Having an ill, injured or hospitalized child can create a crisis situation for the family. All members of the family are affected, as are their roles and routines. As a nurse assistant, you can help the family by being an active listener. Allow the parents and siblings to talk about how they are feeling. Sometimes just allowing a person to talk helps to promote positive steps to coping.

Be honest with the family. If they ask you a question who you do not know the answer to, explain that you do not know but will do your best to find out.

Encourage active participation in the child's care. Emphasize to the parents that they are the ones who know their child the best. Ask them to share with you any specifics about the child's likes or dislikes so that you can provide the child with the best possible care. Parents will most likely feel more in control when sharing this information.

Encourage siblings, too, to talk about how they are feeling and what effect the child's condition is having on them. Also encourage frequent visitation, if appropriate (Figure 21-5). Visiting can help correct misunderstandings about the severity of the child's condition and the cause. However, remember to respect a sibling's wishes and feelings if he does not want to visit.

Talk with the nurse about what you observe with the family. It may be necessary to have the family speak with a social worker or counselor or be referred to a support group.

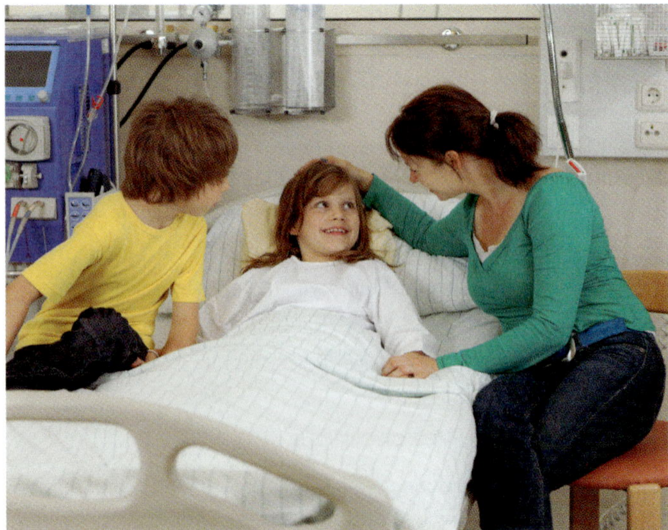

Figure 21-5 Visits from siblings can benefit both the ill child and the sibling. © *iStockPhoto.com/amriphoto*

SPECIFIC CARE RESPONSIBILITIES

Obtaining Vital Signs and Other Measurements

Obtaining vital signs of infants and children is similar to that of adults. However, you will likely need to make some modifications for a child. You may need to have the parent or guardian hold the infant or small toddler in his or her lap. If the toddler is fidgety, it may be easier to take the vital sign measurements with the parent sitting on the floor, with the toddler standing between his or her legs. Normal ranges for vital signs by age group are given in Box 21-2.

Temperature

Recall that there are several methods for measuring a person's temperature. The method used for measuring an infant's or child's temperature is often determined by the child's condition and your employer's policies. Check with the nurse to determine the most appropriate method for temperature measurement.

A rectal temperature may be used for any child up to 5 years of age (though other routes may be preferred or more readily accepted in some children). Once the child is about 4 years old, the oral route may be used because most children this age can hold the thermometer under their tongue. Tympanic thermometers should only be used for children 6 months of age and older. Temporal artery thermometers, which are swept across the forehead to obtain a temperature reading, deliver accurate temperature measurement in children over 3 months of age, if appropriately used. The axillary method may also be an option. Be sure to use the least traumatic method possible for the child. For example, a 6-month-old infant may be upset, crying and extremely fidgety. Using the rectal route to obtain the temperature would cause further upset. In addition, there is a danger of injury to the infant if the rectal route is used, because of the child's fidgeting. In this case, measuring tympanic temperature may be less traumatic for the child. As with adults, do not take a rectal temperature if a child has diarrhea or has had rectal surgery.

To take an infant's rectal temperature, position the baby on her back. Hold the ankles up with one hand and bend the knees to expose the anus. With the

Box 21-2 **Normal Ranges for Vital Sign Measurements in Children**

Normal Temperature Ranges

Route	Age 0–2 Years	Age 3–10 Years	Over Age 11 Years
Oral	N/A	95.9–99.5°F	97.6–99.6°F
Rectal	97.9–100.4°F	97.9–100.4°F	98.6–100.6°F
Tympanic	97.5–100.0°F	97.0–100.0°F	96.6–99.7°F
Axillary	94.5–99.1°F	96.6–98.0°F	95.3–98.4°F

Normal Pulse Rate Ranges

Age	Normal Range (beats/min)
0–3 months	100–150
3–6 months	90–120
6–12 months	80–120
1–3 years	70–110
3–6 years	65–110
6–12 years	60–95
12+ years	55–85

Normal Respiratory Rate Ranges

Age	Normal Range (breaths/min)
0–3 months	35–55
3–6 months	30–45
6–12 months	25–40
1–3 years	20–30
3–6 years	20–25
6–12 years	14–22
12+ years	12–18

Normal Blood Pressure Ranges

Age	Range (mm Hg)
0–3 months	65–85/45–55
3–6 months	70–90/50–65
6–12 months	80–100/55–65
1–3 years	90–105/55–70
3–6 years	95–110/60–75
6–12 years	100–120/60–75
12+ years	110–135/65–85

other hand, gently insert the tip of the lubricated thermometer probe about ½ inch into the rectum and hold it in place until the digital thermometer beeps. Always hold on to the thermometer while it is in the rectum.

To take a child's rectal temperature, have the child lie on his side with his knees flexed, or have him lie on his stomach. A child may be more likely to cooperate if he is held across his parent's lap while you take his rectal temperature. Be sure to insert the tip of the lubricated probe gently and hold the thermometer in place while the child's temperature is registering.

Whenever possible, use an electronic thermometer to measure the oral temperature of children over the age of 5. Always have the child sit or lie down while taking the temperature and stay with the child to make sure that she remains still.

The normal temperature range for a child is the same as it is for an adult, although a child's temperature may change very rapidly. See Box 21-2 for the normal range of temperatures for different age groups. Young children especially may run very high temperatures. Be sure to report any temperature changes immediately.

Pulse rates

Measure the apical pulse in children younger than 2 years, and be sure to count for 1 full minute (Figure 21-6). The infant or young child is typically afraid of an unfamiliar person, especially a nurse assistant approaching with strange-looking equipment, such as a stethoscope. It is difficult to measure a child's pulse rate when he is crying or upset. Try to enlist the child's cooperation and encourage the parent to hold the child. To help the child relax, let him play with another stethoscope or play a listening game. Because activity can affect the reading, report what the child was doing when you took his pulse. In a child older than 2 years, a radial pulse rate may be obtained. However, it is always more accurate to count an apical pulse for 1 full minute in any child. The average pulse rates for children of different age ranges are given in Box 21-2.

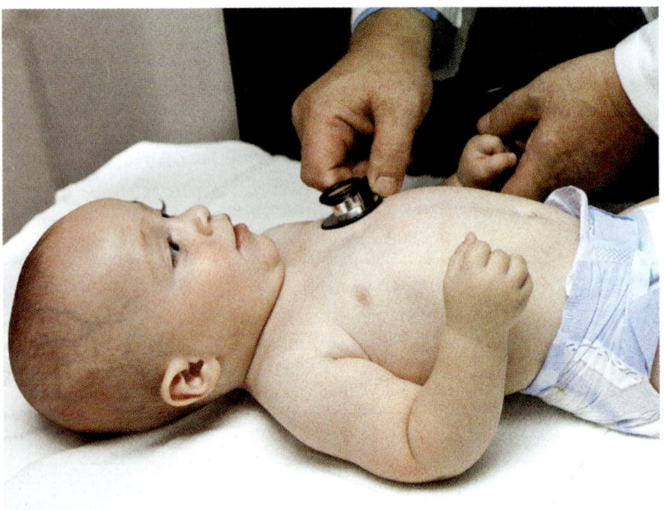

Figure 21-6 An apical pulse is obtained in infants. © *iStockPhoto.com/alle12*

Respirations

For an accurate reading, count a child's respirations while she is quiet or asleep. If you also plan to take a temperature or blood pressure reading, count the respirations *first* in case the child becomes upset and starts to cry. Respiration rates in children are higher than in adults (see Box 21-2) and may be irregular. Be sure to count the respirations for an entire minute. Report any abnormal rate or difficulty breathing.

Blood pressure

In routine health care situations, a child's blood pressure typically is not checked until the child is about 3 years old. However, if the child becomes ill, injured or hospitalized, the child's blood pressure needs to be measured. When you take a child's blood pressure, use the right size cuff. A cuff that is too large gives a reading that is too low. A cuff that is too small gives a reading that is too high. Try to get the child to cooperate during the procedure by using words and concepts that he understands. For example, you may tell the child that the cuff is going to give his arm a "big hug" when you squeeze the black ball. Often it helps if the child sits on his parent's lap or is distracted by a toy. See Box 21-2 for the range of normal or usual blood pressure readings in children. As a group, younger children generally have lower blood pressures than older children do. As with all vital signs in a child, blood pressure readings can change very rapidly. Report even small changes in blood pressure to the nurse. Also, be sure to note the activity of the child while you are taking the blood pressure reading so that the significance of any changes can be evaluated.

Head circumference

Head circumference is another measurement that is routinely obtained in infants and children younger than 3 years. This measurement provides information about the child's brain size and growth. To measure head circumference, you will need a flexible measuring tape that does not stretch. In addition, you need to make sure that the child's hair is unbraided and that decorative hair accessories have been removed. Place the infant or small child in a comfortable position. For example, have the parent hold the infant in his arms, or have the child sit on his lap. Then:

- Position the measuring tape over the biggest part on the back of the head and encircle the head, with the tape positioned just above the eyebrows and ears.
- Pull the tape snugly and read the measurement to the nearest 0.1 cm or 1/8 inch.
- Record your measurement.

Head circumference measurements are usually plotted on a standard growth chart, compared with age and monitored as the child grows.

Meeting Hygiene Needs

When assisting infants and children with personal care, you may need to adapt your skills to meet the child's developmental stage.

Oral care

Many children have six to eight teeth by the time they are 1 year old. If a child's gums are not too tender from teething, use a moist cloth or gauze square wrapped around your finger to gently clean the teeth. If the child is older than 1 year, use a very soft toothbrush dipped in water. Hold the child on your lap to provide comfort and security.

Fluoridated toothpastes are recommended for all children. Keep toothpaste out of reach of young children, and ensure that the child uses the correct amount of toothpaste. For children younger than 2 years, only a smear of toothpaste should be used. Children between the ages of 2 and 5 years may use a small, pea-sized amount. For school-age children at high risk, dentists may recommend daily use of a fluoride mouth rinse to reduce the possibility of tooth decay; however, use of a fluoride rinse is not recommended for all children.

Children usually like to try brushing their own teeth, and it is important to encourage their independence by letting them do so. However, they usually are not able to clean their teeth effectively until the age of 6 to 10 years. Before that age, an adult should brush the child's teeth, and the child should be encouraged to brush his own teeth either before or after the parent's brushing. He should brush for at least 2 minutes. Use a timer to let the child know when the 2 minutes have passed and to make brushing a fun time for him. Children should brush their teeth two to three times a day, making sure to brush just before bedtime.

You can brush a child's teeth when the child is in bed as you would an adult's teeth. You also can position yourself behind a child who is either seated or standing. Use one hand to cup the child's chin and the other to hold the toothbrush.

If a child is NPO (not eating or drinking by mouth), brush his teeth twice each day with a soft toothbrush dipped in water or toothpaste. Because some medicines are heavily sweetened to improve their taste, the teeth should be brushed or the mouth rinsed with water after the child takes these medications. The teeth should also be brushed after vomiting to remove gastric fluids that can wear away tooth enamel. If using the toothbrush causes an ill child to gag, have him rinse his mouth with water and spit it out.

A toothbrush with a large or curved handle or self-adhesive fabric fasteners may be easier for a child with a physical impairment to hold. An electric toothbrush also may be useful.

Bathing

When helping a child to bathe, it is important for you to know the age, developmental stage and capabilities of the child so that you can safely and appropriately provide care. Generally, older and adolescent children are very concerned about privacy, and younger children enjoy playing at bath time.

Safety is the most important thing to keep in mind while bathing children. Never leave a child alone in water. Check the water carefully to make sure that it is between 95° F and 100° F (or just warm on the inside of your wrist). Fill the tub no more than one-third full, and turn the hot water off first. Instruct the child, if it is appropriate, not to turn on the hot water faucet by himself. To prevent falls, make sure nonskid mats are in the tub. Also helpful are safety rails or specially designed seats to support the child who cannot sit by himself. Do not use bath oils in the tub, because they make the tub and the child slippery and hard to hold on to.

If you have to help a child into a tub, be sure to use good body mechanics. If the child is small, bend your knees to squat and lower the child into the tub. Avoid bending over from the waist. If the child weighs more than 35 pounds, an assistive device for lifting the child into and out of the bathtub is recommended.

A large tub may be awkward, uncomfortable and unsafe for bathing a small infant. In a home setting, you may use an infant tub on a table top as an alternative. To hold an infant, place one arm under his neck and back and hold on to the arm on the side farther away from your body. This position gives you a firm grip on the infant and helps to make him feel more secure. Use your other hand to support the buttocks. Gradually lower the infant into the water so that he has a chance to become accustomed to the water temperature and so that he is not startled by the water.

Use one hand to wash an infant or small child who cannot sit without support while holding and supporting him with your other hand. Wash from top to bottom, rinsing each part as you go so that the child does not become too slippery. Also, as with adults, soap is very drying to the skin and may cause vaginal irritation in girls. Use soap sparingly and do not let it soak in the bath water. To keep the child warm, wrap him in a towel as soon as you remove him from the tub. Then help him get dressed.

Toddlers generally enjoy playing with unbreakable cups and toys in the bath. Provide time for play if possible, but do not leave the child alone. Older children and adolescents, on the other hand, may have strong feelings about privacy, and as you would with adults, you should make every effort to give them privacy as long as you can do so safely.

Use the same basic procedure that you would use to bathe an adult in bed when you give a bed bath to an older child or adolescent or help him with a tub bath or shower.

Hair care

Periodically comb a child's hair to remove tangles and prevent them from becoming worse. You may need to comb the hair more often if the child is confined to bed, because lying in bed can cause the hair to become matted and tangled. Some children love to have their hair combed, while others do not want to be bothered. As the child gets older, combing is an important part of building good grooming habits and promoting healthy self-esteem.

You can use a commercial detangling solution to remove tangles from a child's hair. If one is not available, first wet the hair and then apply conditioner to the tangle, which makes the hair shafts slippery. Applying conditioner often enables you to remove the tangle painlessly with combing. Start combing at the ends of the hair and work your way toward the scalp. When you have removed the tangles either rinse the conditioner out of that section of hair or give the child a total shampoo.

Typically a young child needs her hair shampooed once or twice a week. However, specific conditions such as excessive sweating may necessitate more frequent shampooing. Adolescents may wish to shampoo their hair more frequently because the scalp produces more oil at this stage of development. Shampooing can be done during the bath or separately.

For an infant, apply baby shampoo to the scalp with one hand, while you support him as you did when you lowered him into the tub. Tip the infant back so that water and shampoo do not run into his eyes. Rinse out the shampoo by using the washcloth or an unbreakable cup to pour water over his head.

If a child is confined to his bed, wash his hair in the bed using the same procedure you use for an adult. Encourage the child to help by holding a washcloth or towel over his eyes. Wrap the child's head in a towel immediately after the last rinse and follow instructions from the nurse about using a blow dryer to dry his hair. Alternatively, you can use a commercial dry shampoo. The powder-like substance is applied to the hair and then brushed out.

Perineal care

If the child is capable, allow the child to perform her own perineal care and ensure the child's privacy. Provide the child with the necessary supplies and offer assistance as needed.

For children who wear diapers, it is important to clean the perineal area thoroughly to remove all traces of urine and feces from the skin. Be sure to observe the condition of the skin as you clean the area, and report any signs of redness or skin irritation. Wear gloves when you provide perineal care.

If a boy has been circumcised, clean the tip of his penis using strokes moving outward from the urethra. Use only a minimal amount of soap, and rinse thoroughly. If the child is uncircumcised, gently retract the foreskin until you feel resistance (the foreskin usually cannot be retracted fully until about the age of 4), and using a clean section of the washcloth, clean around the tip of the penis, moving from the urethra outward. Rinse in the same pattern and dry well. Be sure to return the foreskin to its original position because leaving the foreskin retracted may interfere with circulation in the head of the penis. After washing and rinsing the penis, clean the scrotum and then the anal area.

When providing perineal care for a girl, wash any skin folds in the groin first. Then, using a separate section of the washcloth, clean the urethral area and then each side of the labia, moving from front to back. Use soap sparingly and rinse thoroughly. After washing and rinsing the urethral area and the labia, clean the anal area. Be sure to remove all secretions, because they can cause skin irritation. Observe the skin for any abrasions or changes in skin color. Report any concerns to the nurse.

Ensuring Nutrition

Good nutrition often is influenced by food habits acquired in childhood. Family food preferences and behaviors strongly influence children's likes, dislikes and eating patterns. Children generally learn to enjoy a wide variety of foods if they are exposed to them in pleasant situations. You can help children in your care establish good eating habits and wholesome attitudes toward food. These attitudes will affect their health throughout their entire lives.

Government food-assistance programs are often available for low-income families. If you provide care for families who are unable to provide their children with a nutritious diet, report this concern to the nurse. The nurse can follow up with appropriate members of the health care team to help the family obtain access to these programs.

In general, healthy infants have good appetites. Children's appetites decrease toward the end of their first year and continue to decrease in their second year as growth slows down. As toddlers, children may show their need for independence by choosing not to eat. Preschool children frequently eat smaller meals and may want to snack between meals. Children who are 3 or 4 years old may eat slowly but generally eat more at one sitting than younger children do. By age 6, most children have developed stable, healthy appetites.

Infants

Infants typically receive feedings of breast milk or formula. Cereal usually is not introduced until the infant is around 5 to 6 months of age. Continue to offer the infant breast milk or formula before any solid meal. Solid food should be a supplement, not a replacement, for breast milk or formula.

When giving an infant cereal, start with 2 tablespoons of rice cereal twice daily and then introduce other single-grain cereals one at a time. Introduce multigrain cereal last. Giving the baby only one new food at a time allows him to get used to the flavor and makes it easier to determine whether he is allergic to any particular type of food. During feedings, the baby may push most of the cereal out of his mouth as a result of the tongue's normal sucking action (Figure 21-7). Use the spoon to gently put the food back into his mouth. To prevent overfeeding or choking, never put cereal into the baby's bottle.

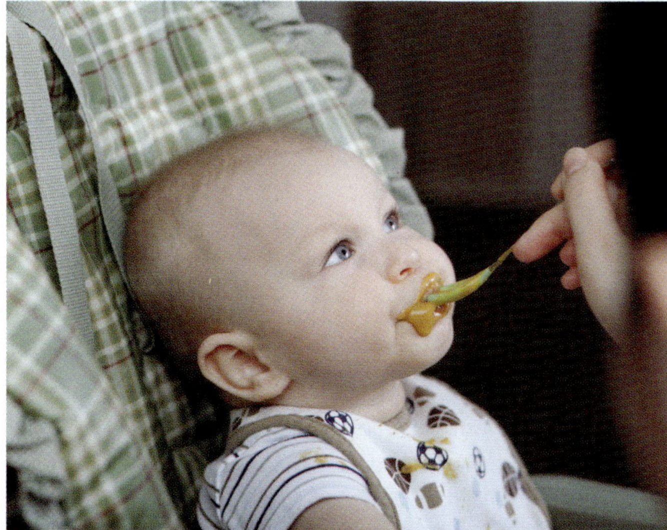

Figure 21-7 Infants often push food back out of the mouth as part of the natural reflex of the tongue. Be patient and gradually put the food back in. © *iStockPhoto.com/ZekaG*

As the infant reaches 6 to 8 months of age, he may begin to hold the bottle of formula. However, you need to continue to hold the infant during feedings to increase his sense of security and to meet his social needs. Gradually, apple and noncitrus juices are introduced one at a time. Solid foods such as strained fruits, vegetables and meats are added. Again, introduce new foods one at a time. When using commercially prepared baby food, spoon a meal-sized portion into a bowl and refrigerate the unused food for up to 24 hours. Feeding the infant directly from the jar introduces bacteria into the jar and contaminates the uneaten portion, which must be thrown away. Never sweeten foods with honey because unpasteurized honey can cause botulism in infants.

Around the age of 9 to 12 months, infants begin to drink liquids from a cup. Continue feeding the child cereal and slowly advance to chunkier toddler foods. During meals, give the child a separate spoon to encourage self-feeding skills. Introduce small finger foods, such as unsugared adult cereals, cooked vegetables and fruits. Avoid giving the child nuts, raw vegetables, popcorn, grapes and hard candy, which can easily lodge in the throat and cause choking. Make sure the child eats foods such as biscuits, toast and crackers while sitting up (never while lying down) to reduce the possibility of choking on crumbs.

Toddlers

Toddlers are beginning to be weaned from bottle or breast-feeding and are getting used to drinking from a cup instead. Remember that the stress of illness or injury can lead a child to regress to a previous behavior. Do not be surprised if a child who was no longer drinking from a bottle begins to do so again.

Milk intake in a toddler typically is limited to 16 to 24 ounces daily to encourage the child to eat solid food. Avoid giving the toddler very spicy foods, which can be hard for a young child to digest. To prevent choking, do not give toddlers small, round or hard foods, such as hot dogs or hard candy. Box 21-3 summarizes the recommendations about foods and choking in children.

Use the child's appetite to gauge how much to serve at mealtime. Typical serving sizes for a 2- to 3-year-old child include 2 to 3 tablespoons of applesauce or cooked vegetables; ¼ of a banana or apple; $^{1}/_{3}$ cup of orange juice; 1 to 2 ounces of meat, fish, or poultry; ½ slice of bread; $^{1}/_{3}$ cup of cooked dry peas, beans or lentils; and 2 to 3 tablespoons of rice or cereal. Make mealtimes fun and encourage the child to use her own cup and spoon while eating. Never force a child to eat or use food as a reward or punishment.

Toddlers are known to be picky eaters. They may eat only one type of food for several days. They also like to "eat

▼ Box 21-3 **Choking in Children: Causative Foods**

The American Academy of Pediatrics (AAP) recommends that young children not be given hard, smooth foods. These foods must be chewed with a grinding motion, which is a skill that children do not master until 4 years of age; therefore, children may attempt to swallow these foods whole. For the same reason, the AAP recommends not giving children peanuts until they are 7 years of age or older. The AAP also recommends that young children not be given round, firm foods such as hot dogs and carrot sticks unless they are chopped into small pieces no larger than ½ inch.

Because food items cause most choking injuries in children, the AAP recommends that these foods be kept away from young children:

- Round, firm food, such as hot dogs and carrot sticks
- Hard, gooey or sticky candy
- Grapes
- Popcorn
- Chewing gum
- Vitamins

and run." Continue to present the child with a balanced diet by offering nutritious between-meal snacks such as cubed cheese and bread or unsalted crackers spread with peanut butter.

Preschoolers

The quality of a preschooler's diet is more important than the quantity. Continue to offer a balanced diet, serving the child approximately 1 tablespoon of each food for each year of age. You may introduce low-fat or skim milk at this time. A preschool child needs the calcium supplied by two to three 8-ounce servings of milk each day but may not be able to drink an entire serving of milk at one time. To make sure the child gets enough calcium, serve milk and dairy products as snacks.

Cheese cut into cubes and served with fruit or crackers makes an ideal snack, as do cheese spreads on crackers or bread. (Avoid serving cream cheese, which is high in fat and is more like butter than cheese.) Cottage cheese with fruit or plain low-fat yogurt with fruit added at home is another good snack choice.

To increase the child's iron and protein intake, include snacks from the meat group. Cut leftover cooked meat into cubes and serve with a fruit or vegetable. Another high-protein snack is hard-cooked eggs served with cheese. Offer sweet, high-fat or salty foods *only* after meeting basic nutrition requirements. Try serving the child yogurt, raisins and graham crackers instead of sweet desserts.

School-age children and adolescents

In the early school-age years, children grow less rapidly than they do in the later school-age years, as they approach puberty. Children's appetites often reflect these differences. Encourage the child to assist with meal planning to promote control and independence. When serving meals, expect to increase the portion size of each food served according to how much the child will eat, and continue to offer a balanced diet.

During the school-age years, a child's food choices and preferences are often influenced by peers and by television commercials. Luckily, most children seem to have an avid interest in food, and this is a good time to teach them how to make healthy food choices. Encouraging a child to choose nutritious snacks is a good way to promote his sense of independence.

When planning meals for an adolescent, be aware that adolescents need more protein and iron, which help the body as it continues to grow and mature. Iron is especially important for adolescent girls who begin to menstruate at this time. Peers and personal body image influence food selection during adolescence. Eating a balanced diet during adolescence is important for promoting good nutrition and maintaining health in the adult years.

CHECK YOUR UNDERSTANDING

Questions for Review

1. **You are providing care to several children of different ages. Which child would you expect to have a fear of the dark?**
   a. A 2-year-old
   b. A 4-year-old
   c. A 6-year-old
   d. A 13-year-old

2. **When providing care to infants and children, you would do which of the following?**
   a. Treat them like miniature adults.
   b. Expect them to react similarly to an adult.
   c. Adapt your care to the child's age and development.
   d. Depend on the parents for most of the care.

3. **A preschooler thinks that he did something to cause his brother's illness. The preschooler is demonstrating:**
   a. Autonomy
   b. Industry
   c. Invincibility
   d. Egocentric thinking

4. **You are caring for a 3-year-old child who has had surgery. Which action demonstrates that you are providing family-centered care?**
   a. Encouraging the parents to visit at any time
   b. Asking the parents to keep the child's brother at home
   c. Discouraging the parents from assisting in the child's care
   d. Keeping the parents away from the child during a procedure

5. **You are caring for a 14-year-old girl who has been injured in a car accident. Which of the following would be most important for you to do?**
   a. Provide for the girl's privacy.
   b. Focus on completing tasks.
   c. Encourage the girl's imagination.
   d. Use simple, concrete terms when talking with her.

6. **You are preparing to check a 10-year-old's temperature. Which method would you most likely use?**
   a. Rectal
   b. Oral
   c. Tympanic
   d. Axillary

7. **You are providing a snack to a 3-year-old. Which of the following would be appropriate to give the child?**
   a. Peanuts
   b. Carrot sticks
   c. Grapes
   d. Applesauce

8. **You ask a 5-year-old boy what color bandage he wants to put on the site where he had a blood specimen drawn. This action helps to address which of the following?**
   a. Separation anxiety
   b. Loss of control
   c. Fear of injury
   d. Fear of change in body image

9. **You are measuring the vital signs of a 13-month-old infant. Which pulse would you count?**
   a. Radial
   b. Femoral
   c. Brachial
   d. Apical

Questions to Ask Yourself

1. *You are assigned to care for two children: a 6-month-old and a 4-year-old. Explain how you would perform mouth care for each of these children. How would it be the same? How would it be different?*
2. *A 6-year-old boy was hit by a car while riding his bicycle. You are assigned to care for him. How would you expect a child of this age to react?*
3. *Create a list of foods that would be appropriate to give a 2-year-old child as a snack.*
4. *How would your care for a toddler be similar yet different from that for a preschooler?*

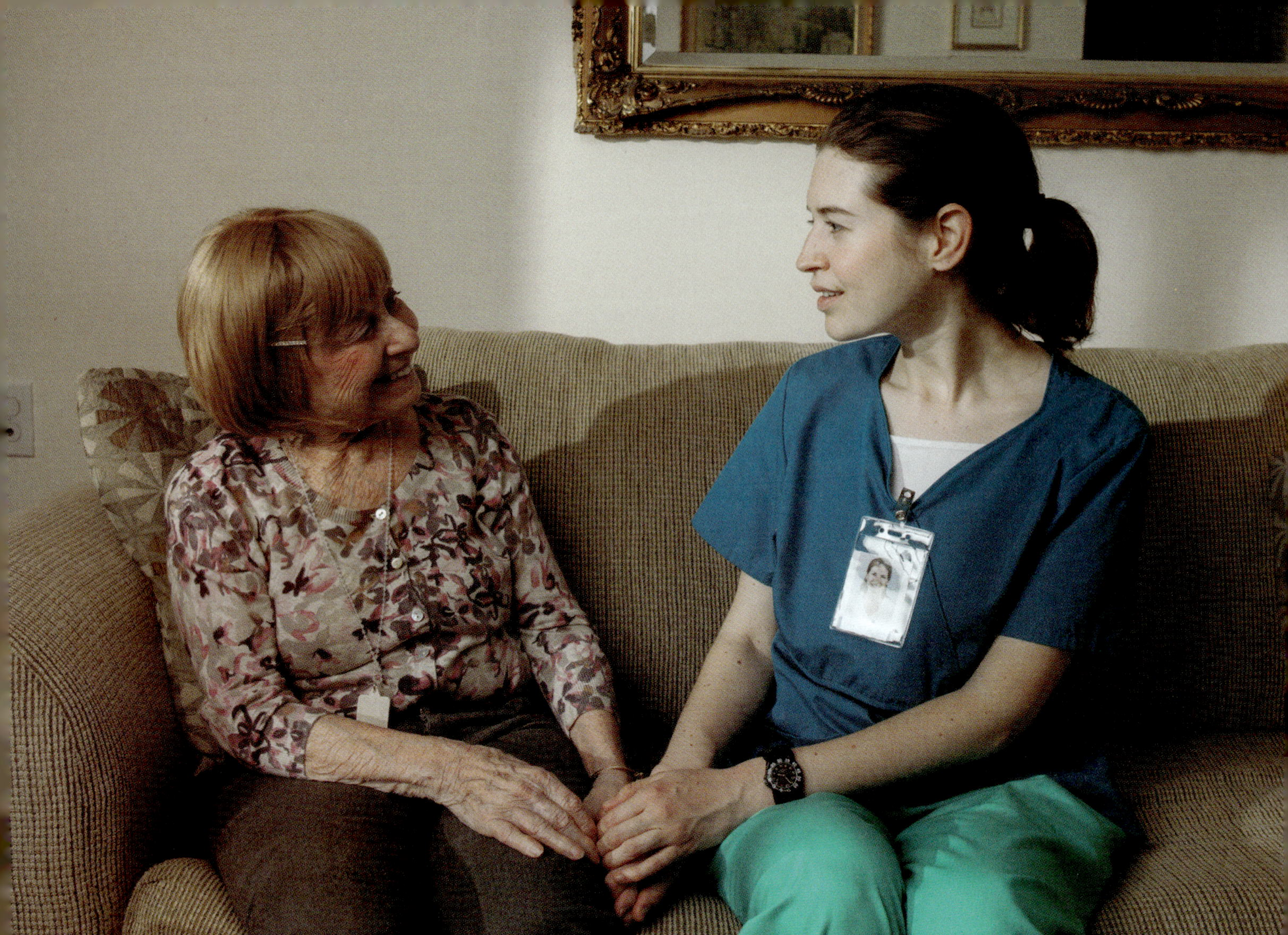

CHAPTER

22 Providing Care for People in Their Homes

Goals

After reading this chapter, you will have the information needed to:

- Define home health care.
- List the members of the home health care team.
- Explain the characteristics needed to be a home health aide.
- Describe how to maintain your personal safety while working as a home health aide.
- Describe how to maintain safety in the home.
- Explain the measures used to control infection when providing care in the home.
- Identify the responsibilities of the home health aide when providing personal care for a client in the home.
- Discuss the role of the home health aide in assisting with home management.

Goals

- Describe ways that a home health aide may assist with nutrition for a client receiving home health care.
- Explain the rules for assisting with medications in home health care.

Key Terms:

homebound **abandonment**

Mrs. Fielding has spent several weeks in the rehabilitation facility receiving physical therapy for injuries from a catastrophic car accident that killed her sister. She has finally arrived home. The home health care nurse has completed Mrs. Fielding's assessment and determined that she needs assistance with personal care and home management. Mrs. Fielding will also be receiving home physical therapy twice a week.

Mrs. Fielding lives in a two-story home with her dog. The bathroom is on the second floor. Although she is able to climb the stairs, she does have some difficulty going up and down the stairs by herself and gets fatigued easily. She plans to stay upstairs until she has bathed and then come downstairs for the rest of the day until bedtime. Mrs. Fielding has a close friend who stays with her during the day and helps her get ready for bed at night. You are assigned to care for Mrs. Fielding.

As a nurse assistant, you have the opportunity to practice your caregiving skills in a wide range of settings. One such setting is home health care. In some states, nurse assistants wishing to work as home health aides must receive additional training. Home health care services are provided to people with an acute illness, a long-term health condition, a permanent disability or a terminal illness who need treatment or support to function effectively in the home environment. It is important to understand that not all home health care clients are elderly.

All of the caregiving principles and skills you learn in this book will be valuable should you become a home health aide. However, there are additional things you will need to know.

OVERVIEW OF HOME HEALTH CARE

A home health care agency provides the personnel who then provide care for people in their homes. A nurse assistant, often called a home health aide, provides the care based on the care plan developed by the home health care nurse.

The home health care process begins with a referral for care. This referral may be from a discharge planner of a hospital or long-term care facility, nurse, doctor, social worker or therapist. A person's family may also initiate the process by calling the home health care agency for help. In this situation, if the agency determines that the person qualifies for services, the agency will contact the person's primary care provider and request a referral. Usually, when a referral is made, a beginning set of orders is also received.

Paying for Home Health Care

Payment for home health care services (reimbursement) varies. In some cases, individual clients may pay for the services from their personal finances. However, more commonly, insurance companies and governmental agencies, such as Medicare and Medicaid (often called third-party payers) provide payment for some or all of the costs of services.

Insurance companies, Medicare and Medicaid have very strict guidelines about the types of care that they will cover and the circumstances under which they will cover this care. For example, Medicare will pay for home health care costs only if the client is **homebound**. This means that the client requires significant effort to leave his home and cannot leave without receiving a great deal of assistance from another person.

The insurance companies can also control the length of time allotted for each visit and the frequency of visits per week. For example, one client may be allowed three visits per week, with each visit lasting only 1 hour, whereas another client may be allowed five visits per week, with each lasting 2 hours.

Home Health Care Team Members

The home health care team consists of various people who work together to provide the best possible client care. As in any other setting, the client is at the center of the team. The client's family members also play key roles because they are often caregivers. Other members of the home health care team typically include the registered home health care nurse, the client's primary care provider, a case manager and a home health aide. Other specialists (such as physical therapists, speech therapists, occupational therapists and medical social workers) may be involved. Regardless of the members involved, communication among team members is essential.

Home health care nurse

The home health care nurse is typically a registered nurse who provides skilled care to the client and family. The home health care nurse is responsible for initially evaluating the client and family and determining their needs. This nurse is also responsible for assessing, teaching, managing resources (either directly or indirectly), developing the care plan and communicating with other members of the home health care team.

Primary care provider

The person's primary care provider, usually a doctor or advanced practice nurse, is the person responsible for certifying that the client needs home health care services and that those services are medically necessary. In addition, the primary care provider is responsible for signing the care plan that specifies which services will be provided. If the client must be homebound to be eligible for services, the primary care provider confirms the person's homebound status.

Case manager

The case manager in home health care is the person responsible for overseeing all aspects of the client's care. The case manager may or may not be the registered home health care nurse who is providing skilled care to the client. The case manager is involved in assessing, planning, facilitating communication with all team members and advocating for the client and family.

Home health aide

A home health aide is responsible for providing personal care for the client, for obtaining measurements that are useful in monitoring the client's status (such as vital signs and weights) and for reporting any observations related to changes in the client's condition or environment to the home health care nurse. A home health aide may also be assigned to perform some light housekeeping duties such as cleaning, preparing meals and doing laundry. In addition, the aide may support the skilled care provided by other team members. For example, if a client is receiving physical therapy, the aide may assist the client to perform range-of-motion exercises based on the physical therapist's instructions (Figure 22-1).

Other specialists

Other specialty personnel may be involved, depending on the person's and family's needs. Physical therapy may be needed to improve the client's strength, functioning and mobility. Services may include therapeutic exercise programs, gait training, range-of-motion exercises and special treatments such as hot packs, ultrasound and whirlpool baths.

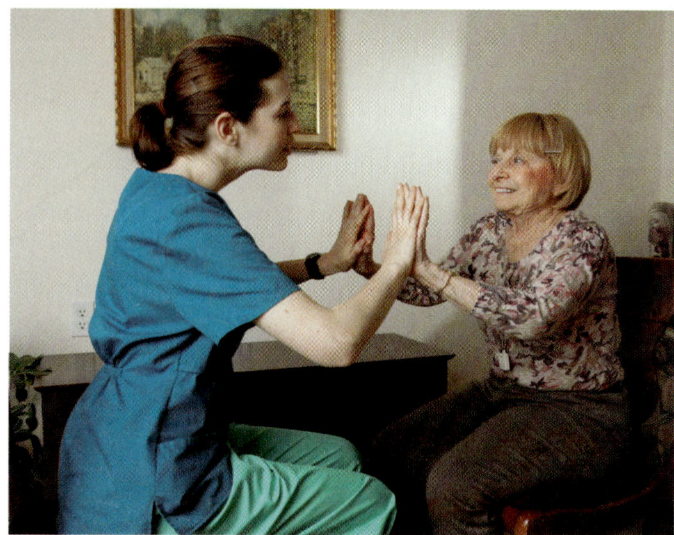

Figure 22-1 A home health aide assists the client to perform strengthening exercises prescribed by physical therapy.

Speech therapy may be needed to assist the client who has difficulty communicating or swallowing. Examples of speech therapy services may include teaching swallowing techniques, performing hearing screening and instructing the client to use prosthetic or assistive devices.

Occupational therapy may be needed to assist the client to regain the ability to perform activities of daily living (ADLs) as independently as possible. This therapy often includes the use of assistive devices. In addition, the occupational therapist may be involved in assisting the client and family with activities such as transportation, home safety awareness and homemaking.

A medical social worker may also be part of the home health care team. Services include helping the client and family adjust to the illness or changes in the ability to function, counseling the client and family, obtaining the necessary resources for the client to improve functioning and assisting with financial issues and problems.

Home Health Care Process

Home health care services begin when the home health care agency receives a referral. Next, the home health care agency determines whether the agency can meet the client's needs in the home and verifies that the client is eligible for services according to the insurance company's policy.

A home health care nurse visits the client's home and evaluates the client's needs and, based on the orders from the client's primary care provider, develops a care plan. The nurse then discusses the plan with other members of the health care team, and together they coordinate their activities. For example, based on the nurse's assessment, the client needs a registered nurse for dressing changes and teaching about new medications, a home health aide for personal care and meal preparation, a physical therapist to assist with ambulation and gait training and a medical social worker to arrange for community support services.

Communication is one very important aspect of home health care that makes it different from care in other settings. Typically in other settings, team members communicate face-to-face. However, in home health care, team members visit the client according to their individual schedules and may rarely see each other. For example, the home health care nurse may see the client at 9:30 a.m. on Mondays, Wednesdays and Fridays. The physical therapist may see the client at 1:30 p.m. on Tuesdays and Thursdays. The medical social worker may see the client at 3:00 p.m. on Thursdays. The home health aide is scheduled from 10:00 a.m. to 12:00 p.m. on Mondays, Tuesdays and Fridays. Thus, communication through documentation is extremely important.

THE HOME HEALTH AIDE'S ROLE

Have you ever had someone come into your home to do repairs? What did it feel like to have a stranger in your home? Were you afraid that he might break something? Were you concerned that he would leave a mess from his work? Did you feel that your home was no longer private? Thinking about your own responses to these questions may help you understand what people experience when they receive home health care and have new people help them in their own homes.

Most people consider the home to be a safe and secure place that has personal meaning and value. The client and her family control the setting, unlike in a facility or other setting. Also, the client does not come to you. You go to the client. Remember this when you provide care in the home.

Just as each client is different, so too are homes and families. At times, you may visit a client with a limited income who lives alone in a small, one-bedroom apartment that is cluttered; at other times, you may provide care for a client who lives in a large home with a spouse and children. Some homes may be spotlessly clean; others may not be as clean as you would prefer. Remember, this is the client's home and *you are a guest in that home*. Treat the client with respect and do not let your view of how the person lives influence your care.

Home Health Aide Characteristics

Working as a home health aide requires that you possess some unique personal characteristics. First, you need to be able to work independently. In most cases, you will be at the client's home without any direct supervision from other team members. You need to feel confident in your caregiving and problem-solving skills. You will not have someone readily available to ask, "What should I do?" No one will be there to tell you what to do.

Second, you need good organizational skills so that you can manage your time efficiently. You have specific assigned care activities that should be completed in a specific block of time. In addition, you need to allow time for documentation as well as travel from one client's home to another. Planning is essential for organization. Make sure that you have all your supplies for each client together, ideally before you leave for the visit but at least before you enter the client's home. This way you can provide care without interruptions. In addition, create a schedule that makes the best use of your travel time. If possible, plan your day so that travel time is minimized. However, always keep in mind that your clients' preferences and needs take precedence when you arrange your schedule.

Third, you must be reliable. Clients receiving home health care services depend on you to arrive on time, at the time scheduled, and remain for the specified amount of time to provide appropriate care (Figure 22-2). Being unreliable is inconsiderate but, more important, it can cause the client harm. For example, you are caring for a client who has diabetes and takes insulin every morning. You are supposed to arrive at the client's home at 8:00 a.m. so that you can help prepare breakfast for her. Breakfast is important for the client so that he does not have low blood-glucose levels after taking his insulin.

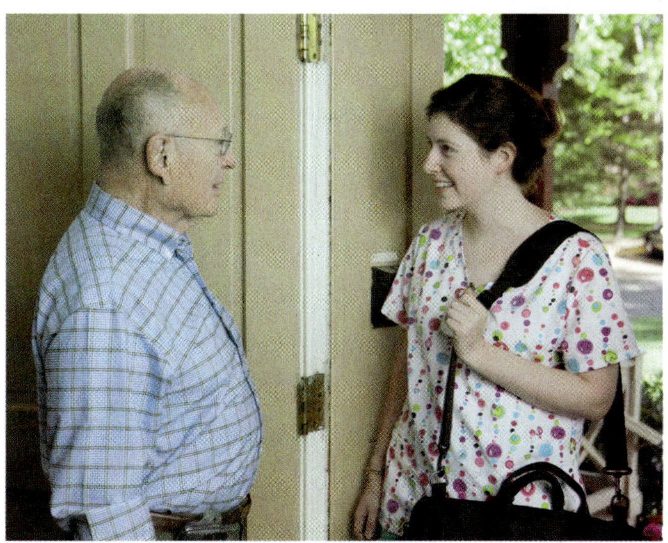

Figure 22-2 Home health aides must be reliable.

Arriving late would put the client at risk for developing a problem with his blood-glucose levels.

Being reliable also means showing up at a client's home to provide the scheduled care and completing all aspects of that care. Clients depend on you to arrive and provide the scheduled care. Failing to do so is called **abandonment** (withdrawal of one's support or help from another person, despite having the responsibility to provide this support or help). Imagine that you decide to leave a client's home about one-half hour earlier than your scheduled time. Typically, when you leave, the client's son has arrived to continue caring for his father. However, when you leave this time, the son has not yet arrived. Leaving a client alone without appropriate assistance is considered abandonment.

However, situations do arise that are out of your control and that cause you to be late or unable to keep a scheduled appointment with a client. In these situations, communication is key. Call your agency to inform the agency that you are running late. Also, call the client who is expecting you so that she will be informed. If you cannot work (for example, because you are sick) call the agency as soon as possible so that the agency can arrange for another home health aide to care for your clients. If a personal emergency arises during your workday that requires you to leave the client before completing your scheduled care or visit, call the agency. Then follow your agency's policies for handling these types of situations so that the client continues to receive the care that she needs without delay.

Fourth, you must have two other characteristics—flexibility and adaptability. Working in the home is quite different from working in an agency or facility. Equipment such as shower chairs and adjustable beds that allow the head of the bed to be raised with the push of a button may not be available. As a result, you will have to improvise and use items that are readily available in the home. For example, you can use pillows or backrests to raise the head of the bed for a client. A bell, whistle, noisemaker or even a portable phone can become an efficient call signal. In some cases, you may need to make a cleaning solution from bleach and water. Regardless of the situation, you need to be flexible and adapt to using whatever is available. Sometimes, you may need to talk to the home health care nurse or case manager to obtain the necessary equipment. Some insurance companies will cover the rental of a piece of equipment for a specified period of time. Other times, the client can rent or purchase the equipment from a medical supply company, or the case manager can arrange for the equipment at minimal to no cost.

Last, a home health aide needs to be able to maintain professional boundaries. As a home health aide, you interact with the client and family in their home. You spend a great deal of time there and, as a result, develop a special trusting relationship. At times, the client and family may come to view you as a friend or part of the family rather than someone who provides care. You need to maintain a professional relationship with the client and family at all times. Visiting the client and family socially is inappropriate. You should also refuse any gift, including gifts of money or food, that are offered. Always follow your agency's policies about accepting gifts.

Maintaining professional boundaries helps prevent the client and family from taking advantage of you, such as asking you for favors. For example, the client may ask you to do something that is not part of the care plan or may ask you to stay an extra half hour because the client's spouse is running late. Always check with your supervisor and agency about whether you can accept specific requests.

Home Health Aide Responsibilities

As a home health aide, you will be primarily responsible for providing personal care. Light housekeeping chores may also be among your responsibilities. How much cleaning you do depends on the availability of family members, the amount of time you spend in the home and the requirements of the client's care plan.

In your role as a home health aide, you are the eyes and ears of the home health care team. Clients and their families may share information with you that they would not share with others. For example, while you help a client get washed and dressed, she may tell you she is really down about not being able to do what she used to do for herself and hates depending on her husband. This information helps shed some light on the client's emotional status. You may also identify subtle changes in the client's condition. You need to communicate this information in writing, using the client's exact words or your direct observations, as well as verbally to the home health care nurse. You fill the role of communicator, informing the home health care nurse or case manager of your observations. In doing so, you act as an advocate to protect the client's rights.

THE HOME HEALTH CARE ENVIRONMENT

Dignity

In any setting, respecting the client and promoting the client's dignity are important. However, these duties take on even greater emphasis in the home environment. The setting is the client's home, a place of safety and security. When you visit the client, you are entering her space. You are a guest in the client's home. Always observe the client's rules for the home and ask permission when touching or using any personal items.

Whenever you receive an assignment, call ahead of time (usually the day or night before the first visit) to let the client know that you are coming and when. Also find out about any specific instructions for getting into the home. For example, you may need to look in a special location for the front door key, or you may need to ring the outer doorbell to be buzzed in.

Be sure to wear the proper agency attire and have your identification badge or name tag readily visible so that the client can identify you. Greet the client and address him by the proper name. Allow the client to guide the conversation.

Safety

Ensuring safety is a more complex task in the home environment than it would be in a facility or agency. Not only must you think about the client's safety, you must also ensure your personal safety, before, during and after a visit. In addition, you have less control over the home environment, and situations can change quickly. You also need to know how to handle emergencies should they arise because, in most cases, you will be in the home without other team members.

Personal safety

Some safety issues you face are unique. Consider this. You do not spend your entire workday in one building. Rather, you travel from one client's home to another. As a result, you are at risk for traffic accidents or car trouble. In addition, some homes that you may visit may not be in the safest of neighborhoods, which places you at risk for being a victim of an attack.

Always trust your own instincts. Be ever mindful and observant of your surroundings. If something does not seem right, it probably is not. Guidelines for maintaining personal safety are given in Box 22-1.

Client safety

Unlike health care facilities, a person's private home is not necessarily designed with safety in mind. There may be many hazards in a home setting that affect the client's safety. For example, the home may be older with wood floors that are uneven or warped or electrical wiring that is outdated. Carpets may be worn. Throw rugs may be loose. Lighting in the hallways, stairways and bathrooms may be dim. The person may have a great deal of furniture in a small space, which makes it hard to move around. Hallways may be narrow or cluttered as well. Regardless of the situation, your role as a home health aide is not to change the client's home environment but rather to maintain the safety of that environment for the client (Box 22-2). If you find any cause for concern, be sure to report your findings to the nurse. Often the nurse can assist with modifications and arrange for equipment if necessary.

ELDER CARE NOTE. Safety issues involving hazards that can affect mobility are especially problematic for the older client. Falls in the home are a major concern with older clients. With aging, bone structure changes, so bones are more vulnerable to even minimal stress, which can lead to fractures. Healing time is also prolonged, which makes recovery from a fracture longer. With prolonged healing, the risk for complications increases.

Box 22-1 Nurse Assistant DO's and DON'Ts

Ensuring Personal Safety

DO plan ahead and check addresses for accuracy.

DO map out your route and identify the locations of police stations, public buildings, gas stations or other structures that may be helpful in an emergency.

DO inform the agency of your schedule and check in several times a day.

DO prepare for the weather, such as snow or ice.

DO keep car doors locked.

DO park in well-lighted areas as close to the client's home as possible.

DO carry a fully charged mobile phone with you at all times.

DO be aware of other people, animals and your surroundings when walking to the client's home.

DO check for immediate hazards such as obstacles or poor lighting, hostile pets, hostile family members or weapons when you enter the client's home.

DON'T walk or drive through unknown areas or alleys.

DON'T carry large amounts of cash or expensive items with you or have them in plain view in your car.

DON'T keep your handbag readily visible in your car.

Box 22-2 Nurse Assistant DO's and DON'Ts

Maintaining a Safe Home

DO keep walkways and steps clear of clutter.

DO encourage the client to remove throw rugs.

DO note whether repairs are needed (for example, loose floorboards, broken steps) and report this need to the nurse.

DO look for safety devices such as smoke detectors, carbon monoxide detectors and fire extinguishers. Make sure that detectors work (by pushing the test button on the device) and that the fire extinguisher is full and ready to use. If these devices are missing or not operational, report this to the nurse.

DO check the house for security features (for example, working locks on exterior doors and windows). If security features are missing or not used, report this to the nurse.

DO note whether safety equipment (such as grab bars) is needed and report this need to the nurse.

DO note whether special equipment (such as a portable commode) is needed to make care safer and report this need to the nurse.

DO ensure good lighting.

DO clean up any spills promptly.

DO keep chemicals, cleaning solutions, medications and other poisonous items in a secure storage area.

DON'T run electrical cords across areas where people walk.

DON'T overload electrical outlets.

DON'T use extension cords, other than on a short-term basis.

Dangers and emergencies

Despite your best efforts to maintain safety, emergencies, including accidents, fires and medical problems, do occur. Regardless of the type of emergency, you must remain calm and use good judgment. For example, if you smell smoke or gas, assist the client and other family members to leave the home, and then call 9-1-1 or the local emergency number from outside of the home. In addition, hostile family members or pets and the presence of weapons in the home may pose a threat to the client's safety as well as your own safety.

Pets

Pay particular attention when a client has a pet. On the surface, the pet may seem calm and friendly. However, the pet may become upset or highly protective when you provide care for the client. If providing pet care is not part of your duties, be proactive and ask the client or a family member to move the pet to another room while you are there. If this is not possible, avoid interacting with the pet, even if it appears friendly. The pet may view you as a threat.

Many people have dogs. If moving the dog to another room is not possible and the dog becomes hostile, do not look the dog in the eye. Rather, look down and to the side to avoid making eye contact while keeping the dog in sight at all times. Talk to the dog in a firm but calm voice and try giving the dog a command (for example, "Sit!"). Try to distract the dog by using an object such as a box of tissues while you slowly move toward a safe area or an exit. If you get bitten by a dog, make sure to get immediate treatment for your injury and report the incident to your agency.

Cats can also pose a threat to your safety. They can scratch you, which places you at risk for infection. If you get scratched, be sure to wash the area immediately with soap and water at the client's house. If a cat bites you, seek medical attention and report the incident to your agency.

Hostile client or family members

Not all clients may be happy to see you. Clients may be angry or upset by the fact that their illness has left them dependent on others for their needs. Family caregivers may feel angry or upset by having to provide the necessary care. Sometimes hostile behavior is a result of fear (such as the fear of one's own declining health, or the declining health of a loved one.) Substance use issues can also cause people to feel threatened by your presence and to act in a hostile manner.

Whenever possible, prevent a problem situation from developing. If a client or family member seems hostile, think about the possible reason for the hostility and then determine how severe the level of threat is. If the threat is low, attempt to calm the client or family member by using caring, supportive statements, such as "How can I make you more comfortable now?" Be aware of what your body language is saying. On the outside, be calm and confident, even though you may be tense and anxious on the inside. Be assertive (but not aggressive, because aggression can fuel hostility). If the hostility increases, work your way to a safe exit and notify your agency once you are out of the home.

Weapons

Many people choose to keep weapons, such as firearms, in their homes. Always ask the client and family about weapons and follow your agency's policy about what to do if there are weapons in the home.

To ensure the safety of everyone in the home, ask the client to move a weapon to a room other than the ones in which you are giving care. This is especially important if the weapon is a loaded firearm. If the client agrees, make a verbal or written agreement that the client will store the weapon in that location while you are in the home. If at any time you feel unsafe or threatened or the client refuses to store the weapon, immediately stop the visit, leave and make sure to explain to the client why you are leaving. Report this information to your supervisor and the agency.

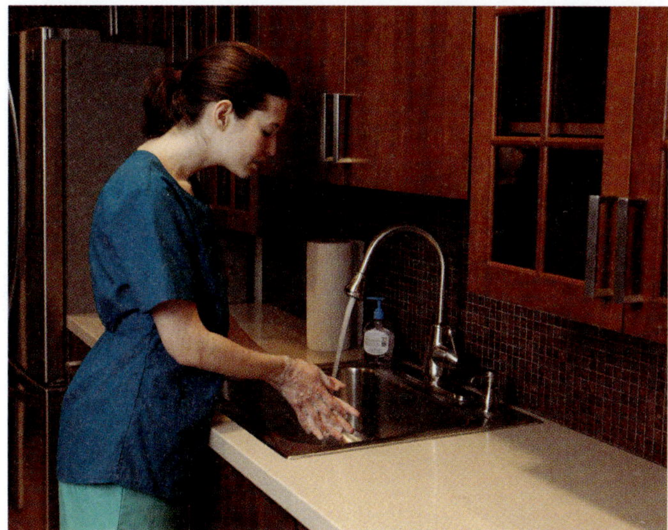

Figure 22-3 Hand washing is important for infection control in all health care settings.

Infection Control

In your role as a home health aide, you move from one home to another as you give care to several clients each day. As you go from one client to the next, you are at risk for transmitting pathogens on your hands, clothes or equipment. Therefore, infection control is as important a concern in home health care as it is in any facility.

Infection control in the home involves much more than just hand washing and standard precautions. It also involves keeping the client's environment clean. Your agency will have infection control policies and procedures that relate to client care, housecleaning and laundering. You need to understand and practice these policies and procedures. You will learn more about your responsibilities related to maintaining a clean environment later in this chapter.

Hand washing and standard precautions

Infection control begins with proper hand washing. You may have to carry your own soap and paper towels or alcohol-based hand rub for hand washing. Wash your hands when you enter a client's home, when your hands become visibly soiled, when you remove your gloves and after you complete each task or procedure (Figure 22-3). If hand-washing facilities are not available and your hands are not visibly soiled, use an alcohol-based hand rub. Then wash your hands with soap and water as soon as you can.

In addition to hand washing, you should follow standard precautions and use personal protective equipment (PPE) as appropriate. You may need to bring PPE with you or it may be stored at the client's home. Be knowledgeable about your clients and be prepared with the necessary PPE before setting out for the day.

If your client uses any sharps (such as needles or lancets) on a routine basis, be sure that the client knows how to dispose of them properly. If necessary, speak to the nurse about obtaining a commercial sharps container. Check with the client's municipality for instructions on proper disposal of the container with used sharps.

Handling supplies and equipment

Because you travel from home to home, you often carry your important equipment and supplies in some type of bag, such as a tote bag or backpack. This bag is a potential source for infection transmission. Therefore, when you enter a client's house, be sure to place your bag on a barrier (such as a piece of newspaper or plastic) to prevent microbes on the outside of the bag from contaminating the client's environment and to prevent microbes from the client's environment from contaminating your bag. When you leave, be sure to discard the barrier in the appropriate trash container.

During your visit, you will most likely be required to use equipment and supplies that travel with you, such as a thermometer, stethoscope and blood-pressure cuff. The client may have his own thermometer to use, but if not, be sure to use individual thermometer covers and clean the thermometer after each use. You will probably need to use your own stethoscope and possibly blood-pressure cuff with all your clients. Therefore, be sure that you properly clean and disinfect your equipment before storing it in your bag and transporting it to another client's home.

Supplies and equipment may also be stored in the client's home. For example, dressings for wound care, which need to be sterile and kept in their original packaging, should be stored in a safe location where the outer wrapping will remain clean and dry and not become torn. Equipment you use for client care during your visit (for example, a bedpan, portable commode or emesis basin) should be cleaned and disinfected according to your agency's policy before returning the equipment to its storage area.

Any disposable equipment or supplies contaminated with blood or body fluids should be placed in a plastic bag for disposal. Secure the bag tightly before placing it the household trash. If necessary, place the first plastic bag into another plastic bag and seal it (this is called double-bagging) and then dispose of the bag with the household trash.

Monitoring for signs and symptoms of infection

Your role as a home health aide puts you in a unique position to monitor the client and family for signs and symptoms of infection. A key responsibility is monitoring the client's vital signs (Figure 22-4). In addition, you have the opportunity to watch for any situations or conditions that may increase a client's risk for developing an infection.

Observations Into Action!

When you work as a home health aide, be sure to report any of the following observations to the home health care nurse:

- **The client or a family member has a fever or other potential signs of an infection (for example, reddened skin, coughing with mucus, thick nasal discharge, vomiting, diarrhea).**
- **Conditions in the home are unsanitary (for example, spoiled food is in the refrigerator, rodent droppings are in areas where food is prepared, accumulated trash or soiled linens are lying around the house).**
- **The home lacks toilet facilities or running water.**

Confidentiality, Privacy and Communication

All people receiving health care have the right to privacy and confidentiality. Think about the home setting. Other people often live in the home. Visitors may come and go. The client may prefer that others, even relatives, do not have information about her health status. Always ask the client's permission before sharing any information about the client. Both written and oral communication must be kept private and confidential.

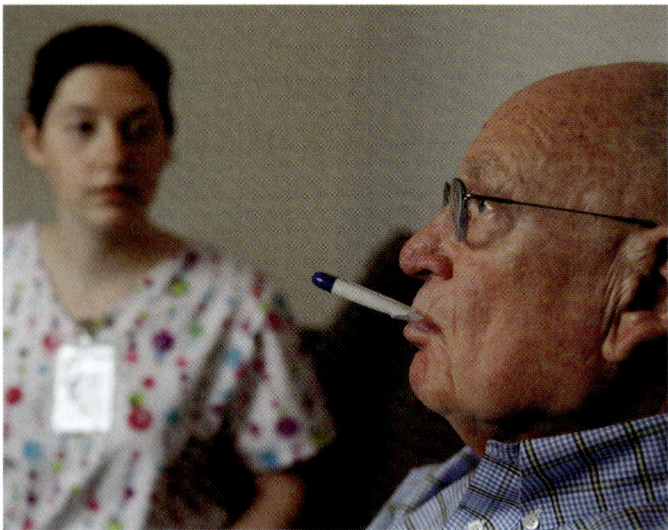

Figure 22-4 A home health aide monitors a client's vital signs. Changes in vital signs may suggest that a client is developing an infection.

If you need to make a phone call to discuss the client's care or status with another member of the health care team, try to avoid doing this where others may overhear you. However, if this is not possible, and others are around to hear the information, then check with the client before calling to make sure he agrees that others who are present may hear the information. In addition, ensure that paperwork and forms (such as the client's care plan) are kept in a secure location that is not in direct view of others in the home. For example, it might be better to keep the care plan in a folder next to the client's bed or on the client's nightstand, instead of placing it on the client's refrigerator. Follow your agency's policy with regard to how documents relating to client care should be stored in the home.

CAREGIVING SKILLS IN THE HOME

Much of the care that you provide in a client's home as a home health aide centers around the client's personal care. That is, you will assist the client with bathing, dressing, preparing and eating meals and moving safely in the home. In addition, you may assist the client with activities related to meeting nutrition needs, such as planning meals, going grocery shopping or providing a specialized diet. You may also be involved in helping the client manage the home, and in many situations, you may be the person who helps make sure that the client is taking her prescribed medications properly.

Assisting with Personal Care

Assisting a client with personal care may require you to adapt the skills that you would use when caring for a client in a facility. For example, the client may not have safety grab bars in the shower, so you may need to have the client sit on a sturdy folding chair for showering. You may also have to work around the schedule of others in the home to use the bathroom. In addition, the client may be staying on the first floor of the home, but the bathroom may be on the second floor. If the client uses a portable commode, there will probably not be a curtain that you can pull for privacy, as in a room in a health care facility.

You will need to determine where the client prefers to complete his personal care. The bathroom may be the best place if the client can walk and the bathroom is readily accessible. However, if the client cannot get to the bathroom, you may have to assist the client with personal care in the area where he is most comfortable, such as a bedroom. Sometimes the need to set up special equipment or a client's inability to manage stairs means that a room on the first floor, such as the dining room or living room, becomes the client's bedroom. Regardless of where you assist with personal care, you need to ensure the client's privacy.

Organize your time and thoughts before beginning each day because your time spent with each client is limited. Your primary responsibility is helping the client with basic personal care (Figure 22-5). However, you also need to consider the areas of the client's home that you must address after you provide personal care. This includes making sure that the bedroom (or the room where the client spends most time), the bathroom, and the kitchen are clean because these areas are important for the client and the care that you provide. In addition, you may also have to do the client's personal laundry and wash the bed linens. The specific cleaning and laundry duties for which you are responsible are included in the client's care plan.

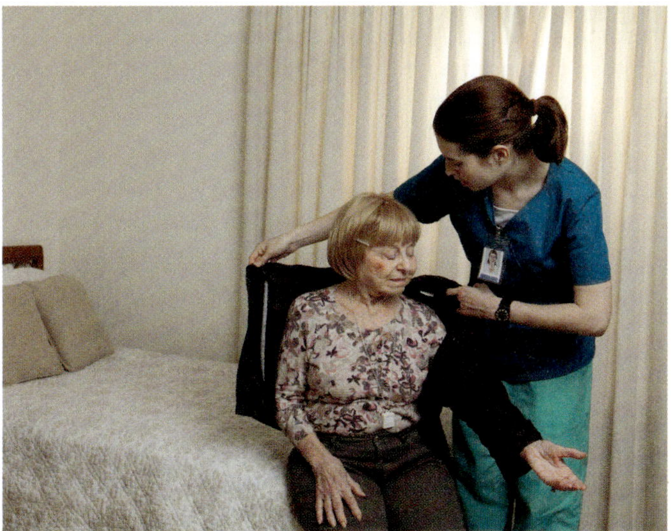

Figure 22-5 Assisting with personal care helps promote the client's self-esteem and dignity.

During your visit, Mrs. Fielding says, "It's so good to be home finally. I'd really love to take a shower." You check the bathroom and note that there is a bathtub and a walk-in shower, but neither has grab bars installed. You know that Mrs. Fielding gets tired really easily.

How will you ensure Mrs. Fielding's safety and still meet her needs?

Maintaining clothing and linens

Some care that you may have to provide for your client is cleaning and maintaining her linens and clothing. If the client has urinary or bowel incontinence, you may have to do laundry more frequently. When you wash a client's linens or clothing, check with the client or an appropriate family member about any preferences for laundry, such as using a special detergent or water temperature. You may need to check clothing labels to determine how to wash certain items.

You may come in contact with body fluids on soiled linens. Always observe infection control precautions, such as keeping dirty linens away from your own clothing and wearing gloves (see Chapter 10). If the linens are soiled with body fluids:

- Immediately remove the soiled linens from the bed and follow infection control precautions.
- Flush solid waste down the toilet.
- Put the contaminated linens in a plastic bag and take them to the washing machine.

Maintaining the bed

The client's comfort is an important consideration when you provide care in the home, especially if the client spends long periods in the bed. Typically, a bed in the home is unlike a hospital bed. It cannot be raised to a comfortable working height, nor is it always a single bed. When you make a bed in a home setting, remember to use good body mechanics. Protect your back by squatting instead of bending over and by moving around the bed instead of reaching across it.

Assisting with Home Management

Maintaining a clean living environment promotes the client's dignity and helps prevent the spread of infections. However, your duties as a home health aide differ greatly from those of a housekeeper. You focus your cleaning on eliminating pathogens, controlling the spread of infections and keeping the house free of safety hazards. Under the home health care nurse's direction, you may help teach family members proper techniques to maintain a clean household.

Always wash your hands before beginning and after completing home maintenance tasks to prevent the spread of pathogens. Wear disposable gloves whenever the possibility exists that you may come into contact with body fluids such as blood, urine or feces. Dispose of your gloves in a covered trash can or a plastic trash bag, and wash your hands when you finish the task. If necessary, put on new gloves for the next job.

Performing general housekeeping tasks

You may be responsible for completing some general housekeeping tasks such as light dusting and vacuuming (Figure 22-6). The client's care plan will specify the specific tasks that you are responsible for completing.

When taking care of a client's home, you must always remember that, just like you, the client may feel very strongly about her home and the things in it. Discuss your cleaning duties with your supervisor and the client so that you know how much you should do, as well as what the client wants and needs to have done. The way that you do things may be different from the way the client does things. If you must do things a certain way to maintain safety or infection control, you may have to explain why. At times, you may have to alter your procedure (if doing so will not cause you to violate a basic principle of care) if the client asks you to handle things differently.

Using cleaning products

In your job as a home health aide you must use cleaning products safely and store all cleaning products in a safe place. You must also know when to use various cleaning agents, including the four basic kinds of household cleaning products:

1. All-purpose cleaning agents for general cleaning of many kinds of surfaces
2. Soaps and detergents for bathing, laundering and washing dishes
3. Cleansers for scouring areas that are hard to clean
4. Specialty cleaners for specific tasks and surfaces such as cleaning glass or ovens

Cleaning products can contain harsh chemicals. Always wear gloves when using cleaning products. Depending on the cleaning product, you may need to wear eye protection as well. Try to ensure good air flow in the room (for example, by opening a window or door). Before using a cleaning product on a surface, test a small area to make sure that the product does not affect the color of the surface. After verifying that the product is safe to use on the surface, apply the product and let it sit for the recommended amount of time.

If you need to disinfect surfaces such as bathroom fixtures, floors and counters, but the cleaners you have are not effective for killing microbes, use a bleach solution. Because full-strength bleach has a very strong odor and is harsh on the skin, always mix it with water. At the beginning of each visit, prepare the solution by mixing 1-1/2 cups of bleach with 1 gallon of water. Make a fresh solution of bleach and water each day, because the disinfecting power of bleach fades if the solution sits too long.

Be sure to work in a well-ventilated area, and wear gloves and eye protection. Put the water in a bucket or other container first and then pour the bleach into it. Mix bleach *only* with water, because mixing it with anything else, especially any product containing ammonia, can create a dangerous gas.

In some situations, you may be required to sterilize an item. Boiling the item for 20 minutes will kill most pathogens. Talk with your supervisor about any specific instructions for sterilizing items.

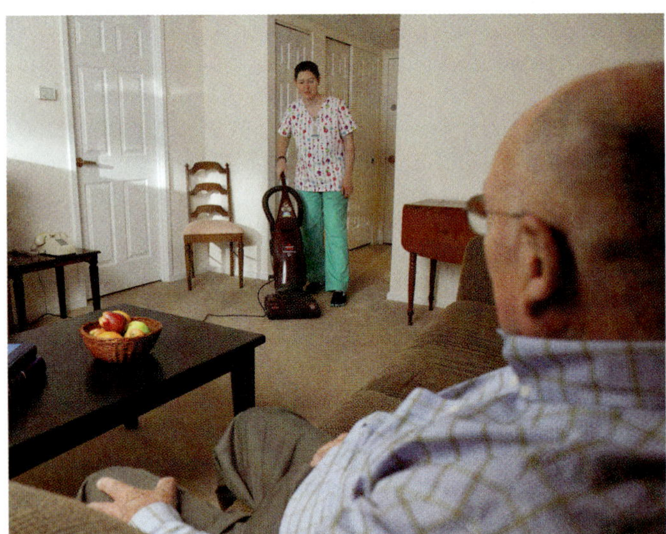

Figure 22-6 A home health aide may perform tasks related to ensuring a clean living environment for the client.

Disposing of trash

You must dispose of any trash that you create while providing care for your client. If time allows, you may also dispose of household trash and may teach family members proper techniques for trash disposal. You may have to wash trash cans periodically with hot soapy water when they are dirty and rinse them with a bleach solution. Washing reduces odors and microbes that grow in trash containers and discourages insects and rodents. Always wash your hands after disposing of trash. Box 22-3 summarizes the methods for disposing of different types of trash.

Box 22-3 Disposing of Different Types of Trash

- **Food**
  - If the client has a garbage disposal, put only soft foods in it. Never put hard or stringy foods in the garbage disposal because they may damage it.
  - If the client composts, place food and kitchen waste (such as coffee grounds and vegetable peels) in the appropriate container for composting.
  - If food items must be disposed of in the trash, drain off any liquid before disposing of the food in a plastic-lined trash container.
- **Grease**
  - Pour cooled grease into a disposable container, never down the sink drain or into a garbage disposal. Put a lid on the container before disposing of it with the trash.
- **Recyclable Items**
  - Rinse cans and bottles to prevent odors that might attract insects, rats or other pests, and then place them in the appropriate containers for recycling.
  - Follow the municipality's guidelines for preparing other items, such as newspapers and cardboard, for recycling.
- **Contaminated and Wet Items**
  - Place contaminated, wet items (such as used tissues, sanitary napkins, disposable briefs or dressings) in a plastic bag. Place this plastic bag inside another plastic bag, and then place the bag in a covered trash container.
  - Always wear disposable gloves when handling these items, and dispose of the gloves properly in a plastic trash bag or covered container.

Assisting with Nutrition

Your responsibilities related to ensuring that the client receives adequate nutrition may include planning meals, shopping for groceries, storing food, and preparing and serving meals (Figure 22-7). You will also be responsible for keeping the kitchen clean.

Planning meals

To plan nutritious meals, you first must learn about the client's eating habits and his likes and dislikes. You also must learn whether the client has any religious or cultural preferences relating to food. In addition, you will need to know if the client has any prescribed diet restrictions, such as a low-salt or low-fat diet. You can find out about the client's nutritional status and needs by checking the client's care plan and talking to the home health care nurse. In addition, you can ask the client questions, such as:

- What do you like to eat?
- How do you like each food prepared? (This question should be specific to the foods the client prefers.)
- Do you follow a special diet or have certain preferences related to your health issues?
- When do you like to eat? How much do you like to eat at each time?
- Do you like to drink liquids with your meals? If so, what types of liquids? Do you prefer hot or cold liquids?
- What kinds of snack foods do you like to eat?
- Is there any food that you do not like or cannot eat?
- Are there foods that you are allergic to? (Allergies should also be documented in the care plan.)

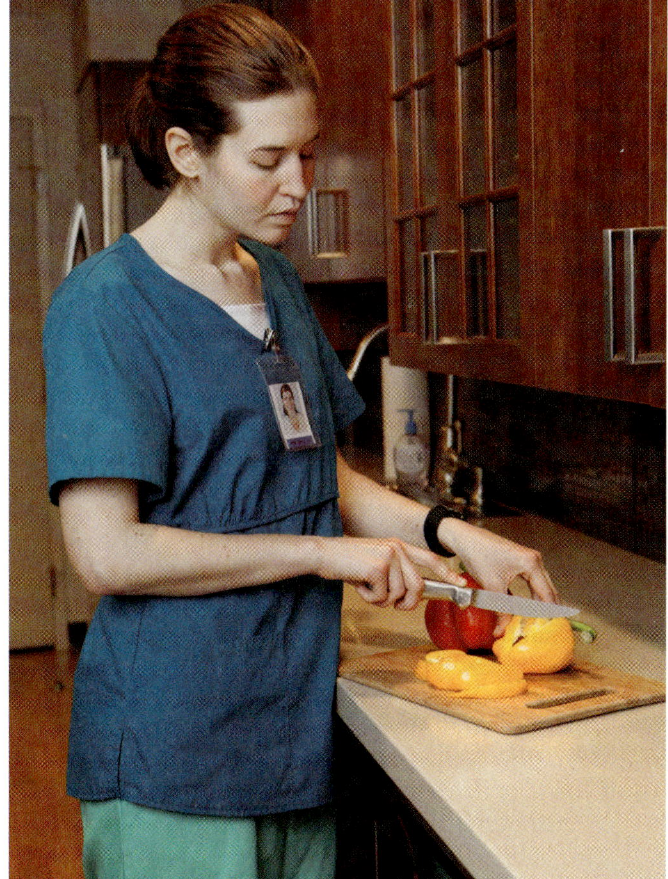

Figure 22-7 A home health aide may be required to prepare meals for the client.

- Do you have any preferences about food storage or handling?
- What foods or brands do you usually buy at the grocery store? (You should ask this question of the person who usually does the shopping for the household.)

Work with the client and family when you plan the desired number of meals. Refer to MyPlate (p.230) for guidance in food selection and meal planning. Include some meals that are based on leftovers. Using leftovers cuts down on the time spent preparing meals and lets you buy larger quantities of items such as meat, rice and pasta, if necessary. Doing so can help save your client money.

Grocery shopping

You may need to shop for groceries for some clients. Effective meal planning lets you shop for everything you need at one time. Use the information you obtained from the client and family to start your shopping list. Then check to see if the client needs any staple items (such as sugar and flour).

Shopping wisely saves money. Money-saving tips include the following:

- Watch newspaper ads for food specials and collect money-saving food coupons.
- Keep an ongoing shopping list. Jot down items to be replaced as you use them, review the list with the client and complete the list before you go shopping. Follow the list carefully as you shop.
- Use the unit price (printed on the shelf label under the product) to select the best buy. The largest package is not always the best value. Unit pricing tells you the cost per pound, quart, ounce or other unit of measure.
- Select less expensive, leaner cuts of meat. These cuts are less expensive because they require long, slow cooking (such as braising or stewing) or overnight marinating to tenderize them.

Handling and storing food

Proper food handling and storage is important to preserve the quality of the food and prevent the spread of infection. Food that is not stored properly can become a breeding ground for microbes, which can lead to illnesses such as food poisoning. To handle and store food properly:

- Wash your hands often with soap and water when you handle food.
- If you suspect that food has become contaminated or has not been handled or stored properly, wrap it in plastic or aluminum foil and throw it away in a covered trash container. Tell your client what foods you are throwing away and why.
- Discard any items that have passed the sell-by date on the container.
- Before and after each use, clean and sanitize food preparation surfaces and utensils, especially any surfaces and utensils that come into contact with raw meats, poultry or fish.
- Defrost any frozen items by placing them in the refrigerator, running them under cold water or using a microwave on the defrost cycle. Avoid defrosting foods at room temperature.
- Keep hot foods hot; make sure that they stay above 140° F or higher before serving.
- Keep cold foods cold; store them in the refrigerator at temperatures of 40° F or lower.
- Wash fresh vegetables and fruit carefully before using them.
- Discard any uneaten portion of a client's meal. The food is unsafe to use again and should not be eaten by anyone else.
- Divide leftovers (such as the uneaten part of a casserole or soups) into smaller containers and refrigerate or freeze them within 2 hours. Label the containers with the contents and the date.

Preparing food

Before you start cooking, review the client's care plan to see whether there are any special restrictions. For example, you may need to mash the client's food or use a blender or food processor to puree it. Next, get to know your way around the kitchen. If no one can give you a tour, take one yourself. Find out where pots, pans, dishes and utensils are kept so that you can readily find the items you need. Ask questions if you are unsure about how an appliance or piece of equipment works. Because you are a guest in the client's home, always obtain permission to use the kitchen or a piece of equipment.

Read through the recipe (if you are following one) and gather all the equipment and ingredients you will need. Prepare all the ingredients (for example, chop the vegetables or grate the cheese) before you begin cooking. Remember to use a separate cutting board for preparing fruits and vegetables and another cutting board for meat, fish and poultry. Wash your hands and your utensils frequently, and try to clean up as you go along. Cook foods carefully to destroy microbes and to retain flavor and nutrients. Basic cooking methods that you may use include baking, roasting, broiling, pan-frying, steaming, slow cooking (or braising) and microwaving. Most general cookbooks provide instructions for cooking using these basic methods.

Serving meals

For many clients, food will not be very appealing. You can help encourage the client to eat by making food look as appetizing as possible and by making meal time as enjoyable as possible:

- Try to set up a meal time schedule and stick to it. However, if the client is not hungry at meal time and wants to eat at another time, be as flexible as possible.

- Set the table properly, or make an effort to make the meal tray attractive. Always use clean utensils and fresh napkins. Some clients may like to use special table linens, plates or utensils.
- Plan colorful meals (Figure 22-8). For example, a meal of mashed potatoes, cauliflower and chicken breast is all white and will not be visually appealing. However, if you serve carrots instead of (or with) the cauliflower, you add some color to the plate. Serving brown rice instead of mashed potatoes would add even more color.
- Allow enough time for the client to use the bathroom before eating.
- Serve hot foods hot and cold foods cold. Test the temperature of hot liquids and foods to prevent burns.
- Make sure that the client is seated comfortably.
- Sit down and talk with the client during the meal.
- Encourage the client to do as much as she can independently. If the client uses assistive devices for eating, make sure that these are available.
- Do not hurry the client while she eats.
- Clear the table or remove the plate as soon as the client has finished eating.

The care plan for Mrs. Fielding includes preparing a meal for her. Because you visit her in the morning, you will need to prepare breakfast. Would you give her breakfast before assisting her with personal care? Or would you assist her with personal care before giving her breakfast? Explain how you would decide.

Assisting with Medications

In the home setting, you may provide some assistance with medications. Only doctors and licensed nurses may actually *give* medications to people. It is illegal for you, as a home health aide, to give any medication to a person in your care—this includes over-the-counter and prescription medications. However, in the home setting, you may be allowed to *help* the client take his medications by reminding him to take the medication, and by reading the label on the medication container to him. Other ways that you can help vary depending on the type of medication:

- **Tablets, capsules or liquids that are taken by mouth.** You can bring the medicine container to the client and you can open it for him. However, you cannot pour out the medicine or remove it from the container in any way (Figure 22-9). You can hand the client a glass of water to assist with swallowing the medication. If necessary, you can also steady the client's hand to keep liquid medicine from spilling.
- **Eye drops.** You can help the client tilt his head back and support his hand as he administers the medication. (Usually, eye drops are placed between the lower eyelid and the eyeball.) After the client has used the eye drops, ask him to close his eyes to distribute the medication.
- **Ointments and lotions.** You may help the client remove a dressing, if necessary. Follow the nurse's instructions for washing the area and then have the client apply the medication. Help the client wash her hands.
- **Transdermal patches.** A transdermal patch contains medication that is absorbed through the skin. You may help the client remove the old patch. Wash the area with soap and water,

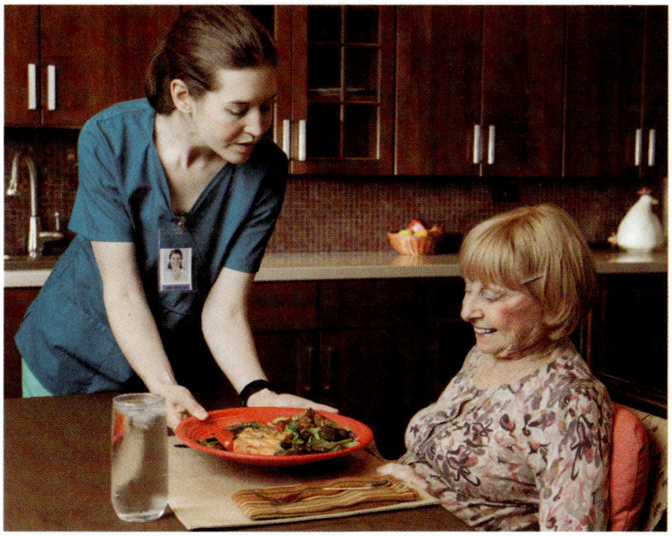

Figure 22-8 Serving a colorful meal can help stimulate the client's appetite.

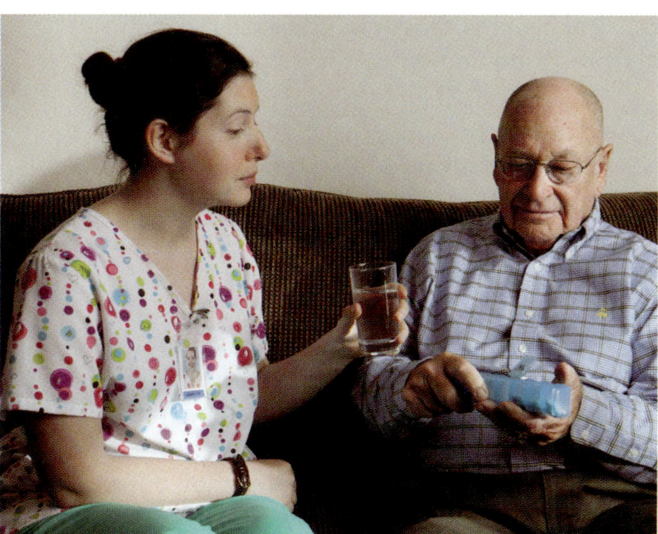

Figure 22-9 A home health aide watches as the client takes his medications out of the container.

and pat it dry. Help the client to apply the new patch in a different area, according to the nurse's instructions.

- **Rectal suppository.** Help the client into a side-lying position and help her unwrap the suppository, if necessary. Have the client put on a glove, and guide the client's hand to the rectal area, if necessary. After the client inserts the suppository, hold the buttocks together for a few minutes to help the client retain the suppository. Help the client back into a comfortable position.

After you assist a client with taking a medication, be sure to document the medication that was taken, the amount, the time and the route.

In some cases, you may need to perform some type of monitoring when a medication is being taken or to make sure that the client has done the necessary self-monitoring. For example, when a client is taking certain types of heart medications, you will need to take the client's pulse before she takes her medicine. A client with diabetes may need to check his blood-glucose level before he takes his dose of insulin.

If a person asks you to fix some special kind of tea or home remedy, check with the home health care nurse first. Herbal products are considered medications. In addition, some herbal products can interact with medications and cause side effects.

Observations Into Action!

When you assist a client at home with medications, notify the home health care nurse of the following:

- **The client is not taking medication as prescribed.**
- **The client is taking more or less than the prescribed amount.**
- **The client is taking medicine other than what was prescribed, including over-the-counter medicine.**
- **The client is taking medication at times other than those ordered.**
- **The client has side effects after taking medications.**
- **The client is having difficulty taking the medication independently (for example, tremors cause her hand to shake, or the client is having difficulty swallowing).**
- **The client says that the medication does not seem to be working.**
- **The client has questions concerning medications.**
- **The medication container is missing a label or the label is hard to read.**
- **The prescription needs to be refilled.**
- **The expiration date on the medication container has passed.**
- **You suspect that someone in the household is misusing any medicine.**

CHECK YOUR UNDERSTANDING

Questions for Review

1. Home health care begins with which of the following?

a. Reimbursement
b. Referral
c. Call from the client's family
d. Case manager

2. Which statement about home health care is true?

a. Most clients pay for the service from their personal finances.
b. A home health aide is responsible for performing cleaning and household maintenance tasks at the client's request.
c. The client must be homebound for Medicare to pay for the service.
d. Home health aides spend the same amount of time with each client.

3. You are considering employment with a home health care agency as a home health aide. You evaluate yourself for the characteristics needed to be a home health aide. Which of the following would most likely interfere with your ability to perform your duties?

a. Rigidness
b. Organization
c. Adaptability
d. Reliability

4. The spouse of one of your home health care clients offers you a check as a thank-you for all your help and support. Which of the following should you do?

a. Say thank you and accept the check.
b. Ask for cash instead.
c. Refuse the gift gracefully.
d. Give the check to your supervisor.

5. **You arrive at a client's home and find that the client has a small dog. The dog seems friendly. Which of the following should you do?**
   a. Allow the dog to approach you to get to know you.
   b. Pet the dog gently to introduce yourself.
   c. Look the dog in the eye to assume control.
   d. Have the client move the dog to another room.

6. **You are providing care to a client in her home. Which of the following would you do first to address infection control in the home?**
   a. Put on gloves.
   b. Wash your hands.
   c. Clean your stethoscope.
   d. Clean the client's environment.

7. **You are performing general housekeeping tasks and need to clean the bathroom after assisting a client with bathing. Which of the following would be best to use?**
   a. Full-strength ammonia
   b. A solution of bleach and water
   c. Hydrogen peroxide
   d. A solution of alcohol and water

8. **You are reviewing the care plan for a client and find that you are to prepare a meal for him. Which of the following would you do first?**
   a. Question the client about what he likes to eat.
   b. Check the refrigerator to see what food is available.
   c. Look for any meals that may be in the freezer.
   d. Call the home health care nurse for more information.

9. **When serving a meal to a client, which action would be least helpful in making mealtime enjoyable?**
   a. Making sure the client is comfortable
   b. Serving hot foods hot and cold foods cold
   c. Varying the meal time schedule
   d. Including foods that are different colors

Questions to Ask Yourself

1. *You and a friend who is also a home health aide meet for coffee after work. You are both talking about your day when your friend says that she "gave" her client his medications today. Is this legal? What might she mean by her statement?*
2. *A client is currently staying in the dining room on the first floor of the home because he cannot go up the stairs. He has a hospital bed and uses a portable commode. How would you provide privacy for the client?*
3. *A client asks you to wipe up the bathroom with her special brand of cleaner. You read the label on the container and find that it is not a disinfectant. How can you respect the client's wishes and still maintain infection control?*
4. *Explain how you demonstrate the characteristics needed for working as a home health aide (be able to work independently, organized, reliable, flexible, adaptable, able to maintain professional boundaries).*
5. *You have been the home health aide for a client for several weeks and you have grown very fond of the client and family. The client is now ready to be discharged and your services will no longer be needed. On one of your last visits, the client hands you an envelope containing a large sum of money. What would you do?*

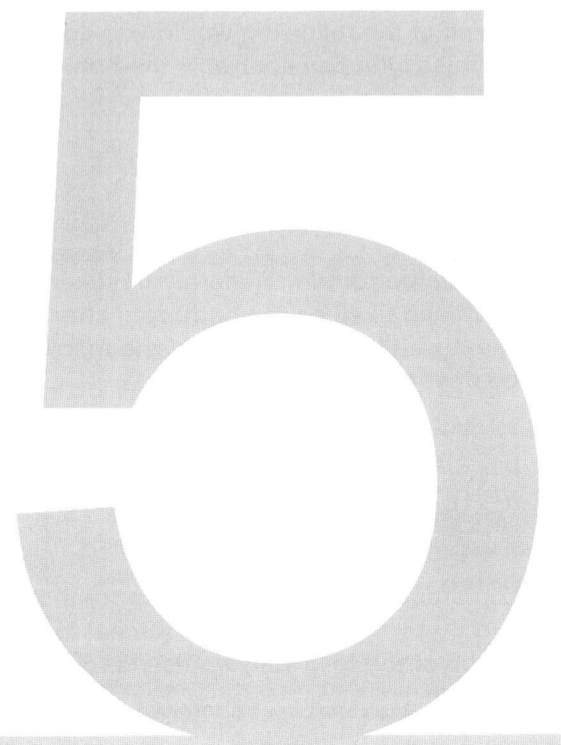

UNIT 5

TRANSITIONING FROM STUDENT TO EMPLOYEE

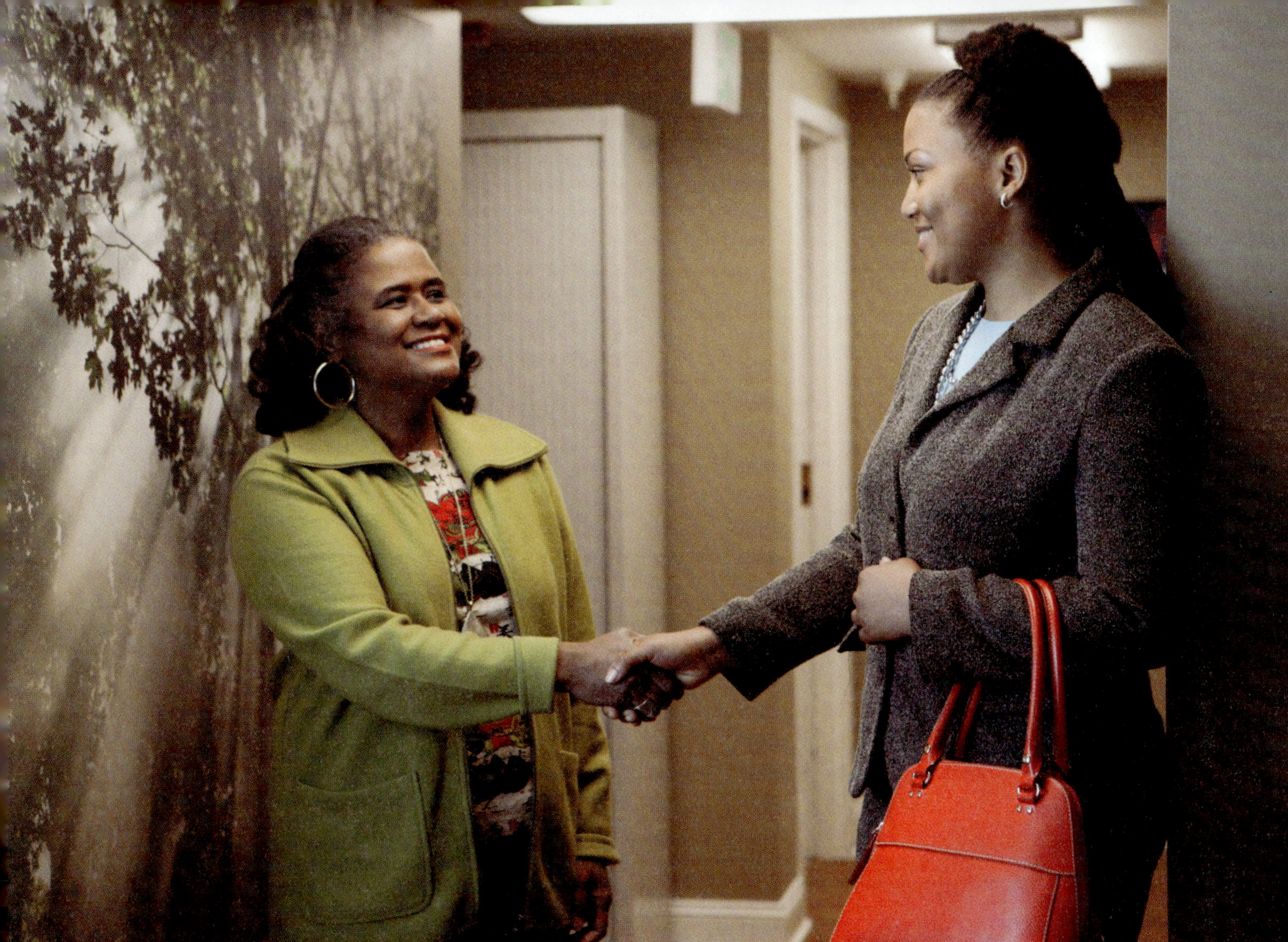

CHAPTER

23

Entering the Workforce

Goals

After reading this chapter, you will have the information needed to:

- Plan a job search.
- Prepare a résumé, reference list and cover letter.
- Describe the job application process.
- Interview effectively.
- Accept or decline a job offer.
- Know what to expect during your first few days on the job.

Key Terms:

résumé
reference list
job application
cover letter
job interview
pre-placement health evaluation
employee orientation
probationary period

You are sitting at lunch with a few of your classmates talking about your classes. Suddenly your friend Jenny says, "Can you believe it? You know, in just about two months, we will all be working somewhere. That's incredible. I don't even know where to start." As the discussion continues, your instructor Ms. Howard walks by. She overhears your conversation and sits down to join you. She says, "You know, with everything going on in our country today, the demand for well-trained, hard-working nurse assistants is very high. More people are living longer lives, many with chronic health conditions. Employers at health care facilities and agencies are looking to use staff members effectively to maximize efficiency while maintaining an excellent quality of care. You are a great group of students, and I think you are going to have lots of choices and opportunities once you are ready to enter the job market!"

PLANNING YOUR JOB SEARCH

Once you graduate from your program and pass your state certification test, you will start looking for a job. Most people start looking for a job without a plan, which can result in wasted time and a feeling of frustration. You can avoid this—and increase your chances of success—by making a plan. Being organized will help you make the most of your search and find the job that is right for you.

Identifying the Right Job for You

Your training qualifies you to work in many different types of health care settings and with many different types of clients. Before beginning your job search, it is a good idea to think about what sort of job situation best suits your interests and lifestyle. Asking the following questions can help you identify job opportunities that will appeal to you:

- In what type of setting do you want to work? For example, would you be more comfortable working in a facility or in a person's home? Do you prefer the fast-paced environment of an acute care setting, such as a hospital or clinic, or would you like to have time to get to know the people in your care over a longer time?
- Is there a particular type of client you enjoy caring for? For example, if you enjoy working with elderly people, then maybe a long-term care setting would be most appealing to you. If you find it satisfying to help people at the end of life, perhaps a hospice organization would be the right fit.
- Would you prefer to work the day, evening or night shift? Do you need to take a spouse's or child's schedule into consideration?
- How will you get to work? If you plan to take public transportation to work, you will need to look for job opportunities in areas that are well-serviced by your desired mode of transportation.

Identifying Job Opportunities

Many resources are available to help people who are looking for a job. One of the best resources is people you already know. Your instructors and the nurse assistants and nurses you worked with during your clinical training may know of job openings for nurse assistants. The Internet is also a very useful tool for looking for job. You can visit the websites of health care facilities and agencies in your area that interest you. Many websites list job opportunities and allow people to apply for them online. Websites such as CareerBuilder.com and Monster.com allow you to search for job opportunities and post your résumé so those who are interested in hiring can find you. Websites such as LinkedIn.com allow you to promote your skills, network with other people and announce your availability. Newspaper ads are also a good source of information about employment opportunities.

You decide that if what Ms. Howard told you about the many opportunities for nurse assistants is true, you better start thinking about what job situation would best suit your needs and make you happiest. You think that the opportunity to work with lots of different clients of all ages would be exciting, and you like the idea of never knowing exactly what the day will bring. You also like the idea of working as part of a team and having co-workers and supervisors close by. You begin to think that maybe a hospital setting would be right for you. You will be driving to work, but you would like to spend no more than 20 minutes commuting each way.

What are the benefits of thinking about your ideal job situation in advance?

What will be your next steps in planning your job search?

APPLYING FOR JOBS

Once you identify job opportunities that interest you, you need to apply for those jobs. Many employers require you to submit a résumé, reference list and cover letter as part of your job application.

Preparing a Résumé

A **résumé** is a document summarizing your contact information, education and previous experience (Figure 23-1). Your résumé should be limited to one page, if possible. Type your résumé using a plain, simple font, and print it out on plain white paper. Résumés usually have several standard parts:

- **Contact information.** Place your contact information at the top of the page, either in the upper left corner or centered. Include your name, mailing address, e-mail address and phone number. When choosing an e-mail address, make sure that it is professional (for example, your first initial and last name).
- **Objective.** Provide a one-line description of your qualifications and the type of job you are seeking (for example, "To obtain a position as a certified nurse assistant in an acute care setting").
- **Education.** List each school or training program that you attended, the dates you attended the program and the degree that you graduated with. Start with your most recent training and work backward to your high school education.
- **Employment.** List the jobs that you held, starting with the most recent and working backward. Include your job title, the dates that you held the job, and a brief description of your duties and accomplishments. Remember that even if the jobs that you held in the past are not directly related to the type of job you are seeking now, you probably still gained experience and skills that are applicable to your current job search. For example, working as a cashier in a retail store demonstrates that you have experience providing customer service, a skill that is very applicable to working in health care.
- **Additional experience.** If applicable, you can include a section listing additional experience that is relevant to the job that you are applying for. For example, if you have done volunteer work or community service, it would be appropriate to list those activities here. Similarly, if you are fluent in another language, be sure to mention that on your résumé.
- **References.** At the end of the résumé, indicate that "References are available on request."

Some information is not appropriate to include on a résumé, including your age, your religion, your sexual orientation, whether you are married and whether you have children. This kind of personal information should have no bearing on whether a potential employer decides to hire you.

Preparing a Reference List

A **reference list** is a document providing the contact information for three to five people who know you well enough in a professional capacity to speak to a potential employer about your experience and suitability for a job. When you think about people to ask to be a reference for you, think about people who know firsthand what your strengths are and what you will bring to a job. Former supervisors, teachers, coaches and clergy members are people you may want to consider asking to serve as a reference for you. Before listing a person on your reference list, contact the person and ask whether he would be willing to serve as a reference for you. Make sure that you have complete contact information for the person, including the person's full name, mailing address, e-mail address and telephone number. Type your reference list neatly, using the same font you used for your résumé, and print it out on a piece of plain white paper.

Submitting Job Applications

Now that you have identified jobs that you would like to apply for and prepared your résumé and reference list, it is time to start submitting applications. A **job application** is a form that employers use to collect basic information about you, such as your contact information, your employment history, your educational history, your additional experience and skills, the hours you are available to work and your references. Much of this information is the same as the information provided on your résumé and reference list, so having these documents on hand will make it much easier to complete the job application. Because a job application is considered a legal document, it is important to be honest and accurate when completing it.

Today, many employers have job candidates complete the job application form online. The online job application is then submitted electronically, along with a copy of your résumé and a **cover letter**. A cover letter is a brief letter to a potential employer that explains why you are interested in the job and organization. In addition, the cover letter is an

Jacalyn Jacinto
123 South Street
Big City, US 12345
(123) 456-7890
jjacinto@speedymail.com

Objective

A position as a certified nurse assistant in a long-term care facility

Education

Big City Chapter, American Red Cross Big City, US	September–October 2012 Nurse Assistant Training CNA certification: November 2012
Community Junior College Big City, US	August–December 2010
Big City High School Big City, US	Graduated: June 2010 High school diploma

Employment

Modern Style Clothing — January 2011–August 2012

Sales Associate. Provided customer service on the floor. Operated cash register. Maintained and restocked merchandise.

Super Savings Supermarket — June 2009–December 2010

Cashier. Provided customer service by scanning and bagging items for check out; operated cash register.

Additional Experience

Big City Chapter, American Red Cross Big City, US	October 2012 CPR/AED for Professional Rescuers and Health Care Providers Red Cross certification: October 2012
Big City Food Bank Volunteer	January 2012–present

Fluent in Spanish

References

References available on request.

Figure 23-1 Sample résumé for a nurse assistant.

opportunity for you to briefly describe the qualifications and experience you have that make you an appropriate candidate for the job that you are applying for (Figure 23-2).

If you are applying for a job that was advertised in the newspaper, you will send your résumé and cover letter to the employer through the mail. If the employer is interested in interviewing you, you will be asked to fill out the job application when you arrive for your interview. Again, having copies of your résumé and references on hand will make it easier to complete this paperwork. Because you will be completing a paper form, be sure to write neatly.

You may also apply for jobs by going to facilities or agencies where you are interested in working and asking at the front desk if you may fill out an application and leave a résumé. The employer will keep your application and résumé on file and may call you if a suitable job opportunity opens up.

You identify openings for nurse assistants at three local hospitals and decide to apply. But first, you know that you need to get your résumé and reference list together and write cover letters to accompany your applications. Before deciding to become a nurse assistant, you held various part-time jobs, including driving a school bus and working as a server at a local restaurant.

What experience from your previous jobs would be valuable and applicable to your role as a nurse assistant? How would you describe this experience on your résumé?

What information will you gather to help you write a cover letter to accompany each application you submit? Why is it important to write a cover letter specific to each job that you are applying for?

Jacalyn Jacinto
123 South Street
Big City, US 12345
November 3, 2012

Patricia Patterson, RN
Director of Nursing
Independence Village
3 Independence Way
Big City, US 12345

Dear Ms. Patterson,

I am writing to express my interest in applying for the certified nurse assistant position I saw advertised on your company's website. Last month, I completed the American Red Cross Nurse Assistant Training course, and I have passed the state certification exam.

During my clinical training at Springhill Manor Rehabilitation, I discovered that I really enjoy caring for older clients and helping them achieve their best possible level of functioning. I understand from looking at your website that Independence Village is known for providing quality restorative care, and I would really like to be part of your team!

Thank you for taking the time to review my résumé. I am available for an interview at your convenience, and I look forward to hearing from you soon.

Sincerely,

Jacalyn Jacinto

Figure 23-2 Sample cover letter.

GOING ON JOB INTERVIEWS

A **job interview** is a meeting between a job candidate and an employer that allows both parties to find out more about each other. During the job interview, the employer will talk with you to learn more about you and your suitability for the job. You can also use the interview as a time to find out more about the organization and the job.

Doing a little research before the interview can help you to feel more confident and prepared. Visit the organization's website. Often, there is a great deal of information on the website about the company's history, mission (that is, its statement of purpose), ownership and the services that it provides. Being knowledgeable about the organization and the job you are applying for demonstrates to the employer that you are serious about your job search and that you are genuinely interested in working for the organization.

Think about questions that you might be asked during the interview and how you will answer them. Examples of questions you may be asked include:

- Why do you want to work as a nurse assistant?
- What do you find most satisfying about working as a nurse assistant?
- Why did you choose to apply for a job at our organization?
- What are your career goals for 5 years from now?
- Tell me why you are the best candidate for this job.
- Tell me about a time that you had a problem at work. How did you solve it?
- Describe your ideal work environment.
- Why did you leave your last job?

Remember that the interview is also a chance for you to ask questions. Think about these questions in advance. Your goal is to get a better understanding of what would be expected of you as an employee and what the work environment will be like. Examples of questions you might ask include:

- What do the nurse assistants who work here like best about working here?
- May I talk with one of the nurse assistants who works here?
- On average, how many people would I care for during a shift?
- How does the organization support professional advancement for employees? For example, will I have the opportunity to receive ongoing training as part of my job?
- May I have a copy of the job description?
- How often are employee reviews conducted, and what standards will I be held to?

Although you may be interested in learning more about what the organization can offer you in terms of pay, vacation time and health benefits, the interview is not the time to ask these questions. Save these questions for when you receive a job offer!

Before your interview, make sure that the clothes you intend to wear are clean, pressed and in good repair (Figure 23-3). Women should wear a blouse and dress slacks or a skirt, or a dress. Avoid clothing that is overly revealing, such as mini-skirts, tops with low-cut necklines and open-toed shoes. Men should wear a button-down shirt and tie and a pressed pair of khakis or dress slacks. Pay attention to grooming as well. You want to help the employer see you as a member of the staff and a representative of the organization, so the same guidelines you learned in Chapter 1 about maintaining a professional appearance apply here. Make sure that your hair and nails are neat, clean and trimmed. Avoid strong perfume or cologne. Any jewelry you choose to wear should be minimal.

Put together all the paperwork that you will need for your interview and have it organized and ready to go with you. The person who is interviewing you may request a hard copy of your résumé and reference list. Even if she does not ask for a copy of these documents, having them on hand will make it easier to complete the job application.

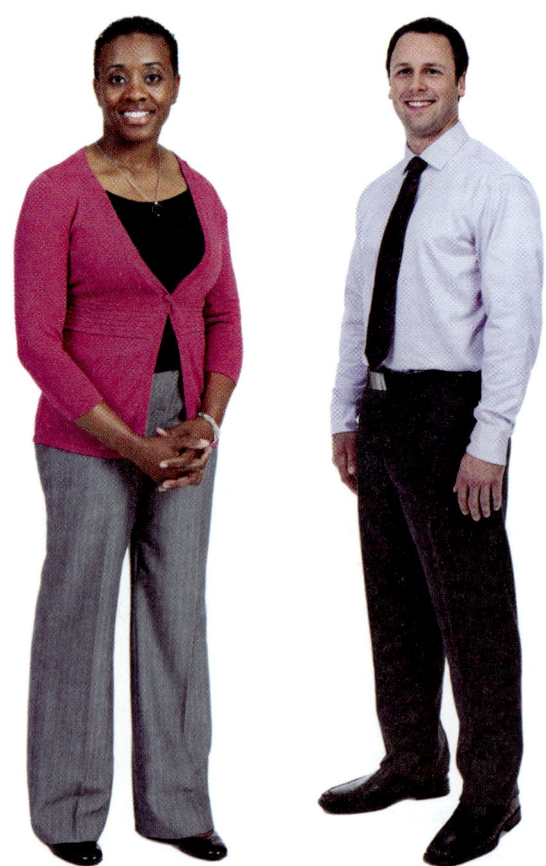

Figure 23-3 Help potential employers see you as a member of their staff by dressing neatly and professionally for the interview.

Also bring along the list of questions that you would like to ask the interviewer.

Plan your route to the interview and leave early enough so that you get there 10 to 15 minutes before you are expected. When you arrive at the interview, turn off your cell phone. You do not want a call to interrupt your interview. When you meet the person who will be interviewing you, remember that manners count. Employers need to know that you will treat your clients and their family members, as well as your co-workers and managers, with dignity and respect. A firm handshake is a great introduction. Although it is natural to be nervous, try to appear calm and at ease, and try to smile!

The interview usually begins with the interviewer asking you a few questions about yourself and why you are interested in the job. This is when your advance preparation will pay off! Answer questions honestly and to the best of your ability. Keep your answers brief and to the point. If you do not know the answer to a question, it is fine to say that you do not know. When you speak about past employers, always be as positive as possible, even if the experience was a negative one. If you were fired from a previous job, be honest. It is better that the employer find this out from you firsthand.

At the end of the interview, thank the interviewer for his time and ask when he expects to make a hiring decision. Within one day of your interview, send a written note by mail or email to the interviewer to thank him again for the opportunity to interview. In your note or email, express your interest in working for the organization and include a brief statement about why you find the job appealing and think it is a good fit for you (Figure 23-4). If the employer has narrowed the choice down to you and one other candidate, this follow-up email or card may make the difference. If you do not hear back from the interviewer within the time frame he gave you at the end of the interview, it is appropriate to call and ask whether the job has been filled or whether you are still being considered for it. Calling shows initiative and demonstrates to the employer that you are genuinely interested in the job.

Your hard work and preparation paid off, and you have been asked to come in for two interviews.

What will you do to prepare for your interviews, and make a good impression on your potential employer?

RESPONDING TO A JOB OFFER

Job offers are usually made over the telephone. Now is the time to ask about the pay and benefits offered by the company! It is all right to ask the person making the offer if you may have some time to think about the offer before accepting or declining it, but be sure to get back to the person within a day. You may be lucky enough to receive several job offers at once. This is where all of the thought that you have put into your job search and all of the information that you gathered will be very useful, because it will help you choose the job that fits you best.

In some cases, you may not receive a job offer. Take a little time to think about how you felt the interview went and whether you can do certain things better next time. And remember, each interview you do will add to your experience and will make you better at the next interview.

November 15, 2012

Dear Ms. Patterson,

Thank you so much for your time today and for considering me for the nurse assistant position. I really enjoyed meeting you and learning more about Independence Village. I am very interested in working for your organization, because I think it would be very satisfying to help people achieve or maintain their highest level of functioning.

Sincerely,

Jacalyn Jacinto

Figure 23-4 Sample thank-you note.

BECOMING A NEW EMPLOYEE

Pre-placement Health Evaluation

After you receive and accept a job offer with an organization, you will be required to complete a **pre-placement health evaluation** to ensure that you are physically and emotionally capable of meeting the job requirements and to identify any accommodations that may need to be made so that you can perform the job competently and safely. As part of the pre-placement health evaluation, you will be required to complete several health screening tests, such as a physical examination, a tuberculosis (TB) screening test and a drug screening test, and to verify that necessary immunizations are up-to-date. The pre-placement health evaluation is done after a job offer is made because it is illegal for an employer to ask during the interview process about disabilities that may affect your ability to perform your duties. This is in accordance with the Americans with Disabilities Act and is done to prevent discrimination against people who may have disabilities but can perform the job (with or without accommodations). Depending on the results of the pre-placement health evaluation, however, employers do have the right to withdraw a job offer that has been made, if it is determined that reasonable accommodations cannot be made to allow you to perform the job competently and safely.

Orientation

When you become a new employee of an organization, you will receive an **employee orientation**. During employee orientation, you will receive information about:

- The benefits you are entitled to as an employee
- Your employer's expectations relative to your job performance
- Your employer's policies and procedures related to subjects such as attendance and dress code
- Your employer's emergency and disaster response protocols

During orientation, you should be provided with a written job description and a written "policies and procedures" manual. Receiving this orientation to your new workplace, along with any related documentation, is one of your rights as an employee.

Probationary Period

Some employers have a policy of considering the first few months to 1 year of an employee's employment with them to be a **probationary period**. During this time, the employer closely evaluates the job performance and potential of the employee. At the end of the probationary period (which usually lasts from 3 months to 1 year), the employee's supervisor completes a formal performance evaluation and discusses the employee's job performance to date with the employee. Some employers may not offer employee benefits until the probationary period is over and the employee is found to be performing the job to expectations.

CHECK YOUR UNDERSTANDING

Questions for Review

1. **Which document is used to summarize your education and employment history for a potential employer?**
   a. Cover letter
   b. Orientation document
   c. Résumé
   d. Reference list

2. **Which of the following should NOT be included on a résumé?**
   a. Your email address
   b. Your telephone number
   c. Your marital status
   d. Your volunteer work

3. **A job interview is your opportunity to:**
   a. Tell the employer your requirements related to salary, vacation and health benefits.
   b. Find out as much as you can about the organization and what it would be like to work there.
   c. Receive feedback on your job performance to date.
   d. Receive feedback on your résumé.

4. **Which of the following people would make a good professional reference for a person applying for a job as a nurse assistant?**
   a. A best friend
   b. A grandparent
   c. Your youth group leader
   d. All of the above

5. **What is the goal when dressing for an interview?**
   a. To impress the interviewer with your fashion sense
   b. To present a neat, clean, professional appearance
   c. To give the interviewer insight into your personality
   d. All of the above

6. **During a job interview, the employer's goal is to:**
   a. Determine whether you are the best person for the job.
   b. Make you nervous by asking you a series of questions.
   c. Orient you to the organization's policies and procedures.
   d. Verify that the information that you provided on your résumé and application is accurate and correct.

7. **What is the purpose of the pre-placement health evaluation?**
   a. To inform new employees of the organization's procedures and policies
   b. To discriminate against employees with health issues or disabilities
   c. To ensure that employees are physically and emotionally capable of meeting the job requirements and to identify any accommodations that may need to be made so that the employee can perform the job competently
   d. To make sure the employee is performing up to the employer's standards before benefits are offered

Questions to Ask Yourself

1. *Think about jobs that you have held (paid and unpaid) to date. What skills or experiences from these jobs could apply to your practice as a nurse assistant? What other talents do you have that might serve you well when you are working as a nurse assistant?*
2. *Who could you ask to serve as a professional reference for you? What do you think the people you have selected as references would say about your professionalism, your work ethic and the personal qualities that will allow you to excel as a nurse assistant and an employee?*
3. *Think about the image you present to the public (for example, on social networking sites such as Facebook or Twitter, or through the message on your answering machine or cell phone). What impressions do you think a person who does not know you well would form about you by looking at your profile on a social media site, or listening to the message on your answering machine or cell phone? Do you think that this impression may help or hurt your chances of being offered a job?*
4. *You want to make a good first impression on a potential employer. What are some actions you can take?*
5. *What job situation would be most appealing to you? How will you go about organizing your job search?*

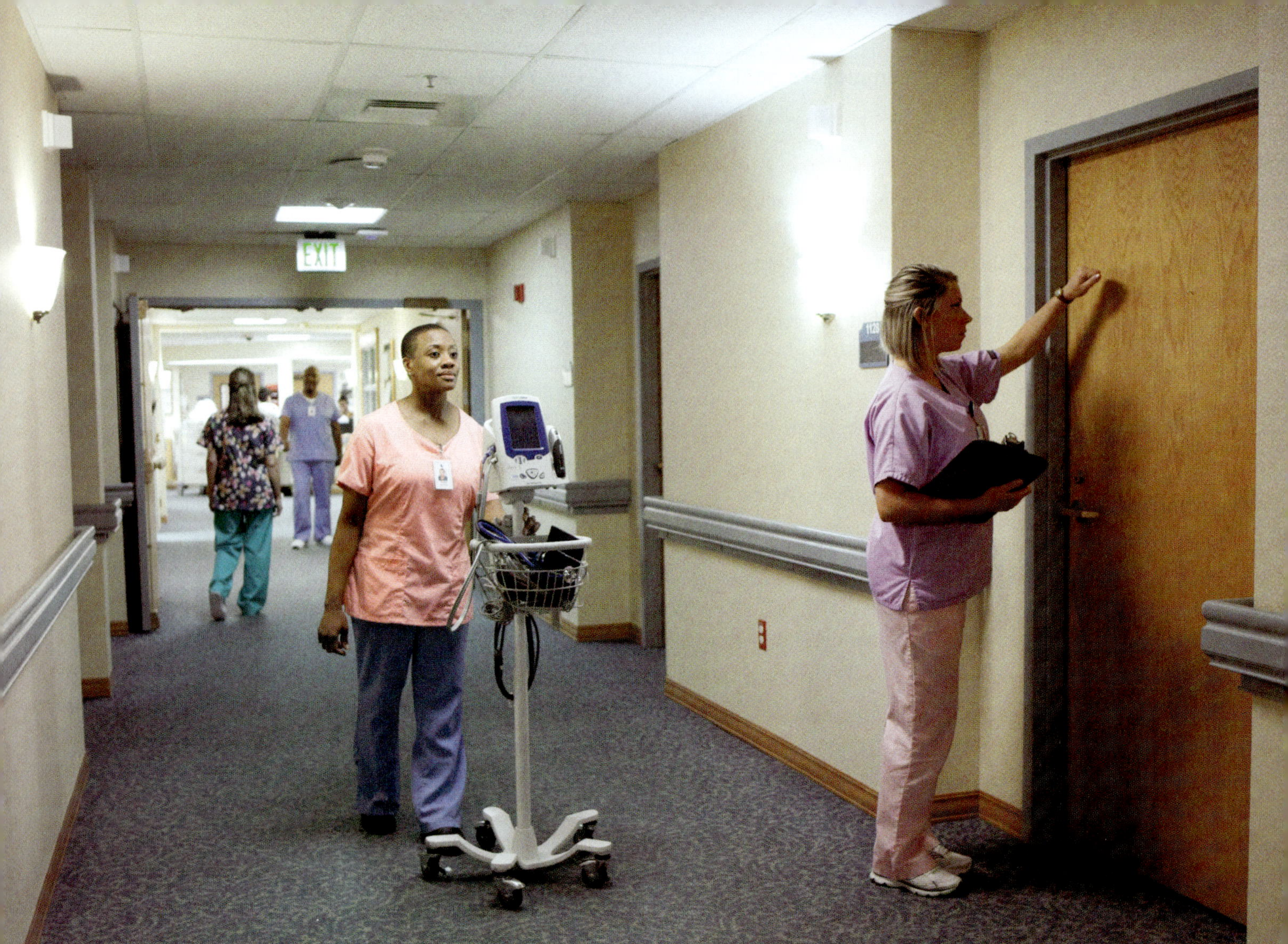

CHAPTER

24 Enjoying Professional Success

Goals

After reading this chapter, you will have the information needed to:

- Describe the basic expectations employers have for those wishing to be employed as nurse assistants.
- Describe the ways a nurse assistant can manage violence and harassment in the workplace.
- Describe the interpersonal skills a nurse assistant can use to manage difficult situations at work and contribute to a healthy work environment.
- Describe how to manage your time and prioritize your responsibilities.
- Describe the importance of caring for yourself, as well as others.
- Describe opportunities for career development and advancement for nurse assistants.

Key Terms:

harassment
in-service training
assertive
prioritize
schedule

You have just arrived at Morningside Nursing Home after a crazy morning at home. Your 8-year-old daughter told you that she needed to pick out another outfit for school because her shirt didn't match her pants. Then your 6-year-old son told you that he needed to bring in something for snack time at school today. And after all this, you realized that you needed to get gas in the car to get to work. As you enter the doorway at Morningside, you think to yourself, "I woke up feeling great about beginning my second month as a nurse assistant. I sure hope I can manage my day at work better than I've managed my time at home today. It's a miracle that I'm even here!"

BASIC EXPECTATIONS FOR THOSE EMPLOYED AS NURSE ASSISTANTS

Adhering to Employer Policies

The first step to being successful in the workplace is to learn about and adhere to your employer's policies. Although you will learn about your employer's specific policies and procedures during your employee orientation, most employers have common basic expectations for employees. These include the following:

- Show up on time and ready to work.
- If you will not be at work, call your supervisor or the designated person as soon as you know that you will not be coming in—at least 2 hours before your shift begins.
- Take breaks only when assigned. Before going on break, ensure the safety of those in your care. Tell your supervisor where you are going and when you will be returning, and return by the agreed-upon time. When your shift is over, report to your supervisor before leaving the floor.
- Clock in and out only on your time card. Do not clock in and out for anyone else.
- Follow directions. If you do not understand something, ask for clarification.
- Complete tasks. If you are not able to complete something, tell your supervisor.
- Document your actions. Remember: *It is not done if it is not documented.*
- Be aware that certain actions are never tolerated in the workplace. Violence or the threat of violence, abuse, harassment, possession of weapons or illegal drugs, intoxication and theft are each considered grounds for immediate termination by most employers. Should you either witness or be subjected to any of these circumstances, report them immediately to your supervisor or human resources department and complete an incident report.

Keeping Your Certification Up to Date

Keeping your nurse assistant certification up to date is also essential to keeping your job. Although each state has different renewal requirements, the following documents and information are most commonly needed to renew your certification:

- **Proof of employment.** To renew your certification, you must show that you are working or have recently worked as a nurse assistant. If you allow your certification to lapse, you will be required to take the training course and pass the certification evaluation again in order to be recertified.
- **Proof of completion of in-service requirements.** OBRA (the Omnibus Budget Reconciliation Act of 1987) requires nurse assistants to complete at least 12 hours of in-service training each year. **In-service training** is additional training offered by your employer with the intent of keeping employees' skills and knowledge up to date. During in-service training, you may be taught new skills or information, or receive refresher training in existing skills.
- **Renewal fee**
- **Completed application**

The application for certification renewal, as well as directions on where to send the application and fee, can usually be found on the website of the organization that maintains the registry for nurse assistants in your state (for example, the state Board of Nursing).

Time-management skills are important in the renewal process. You have to plan ahead to have your in-service hours completed, your renewal fee saved and your application completed and submitted before your certification expires. Keeping your job means keeping your nurse assistant certification.

DEALING WITH VIOLENCE AND HARASSMENT IN THE WORKPLACE

The risk for experiencing violent or aggressive behavior while on the job is, unfortunately, a very real one for nurse assistants and other health care workers. Although less common, harassment by fellow employees can also occur on the job. Being able to manage these difficult situations appropriately is important for your health and happiness at work.

Violence in the Workplace

As a nurse assistant, you may care for people who display violent or aggressive behavior toward you, such as hitting, kicking, slapping, spitting, biting or making verbal threats or offensive statements. Medication side effects and conditions such as dementia or mental illness can cause a person to act violently or aggressively. Although it is never acceptable for you to respond with violence or to cause harm to the person, it is also not expected that you must tolerate violence or abuse on the job.

The Occupational Safety and Health Administration (OSHA) recommends that employers establish violence-prevention programs. These programs provide training and establish protocols for preventing and responding to inappropriate conduct. The participation of all employees is important to ensure the success of the violence-prevention program.

As a nurse assistant, you can contribute to the success of a workplace violence-prevention program by taking the following measures:

- **Follow your employer's policy for reporting incidents.** Promptly report any incident of violence or aggression, and complete an incident report according to your employer's policy.
- **Communicate with other members of the health care team.** When caring for a person who displays violent or aggressive behavior, it is important to share your observations with the nurse about actions that can provoke this behavior, as well as actions that can reduce this behavior. The nurse can then include these strategies for reducing or responding to inappropriate behavior in the person's care plan, so that all caregivers have access to them.
- **Attend violence-prevention training offered by your employer.** Topics often include how to recognize warning signs (for example, behavioral changes or increasing anger) that could lead to a violent or abusive incident; how to manage an unsafe situation; and what procedures to follow should an incident occur.
- **Know ways of responding to another person's anger or aggression** (Box 24-1). Responding in these ways can help the situation from escalating out of control.

Harassment

Harassment is ongoing behavior that causes significant distress to another person. The behavior is done deliberately and repeatedly to frighten or distress the person. Harassment can be verbal or physical. You may find yourself being harassed by a fellow employee. Actions such as making unwanted sexual advances or comments; making comments about a person's gender, race, sexual orientation, culture, religious beliefs or other unique traits; or discriminating against a person

Box 24-1 How to Respond to and Manage Another Person's Anger or Aggressive Behavior

- Seek causes for the behavior. For example, an undiagnosed infection or an injury can cause a person to respond with anger or aggression when you attempt to give care.
- Do not take the person's anger personally.
- Avoid getting too close to the person or touching the person. This may be threatening to the person and may make him or her angrier or more aggressive.
- If someone is angry about what you are doing or responds with aggression, stop the task and give the person time to cool off.
- Try distracting the person with another activity or change the topic and tone of the conversation to something pleasant.
- Ask for help from a co-worker when you must provide care to a person who is known to behave in a violent or aggressive manner.

because of the person's unique traits are all forms of harassment. If you feel that you are being harassed at work, you should bring the matter to the attention of your supervisor, the human resources department, or both.

CONTRIBUTING TO A POSITIVE WORK ENVIRONMENT

Working in health care can be stressful. As a nurse assistant, you have a great deal of responsibility to provide safe, compassionate care. There will be multiple demands on your time, and it can be challenging to balance all of your responsibilities and make sure that everyone's needs are met. In addition, health care is a people-focused profession. Where there are people, there are emotions. Especially in health care, these emotions can be very strong. If not managed well, they can lead to increased stress and burn-out.

A positive work environment is one where staff members support each other and feel supported. Every employee can contribute to a positive work environment. To succeed in the workplace and help contribute to a positive work environment, you must know how to manage stress and other strong emotions, such as anger. You must also have strong interpersonal skills, including skills related to resolving conflicts and advocating for yourself and others. Guidelines for contributing to a positive work environment are given in Box 24-2.

Managing Feelings of Anger

Anger is a natural human response to stress. Anger is neither better nor worse than any other human emotion. Feelings of anger are often accompanied by physical symptoms, such as increased heart and respiratory rates, increased blood pressure and flushing of the cheeks. Some people burst into tears when they become angry. Although anger is a normal response in certain situations, it is important to know how to handle this strong emotion appropriately. Managing anger is crucial to succeeding in your job (as well as in your personal life!).

In your job as a nurse assistant, you may have occasion to feel angry. Sometimes you may not be treated with the dignity and respect you deserve. A person in your care may say inappropriate things, hit you, or spit on you. It is important to look at why the person might be saying or doing these things. Often, these inappropriate behaviors are part of the disease process, and the person cannot help his or her behavior. Understanding this might help to reduce some of the anger you are feeling in response to the person's behavior.

Co-workers may not treat you with the dignity and respect that you deserve, either. Some staff members may focus more on your job title than your contributions, and treat you in a dismissive or condescending way. Staff members who are stressed may also show negative behavior. Stress makes people less tolerant, and they can become angry more easily. Sometimes you will be the target of another person's anger, even when you do not deserve to be.

The natural response when someone treats you badly or unfairly is to become angry. Unchecked anger may cause you to say or do something that you will regret. To prevent this from happening, take deep breaths, and try to regain control of your emotions. Think about reasons why the other person might be behaving in the way that is making you angry, and try to practice empathy. If necessary, remove yourself from the situation until you can regain control. (Of course, if the situation involves a person in your care, arrange for the person's safety before leaving.)

Managing Conflict

Conflict, or disagreements, can arise when two people have differing viewpoints. Health care is people-focused, and as a result, it can be emotionally charged. There are many opportunities for conflict to arise. Conflicts may arise between two staff members, or between a staff member and a person in his or her care (or a family

Box 24-2 Nurse Assistant DO's and DON'Ts

Contributing to a Positive Work Environment

DO support your co-workers. Be willing to pitch in to help others when needed.

DO use good communication skills to prevent misunderstandings from occurring and to resolve misunderstandings that do occur.

DO treat everyone courteously.

DO smile!

DON'T gossip. Gossip is usually negative and not factual, and it can distract you and others from the work you need to do. Avoiding gossip helps to keep stress and other unnecessary negative emotions out of your life.

DON'T call out absent from work unless you are really unable to attend because of illness or a family emergency. When one staff member is absent, others have to pick up that person's workload for the shift.

member of a person receiving care). Conflicts can also arise between two people receiving care.

No matter when it arises or who it involves, conflict always has a negative impact in the workplace. It is always best to resolve conflict as quickly as possible so that both parties have a more positive attitude about the future (Figure 24-1). It is also best to confront the source of the conflict directly, but this does not mean attacking the other person. Even if a team member is rude to you, it is not appropriate for you to be rude in return. Rather, try saying something such as, "When you talk to me like that, it makes me feel bad, and it is difficult for me to want to work with you. I really don't like feeling this way." This statement expresses how the other person's behavior affects you. It is nonthreatening, and it invites conversation, which can lead to settlement. The two of you can discuss what is not right and decide how you can work together to make the situation better for both parties. Guidelines for resolving conflicts are given in Box 24-3.

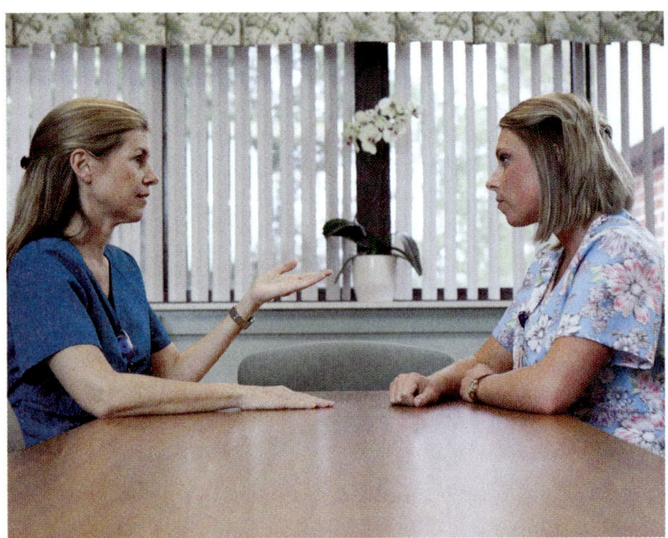

Figure 24-1 Resolving conflicts that arise is essential.

Most conflict can be resolved between the two parties involved. If you believe you have honestly tried, but failed, to resolve the conflict, you should bring the problem to the attention of your supervisor. Because unresolved conflict can be very disruptive to the workplace and it can affect the quality of care that is provided, it is very important to work together to find a solution to the problem. And, once the conflict is satisfactorily resolved, it is important for both parties to put the conflict behind them and move on.

Practicing Assertive Communication

The ability to be **assertive** is another important interpersonal skill to practice in the workplace. Being assertive means that you are able to make your needs and feelings known in a respectful way. An assertive person communicates his or her needs and feelings in a direct way, while still respecting the needs and feelings of others. This is different from an aggressive person, who communicates his or her needs and feelings directly, but without regard for the needs and feelings of others. An aggressive person comes across as threatening or a bully. An assertive person is also different from a passive or passive-aggressive person, who fails to communicate his or her needs and feelings at all, but instead becomes stressed, resentful or angry about the situation. Instead of facing the issue directly, a passive person internalizes his or her anger and dissatisfaction. A passive-aggressive person internalizes his or her anger and dissatisfaction and also may act out in inappropriate ways (for example, by making sarcastic comments).

Consider this situation: A co-worker asks if you can come help her in 15 minutes, because she needs help

Box 24-3 Nurse Assistant DO's and DON'Ts

Resolving Conflict

DO ask to speak with the person privately.

DON'T use accusatory language that assigns blame to the other person. Instead, take responsibility for your own emotional response to the situation. For example, instead of saying, "You should have known better!" say, "I'm concerned by what I saw you doing yesterday."

DO allow the other person to express his or her feelings about the situation, and try to understand the other person's viewpoint.

DO ask the other person to work with you to find a solution to the problem that meets everyone's needs.

DO understand that sometimes in order to move beyond the conflict, you may just have to "agree to disagree" about certain points.

DO apologize for any role you may have played in the conflict.

DO seek help from a supervisor if it is impossible to resolve the conflict on your own. Unresolved conflicts affect the quality of the work environment and the care that you provide, and therefore cannot be allowed to continue.

getting a person in her care out of bed. It is near the end of your shift, and you really need to leave work on time today because you have to pick up your daughter at school. A passive response would be "Sure!" (while you become stressed and silently resent the fact that now you will be late to pick up your daughter). An aggressive response would be "No way! I told you earlier today that I had to leave on time today. Why don't you ever listen to me?" This type of response does nothing to help your co-worker and, in addition, will probably make her feel bad. But an assertive response would be "My shift is over in 15 minutes, and I need to leave on time today to pick up my daughter at school. I can help you now, or maybe Mary is available to help you later." The assertive response helps you to meet your needs, while also helping your co-worker to solve her problem.

When using assertive communication skills, what you say is as important as how you say it. Speak confidently, but without aggression or blame. Maintain a pleasant facial expression. Acknowledge that you understand the situation and the other person's point of view. Then, explain your point of view or position, using "I" statements. Finally, try to offer a suggestion for reaching a solution.

Being able to assert yourself helps to reduce stress, because it can help you to manage your time and your workload and prevent feelings of resentment and anger that can occur when you take on more responsibility than you can handle. Being assertive also helps you to gain the respect of others, because they see that you are direct about communicating your needs but also are understanding of their needs. Finally, the ability to speak up is important to protect yourself, those in your care and even your employer. For example, suppose another staff member asks you to do a procedure that you are not legally allowed to do. You may not be comfortable denying the person's request, especially if the person is senior to you in the organization. However, to protect yourself, the person in your care and even your employer, it is important for you to speak up in a respectful manner and tell the person that you cannot do the task and explain why.

MANAGING TIME

As you move from the role of student to employee, you move into areas of greater responsibility. You can make this transition smoothly if you know how to:

- Plan your time, using critical thinking skills to assess situations.
- Balance your scheduling needs and the needs of the people in your care.
- Stay in control of your time.

Using Critical Thinking Skills to Manage Your Time

The ability to think critically about situations and problems will help you in your everyday life and at work. Critical thinking is a five-step process:

1. Identify the problem.
2. List alternatives to solve the problem.
3. List the pros and cons of each alternative solution.
4. Decide on the solution.
5. Evaluate: Is the problem solved?

When you think critically about a situation, you are able to see the impact various courses of action may have. For example, you are on your way to help Mrs. Symington transfer from bed to the bathroom when you see Mr. Shilling's call light go on. You know that Mr. Shilling is impatient and will try to get out of bed without help, risking a fall. Mrs. Symington is less inclined to get out of bed without assistance, but she may have an episode of incontinence if she needs to wait too much longer. You look around and do not see anyone who is immediately available to help you. You decide to help Mr. Shilling first, since the consequences of a fall could be potentially much worse than having to change Mrs. Symington's clothing and linens. Applying critical thinking skills to this problem helped you determine the potential consequences of each course of action and make a decision.

Critical thinking skills also allow you to solve problems that may arise because each person in your care, and each situation, is unique. For example, you are a home health aide and Mr. Tripp, one of the clients in your care, has trouble standing at the sink to shave. It is not possible for Mr. Tripp to sit at the sink because there is nowhere for him to put his knees. You could shave Mr. Tripp in bed, or you could set him up with his shaving supplies at the kitchen table. You decide to set Mr. Tripp up to shave at the table, so that he can still maintain his independence. In this way, you used your critical thinking skills to determine the best solution to the problem.

Developing Time-Management Skills

Your personal life

Time management is one of the most challenging tasks you face as a busy adult—particularly if you are a parent. It can be difficult to juggle job and family responsibilities, as well as time for yourself. Completing the time-management checklist in Box 24-4 can help you get an idea of where your current strengths and weaknesses are when it comes to time management.

Box 24-4 **Time-Management Checklist**

Answer *yes* or *no* to each statement in this time-management checklist.

	Yes	No
1. I get to work 15 minutes early so that I can plan my workday before it begins.		
2. I know what I want to accomplish each day.		
3. I list tasks that need to be done each day and check them off as they are completed.		
4. I take big jobs and break them into smaller pieces.		
5. I do not take too much time away from my work by continually listing and planning.		
6. I do the most difficult and least interesting jobs first thing in the morning.		
7. I do not put off tasks; I do them *now*.		
8. I avoid letting one day's work carry over to the next day.		
9. I make full use of each day to complete that day's work.		
10. I sometimes evaluate myself to find out where I lose time.		
11. People compliment me on my use of time.		
12. I do not spend too much time on the phone.		
13. I watch and learn from the people around me who always seem to be ahead of schedule.		
14. I look for ways to use my time wisely each day.		
15. I group tasks logically.		
16. I listen carefully when someone gives me directions or other information.		
17. I set deadlines and strive to meet them.		

Now, look at the statements where you checked "yes." These are areas where you are already practicing good time-management skills! Next, look at the statements where you checked "no." These are areas that you will want to work on improving, to improve your time-management skills.

Good time-management skills are essential in helping you keep your job and reduce your stress levels. Here are some strategies you can use to help you manage your time effectively:

- Plan ahead for each day. **Prioritize** (list in order of importance) the things you must accomplish each day. Allow a realistic amount of time to complete each item.
- Have back-up plans in place (for example, for child care and transportation).
- Always plan to report to work at least 15 minutes before your shift starts.
- Make sure you have a reliable alarm clock.
- Have a reliable form of transportation.
- Keep a monthly calendar noting personal and family activities and appointments. Record all activities and appointments and coordinate them with your work schedule.
- Share household duties with your spouse and children.
- Establish set times for daily activities such as homework, baths and bedtime.
- Check your phone messages and write them down. Open mail daily.
- Pay bills twice a month (for example, on the 1st and the 15th of each month).
- Keep an ongoing grocery list, noting items that need to be replaced as they are used up, and shop once a week for the entire week.

Think back to your crazy morning. What time-management skills could you have used to make your morning easier?

Your work life

The world of learning and the world of work are different. When you learn new ideas and skills in a training program, you learn to perform every step of a task—such as giving a complete bed bath—in a specific, uninterrupted way. By learning the ideal way to perform these skills, you master how to perform each step. However, in a real-life setting, the situations are not as ideal, nor are they as specific. You may need to modify the skills you have learned to meet the specific needs of each person in your care. In addition, you will be required to provide care for many more people at once.

In the real world, other people and situations influence how you use your time. For example, someone else makes decisions about how many people are in your care. How much time you spend caring for each person is also determined by factors outside your control, such as the person's medical condition and level of mobility. Finally, unplanned events happen when you least expect them. For example, you may be giving a bed bath when the person you are bathing begins to vomit. You have to stop what you are doing and sit the person up or turn his head to the side. Then, once the person is no longer vomiting, you must make sure he is all right, report the situation to the nurse and decide what new actions to take. In addition, the person may have to be bathed again, and the linens may have to be changed. You must make new decisions based on each new situation. No matter what you decide, this bed bath will take longer than usual.

Box 24-5 describes a typical day in the life of Nora, a nurse assistant working in a nursing home. Reading about Nora's day can help you to see some of the time-management challenges that arise during a typical day and effective ways of handling them. Learning to make the most of your time enables you to give people the best care possible.

Planning your day

Every day on your new job, you have many tasks to complete and details to remember. So far, you have been learning specific skills. Now you have to know how to put them all together. You must create a **schedule** (a written plan that lists the time and order of several tasks) to guide you through the day. At first, scheduling your time seems difficult. As you gain experience, it will become easier.

At the beginning of each shift, you find out how many people are in your care and who they are. The nursing care plan and a verbal report from either the caregivers who worked on the previous shift or from your supervisor give you information about the kind of care that each

Text continues on page 394.

▼ Box 24-5 **Nora's Day**

In the following account of a typical day in the life of a nurse assistant, Nora Fuentes, you will see how a nurse assistant plans her day and controls her time, yet responds to the needs of the people in her care. If you try to stay organized and plan your day, as well as remain flexible and responsive to unexpected situations as they arise, you too can manage your time effectively. As you are reading about Nora's day, remember the five principles of care—safety, privacy, dignity, communication and independence—and look for examples of how Nora practices these principles.

Planning the Day

Nora arrives for work promptly at 7 A.M. In morning report, Nora learns that she has five residents in her care: Rachel Morgan, Victor Rivera, Jake Wilson, Shirley McDay and Rodney Britten.

Nora already knows four of these residents well, but Mr. Britten has been at the nursing home just a few days. She looks at the quick, abbreviated notes she has written during report and reads:

Rm. 121 *R. Morgan,* 45, MS (un-bed)

- Can feed self (DR)
- Help with: bed bath—dressing—bedpan—transfer to w/c—ROM
- Blurred vision—tires easily
- *PT—1 P.M.

Rm. 114 *V. Rivera,* 78, stroke (un-bed)

- Help with: bed bath—dressing—elec razor—urinal (7, 9, 11, 1)—feeding (DR)—transfer to w/c
- L-sided weakness—*ROM in A.M.
- *PT—1 P.M.

Rm. 120 *J. Wilson,* 79, diabetes (un-bed)

- Can: dress—feed self (DR)—walk/cane—tub
- Help with: dentures—elec razor
- Sight—light perception—sensation: hands & feet
- *PT—10:30 A.M. RecT—2 P.M.
- *Urine S&A early A.M.—diabetic diet

Rm. 119 *S. McDay,* 55, Alzheimer's (un-bed)

- Can: feed self (DR)—OOB bathroom—walk with assist
- Help with: tub—remind her to use the toilet—incont. care—dressing
- Wanders A.M. & P.M.—rummages and hoards

Rm. 124 *R. Britten,* 41, AIDS, wound isolation (oc-bed)

- Help with: bed bath—soft foods and liquids—bedpan
- Vomiting and diarrhea
- *VS in A.M.

* Indicates that the task must be done at a particular time.

Continued on next page

▼ Box 24-5 **Nora's Day** *Continued*

After reading the morning report, Nora creates a schedule for the day's activities similar to the one shown here:

	Rachel Morgan	**Victor Rivera**	**Jake Wilson**	**Shirley McDay**	**Rodney Britten (Reverse Isolation)**
7:00 A.M.	Bedpan	Urinal	Urine S&A Tub 7:15		VS
	Set up A.M. care, bed bath, help dress		Assist dentures/ shave	Tub 7:45 Help dress	A.M. care (gown/ gloves)
8:00 A.M.	Rest				Tray setup
	Up to w/c to DR (need help)	Tray setup/assist feed	Assist walk to DR	Assist walk to DR	Assist feed Oc-bed
9:00 A.M.	Un-bed	Urinal			Rest
	DR—back	A.M. care, help dress, ROM	DR—back	DR—back	
10:00 A.M.	Rest in bed (need help)	Up to w/c (need help)	*10:30 PT Un-bed	Un-bed	
	ROM	Un-bed			
11:00 A.M.	Rest	Urinal		Check incont.	Check diarrhea
11:30 lunch					
12:00 noon	Up to w/c to DR (need help)	Tray setup Assist feed	Assist walk to DR	Check incont. Assist walk to DR	Tray setup Assist feed Rest
1:00 P.M.	*1:00 w/c DR to PT	Urinal *1:00 PT	DR—back	DR—back	Check diarrhea
2:00 P.M.	Rest in bed (need help)	Rest in bed (need help) Wife visits	*2:00 RecT	Check incont.	VS
3:00 P.M. Report Charting		Urinal			Check diarrhea Remove trash and linens (need help)

* Indicates that task is to be done at a specific time.

Nora looks over her schedule and notes that she needs help transferring Rachel Morgan and Victor Rivera into and out of bed. Nora decides to talk to her co-worker Arthur to see whether he might be able to help her. Arthur and Nora compare assignment sheets and realize that they are working in nearby rooms and that they both will need help with transferring their assigned residents, so they arrange to work together. They also realize that they have the same lunch break.

Following the Schedule

Nora's first stop is Room 121, where she offers Rachel Morgan the bedpan. "I'll be back shortly to help you with your bed bath and dressing," Nora says before she leaves the room.

Nora's next stop is Room 114. She offers Victor Rivera his urinal. Because Mr. Rivera has had a stroke and is on a bladder training program, he must be offered his urinal every 2 hours. "I'll be back with your breakfast tray, Mr. Rivera," Nora says. Nora washes her hands after exiting Mr. Rivera's room.

She then heads to Room 120. Because Jake Wilson is diabetic, he has to have his urine checked for glucose and acetone daily. He knows the routine well, so he urinated once earlier in the morning and then again later to provide a sample.

▼ Box 24-5 **Nora's Day** *Continued*

Nora thanks him before asking how his favorite football team did in the game last night.

"The Dolphins beat the Cardinals 34 to 10! You should have seen it!" Mr. Wilson says, his eyes sparkling. "I played some football myself when I was younger."

Using standard precautions, Nora tests the urine for sugar and acetone and records the results, which she later reports to the nurse.

"How are my levels this morning?" asks Mr. Wilson.

Nora reassures Mr. Wilson that the test results are normal. She washes her hands and then walks with him to the tub room. While Nora helps Mr. Wilson with his dentures and shaving, they discuss his activities for the day.

"Today's my session with the physical therapist," he says. "I want to be on time for her."

"Don't worry, Mr. Wilson," says Nora, as she walks him back to his room. "You'll be there on time." She then goes to Rachel Morgan's room to set up her A.M. care.

"I think I can wash myself today, but it may take me awhile," Mrs. Morgan says.

Nora smiles at her. "You just do what you can, Mrs. Morgan," she says at the door, "and I'll be back to help you finish your bed bath."

Nora puts on a gown and gloves before going into Mr. Britten's room to take his vital signs and provide A.M. care. Mr. Britten, who has AIDS, has developed a staph infection in an open wound on his arm and must remain in wound isolation until the infection is gone.

"Hello, Ms. Fuentes," Mr. Britten says quietly. Nora greets Mr. Britten and begins wrapping the blood pressure cuff around his unaffected arm. She asks him about his partner's upcoming trip to Australia.

A smile tugs at the corners of his mouth. "Owen leaves for Sydney today," he says. "Would you believe I already miss him? He'll be gone for 2 whole weeks." Nora records Mr. Britten's vital signs, which are normal.

"Maybe he'll bring you a kangaroo," she says.

"If he does, I'll name it 'Nora,'" he says with a grin.

Nora discards her gown and gloves and washes her hands before going to Room 119, where she greets Shirley McDay, who has Alzheimer's disease.

"Hello, Mrs. McDay, I'm Ms. Fuentes, your nurse assistant. Today is Tuesday, it's 7:45, and it's time for your morning bath," says Nora. After the bath, Nora helps Mrs. McDay get dressed.

"I think I'll wear this outfit today," says Mrs. McDay, selecting a green blouse and an orange skirt from her closet. The blouse and skirt do not match, but Nora knows that green and orange are Mrs. McDay's favorite colors.

Wanting to say something positive, Nora says, "That blouse looks so nice on you." Mrs. McDay smiles shyly.

Then Nora returns to Mrs. Morgan's room to help her finish her bed bath and get dressed. Because Mrs. Morgan tires easily, Nora helps her get comfortable in her bed so that she can rest before going to the dining room for breakfast.

Next, Nora puts on a gown and gloves and enters Mr. Britten's room with his breakfast tray. She suggests that he start eating the breakfast himself while she helps the other residents to the dining room for breakfast. Nora assures him that she will come back to help him finish his breakfast.

Nora removes and discards the gown and gloves and washes her hands before enlisting Arthur's help with getting Mrs. Morgan out of bed and into the wheelchair. As she pushes Mrs. Morgan to the dining room, she stops along the way and invites Jake Wilson and Shirley McDay to walk with her and Mrs. Morgan to the dining room.

After getting the three residents settled in the dining room, Nora takes a breakfast tray to Mr. Rivera who, until his condition worsened this week, had been eating regularly in the dining room. She helps him with his breakfast by placing her hand over his hand on the spoon. He has difficulty chewing and swallowing, so it takes a long time to help him eat. "My wife is coming to visit me today," says Mr. Rivera, dribbling oatmeal out of his mouth. "I can hardly wait." Nora gently wipes his chin and discusses the visit with him.

Observing contact precautions when she returns to Mr. Britten's room, Nora apologizes for taking so long. Much to her surprise, she finds that Mr. Britten has eaten all his breakfast by himself.

"I'm so tired, I just want to sleep now," he says. Nora leaves Mr. Britten's room. She removes and discards the gown and gloves and washes her hands.

While Mrs. Morgan eats breakfast in the dining room, Nora changes the linens on her bed. Then she goes into Mr. Rivera's room and offers him the urinal.

"One of these days I'm going to be regular like a clock," Mr. Rivera jokes. Nora helps him with his bed bath and helps him brush his teeth. While helping him dress, Nora encourages Mr. Rivera to fasten as many buttons as possible with his "good hand."

"You did more buttons today than you did yesterday," she says when he becomes tired. "You're really making good progress."

Continued on next page

▼ Box 24-5 **Nora's Day** *Continued*

Mr. Rivera beams. When Mr. Rivera is dressed, Nora helps him slowly complete his range-of-motion exercises. Nora washes her hands after leaving the room.

On her way to the dining room, Nora smiles at Arthur, who is leading a resident back to her room. In the dining room, Nora greets Rachel Morgan and wheels her to the elevator.

"How was breakfast?" Nora asks.

"Today they had pancakes, which I just love," says Mrs. Morgan. When they reach Room 121, Nora tells Mrs. Morgan that she will be right back with someone to help transfer her into her bed.

"All right, dear," says Mrs. Morgan. Nora steps into the hall and sees Arthur carrying bed linens.

"Arthur, could you please help me transfer Mrs. Morgan into her bed?" she asks.

"Comin' right up," says Arthur. "Let me just put these linens down in Mr. Lightfoot's room, and I'll be right there." After Mrs. Morgan is comfortably settled in bed, Nora heads back to the dining room, where Mr. Wilson and Mrs. McDay have finished breakfast. As the three near the elevator, Mr. Wilson mentions that he is going to visit a friend on the second floor. Nora glances quickly at her watch and reminds him about his physical therapy appointment.

"I'll be back in time," says Mr. Wilson. Nora walks Mrs. McDay back to her room.

"Is this my room?" Mrs. McDay asks as they near the supply closet.

"No, here we are," Nora says at the door to Room 119. She encourages Mrs. McDay to sit in a chair while Nora changes the linens on her bed. After the bed is made, Mrs. McDay climbs onto the bedspread and reaches for a magazine.

Nora sighs as she walks to Mr. Britten's room. She puts on a gown and gloves and enters the room. Mr. Britten is awake and is glad to see her. Nora gives him his bed bath, moving him as gently as possible to protect his fragile skin. She makes sure he is comfortable before leaving the room.

Getting Assistance

Nora heads toward Room 118 to see whether she can find Arthur. He is in the room finishing Stephen Lightfoot's personal care. Arthur is ready to move Mr. Lightfoot out of bed, and he needs Nora's help.

"Arthur, I'll help you move Mr. Lightfoot *and* change his bed if you will help me move Mr. Rivera and change his linens," Nora says.

"You've got a deal," says Arthur.

As Nora and Arthur lift Mr. Lightfoot into the bedside chair, he complains of extreme shortness of breath. First, Arthur makes sure that Mr. Lightfoot's oxygen tubes are not kinked anywhere. Then, so that Mr. Lightfoot doesn't hear, he quietly consults with Nora to see whether she also noticed the blue color around his lips. Arthur decides to report Mr. Lightfoot's condition to the nurse. He measures Mr. Lightfoot's pulse and respirations and asks Nora to stay with him while he reports Mr. Lightfoot's vital signs and change in color to the nurse.

After the nurse checks on Mr. Lightfoot, Nora and Arthur go to Mr. Rivera's room. It is now about 10:15 A.M. They move him into his wheelchair and change his bed.

After leaving Mr. Rivera's room, Nora passes Mr. Wilson in the hall on the way to his physical therapy appointment. She then goes directly to Room 121 to help Rachel Morgan with her range-of-motion exercises.

"Both of my arms are kind of stiff today," says Mrs. Morgan, as they begin the exercises. Nora gently moves her wrists back and forth.

"We'll do everything slowly," she says, "and you tell me when to stop."

After completing the exercises, Mrs. Morgan rests in her bed.

Adjusting the Schedule

At 11:00 A.M., Nora finishes changing the linens on Mr. Wilson's bed when she remembers that it is time to offer Mr. Rivera the urinal again.

"Gosh, I've got to go check on Mr. Britten, too," she thinks to herself as she rushes toward Mr. Rivera's room.

Halfway down the hallway, Nora notices that Mrs. McDay's call signal is on. "I'll be right there," she calls to Mrs. McDay. In her nervous state, Nora bumps into Arthur in the hall.

"Arthur," she says, "I don't know what to do first! Mr. Rivera, Mrs. McDay and Mr. Britten all need my help at the same time!"

"Calm down, Nora," says Arthur. "Let me see your schedule."

Down the hallway, Mrs. McDay cries out for her mother.

"I'll offer Mr. Rivera his urinal and then check on Mr. Britten while you take care of Mrs. McDay. Sounds like she really needs you," says Arthur.

"I don't know what I'd do without you!" Nora calls over her shoulder.

When Nora steps into Room 119, she sees that Mrs. McDay has wet the bed. Mrs. McDay rocks in her bed, scolding herself and picking at her bedspread. "I'm nothing but a baby! A baby!" she mutters under her breath.

Box 24-5 **Nora's Day** *Continued*

Nora sighs to herself as she helps Mrs. McDay out of bed, removes the wet linens and puts them in the hamper. As she helps Mrs. McDay wash and dress, she reassures her that the incontinence is not her fault and tells her that she doesn't mind helping her clean up. She continues to comfort Mrs. McDay as she makes her bed.

After a few minutes, Mrs. McDay asks, "Can I go to the dayroom?"

After helping Mrs. McDay to the dayroom, Nora goes to Room 124 and changes Mr. Britten's bed linens. She knows that he feels lonely in isolation and that he enjoys visiting with her while she provides care. However, Nora is scheduled for lunch at 11:30, and she is very hungry. She doesn't know how she is going to make it.

Controlling Time

After heating her soup in the microwave, Nora joins Arthur at a table where he is sipping a cup of coffee. It is 11:40 A.M., and Nora has just 20 minutes to relax before she will have to begin taking residents to the dining room and helping with lunch.

"I always seem to be running late," Nora says.

"Some days are like that," Arthur agrees. Then he suggests that they review Nora's schedule to see whether she could have made any changes.

Arthur looks over Nora's schedule. "It seems to me that you have everything well organized," he says. "But people aren't like puzzle pieces, you know, that always fit into place. They don't always fit into our plans." Nora smiles.

"What do you do at home when things don't work out as planned with your kids' schedules?" Arthur asks.

Nora laughs and confesses that she tries to stay flexible and roll with the punches. "Eventually everything works out, most of the time," Nora says.

Arthur laughs. "That's what they mean by experience being the best teacher," he says. "It takes a while to learn how to balance the needs of each person with all the things that you have to get done. Do you think you could have done anything differently this morning?"

Nora thinks back on her morning. "I guess I could have checked on Mr. Britten before I did Mrs. Morgan's range-of-motion exercises. But I didn't know that Mrs. McDay would need me just when I had to offer Mr. Rivera his urinal. I was so worried that I would mess up his bladder training program. I can't thank you enough for helping me today."

When Nora finishes talking, Arthur asks her what she has accomplished that morning. As Nora begins to list the many things that she accomplished, she begins to relax, realizing that she has successfully completed all her morning tasks. Feeling renewed, she goes back on the floor and helps everybody get lunch.

Focusing on Each Person

It is 12:30 P.M. when Nora brings Mr. Britten his lunch tray. Instead of hurrying out, she stops to talk for a few minutes. Mr. Britten tells her about how hard it is for him to be in the nursing home while his partner is traveling on business.

"I worry about him, and I would feel better if I were at home," he says. "He's the only friend and family I have."

"Owen sounds like a very special person. I hope I get to meet him," says Nora. She tells Mr. Britten that she will be back later to check on him.

Nora stops by Rachel Morgan's and Victor Rivera's rooms to make sure that they are ready for their physical therapy appointments at 1:00 P.M. She offers Mr. Rivera his urinal before leaving.

At 1:15, Nora finds Mrs. McDay sitting by the window in her room. Nora asks her whether she would like to talk for a while. Mrs. McDay looks up at Nora and yells, "I just want to be alone!" Then she begins to cry. Nora recognizes that the earlier incontinence has upset Mrs. McDay more than Nora realized.

Nora walks over to Mrs. McDay, sits next to her and speaks to her in a calm voice. After a while, Nora comments to Mrs. McDay that the brightly colored afghan spread across her lap is very pretty. Mrs. McDay smiles a little. "My sister made this afghan for me when I got married," she tells Nora.

At a few minutes before 2:00 P.M., Nora stops in Room 120 to check on Mr. Wilson before his recreational therapy appointment. A physical therapy aide brings Mr. Rivera into his room and helps Nora move Mr. Rivera into his bed so that he can rest before his wife comes to visit. The physical therapy aide returns to the hall with Mrs. Morgan and again helps Nora as they transfer Mrs. Morgan out of the wheelchair and back into bed.

"Those physical therapy sessions always wear me out," Mrs. Morgan says as Nora tucks the sheet around her shoulders. A few minutes later, Mrs. Morgan is fast asleep.

Nora's shift is over at 3:00 P.M. Before leaving, Nora and Arthur go to Mr. Britten's room. Nora checks his vital signs, and then she and Arthur double-bag and transfer his soiled linens and trash. After saying good-bye to everyone, Nora completes her charting and makes her report to the team for the next shift. She includes a description of Mrs. McDay's catastrophic reaction in her report.

As she leaves the floor, Nora waves to Mr. Wilson, who is returning from recreation therapy. She smiles and feels very satisfied with herself.

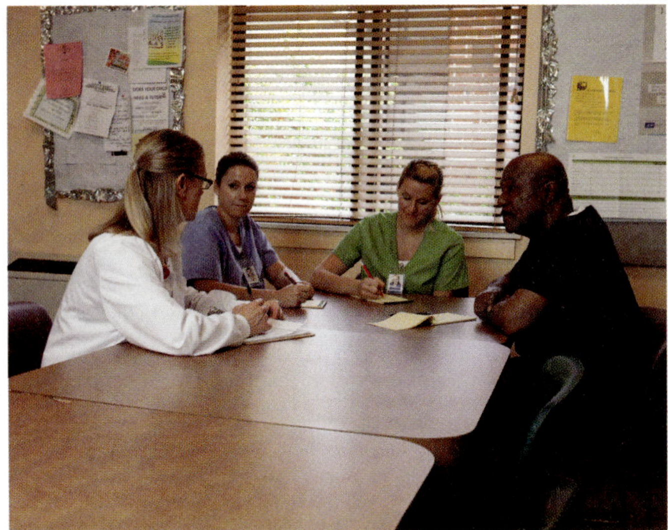

Figure 24-2 During the change-of-shift report, you will receive updates and instructions that help you plan your day.

person needs or about changes to the existing care plan (Figure 24-2). You also learn about prescheduled activities or treatments. As you listen to the report, take notes, being careful to write down the following:

- Daily tasks that have to be done at specific times, such as measuring vital signs, providing treatments, serving meals, and turning and positioning
- Daily tasks that must be done but have no set time, such as bathing, dressing and mouth care
- Special things that have to be done or considered that day for the people in your care, such as a appointments for physical therapy or a diagnostic test or procedure
- Your assigned break and lunch times

After listing the tasks that you must do that day, think about the order in which to do things and write down a tentative schedule. Some tasks might involve important preparation steps. For example, you may have to schedule time to use the tub room before you can give a person a tub bath. Other tasks may require help from another co-worker or supervisor. When you make your schedule, be sure to think about these needs and include time for them in your schedule. Also think about what you know about each resident in your care. For example, you may have learned that Mrs. Wiggins, who has dementia, becomes agitated if she is rushed through her morning care or if her usual routine is changed. In addition, you know that when Mrs. Wiggins becomes agitated, it takes much longer to provide care for her. Take this knowledge into account when planning your schedule, by planning to follow Mrs. Wiggins's routine as much as possible and allowing plenty of time for care so that she is not rushed.

After you finish your schedule, put a star next to each task that must be done at a specific time. Then prioritize the remaining tasks by marking the most important ones to remind you to do them first, if possible. Now, when you look at your schedule, you know *what* must be done and *when* it must be done. Unscheduled events always occur. But when you know what *must* be done, it is easier to readjust your schedule.

Working in a health care setting is much like traveling by car. No matter how well you map out your trip, you are bound to make some detours along the way. Your schedule is like a road map that helps you find an alternate route to your destination. Every day, no matter how well you plan things for yourself, people's needs change—and so does your schedule. You may ask, "Why bother to make a schedule if I can never stick to it?" The answer is that the schedule is an important tool that reminds you of *what* you have to do, *when* you must do it and *which* things are most important for you to do. Often you will feel pressured to begin the day's activities without planning, but it will save you time in the end if you take a few minutes to create a plan at the start.

During report, you learn that you will be caring for six residents today. Two of the residents, Mrs. Quillen and Mr. Short, require complete assistance with bathing, dressing and eating. Mr. Short is also scheduled for physical therapy at 10 a.m. Two other residents assigned to your care, Mr. Fernandez and Mrs. Lewis, also need help with personal care and ambulation. Mrs. Lewis has an appointment to have her hair cut after lunch. The fifth resident assigned to you, Mrs. Langdon, has Alzheimer's disease and requires frequent supervision because she often is seen wandering and hoarding throughout the day. Your last assigned resident, Mr. James, has just been transferred to Morningside after having had a stroke that left him paralyzed on his left side. He is extremely weak and is allowed out of bed to the chair for short periods of time three times a day. The nurse from the previous shift tells you that Mr. James was up all night.

What tasks would you write down on your schedule for the day, and how would you prioritize them?

What issues would you need to consider when developing your schedule for the day to ensure that you are practicing the five principles of care (safety, privacy, dignity, communication and independence) with each of the people in your care?

Working as a team

What do you do when you need additional time to meet the needs of a person in your care? How do you cope when an assignment is too risky for you to handle alone or too time-consuming for you to do your best job? What do you do when several people need your attention at once? These questions are difficult to answer, but in the real world these situations do happen.

Teamwork is essential in health care (Figure 24-3). It may be difficult to ask for help from co-workers who are just as busy as you are, but often two people can accomplish a task more quickly and more safely than one person can. Try to accommodate co-worker's requests for help as much as your schedule allows. This fosters a spirit of teamwork and will make others more willing to help you when you need it.

When an assignment seems too risky to handle alone or too time-consuming for you to do a thorough job, it is important that you discuss this problem with your supervisor. Perhaps your supervisor does not realize how much time is required to meet the special needs of a certain person in your care, or perhaps you do not realize that another member of the team has just called out sick. Sharing information with your supervisor and other members of the health care team helps the health care team work well together so that everyone can enjoy a sense of satisfaction from a job well done.

Staying in control of your time

You have just finished helping Mr. Wilson brush his hair and shave. You are ready to leave his room to attend to the next thing on your schedule when he says, "Before you leave, could you do one quick favor for me?" You say that you would be happy to do something for him. Then he says, "Could you please make me a cup of tea and some toast? I'm hungry now, but I just couldn't eat breakfast earlier. I don't want to wait for an order to come up from the kitchen."

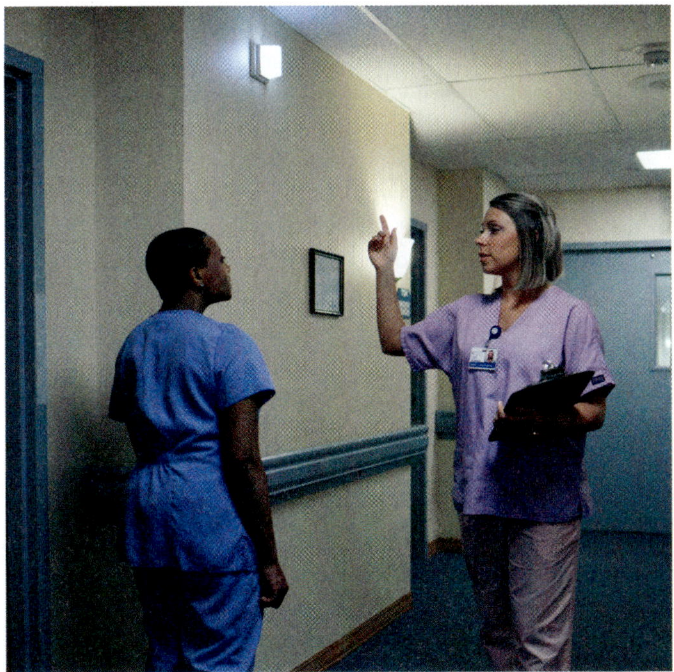

Figure 24-3 Teamwork is essential in a health care setting. Accommodate your co-workers' requests for help as much as you can, and they should do the same for you.

You want to be able to do this special task for Mr. Wilson, but you think to yourself that his quick favor is not going to be quick at all. You know that this task may take 10 minutes of your time. What can you do now? What could you have done to anticipate this situation?

Sometimes, unplanned events can be handled by taking charge of your time from the beginning. When you first go into Mr. Wilson's room, check to see what has to be done and let him know how long you are going to be there this time. Also, let him know when you plan to come back. Before you start your tasks in Mr. Wilson's room, ask him whether he thinks he might need anything special. If, at the beginning of your time with Mr. Wilson, he says he wants tea and toast, you can adjust the time that you spend on other planned tasks to include his special request. If you wait until the end of your time with Mr. Wilson to find out that he has special needs, these last-minute requests may affect the rest of your schedule.

If you communicate your plans clearly to the person in your care, you may lessen the number of unplanned events during the day. What you say through verbal communication is just as important as what you say though nonverbal communication (such as your facial expressions or body language). The following tips will help you remember to communicate your message clearly and, in the end, may save time:

- When you assist a person, even on a very busy day, try to be relaxed. Remember that the person in your care is your reason for being there. If you seem to be hurried and stressed, the person also may become stressed, which may require you to spend more time with her.
- If touching is acceptable to the person, use touch to reassure and comfort the person while you provide care. Placing a hand on the person's shoulder or holding his hand is calming and helps him know that you care. Showing the person that you care about him may help him feel more secure and help you spend your time more efficiently and effectively.
- When you help a person, take time to speak with him and really listen to what he has to say. Sometimes the simple act of stopping and listening to the person shows that you are available. This action can reduce his anxiety and perhaps even save you time in the long run.
- Before you leave a person's room, always ask if there is anything else the person needs before you

leave. This helps to improve efficiency by allowing you to handle (or make arrangements for someone else to handle) the person's requests before you leave, thereby minimizing interruptions later. This also leaves the person with the satisfaction of knowing that you are concerned about meeting her needs and want her to be comfortable.

Co-workers may also place demands on your time. While it is important to try and accommodate co-workers' requests for help whenever possible, remember what you learned earlier about assertive communication. Review your schedule, and think about where you might be able to rearrange some of your responsibilities to help your co-worker. If you cannot shift some of your responsibilities without negatively impacting your schedule, then tell your co-worker you are not available to help and explain why. But try to offer another solution to the problem, such as suggesting someone else who might be able to help, or seeing how the two of you might be able to coordinate your schedules and work together to make sure both of you are able to complete your tasks for the day.

As you go through the day, your schedule seems to be working. You breathe a sigh of relief. So you proceed with your next task and decide to get Mr. James out of bed. As you enter his room, you notice that he is sleeping soundly. You know that you need to get him out of bed, but you also know that he didn't sleep well the night before. You also know that you need to get Mrs. Lewis ready for her haircut appointment.

What would you do? What would be your priorities?

How would this situation affect your stress level?

CARING FOR YOURSELF

While you are at work, you are dedicated to taking care of others. In your personal life, you may also be responsible for caring for others, such as children or your own aging parents. It can be hard to make sure your own needs are met, when you are so busy meeting the needs of others. However, in order to do your best for the others in your life, you must take care of yourself too.

Staying Physically Healthy

Being a nurse assistant is very physically demanding work. Taking good care of your physical health gives you more energy and helps to prevent work-related injuries. To maintain your physical health:

- **Get enough sleep.** On average, most people need between 6 and 8 hours of sleep each night to function well. Sleep allows the body to rest and rejuvenate itself and recover from the physical and mental stresses of the day. When we do not get enough sleep, it makes it difficult to think clearly, and we lack energy and stamina. We are less able to tolerate emotional stress, and we are more likely to catch contagious illnesses, such as a cold or the flu. Lack of sleep also puts a person at risk for health conditions, such as hypertension and weight gain.
- **Eat a healthy diet.** In Chapter 14, you learned about tools you can use to plan a healthy diet, such as MyPlate.gov and nutrition labels on packaged foods. A healthy diet gives your body the nutrients it needs to function properly and helps to maintain a healthy body weight.
- **Incorporate exercise into your life.** Find a physical activity (or activities) that you enjoy, and make a "date" with yourself to exercise several times a week. Try to mix up activities that get your heart pumping ("cardio") with activities that strengthen your muscles (such as weight training) and increase flexibility (such as yoga). Regular exercise helps to keep your heart, lungs and bones healthy and is essential for maintaining a healthy body weight. In addition, exercise is a great way to relieve mental and emotional stress.
- **Avoid habits that can harm your health.** Habits such as smoking, excessive alcohol use or the inappropriate use of drugs (legal and illegal) can have a very negative impact on your health. If you smoke, or if you think that you might use alcohol or drugs excessively or inappropriately, take steps to break these habits. For example, share your concerns with your primary care provider, a clergy member or other trusted person in your life. Acknowledging the problem is the first step in solving the problem and developing new, healthier habits.
- **Practice preventive health care.** See your primary care provider at least once a year. Routine physical examinations and screening tests can help to detect health problems early, before they become more difficult to treat or cause permanent harm to your body. Also see your dentist twice a year for routine teeth cleaning and a dental exam.

Staying Mentally Healthy

As you have learned, working as a nurse assistant can be stressful. The multiple demands on your time, having to care for people who may not seem appreciative of your efforts and facing the loss of people in your care who you have grown close to are just some of the situations that can make your job emotionally stressful. To stay healthy, you must find positive ways of managing this stress (Figure 24-4). Examples of positive ways to relieve stress include:

- Engaging in prayer or meditation
- Engaging in physical activity
- Enjoying a hobby
- Spending time with friends and other people you enjoy being with

Although it can be difficult, it is important to make time for yourself to do what you enjoy doing. This time away from the pressures of work and family can help you to relax and recharge, so that you are better able to handle stressful situations when they do arise. If stress becomes too great and you find that your usual methods of managing stress are not working, or if you find yourself turning to unhealthy methods of managing stress (such as drinking too much alcohol or using drugs inappropriately), talk to your supervisor. Many employers have stress management or employee assistance programs available to help employees manage the stress in their lives.

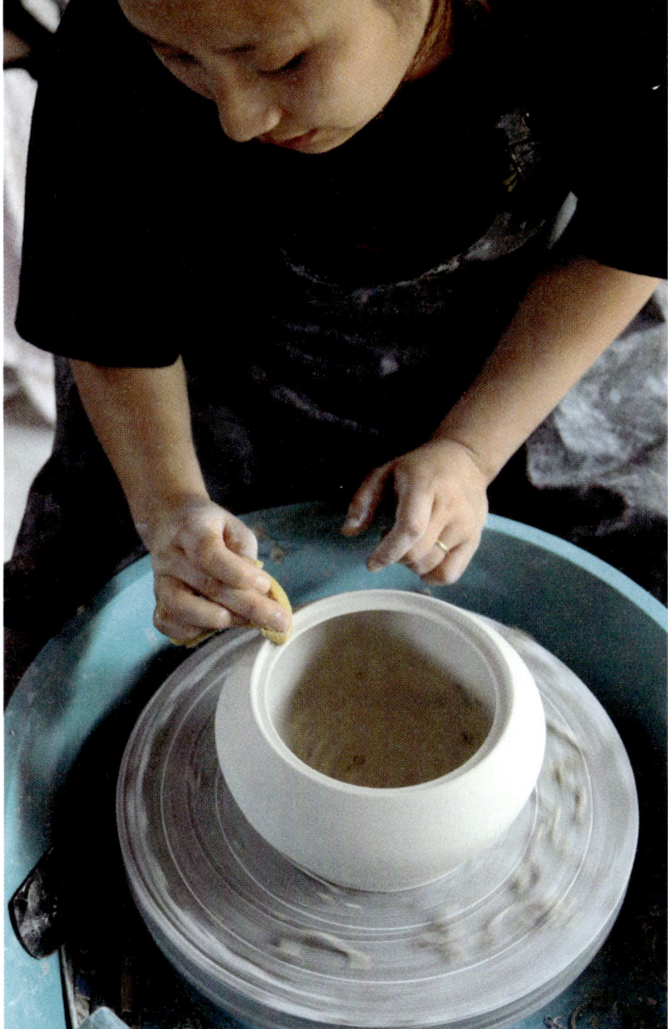

Figure 24-4 It is important to take time for yourself to do things that you enjoy doing. © *iStockPhoto.com/MoMorad*

DEVELOPING YOUR CAREER

Lifelong Learning

Now that you have completed this training course, you have learned the basic skills and techniques needed to become a certified nursing assistant. However, your training does not end on the last day of class! Once on the job, you will have the chance to learn new skills, new methods of providing care and new reasons for doing things a certain way. It is crucial to keep up to date with new information and to incorporate this information into your practice as a nurse assistant. Make an effort to continuously increase your knowledge. Ask the nurse about new techniques or equipment that you see being used, or for more information about specific disorders that the people in your care may have. Become a member of professional organizations for nurse assistants, such as the National Network of Career Nursing Assistants and the National Association of Health Care Assistants (NAHCA), to stay on top of new developments that affect the profession. Learning is truly a lifelong endeavor.

Opportunities for Professional Growth

Although many people enjoy long and fulfilling careers as nurse assistants, training and working as a nurse assistant is excellent preparation for other careers in the health care field as well. For example, you may decide that you want to go back to school to become a licensed practical/vocational nurse or a registered nurse. Or, maybe you will want to receive additional training to work in one of the emerging roles in health care. Because of changes in our health care system, new roles are emerging as employers seek ways to deliver quality care in a cost-effective, efficient manner. Examples of some of these emerging roles include patient care technician (PCT) and medication aide:

- **Patient care technician (PCT).** In addition to the basic skills needed to be a nurse assistant, PCT training may include training in more advanced nursing skills (such as checking blood-glucose levels and inserting or removing indwelling urinary catheters), skills related to drawing blood samples (phlebotomy), and skills related to obtaining and monitoring electrocardiograms (ECGs).

- **Medication aide.** Medication aide training builds on nurse assistant training to provide additional instruction in how drugs work in the body and the safe administration of drugs. Medication aides who complete the training are qualified to administer certain drugs in certain settings under the supervision of a licensed nurse.

Or perhaps you may decide to pursue another career in health care that is not related to nursing at all. Learning about the job responsibilities of other members of the health care team can help you to define goals for your own career, should you decide that you want to branch out from nurse assisting.

Leaving a Job

You will likely hold many jobs over the course of your career. When you decide to leave a job, first speak with your supervisor about your intention to leave and let him or her know when your last day will be. It is courteous to give your employer a minimum of 2 weeks' notice so that arrangements can be made for someone else to take on your responsibilities after you are gone. Submit a formal resignation letter thanking your employer for the opportunity to work at the organization and stating your intention to end your employment and your intended last day.

Some employers will conduct an exit interview with you before you leave. The purpose of this interview is to help employers understand why employees leave, so that they can reduce employee loss and turnover. Although it is important to be honest about your reasons for leaving, try to avoid speaking negatively or in an accusing way about the organization, your supervisor, or your co-workers. You never know who you will find yourself working with again in the future.

MAKING A DIFFERENCE

"After the verb 'to love,' 'to help' is the most beautiful verb in the world!" This quote is from Bertha von Suttner, an Austrian novelist and the first woman to receive the Nobel Peace Prize. By deciding to enter the health care field, particularly in the role of nurse assistant, you have made a choice to make a career out of helping others. This is truly a wonderful choice. Along the way, you will discover just how rewarding caregiving can be. It might happen when you are discharging a person home. It might happen after giving a distressed family member some time and comfort. It might happen when a person you took care of comes back just to see you. That person may look into your eyes and take your hand. Then the most wonderful thing that can happen to a nurse assistant will happen to you. The person will say, "Thank you. You made it easier. You are a great nurse assistant." You have the ability to make a significant difference in the lives of those in your care and their family members. Always remember this, and try every day, with every person in your care, to be the best nurse assistant you can.

CHECK YOUR UNDERSTANDING

Questions for Review

1. **When a co-worker asks for your assistance, you should:**
   a. Stop whatever you are doing and help your co-worker.
   b. Refuse to help if your schedule does not allow time for such an interruption.
   c. Work this request into your schedule as well as possible.
   d. Report the request to the nurse.

2. **How can making a schedule help you to manage your time?**
   a. It can help prevent unexpected requests from those in your care.
   b. It can be used to show the nurse and your co-workers how busy you are, so that they do not ask you to take on additional responsibilities.
   c. It can help you see what needs to be done and when.
   d. It can help to manage conflicts that may arise.

3. **What is the best way to handle unexpected events?**
   a. Rearrange your schedule the best you can to accommodate the unexpected event.
   b. Ignore the unexpected event and stick to your planned schedule.
   c. Report the unexpected event to the nurse so that he or she can manage the situation.
   d. Ignore your schedule for the rest of the day.

4. **You are a home health aide. When you arrive at your client's home, her son greets you at the door and asks if you would not mind running to the store to pick up some milk, since they are out. Which of the following is an example of an assertive response?**
   a. "You should have seen to this before I got here. I'm much too busy to be running to the store!"
   b. "I can't go to the store because I only have 45 minutes with your mother, and there's a lot

we need to get done in that time. How about you go to the store while I'm here with your mother?"

c. "Okay. Hopefully I can make up some time so that I'm not late to my next client's appointment."

d. "You should have called me. I could have stopped for the milk on the way here, but now it's too late for me to help you."

5. Which of the following is a positive way to deal with work-related stress?

a. Get a prescription for an antidepressant medication.

b. Engage in an activity that you find enjoyable, such as knitting or woodworking.

c. Drink excessive amounts of alcohol to make it easier to forget about problems at work.

d. Take out your work-related stress on others, such as your co-workers.

6. Mr. Gordon has dementia. Today, while you were assisting Mr. Gordon with dressing, he slapped you across the face. An appropriate response would be to:

a. Slap Mr. Gordon back to get him to stop behaving in this way.

b. Report Mr. Gordon's behavior to the nurse, and complete an incident report.

c. Tell Mr. Gordon that if he does not stop behaving in this way, you will have him removed from the facility.

d. Ignore Mr. Gordon's behavior. He cannot help his behavior because of his disease.

7. All of the following are effective strategies for managing another person's anger EXCEPT

a. Standing very close to the person and making yourself appear taller so that the person knows who is in charge.

b. Stopping the task and giving the person an opportunity to cool down.

c. Ensuring the person's safety and leaving the area.

d. Using distraction techniques, such as changing the subject or activity.

Questions to Ask Yourself

1. *You are serving dinner to the residents of a nursing home. You realize that Mr. Harris and Miss Yarnell both need a lot of assistance with eating tonight. You provide care for both of them and for one other person who also needs help with eating. What would you do so that each of these residents has the chance to eat a hot dinner?*

2. *You are on your way to answer a resident's request for help when the daughter of another resident on the unit, Mr. Ipswitch, stops you in the hallway. You can tell by her body language that she is very angry. She says to you, "We are paying an incredible amount of money for my father to be here, and the service is terrible! He just told me that he has made repeated requests to have his baths in the evening instead of in the morning, and no one is listening to him. Is it really that hard to reschedule my father's bath?" What should you do? How would you respond to Mr. Ipswitch's daughter?*

3. *Mrs. Greene is a new resident on the unit. She was admitted to the nursing home because her dementia had advanced to the point where her niece could no longer care for her at home. When you are talking with Mrs. Greene's niece, she says to you, "My Aunt Jane has just become so nasty in her old age. She doesn't appreciate anything I do for her, and I do a lot. Good luck dealing with her!" What would you say to Mrs. Greene's niece? How will you respond to Mrs. Greene if she treats you the way she has been treating her niece?*

Appendices

Medical Terminology and Abbreviations

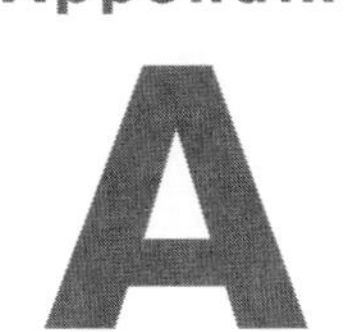

PREFIXES

Prefix	Meaning
a-, an-	without, not
ab-, abs-	away from
ad-	toward, near
anti-	against
brady-	slow
circum-	around
contra-	against, opposite
de-	down
di-	two
dys-	abnormal, difficult, bad
erythro-	red
ex-	out, out of, from
hyper-	over, excessive
hypo-	under, decreased
in-	not
mal-	bad, abnormal
non-	no, not
peri-	around, covering
post-	after, behind
pre-, pro-	before, in front of
re-	again
semi-	half
tachy-	fast, rapid

ROOTS AND COMMONLY USED COMBINING VOWELS

Root	Meaning
arthr/o	joint
bronch/o	bronchus, bronchi
cephal/o	head
cholecsyt/o	gall bladder
col/o	colon, large intestine, bowel
crani/o	skull
cyan/o	blue

cyte	cell
dermat/o	skin
fet/o	unborn child, fetus
gastr/o	stomach
glycos/o	sugar
gynec/o	woman
hemat/o	blood
herni/o	rupture
hyster/o	uterus
lapar/o	abdomen, flank
lith/o	stone
mamm/o, mast/o	breast
men/o	menstruation
my/o	muscle
narc/o	sleep, numbness, stupor
ophthalm/o	eye
oste/o	bone
path/o	disease
ped/o	foot, child
phleb/o	vein
pneum/o	lung, air
proct/o	rectum
psych/o	mind
pulmon/o	lung
rect/o	rectum
ren/o	kidney
sept/o, sept/i	infection
therm/o	heat
thorac/o	chest
thromb/o	clot
tox/o, toxic/o	poison
ur/o	urine
urethr/o	urethra
uter/o	uterus
vertebr/o	spine, vertebrae

SUFFIXES

Suffix	**Meaning**
-al	pertaining to
-algia, -algesia	pain
-cide	kill
-cise	cut
-ectomy	removal
-emia	blood

-esthesia	sensation
-gram	printed record
-graph	device for recording
-itis	inflammation
-iasis, -ism	having the characteristics or condition of
-logy	the study or science of
-meter	measuring instrument
-oma	tumor
-pathy	disease
-phasia	speaking
-phobia	exaggerated fear
-plegia	paralysis
-rrhage, -rrhagia, -rrhea	excessive flow
-rrhaphy	surgical repair
-scopy	examination using a scope
-stomy	creation of an opening
-tomy	surgical cutting

ABBREVIATIONS

Abbreviation	Meaning
abd	abdomen
ac	before a meal
ADLs	activities of daily living
ad lib	as desired
adm	admission, admitted
AM	morning
amb	ambulate, ambulatory
amt	amount
approx	approximately
ASAP	as soon as possible
as tol	as tolerated
ax	axillary
bid	twice a day
BM	bowel movement
BP, B/P	blood pressure
BR	bed rest
cath	catheter
CBR	complete bed rest
cc	cubic centimeter
cl liq	clear liquids
c/o	complains of
CPR	cardiopulmonary resuscitation
dc, d/c	discontinue
disch	discharge

DNR	do not resuscitate
DOB	date of birth
DR	dining room
drsg	dressing
fl (fld)	fluid
h (hr)	hour
H_2O	water
HOB	head of bed
HS, hs	Hour of sleep (bedtime)
I&O	intake and output
IV	intravenous
liq	liquid
meds	medications
mL	milliliter
noc, noct	night
NPO	nothing by mouth
N&V	nausea and vomiting
O	oral
O_2	oxygen
oc-bed	occupied bed
OOB	out of bed
OT	occupational therapy
pc	after meals
PM	afternoon, evening
PRN	as needed
PT	physical therapy
q	every
qd	every day
qh	every hour
R	rectal
rehab	rehabilitation
resp	respiration
ROM	range of motion
SOB	shortness of breath
ST	speech therapy
STAT	immediately
tid	three times a day
TPR	temperature, pulse, respirations
TY	tympanic
un-bed	unoccupied bed
UTI	urinary tract infection
VS	vital signs
WA	while awake
w/c	wheelchair
wt	weight

Body Basics

Our behavior is affected by our bodies and how well they function. If our bodies are strong, we can work and exercise. If our bodies are physically fit, we feel more confident. When our bodies are in proper working order, we can take walks, enjoy meals, attend events and engage in countless other activities. However, when we are ill or our bodies are injured, our behaviors change.

Ten systems of organs work together to allow the body to function. Each system plays an important part in daily activities. The skin, or *integumentary system,* protects the body. The *muscular system* allows the body to move. The bones of the *skeletal system* give structure to the body. The heart and blood work together in the *cardiovascular system* to distribute oxygen and nutrients to every cell in the body and to remove waste materials from the cells. The *respiratory system* brings oxygen into the body and removes carbon dioxide from the body. The *digestive system* processes food to nourish the body. The *urinary system* rids the body of harmful wastes. The *nervous system* controls the function of other organ systems and allows us to engage with the world around us. The *endocrine system* also coordinates the function of other systems, by producing chemical messengers called hormones that regulate a wide variety of ongoing functions. The *reproductive system* allows continuation of the species.

Our bodies change as we age. Aging is an ongoing, natural and expected process. Throughout life, our bodies replace old cells with new ones. As we age, this process of cell replacement slows down, resulting in body systems that do not work as well as they used to. Our body systems grow and change until they reach their peak, and then they start to decline. Different body systems reach their maximum ability at different times during life. For example, the muscular system reaches its peak of ability when we are in our 20s.

Aging is a normal part of life, not a disease. Some people appear to grow older more rapidly than others because of heredity, and others age faster because they live in an unhealthy environment or neglect their health. Positive behaviors like exercise and nutritious eating can slow down the aging process, but nothing can make it stop. You can keep your body healthy by adopting positive behaviors. Also, by encouraging positive behaviors among the people in your care, you can help keep them as healthy as possible.

THE INTEGUMENTARY SYSTEM

The skin, hair and nails, together called the *integumentary system,* protect the body from the outside world. The skin acts as a barrier to microbes, keeps water inside the body, regulates body temperature and contains sensory organs for the sense of touch. When exposed to sunlight, the skin also produces vitamin D, a vitamin that is important for maintaining bone health.

The skin is made up of two layers, the dermis and epidermis (Figure B-1). The skin rests on a layer of fat called the *subcutaneous layer.* The outer layer of the skin, called the *epidermis,* is firm and dry to the touch. Beneath the epidermis, the *dermis* contains sweat

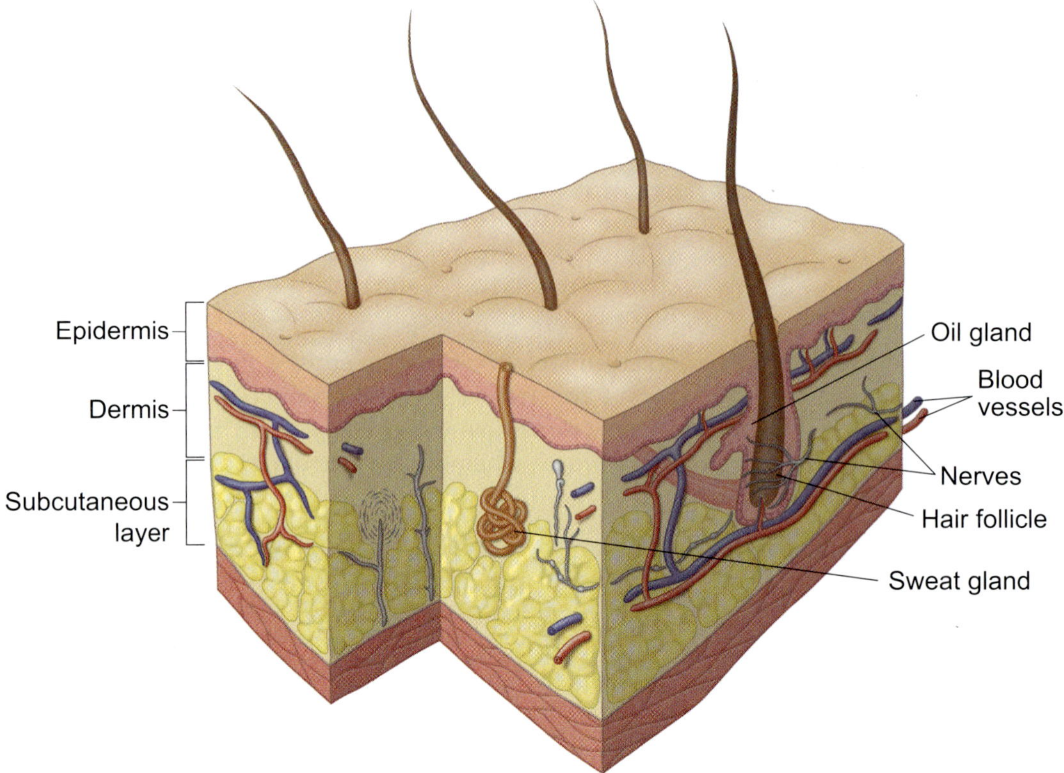

Figure B-1 The skin.

glands (which produce sweat to keep the body's temperature in a safe range), oil glands (which produce oil to keep the skin soft and flexible), hair follicles (which produce the hairs that cover most of our bodies) and sensory receptors (which give us our sense of touch). The blood vessels and nerves that supply the skin start in the subcutaneous layer and send branches into the dermis.

As a person ages, the skin becomes less elastic, the amount of fat under the skin decreases, and the oil glands produce less oil. The skin becomes thinner, dryer and more fragile, making the older person more susceptible to injuries and skin infections. If the skin is injured, it often takes much longer to heal.

THE MUSCULAR SYSTEM

Every movement in the human body, from the blink of the eye to the beat of the heart, depends on muscles (Figure B-2). The body has hundreds of muscles that come in all sizes, from the delicate muscles in the ear to the thick, powerful muscles in the legs.

Muscles do their work by getting shorter, or contracting, in response to electrical impulses sent through nerves. To recover from their work, they relax, or get longer. Some muscles, such as those in the arms and legs, work together in contracting and relaxing teams to ensure that movement is controlled and smooth. For example, when you bend your arm at the elbow, muscles on one side of your arm contract, pulling on the joint and causing it to bend, while muscles on the opposite side relax. When you straighten your arm, the opposite happens. These muscles, which are attached to bones by tendons, are *voluntary*, which means that the person is able to control when these muscles contract and relax. Other muscles, such as the heart muscle and the muscles that line the digestive tract and blood vessels, are *involuntary.* The person is not able to control when these muscles contract and relax. Instead, these muscles contract and relax automatically, in response to signals from the central nervous system.

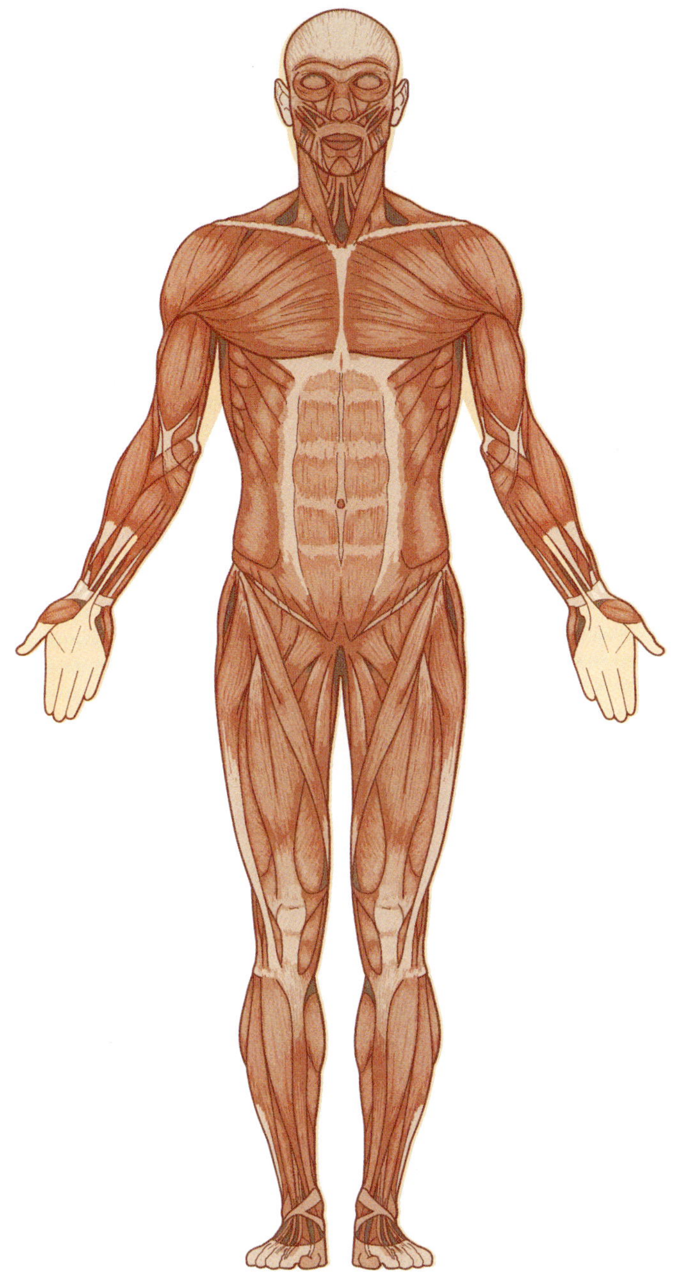

Figure B-2 The muscular system.

As a person ages, the muscles get smaller and less elastic and lose strength. The person's ability to perform activities of daily living (ADLs) or to maintain balance may be affected. Not using the muscles regularly can cause muscle mass to be lost much faster. Regular exercise and a nutritious diet benefit people of all ages by helping to keep the muscles strong and healthy.

THE SKELETAL SYSTEM

The skeletal system consists of 206 bones in various sizes and shapes (Figure B-3). The bones are primarily made of calcium, a hard mineral that gives the bones strength and durability.

In addition to providing structure for the body, some bones protect vital organs. For example, the skull surrounds the brain, the 12 ribs and breastbone (sternum) cover the heart and lungs, and the vertebrae guard the spinal cord.

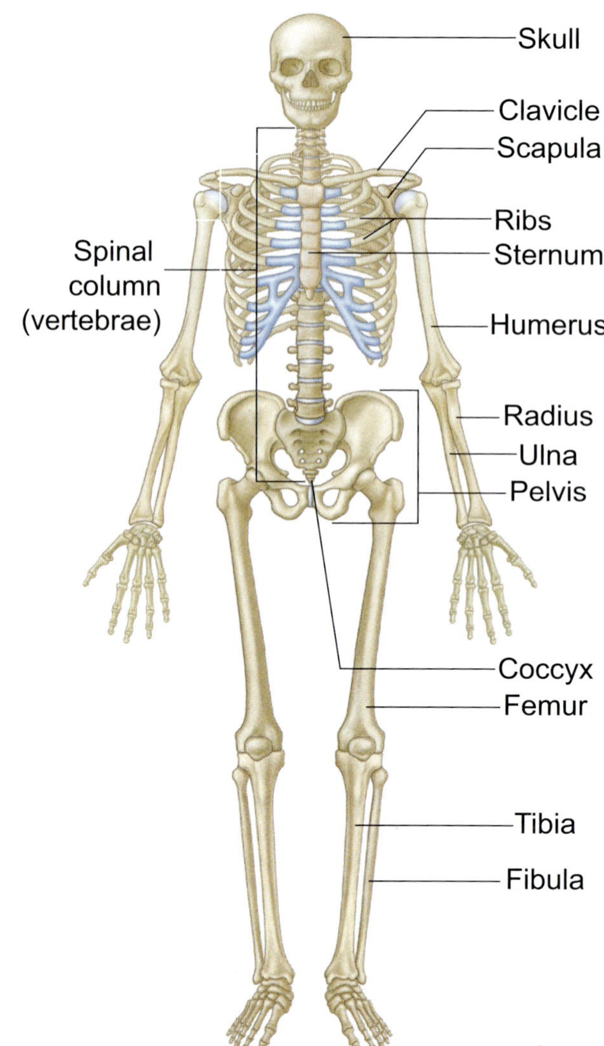

Figure B-3 The skeletal system.

The smallest bones are the ossicles, found inside the ear; they are no larger than the head of a match. The largest bone is the femur, which is the thick, sturdy bone between the hip and the knee. Long bones, such as those in the arms and legs, are not solid structures but have center cavities filled with red marrow (which produces red blood cells) and yellow marrow (which is mostly fat cells).

As a person ages, the body becomes less able to absorb calcium. Calcium regulates many functions in the body, such as muscle contraction and the conduction of electrical impulses by the nerves. When the body cannot absorb the calcium it needs from the food we eat, it starts to draw on the calcium stored in the bones. With time, this causes the bones to become more fragile and puts the older person at risk for fractures. When a person is ill or immobile, this loss of bone tissue can happen much more rapidly.

Normal use of the joints over a lifetime can also cause pain and stiffness in the joints with aging. Over time, the cartilage that cushions the ends of the bones and the ligaments and tendons (which connect the bones to each other and to the muscles) becomes thinner and less elastic, which can lead to joint stiffness and pain. As a result, an older person may have more difficulty walking or standing up and may be more at risk for falling.

THE CARDIOVASCULAR SYSTEM

The cardiovascular system consists of the heart and the blood vessels (Figure B-4). The heart, made mostly of thick muscle, is about the size of a man's fist and weighs about 12 ounces. It is divided into four compartments, called *chambers*, which are separated by small valves that act like swinging doors to keep blood flowing in one direction. When the heart pumps, it sends blood out through the arteries to all of the tissues in the body. When the heart relaxes, it refills with blood that is returning from the tissues through the veins. The blood itself is made of cells and plasma, the fluid that carries the cells. Red cells carry oxygen, white cells fight infection, and platelets help the blood to clot.

Blood vessels called *arteries* carry blood away from the heart to the rest of the body. The largest artery, the aorta, has strong, elastic walls that will not tear under the high pressure of the blood as it is pumped from the heart. As the arteries get further from the heart, they become smaller in diameter. Blood vessels called *veins* carry blood back to the heart. Veins are thinner than arteries because they carry blood under less pressure. As the veins get closer to the heart, they become larger in diameter. Tiny blood vessels called *capillaries*

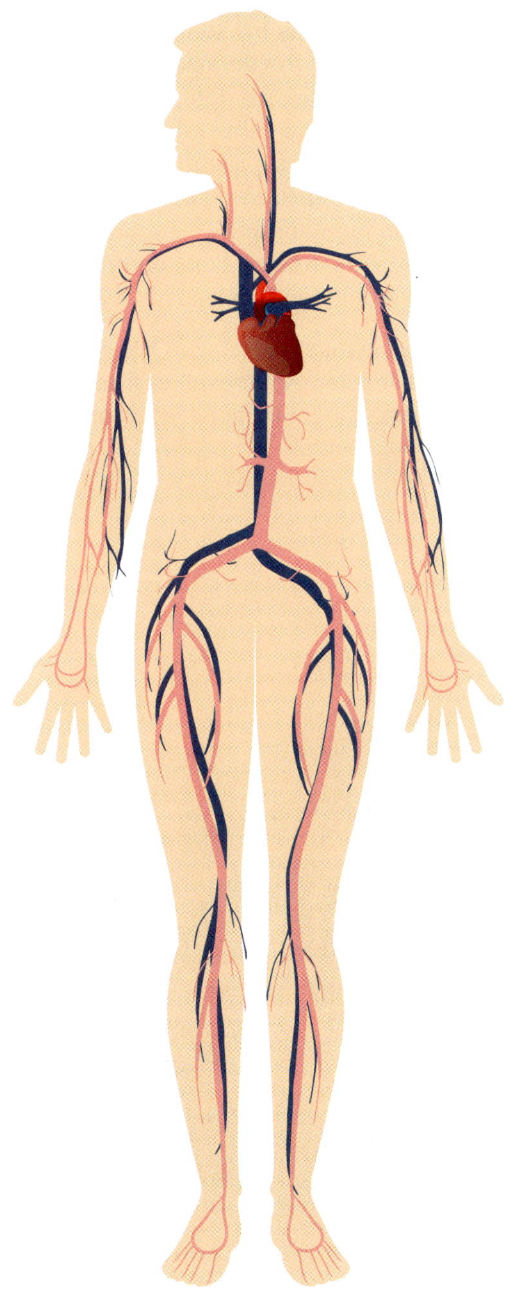

Figure B-4 The cardiovascular system.

connect the arteries to the veins. Capillaries are so small that red blood cells, visible only through a microscope, have to squeeze through them single file.

As a person grows older, the veins and arteries lose some of their elasticity. When the walls of the arteries do not expand as easily, it becomes harder for blood to flow through them, and the person's blood pressure may increase. The person may also experience *orthostatic hypotension* (dizziness caused by a sudden decrease in blood pressure that occurs when the person stands up from a seated or supine position). Orthostatic hypotension occurs because the arteries are not able to constrict quickly, and as a result, it takes more time for the blood to reach the brain. Decreased elasticity in the veins slows down the return of blood to the heart.

THE RESPIRATORY SYSTEM

The respiratory system (Figure B-5) brings oxygen into the body and removes carbon dioxide from the body.

When a person inhales, air enters the body through the mouth and nose. It passes through the *nasal cavity*, into the *pharynx*, through the *larynx* and into the *trachea* (the "windpipe"), the thick tube that leads to the lungs. On its trip to the lungs, tiny hairs called *cilia* warm and clean the air. The air continues along the trachea, which splits into two slightly smaller tubes called the *bronchi*. The bronchi enter the right and left lungs and then divide like the branches of a tree, becoming smaller and smaller tubes (called *bronchioles*) that end in little air spaces called *alveoli*. Each lung has millions of alveoli, which look like bunches of grapes. The alveoli are surrounded by capillaries. Life-giving oxygen passes through the walls of the alveoli into the blood in the capillaries, where it is taken back to the heart for distribution to the rest of the body. At the same time, carbon dioxide, a waste gas, passes from the blood into the alveoli so that it can be exhaled when the person breathes out.

As a person ages, the lungs become less elastic, and the muscles that assist with breathing and coughing become weaker. As a result of these changes, the older person has an increased risk for developing lung infections, such as pneumonia.

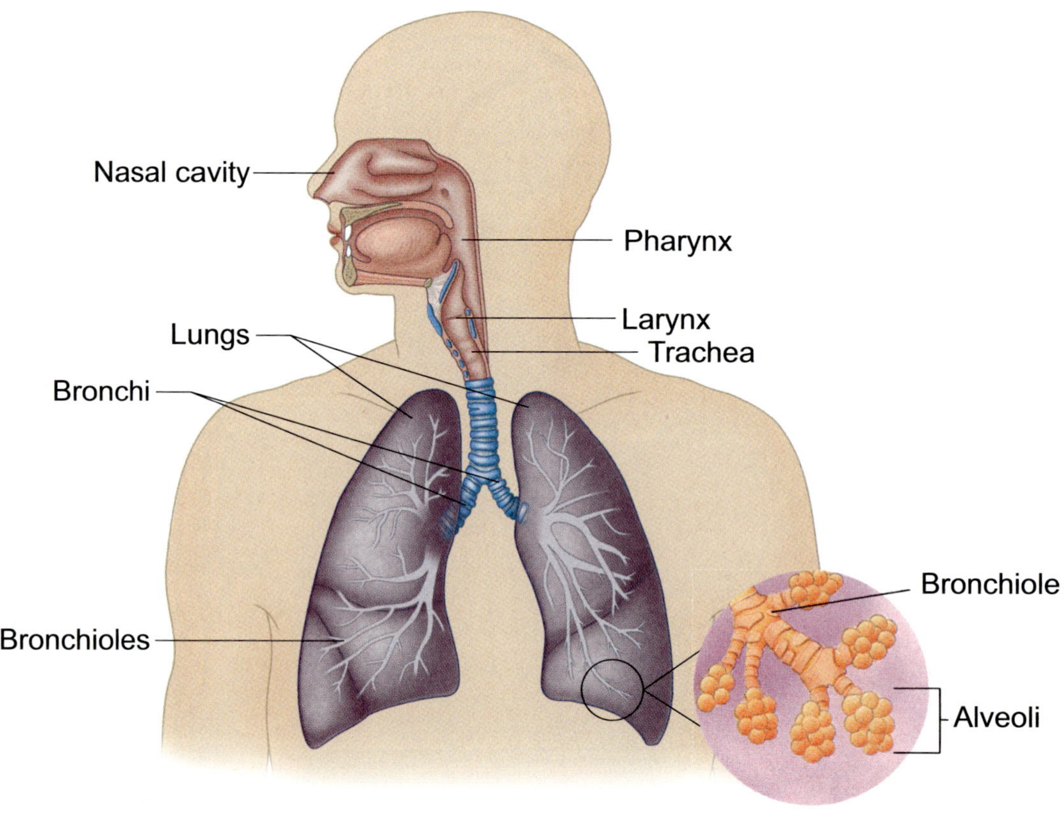

Figure B-5 The respiratory system.

THE DIGESTIVE SYSTEM

The digestive system consists of organs that break down food, absorb nutrients and eliminate the solid waste produced by the digestion process (Figure B-6). The process of breaking down food is called *digestion*. Digestion begins in the mouth. Chewing with the teeth breaks the food down into smaller pieces, and chemicals in the saliva help to break the food down further. The tongue contains sensory receptors, called taste buds, that allow us to taste the food that we eat. The tongue is also used to push the food to the back of the mouth. Swallowing causes the food to travel down the *esophagus*, a muscular tube that connects the mouth to the *stomach*. Once in the stomach, the food mixes with chemicals produced by the lining of the stomach, helping to break the food down even more. From the stomach, the partially digested food enters the small intestine. Contraction of the muscular lining of the intestine causes the partially digested food to move through the small intestine and then through the large intestine. As the partially digested food moves through the intestines, or "bowels," water and nutrients are absorbed through the walls of the intestine into the bloodstream. By the time the digested food reaches the end of the large intestine, all usable materials have been removed, and all that is left is the waste product of digestion, or feces. The feces leave the body through the rectum and anus.

Other organs play a role in digestion as well. The *pancreas*, which is located in the abdomen near the stomach, produces enzymes and hormones that aid digestion and affect how the body uses the nutrients it obtains from food. The *liver*, a large organ located above the stomach, produces and secretes *bile*, a substance that helps the

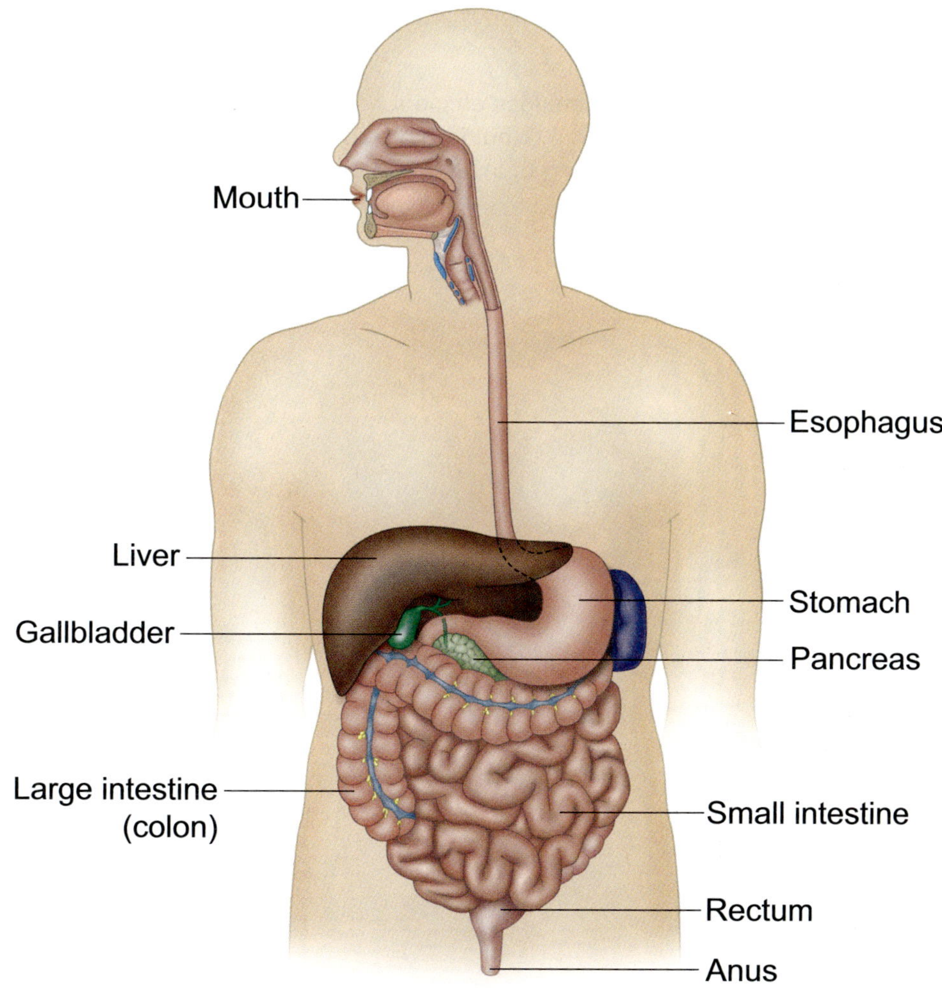

Figure B-6 The digestive system.

body break down fats. Some of the bile the liver produces is excreted directly into the small intestine, and the rest is stored in a small pouch attached to the liver, called the *gallbladder*. (The liver also performs many functions that are not related to digestion. For example, it helps to clean the blood, and it plays a role in producing the proteins that help the blood to clot.)

As a person ages, the taste buds become less sensitive, which may result in a decrease in appetite. Saliva production decreases, resulting in a dry mouth and an increase in plaque on the teeth. Intestinal muscle tone decreases, which may lead to constipation. The body produces less of the chemicals that aid in digestion, causing digestion to become less efficient. As a result, the older person may experience weight loss and vitamin and mineral deficiencies.

THE URINARY SYSTEM

The urinary system, which consists of the kidneys, ureters, bladder and urethra, removes waste products from the blood and eliminates them as urine (Figure B-7). The two *kidneys*, bean-shaped organs about 4 inches long, are located at waist level, one on each side of the body. As blood passes through the kidneys, the kidneys filter out waste products and excess fluid to form urine. The urine passes from the kidneys through the *ureters*, where it is stored in the *bladder*. Urine collects in the bladder until it fills to about 2½ cups. At this point, the person feels the urge to urinate, or pass urine from the body.

Urine passes from the bladder to the outside of the body through the *urethra*. In women, the urethra is separate from the reproductive system, with the opening located in front of the vagina. In men, both urine and semen pass through the urethra, but never at the same time.

As a person ages, the kidneys become less efficient. Muscle weakness can reduce the amount of urine the bladder is able to hold before the person feels the need to urinate, and may contribute to dribbling of urine when the person coughs, sneezes or

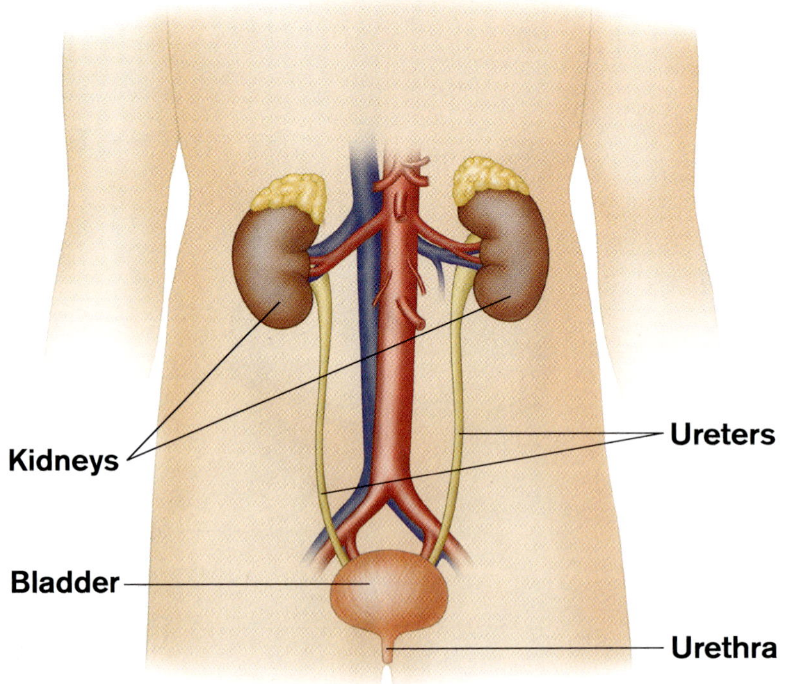

Figure B-7 The urinary system.

stands up. In men, the prostate gland (a gland located near the urethra that plays a role in the production of semen) may enlarge. This puts pressure on the urethra, making it difficult for the man to empty his bladder completely. As a result, the man may dribble urine. Incomplete emptying of the bladder, due to pressure from an enlarged prostate, decreased muscle tone, or both, can also put the older person at increased risk for urinary tract infections.

THE NERVOUS SYSTEM

The nervous system coordinates our responses to what goes on in the world around us, as well as what is happening inside of us. The nervous system consists of the *brain*, the *spinal cord* and the *nerves* (Figure B-8). Special nerve cells that send and receive information, called *neurons*, form the nervous tissue.

The brain processes and gives meaning to information that it receives from the organs. This information travels from the organs through a network of nerves to the spinal cord (a thick bundle of nervous tissue that extends from the base of the brain to about waist level). The information is carried through the spinal cord to the brain for processing. The brain also sends commands to the rest of the body. In this case, the commands travel from the brain, down the spinal cord and out through the nerves to the organs.

A person is born with as many neurons as he or she will ever have. After age 25, the body experiences a slow, but steady, loss of neurons. As a person gets older, the rate at which

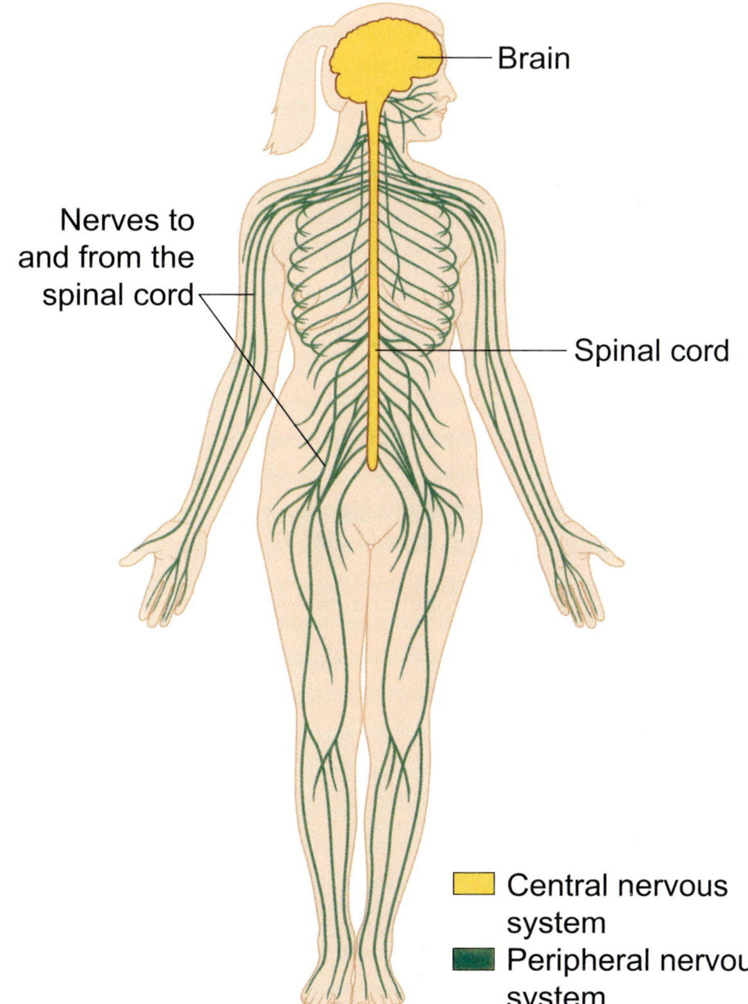

Figure B-8 The nervous system.

messages are sent through the nervous system slows down, causing the body to react more slowly. For example, it may take longer for the brain to receive the message that the hand is touching something hot and send the command to pull the hand away. It may also take an older person longer to learn new information.

THE ENDOCRINE SYSTEM

Many glands located throughout the body make up the endocrine system (Figure B-9). Each gland secretes one or more substances called *hormones*. Hormones travel through the blood or through tubes called *ducts* to their "target" organ. The hormones tell the target organ what to do, when to do it and how much it should do.

The largest gland is the *pancreas*, located in the abdomen near the stomach. Scattered throughout the pancreas are special cells that secrete insulin, the hormone that regulates the amount of glucose (sugar) in the bloodstream. Some forms of diabetes occur when the pancreas does not produce enough insulin.

Four small *parathyroid glands* and the larger *thyroid gland* are all grouped together in the neck, in front of the trachea. The parathyroid glands secrete a hormone that controls the level of calcium in the blood and bones. The thyroid gland secretes a hormone that is key in regulating metabolism (the rate at which the body turns food into energy).

Two other glands that influence metabolism are the *adrenal glands*, located on the top of each kidney. The adrenal glands secrete hormones that control the amount of salt, potassium and water in the body; they also constrict blood vessels and make the heart pump faster.

The *testes* and *ovaries* secrete hormones related to reproduction. In men, the testes secrete androgens, the hormones responsible for male sex characteristics. In women, the ovaries secrete hormones that influence menstruation and pregnancy.

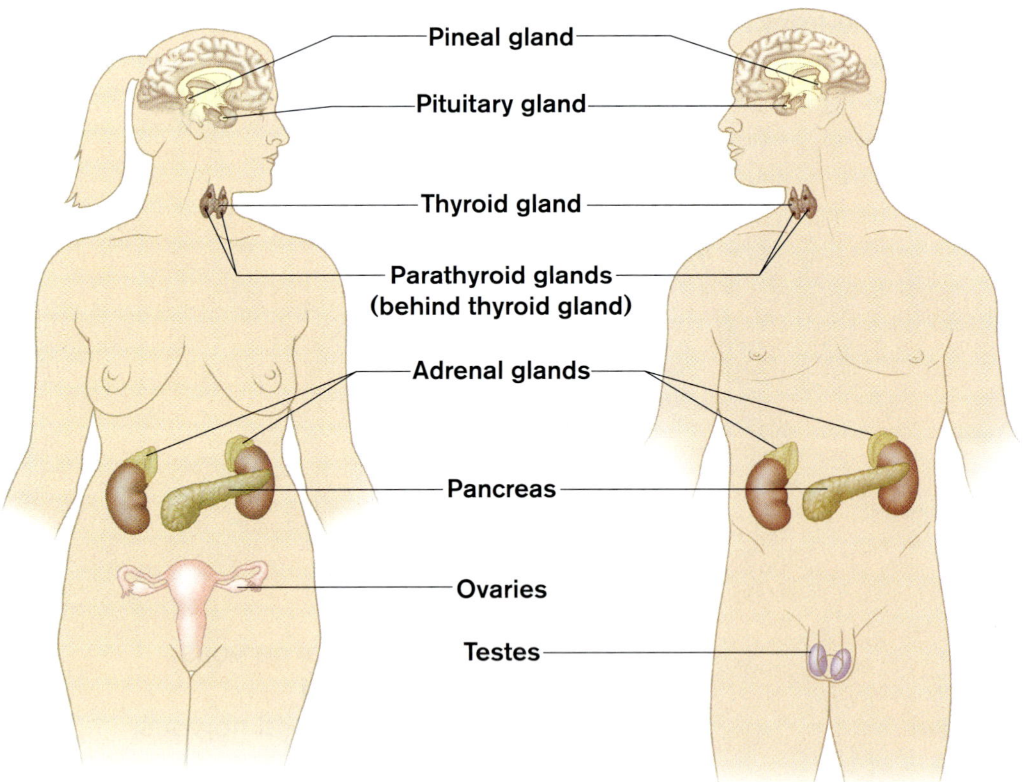

Figure B-9 The endocrine system.

The pineal gland and pituitary gland are located in the brain. The *pineal* gland secretes a hormone that helps to regulate the sleep–wake cycle. The *pituitary gland* is the "master gland." It secretes growth hormone, as well as hormones that control all of the other glands in the body.

In the endocrine system, the most striking effects of aging are seen in women who have reached menopause. At menopause, the ovaries stop producing the hormones estrogen and progesterone, causing menstruation to end. The woman is no longer able to become pregnant or bear children. Androgen production in men slows with aging but does not stop. Most other hormones are not affected by aging.

THE REPRODUCTIVE SYSTEM

The reproductive system consists of the organs involved in producing the cells and hormones that are necessary to create a new life. The female reproductive system also includes organs involved with supporting the baby before and after its birth.

The female reproductive system consists of the ovaries, fallopian tubes, uterus, vagina and breasts (Figure B-10). The *ovaries*, two almond-shaped glands located on either side of the uterus in the abdomen, produce eggs (the female reproductive cell) and hormones during the woman's reproductive years. A girl is born with all of the eggs she will ever have. Each month, hormones released by the ovaries cause one or more of the eggs to develop and be released into the *fallopian tubes*. The fallopian tubes carry the egg to the *uterus*, a hollow, muscular organ. If the egg is fertilized by a man's sperm, it may develop into an embryo and then into a fetus. The uterus serves as the home of the growing fetus for 9 months. If the egg is not fertilized, the lining of the uterus is shed (menstruation) and the cycle begins again. The lower portion of the uterus, called the *cervix*, opens into the *vagina,* the passageway extending from the uterus to the outside of the body. The vagina is the

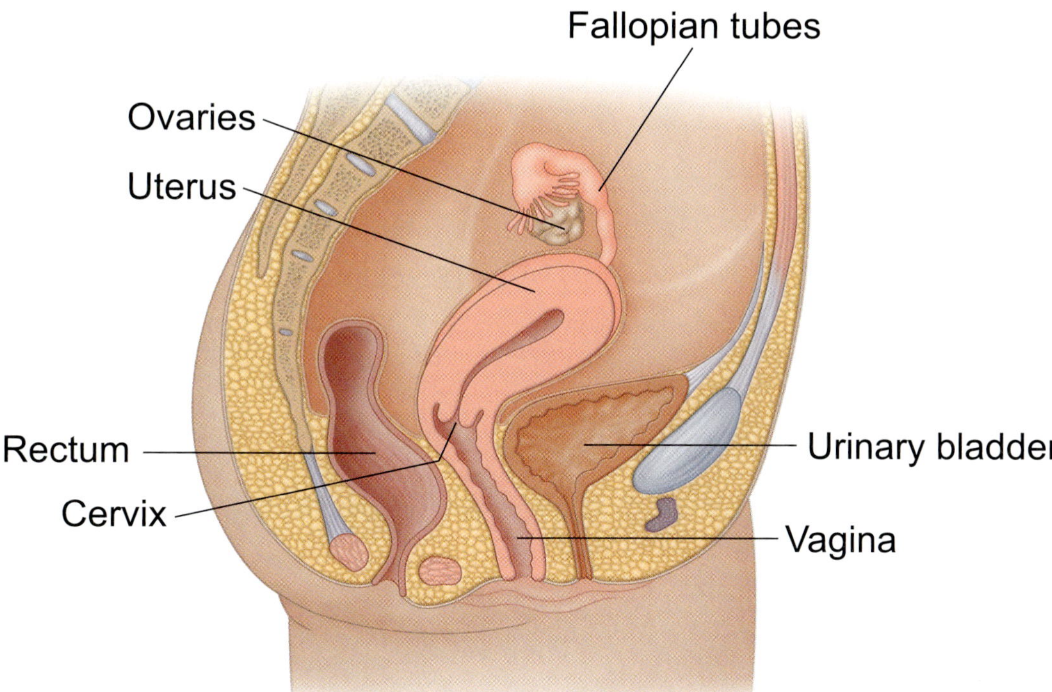

Figure B-10 The female reproductive system.

birth canal and the passage through which menstrual blood leaves the body. The vagina also serves as the organ that receives the man's penis during sexual intercourse. In women, the breasts are also considered part of the reproductive system, because they produce milk that is used to nourish the baby after birth.

The male reproductive organs include the penis, the scrotum and testes (testicles), the epididymis, the vas deferens, the seminal vesicles and the prostate gland (Figure B-11). The *testes*, which produce sperm (the male reproductive cell) and hormones, are housed in the *scrotum*, a pouch of loose skin located behind the penis. Sperm cells begin to develop in the testes, but finish developing as they move through the *epididymis*, a coiled passageway that leads to the *vas deferens.* While in the vas deferens, the mature sperm cells mix with secretions from the *seminal vesicles* and *prostate gland* to form semen. The vas deferens connects to the urethra. When a man ejaculates, semen leaves the body through the urethra.

Although both men and women can enjoy sexual activity well into old age, changes do occur in the way the reproductive system functions. In women, hormonal changes cause the reproductive system to stop releasing eggs and the woman stops menstruating. These changes occur when the woman is in her mid- to late 40s or early 50s. As a man gets older, he may produce fewer sperm and less semen, but he can still father a child in later years.

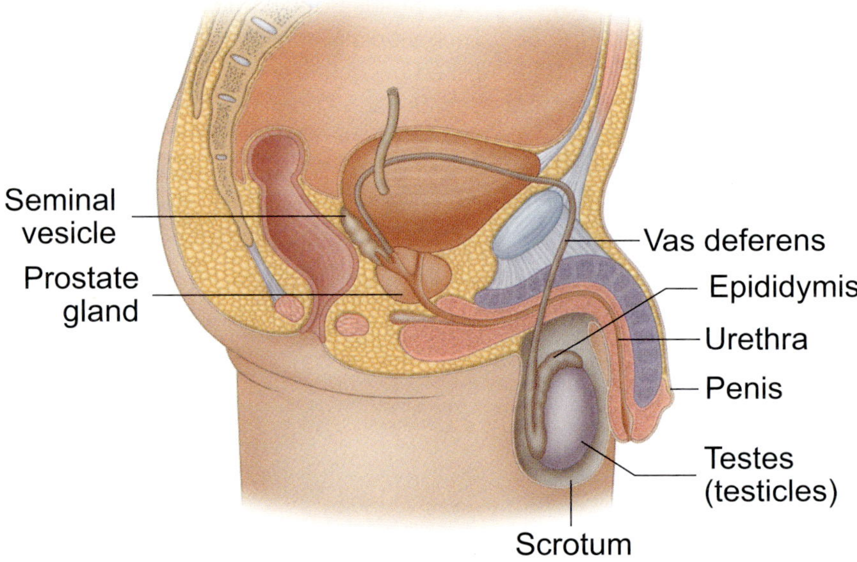

Figure B-11 The male reproductive system.

Math and Measurements Review

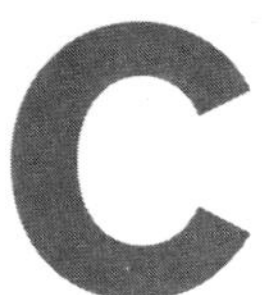

As a nurse assistant, you may need to perform math calculations and use common measurements in your work.

KEY TERMS

Word	Definition	Example
Decimal number	A number that contains a decimal point that separates the whole from its fractional part	3.5
Denominator	The number below the line in a fraction that tells into how many equal parts something has been divided	In the fraction 2/3, 3 is the denominator and tells that the object has been divided into 3 equal parts.
Difference	The answer in subtraction	In the math problem 18 minus 8 equals 10, 10 is the difference.
Digit	One of the numbers 0 through 9	0, 1, 2, 3, 4, 5, 6, 7, 8, 9
Dividend	The number being divided by another number	In the math problem 12 divided by 4 equals 3, 12 is the dividend.
Divisor	The number by which another number is divided	In the math problem 12 divided by 4 equals 3, 4 is the divisor.
Fraction	One or more of the equal parts of a whole	2/3
Minuend	Number from which another number is to be subtracted	In the math problem 26 minus 3 equals 23, 26 is the minuend.
Multiplicand	Number to be multiplied by another number	In the math problem 8 times 73 equals 584, 73 is the multiplicand.
Multiplier	Number by which another number is to be multiplied	In the math problem 8 times 73 equals 584, 8 is the multiplier.
Numerator	The number above the line in a fraction that tells how many parts are in use	In the fraction 2/3, 2 is the numerator and tells that 2 of the equal parts are being used.

Percent	Parts per 100; a fraction where "100" is the denominator	22 percent equals 22/100.
Place value	The position that a digit holds in a number; the place gives the digit its value. ten thousands, tenths, hundredths, hundred thousands, thousands, thousandths, hundreds, ten thousandths, tens, millions, ones **2,547,982.1356** decimal point	The place values of 56.89 are as follows: The numbers to the left of the decimal point (.) are whole numbers. "5" is in the "tens" place and "6" is in the "ones" place. The numbers to the right of the decimal point are a fraction. "8" is in the "tenths" place and "9" is in the "hundredths" place.
Product	The answer in a multiplication problem	In the math problem 8 times 73 equals 584, 584 is the product.
Quotient	The answer in a division problem	In the math problem 10 divided by 2 equals 5, 5 is the quotient.
Subtrahend	Number to be subtracted from another number	In the math problem 26 minus 3 equals 23, 3 is the subtrahend.
Sum	The answer in an addition problem	In the math problem 4 plus 3 equals 7, 7 is the sum.

WORKING WITH WHOLE NUMBERS AND DECIMALS

Addition

When adding decimals, remember to line the decimal points up. A digit that is written in the wrong position will produce a wrong answer when working with decimals. When adding a whole number to a decimal, you may find it helpful to add a decimal point after the whole number and place zeros in the decimal positions to the right of the decimal point. For example, to add 6 plus 0.45, set up the equation this way:

6.00
+ 0.45
6.45

To add, start with the right column of numbers and move to the left.

↓
5.94
+ 2.65
9

Think: 4 and 5 are 9. Write the 9 immediately under the first column.

↓
5.94
+ 2.65
.59

Think: 9 and 6 are 15. Write the 5 immediately under the second column, then "carry" the 1 and add it to the third column. (Remember to keep the decimal points in a straight line.)

↓
1
5.94
+ 2.65
8.59

Think: 1 and 5 are 6, and 6 and 2 are 8. Write the 8 immediately under the third column.

8.59 is the sum and is read "eight and fifty-nine hundredths."

To check addition, cover the sum, then add the columns from bottom to top and write the sum in small figures at the top. The sums at the top and bottom should be equal.

Note: *Use the same method of carrying when adding whole numbers.*

Practice problems: addition

1. 6.83 + 2.98	2. 4.75 + 3.66	3. 3.28 + 2.92	4. 52.94 + 38.66	5. 6.37 + 48.77
6. 78.54 + 14.57	7. 13.96 + 59.57	8. 44.26 + 37.86	9. 67.85 + 28.89	10. 55.47 + 34.73
11. 8.71 + 5.00	12. 75.62 + 14.58	13. 63.48 + 29.61	14. 57.64 + 37.57	15. 38.51 + 46.89
16. 5.27 + .58	17. 65.74 + 36.76	18. 83.25 + 57.28	19. 94.16 + 57.28	20. 97.51 + 68.68

Subtraction

Subtraction problems are set up and approached in the same way as addition problems. Work from right to left, and remember to line up the decimal points. When subtracting decimals and whole numbers, add a decimal point after the whole number and place zeros in the decimal positions to the right of the decimal point to keep the decimal points lined up. When a digit in the minuend (the top number) is smaller than the digit in the subtrahend (the bottom number), then it is necessary to "borrow" from the next digit to the left in the minuend.

To subtract, start with the right column of numbers and move to the left:

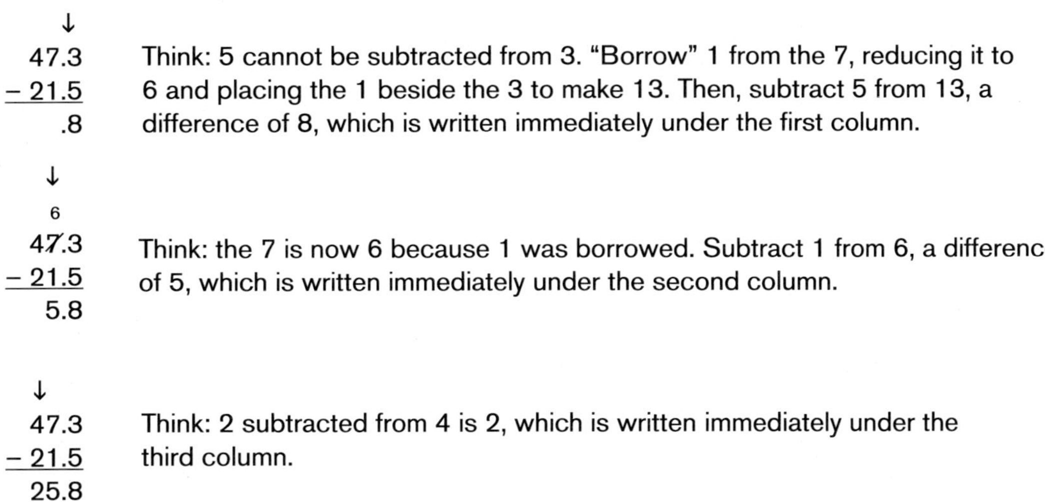

↓
47.3
− 21.5
.8

Think: 5 cannot be subtracted from 3. "Borrow" 1 from the 7, reducing it to 6 and placing the 1 beside the 3 to make 13. Then, subtract 5 from 13, a difference of 8, which is written immediately under the first column.

↓
6
47.3
− 21.5
5.8

Think: the 7 is now 6 because 1 was borrowed. Subtract 1 from 6, a difference of 5, which is written immediately under the second column.

↓
47.3
− 21.5
25.8

Think: 2 subtracted from 4 is 2, which is written immediately under the third column.

25.8 is the difference and is read "twenty-five and eight tenths."

Let's try another problem:

```
     ↓
  9 9
7 10 10 10
8 0 0 0
- 3 7 2 5
  4 2 7 5
```

Think: 5 cannot be subtracted from 0. Because the next two columns contain zeros as well, continue to the next column to the left until a digit other than 0 is available. Borrow 1 from the 8, reducing it to 7. Place the borrowed 1 beside the 0 in the next column to the right to make it 10. Borrow 1 from the 10, reducing it to 9. Place the borrowed 1 beside the 0 in the next column to the right to make it 10. Borrow 1 from the 10, reducing it to 9. Place the borrowed 1 beside the 0 in the first column to make it 10. Now subtract as usual.

Practice problems: subtraction

1.	500 – 475	2.	10,500 – 6,486	3.	4,631 – 1,719	4.	4,273 – 3,615	5.	8,126 – 5,918
6.	45.78 – 24.21	7.	57.08 – 29.26	8.	24.86 – 18.15	9.	30.78 – .25	10.	32.86 – 26.45

11. Bill helped his father plant 375 boxes of strawberry plants. Bill planted 12.5 boxes. How many did his father plant?
12. Eight thousand people are expected for the convention. By 3 o'clock, 2975 people were registered. How many more registrants will be needed to achieve the expected attendance?
13. The Marion Anderson auditorium will seat 1578 people. How many chairs will be needed in the aisle to seat a convention of 2000 people?
14. North Central Christian School had 45 boys in the graduating class of 2001 and only 38 girls. How many more boys did they have than girls?
15. The population of a certain city was 20,040 according to the 1990 census and 29,058 according to the 2000 census. How much had the population increased between 1990 and 2000?

Multiplication

Multiplication is a quicker method of addition. For example, if 15 students each have 12 pieces of fruit, and it is necessary to know how many pieces of fruit the students have all together, add 12 + 12 + 12 + 12 + 12 + 12 + 12 + 12 + 12 + 12 + 12 + 12 + 12 + 12 + 12. The quicker solution is to multiply 15 (the number of students) times 12 (the number of pieces of fruit each student has).

To multiply two numbers together, work from the right to the left. It is important to keep the digits lined up properly as you work:

```
    ↓
   4
 628
× 25
   0
```

Think: 5 times 8 equals 40. Write the 0 immediately under the first column, and carry the 4.

```
   ↓
  1 4
 628
× 25
  40
```

Think: 5 times 2 equals 10. Add the carried 4 to get 14. Write 4 immediately under the second column, and carry the 1.

```
   ↓
  628
×  25
 3140
```

Think: 5 times 6 equals 30. Add the carried 1 to get 31. Write 1 immediately under the third column, and write 3 written immediately under the fourth column.

```
     ↓
     1
  628
×  25
 3140
    6
```

Now think: 2 times 8 equals 16. Write the 6 immediately under the second column (below the 4), and carry the 1.

```
    ↓
    1
  628
×  25
 3140
   56
```

Think: 2 times 2 equals 4. Add the carried 1 to get 5. Write 5 immediately under the third column (below the 1).

```
   ↓
   628
×   25
  3140
 1256
15,700
```

Think: 2 times 6 equals 12. Write the 2 of immediately under the fourth column (below the 3), and write the 1 written immediately under the fifth column.

Then add the products together to get the answer.

If the problem involves a decimal, multiply the numbers as if they were all whole numbers. Then count the number of decimal places in the multiplicand and multiplier, and add them together. This is the number of decimal places that will be in your answer. Starting from the right, count over the total number of decimal places and put the decimal point there. For example, in the following example, the multiplicand has 2 decimal places and the multiplier has 1, for a total of 3, so you will count over three places to place the decimal point in your answer:

```
   6.28
×   2.5
   3140
  1256
 15.700
```

Practice problems: multiplication

1. 276 × 36
2. 35.84 × 45.67
3. 48.96 × 15.94
4. 9.67 × 5.6
5. 602 × 3.66
6. 8563 × 35.79
7. 785.4 × 14.57
8. $ 50.14 × 3348
9. 56.02 × 9.8
10. 67.85 × 2.86
11. Sandy spent 4 weeks at summer camp. How many days was she there?
12. Susie counted the tongue depressors that she uses each day. She uses 750 each day. How many are used in March? How many are used in April?
13. A dentist has 36 boxes of toothbrushes to pass out to his dental patients. Each box contains 24 toothbrushes. How many toothbrushes does he have?
14. An instructor has 50 students in one course. Each course uses 5 notebooks per student. How many notebooks will the instructor order?

Division

Division problems require both multiplication and subtraction. As with other calculations you have done, you will need to line the digits up properly.

Remember that the dividend is the number being divided by another number, called the divisor. The answer is called the quotient:

```
            121    quotient
divisor  3)364    dividend
```

You can check your answer by multiplying the quotient by the divisor. If the product equals the dividend, it is correct.

To set up a division problem, place the dividend inside the bracket and the divisor on the outside of the bracket. Work from the left to the right:

```
  ↓
  4
3)1206
  12
```

Think: 3 cannot divide into 1 (nothing is written over the 1). The 1 must be considered with the 2 as 12. Think: 3 will divide into 12 four times with no remainder. Write the 4 immediately over the 2. Multiply the 4 by the 3, and write the product immediately under the 12 in the dividend.

```
   ↓
  40
3)1206
  12
```

Think: 3 cannot divide into 0, and write a 0 immediately over the 0 in the dividend.

```
  402
3)1206
  12
     6
     6
     0
```

Think: 3 will divide into 6 two times. Write the 2 immediately over the 6. Multiply 3 times 2, and write the product under the 6. Think: 6 subtracted from 6 is a difference of 0. The answer is 402 with a remainder of 0.

When dividing a decimal by a whole number, put a decimal point directly above the decimal point in the dividend. Then divide as you would whole numbers:

Put a decimal point in the answer directly above the decimal point in the dividend.

```
   .
3)5.1
```

```
  1.7
3)5.1
  3
  21
  21
   0
```

Divide as you would with whole numbers.

The answer is 1.7 with a remainder of 0.

Use a zero as a placeholder in the answer between the decimal point and the first digit of the answer if the decimal point comes first in the dividend:

```
  .085
5).425
```

To divide by a decimal, count the number of decimal places in the divisor. Move the decimal point over to make the divisor a whole number, and then move the decimal point in the dividend the corresponding number of places. (If the dividend is a whole number, place the decimal point at the end and add the corresponding number of zeroes after it). Put a decimal point in the answer directly above the decimal point in the dividend, and divide as you would whole numbers:

$.2\overline{)1.42}$

$2\overline{)14.2}$

$$\begin{array}{r} 7.1 \\ 2\overline{)14.2} \\ -14 \\ \hline 2 \\ 2 \\ \hline 0 \end{array}$$

Put a decimal point in the quotient directly above the decimal point in the dividend, and divide as whole numbers.

The answer is 7.1 with a remainder of 0.

When you finish with long division and you have a remainder, you may continue dividing to express the remainder as a decimal. Put a decimal point and a zero to the right of the last digit in the dividend and a decimal point directly above in the quotient. Divide and continue to add zeros until there is no remainder.

$$\begin{array}{r} 14.5 \\ 6\overline{)87.0} \\ 6 \\ \hline 27 \\ 24 \\ \hline 30 \\ 30 \\ \hline \end{array}$$

A repeating pattern may appear. Either stop dividing at this point or show the quotient with a bar (line) across the top of the repeating part of the quotient. In the example below the full quotient is repeating.

$$\begin{array}{r} \overline{.444} \\ 9\overline{)4.000} \\ -\ 36 \\ \hline 40 \\ -\ 36 \\ \hline 4 \end{array}$$

Sometimes it is desirable to round off a decimal. To round off decimals, use the following procedure:

1. Find the place you are rounding off to and underline the digit in that place. Then circle the digit to the right.

   7.<u>3</u> ② round to the nearest tenth

   8.<u>2</u> ⑥ 4 round to the nearest tenth

   7.3 <u>2</u> ③ round to the nearest hundredth

   3.2 <u>5</u> ⑥ round to the nearest hundredth

   4.4 4 <u>4</u> ④ round to the nearest thousandth

   4.4 4 <u>6</u> ⑧ round to the nearest thousandth

2. If the circled digit is 0, 1, 2, 3, or 4, then the underlined digit stays the same. If the circled digit is 5, 6, 7, 8, or 9, then add 1 to the underlined digit. Drop all the digits that follow the underlined digit.

   7.32 becomes 7.3 (rounded off to the nearest tenth).

8.264 becomes 8.3 (rounded off to the nearest tenth).

7.323 becomes 7.32 (rounded off to the nearest hundredth).

3.256 becomes 3.26 (rounded off to the nearest hundredth).

4.4444 becomes 4.444 (rounded off to the nearest thousandth).

4.4468 becomes 4.447 (rounded off to the nearest thousandth).

Practice problems: division and rounding

1. $9\overline{)999}$
2. $8\overline{)692}$
3. $11\overline{)1{,}134}$
4. $4\overline{)5{,}144}$
5. $15\overline{)1{,}286}$
6. $.5\overline{)6{,}329}$
7. $.6\overline{)3.87}$
8. $7\overline{).867}$
9. Betsy bought 6 donuts for $.79. About how much did each donut cost?
10. John bought a box of 8 pens for $3.49. How much did each pen cost?
11. Undershirts are sold in packages at $6.51 per package with 3 shirts to a package. How much does each shirt cost?
12. Mrs. Bates needs to buy some dog food for her dog Clementine. She needs to decide which bag is more economical, the large 20-lb bag for $15.95 or the small 5-lb bag for $3.49. Which bag should she buy? Round your answers to the nearest cent.
13. Round the following numbers.

    To the nearest tenth:

    a. 3.82 ____ b. 8.47 ____ c. 13.95 ____ d. 80.333 ____

    To the nearest hundredth:

    e. 7.893 ____ f. 3.235 ____

    To the nearest thousandth:

    g. 6.7356 ____ h. 8.9532 ____

    To the nearest whole number:

    i. 6.4356 ____ j. 8.9532 ____

WORKING WITH FRACTIONS

A fraction is defined as one or more of the equal parts of a whole.

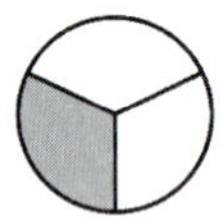

$\frac{1}{3}$ (one-third)

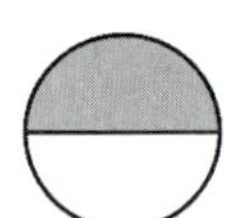

$\frac{1}{2}$ (one-half)

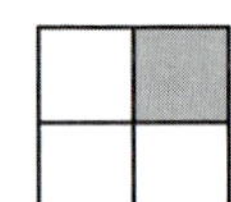

$\frac{1}{4}$ (one-fourth)

The bottom number of a fraction is the *denominator* and tells into how many equal parts a certain object has been divided into. It names the fraction. The top number is the *numerator* and tells the number of parts that are being worked with. The square above has been divided into 4 parts and 1 part is being worked with.

Adding and Subtracting Fractions

Remember, the denominator *names* the fractions. Fractions with different denominators (names) cannot be added or subtracted until they are given the same name.

Be sure the denominators are the same before adding and subtracting, as in the example below.

$$\frac{2}{4} + \frac{1}{4} = \frac{3}{4}$$

$$\frac{5}{9} - \frac{3}{9} = \frac{2}{9}$$

To add or subtract fractions that do not have a common denominator or name, you must first convert the denominators to a common denominator. This process is called finding the least common denominator (LCD). Use the following steps:

Example: Add $\frac{3}{4}$

$+\frac{4}{5}$

1. List the first multiples of the larger denominator, 5: 5, 10, 15, 20, 25, etc.
2. List the first multiples of the smaller denominator, 4: 4, 8, 12, 16, 20
3. Circle the first common, or shared, multiple of 5 and 4. The first one that they share, or have in common, is 20. The LCD is 20.
4. Then convert each fraction to use that LCD.
   Example: $\frac{3}{4} \times \frac{5}{5} = \frac{15}{20}$ $\quad \frac{4}{5} \times \frac{4}{4} = \frac{16}{20}$
5. Now you can add the fractions:
   $\frac{15}{20} + \frac{16}{20} = \frac{31}{20}$

Multiplying and Dividing Fractions

Multiplying and dividing fractions do not require that denominators be the same or have a common name.

When multiplying fractions, multiply the numerators and then the denominators.

$$\frac{5}{4} \times \frac{3}{8} = \frac{15}{32}$$

When dividing, rewrite the problem, inverting the second fraction (turning it upside down), and then multiply.

$\frac{1}{8} \div \frac{5}{6} =$ Rewrite this problem, turning the second fraction upside down and changing the division sign to a multiplication sign.

$\frac{1}{8} \times \frac{6}{5} =$ Now multiply.

$\frac{1}{8} \times \frac{6}{5} = \frac{6}{40}$ Make the answer as small as possible by finding the largest number that both the numerator and denominator can be divided by. In this case, both 6 and 40 can be divided by 2.

$\frac{6}{40} = \frac{3}{20}$ $\frac{3}{20}$ is the correct answer.

Practice problems: fractions

Add

1. $\frac{7}{8} + \frac{1}{2}$

2. $\frac{5}{8} + \frac{2}{3}$

3. $\frac{5}{16} + \frac{3}{4}$

4. $\frac{3}{4} + \frac{1}{6}$

Subtract

5. $\frac{5}{10} - \frac{1}{5}$

6. $\frac{3}{4} - \frac{5}{16}$

7. $\frac{2}{3} - \frac{1}{5}$

8. $\frac{7}{8} - \frac{2}{4}$

Multiply

9. $\frac{15}{16} \times \frac{4}{5} =$ ___

10. $\frac{5}{6} \times \frac{9}{10} =$ ___

11. $\frac{7}{10} \times \frac{1}{4} =$ ___

Divide

12. $\frac{3}{8} \div \frac{3}{5} =$ ___

13. $\frac{5}{16} \div \frac{1}{8} =$ ___

14. $\frac{1}{3} \div \frac{1}{6} =$ ___

WORKING WITH PERCENTS

"Percent" means "parts per 100." A percent is simply a fraction where the denominator is "100." A percent can be written using the symbol "%" (for example, 25%). A percent can also be written as a fraction (for example, 25/100) or a decimal (for example, 0.25). For example:

50% = 50 out of every 100 = $\frac{50}{100}$ = 0.50

16% = 16 out of every 100 = $\frac{16}{100}$ = 0.16

1% = 1 out of every 100 = $\frac{1}{100}$ = 0.01

98% = 98 out of every 100 = $\frac{98}{100}$ = 0.98

To find the percent for any fraction, you can divide the numerator by the denominator to find the decimal. Then you can write the percent.

$\frac{1}{20} = 20\overline{)1.00} = 0.05 = 5\%$

Practice problems: percents

1. 10% of 90 is ____
2. 20% of 90 is ____
3. 30% of 90 is ____
4. 40% of 90 is ____

SYSTEMS OF MEASUREMENT

The Metric System

The metric system is based on units of 10. The basic units used in the metric system are:

	Unit	Abbreviation
Length	meter	m
Mass (weight)	gram	g
Volume	liter	L

Prefixes are added to the basic unit of measure to change the value. For example:

milli- for $\frac{1}{1000}$

centi- for $\frac{1}{100}$

deci- for $\frac{1}{10}$

kilo- for 1000

So, for example, a milliliter (mL) is equal to $\frac{1}{1000}$ of a liter. A kilogram (kg) is equal to 1000 grams, and so on.

The English System

The English system is a historical system that was developed using body parts and familiar objects as units of measure. Eventually, these measurements were standardized. The basic units used in the English system are:

	Unit	Abbreviation
Length	inch	in
	foot	ft
	yard	yd
	mile	
Mass (weight)	pound	lb
	ton	
Volume	ounce	oz
	cup	
	pint	pt
	quart	qt
	gallon	gal

Common equivalents are:

Length	Mass (weight)	Volume
12 inches = 1 foot	16 ounces = 1 pound	16 ounces = 1 pint
3 feet = 1 yard	2000 pounds = 1 ton	2 pints = 1 quart
5280 feet = 1 mile		4 quarts = 1 gallon

ANSWERS TO PRACTICE PROBLEMS

Addition

1. 9.81
2. 8.41
3. 6.20
4. 91.60
5. 55.14
6. 93.11
7. 73.53
8. 82.12
9. 96.74
10. 90.20
11. 13.71
12. 90.20
13. 93.09
14. 95.21
15. 85.40
16. 5.85
17. 102.50
18. 140.53
19. 151.44
20. 166.19

Subtraction

1. 25
2. 4014
3. 2912
4. 658
5. 2208
6. 21.57
7. 27.82
8. 6.71
9. 30.53
10. 6.41
11. 362.5
12. 5025
13. 422
14. 7
15. 9018

Multiplication

1. 9936
2. 1,636.8128
3. 780.4224
4. 54.152
5. 2,203.32
6. 306,469.77
7. 11,443.278
8. $167,868.72
9. 548.996
10. 194.0510
11. 28
12. March: 23,250; April: 22,500
13. 864
14. 250

Division and Rounding

1. 111
2. 86.5
3. $103.0\overline{9}$
4. 1286
5. $85.7\overline{3}$
6. 12,658
7. 6.45
8. .124
9. $.13
10. $.44
11. $2.17
12. 5-lb bag
13. a. 3.8 b. 8.5 c. 14.0 d. 80.3 e. 7.89 f. 3.24 g. 6.736 h. 8.953 i. 6 j. 9

Fractions

1. $\frac{13}{8}$
2. $\frac{31}{24}$
3. $\frac{11}{16}$
4. $\frac{11}{12}$
5. $\frac{1}{2}$
6. $\frac{7}{16}$
7. $\frac{7}{15}$
8. $\frac{3}{8}$
9. $\frac{3}{4}$
10. $\frac{3}{4}$
11. $\frac{7}{40}$
12. $\frac{5}{8}$
13. $2\frac{1}{2}$
14. 2

Percents

1. 9
2. 18
3. 27
4. 36

Appendix

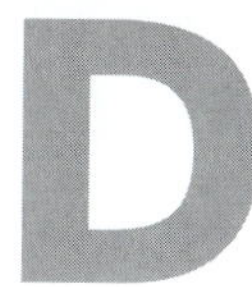

Additional Skills

Skill D-1
Cleaning a Glass Thermometer

PREPARATION

1. Wash your hands.
2. Gather your supplies:
   - Glass thermometer
   - Thermometer holder
   - Cotton balls or tissues
   - Paper towels
   - Gloves (optional)

PROCEDURE

3. Wash your hands. Put on the gloves, if using.
4. Place a paper towel in the sink in case you drop the thermometer while you are cleaning it.
5. Turn on the faucet with a clean paper towel. Adjust the temperature of the water so that it is cool, not hot.
6. Stand over the sink and hold the thermometer by the stem end.
7. Wet a cotton ball or tissue with water and apply soap.
8. Wipe down the length of the thermometer using a twisting motion, starting at your fingers and working downward over the bulb (Figure D-1). Discard the cotton ball or tissue in a facility-approved waste container.

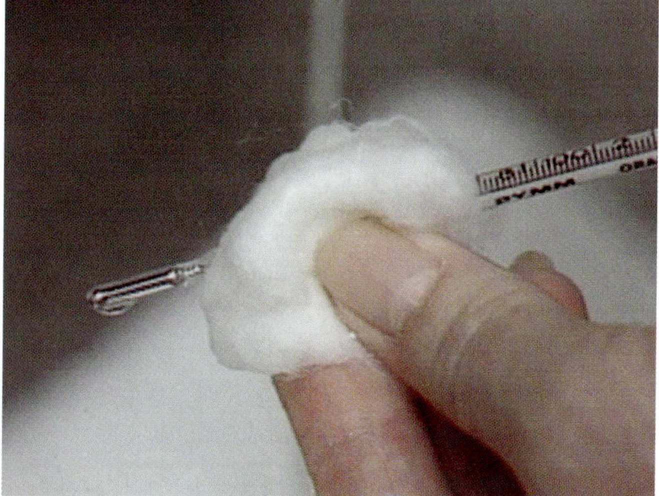

Figure D-1

9. Wet another cotton ball or tissue with only clean water.
10. Rinse the thermometer by using the same twisting motion as before to wipe down the length of the thermometer. Discard the cotton ball or tissue in a facility-approved waste container.
11. Repeat steps 7 through 10 one more time.
12. Dry the thermometer with a clean cotton ball or tissue, using the same twisting motion and wiping down the length of the thermometer. Discard the cotton ball or tissue in a facility-approved waste container.
13. Shake the thermometer down and put it in its holder.
14. Remove the paper towel that you used to line the sink and discard it in a facility-approved waste container.
15. Remove and dispose of your gloves, if worn.
16. Wash your hands.

Skill D-2

Using a Glass Thermometer to Measure a Person's Temperature

PREPARATION

1. Wash your hands.
2. Gather your supplies:
   - Glass thermometer with blue tip (oral or axillary temperature) or red tip (rectal temperature)
   - Thermometer sheath (optional)
   - Gloves (rectal temperature)
   - Cotton balls
   - Tissues
   - Pen and paper
   - Watch with a second hand
3. Knock, greet the person and ensure privacy.
4. Explain the procedure.
5. Adjust equipment for body mechanics and safety: Raise the bed to a comfortable working height. Make sure the wheels are locked.

PROCEDURE

6. Clean the thermometer with cool water and soap (see Skill D-1). Inspect the thermometer to ensure that there are no chips or cracks in the glass.
7. Shake down the thermometer so that the mercury or mercury-like substance is below the 94° mark (if using a Fahrenheit thermometer) or the 34° mark (if using a Celsius thermometer).
8. Place the thermometer sheath, if you are using one, on the thermometer (Figure D-1).

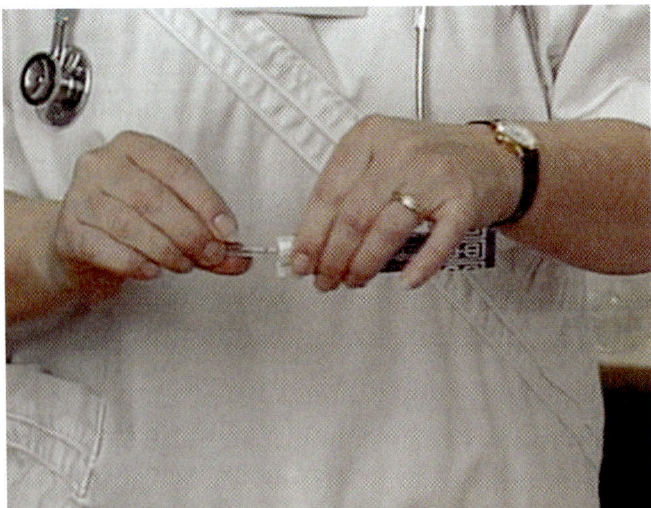

Figure D-1

9. Position the person appropriately.
   - **Oral or axillary temperature:** Position the person in Fowler's position (sitting up with the head of the bed elevated) or the supine position (lying on the back).
   - **Rectal temperature:** Help the person lie on one side with his or her back toward you and the top knee flexed.
10. If taking a rectal temperature, lubricate the tip of the thermometer by placing a small amount of lubricating jelly on a tissue and dipping the tip of the thermometer in it. Put on the gloves.
11. Note the time and place the thermometer.
    - **Oral temperature:** Put the thermometer under the person's tongue and slightly to one side (Figure D-2, A). Ask the person to close his or her lips around the thermometer.

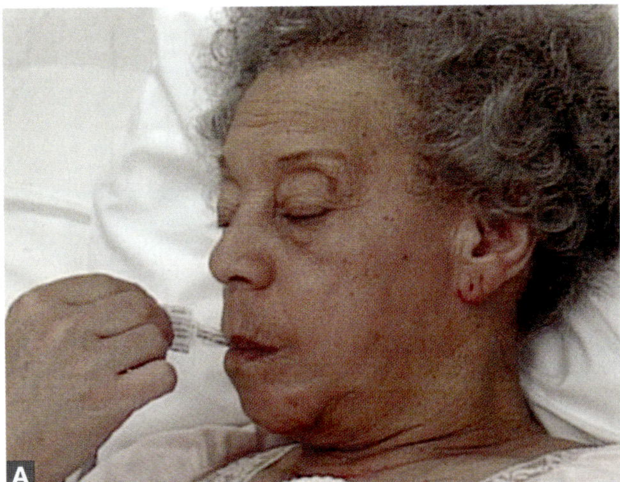

Figure D-2, A

    - **Rectal temperature:** Adjust the top covers and the person's clothing as necessary to expose the buttocks. Lift the person's upper buttock and insert the thermometer into the anus no more than 1 inch in an adult or 1/2 inch in a child (Figure D-2, B). Stay with the person and hold the thermometer in place.

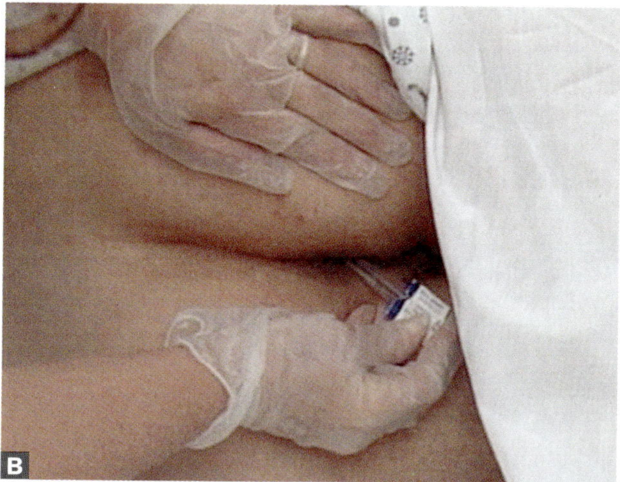

Figure D-2, B

- **Axillary temperature:** Expose the person's underarm and pat the skin dry with a tissue, if necessary. Put the probe in the middle of the person's underarm, and then bring the person's arm across his or her chest to hold the thermometer in place (Figure D-2, C).

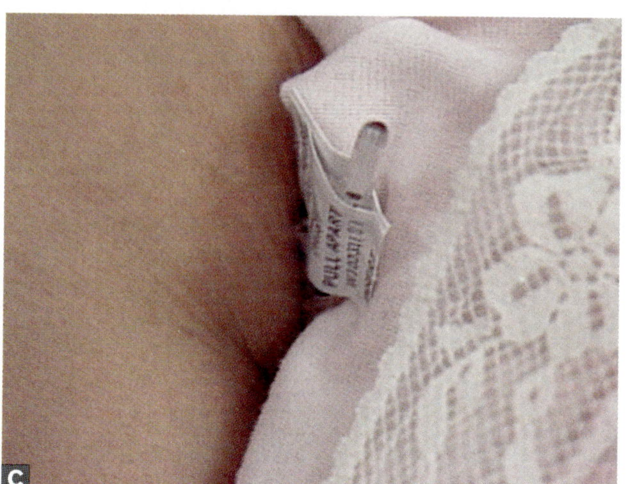

Figure D-2, C

12. Keep the thermometer in place for the specified amount of time.
    - **Oral temperature:** 5 to 8 minutes, or according to facility policy
    - **Rectal temperature:** 3 minutes, or according to facility policy
    - **Axillary temperature:** 10 minutes, or according to facility policy
13. Remove the thermometer. If used, discard the thermometer sheath in a facility-approved waste container. Wipe off the thermometer with a tissue and discard the tissue in a facility-approved waste container.
14. Read the temperature measurement by holding the thermometer horizontally by the stem end at eye level and rotating it until you can see the line made by the substance inside the thermometer (Figure D-3).

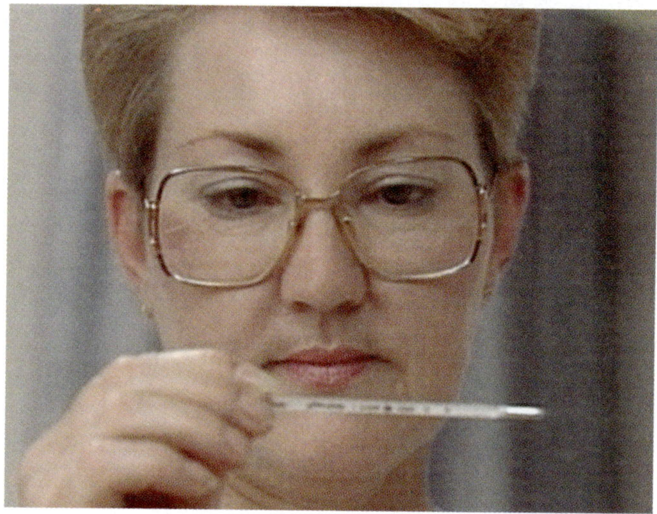

Figure D-3

15. Place the thermometer on a clean, dry tissue or paper towel.

Continued on next page

Skill D-2
Using a Glass Thermometer to Measure a Person's Temperature *Continued*

16. Help make the person comfortable.
    - **Rectal temperature:** Wipe the lubricating jelly from the person's buttocks with a tissue and discard the tissue in a facility-approved waste container. Adjust the person's clothing to cover the buttocks and assist him or her into a comfortable position.
    - **Axillary temperature:** Adjust the person's clothing to cover the underarm area.
17. Remove and dispose of your gloves. Wash your hands.
18. Write down the person's name, the time, the temperature measurement and the method used to obtain the temperature (***O*** for oral, ***R*** for rectal, or ***A*** for axillary).
19. Clean the thermometer, shake it down, and put it back in its holder.
20. Continue obtaining other vital sign measurements, or follow the completion steps.

COMPLETION

21. Ensure the person's comfort and good body alignment.
22. Adjust equipment for safety: Lower the bed to the level specified in the person's care plan. Make sure the wheels on the bed are locked. Place the person's method of calling for help within reach. Lower or raise the side rails according to the person's care plan.
23. Clean up your work area.
24. Wash your hands.
25. Report and record.

Skill D-3
Measuring a Person's Blood Pressure (One-Step Method)

PREPARATION

1. Wash your hands.
2. Gather your supplies:
   - Sphygmomanometer with the correct size cuff
   - Stethoscope
   - Alcohol wipes
   - Pen and paper
3. Knock, greet the person, and ensure privacy.
4. Explain the procedure.
5. Adjust equipment for body mechanics and safety: Raise the bed to a comfortable working height. Make sure the wheels on the bed are locked.

PROCEDURE

6. Position the person appropriately:
   - **In bed:** Position the person in the supine position (lying on the back). Position the person's arm so that it is resting comfortably, palm up, on the bed.
   - **In a chair:** Have the person sit with both feet flat on the floor. Position the forearm so that it is fully supported, palm up, and level with the person's heart.
7. Clean the earpieces and diaphragm of the stethoscope with an alcohol wipe. Discard the wipe in a facility-approved waste container.
8. Turn the screw to the left (down) and squeeze all of the air out of the cuff. Adjust the person's clothing as necessary to expose the upper arm.
9. Locate the person's brachial pulse on the inside of the elbow.
10. Place the cuff on the person's arm, over bare skin, with the arrow directly over the brachial artery. The bottom edge of the cuff should be about 1 inch above the person's elbow. Wrap the cuff around the person's arm snugly and smoothly and secure the cuff. Make sure it is snug enough to stay in place, but not uncomfortably tight.
11. Put the earpieces in your ears with the tips facing forward (toward your nose). Place the diaphragm of the stethoscope firmly over the person's brachial pulse.
12. Turn the screw to the right (up) and pump the bulb to inflate the cuff to between 160 mm Hg and 180 mm Hg. Alternatively, inflate the cuff to 30 mm Hg beyond the person's last recorded systolic pressure.
13. Turn the screw to the left (down) and let the air out of the cuff slowly (about 2 to 4 mm Hg per second). The reading when you first hear the pulse sound is the *systolic* pressure. Remember this number and continue letting the air out slowly.
14. The reading when the pulse sound stops or changes is the *diastolic* pressure. Remember this number and quickly let out the rest of the air.

    Note: If pulse sounds are heard immediately after starting to deflate the cuff, you must completely deflate the cuff. Then re-inflate the cuff to no more than 200 mm Hg, and repeat steps 13 and 14.
15. Write down the person's name, the time and the blood pressure measurement.
16. Remove the cuff from the person's arm.

COMPLETION

17. Ensure the person's comfort and good body alignment.
18. Adjust equipment for safety. Lower the bed to the level specified in the person's care plan. Make sure the wheels on the bed are locked. Place the person's method of calling for help within reach. Lower or raise the side rails according to the person's care plan.
19. Clean up your work area.
20. Wash your hands.
21. Report and record.

Appendix

E Answers to Questions for Review

Chapter 1, **Being A Nurse Assistant**

1-d, 2-c, 3-b, 4-a, 5-d, 6-a, 7-c, 8-b

Chapter 2, **Working in the Health Care System**

1-c, 2-b, 3-c, 4-b, 5-a, 6-c

Chapter 3, **Understanding Legal and Ethical Aspects of Health Care**

1-c, 2-c, 3-c, 4-a, 5-a

Chapter 4, **Understanding the People in Our Care**

1-b, 2-b, 3-b, 4-b, 5-c, 6-b, 7-b, 8-b

Chapter 5, **Communicating with People**

1-b, 2-b, 3-b, 4-d, 5-d, 6-a, 7-d, 8-d, 9-c, 10-d

Chapter 6, **Controlling the Spread of Infection**

1-b, 2-b, 3-a, 4-d, 5-c, 6-a

Chapter 7, **Preventing Injuries**

1-d, 2-c, 3-a, 4-b, 5-b, 6-b, 7-d, 8-a, 9-c

Chapter 8, **Responding to Emergencies**

1-c, 2-b, 3-d, 4-b, 5-a, 6-b, 7-b, 8-b, 9-b

Chapter 9, **Measuring Vital Signs, Weight and Height**

1-b, 2-d, 3-a, 4-a, 5-b, 6-a, 7-c, 8-b, 9-d, 10-d

Chapter 10, **Maintaining A Comfortable Environment**

1-c, 2-b, 3-b, 4-b, 5-a, 6-a, 7-d, 8-d, 9-b

Chapter 11, **Providing Restorative Care**

1-c, 2-d, 3-a, 4-d, 5-c, 6-d, 7-d, 8-d, 9-c

Chapter 12, **Assisting with Positioning and Transferring**

1-a, 2-c, 3-d, 4-d, 5-b, 6-c, 7-c

Chapter 13, **Assisting with Personal Cleanliness and Grooming**

1-d, 2-c, 3-b, 4-c, 5-b, 6-d, 7-d, 8-b, 9-c, 10-d, 11-d

Chapter 14, **Assisting with Meals and Fluids**

1-c, 2-b, 3-a, 4-a, 5-b, 6-d, 7-c, 8-a, 9-b, 10-c, 11-d, 12-d

Chapter 15, **Assisting with Elimination**

1-c, 2-c, 3-c, 4-b, 5-c, 6-d, 7-d, 8-c, 9-c, 10-a

Chapter 16, **Promoting Comfort and Rest**

1-c, 2-a, 3-b, 4-d, 5-c, 6-a, 7-b, 8-b, 9-a

Chapter 17, **Assisting with Admissions, Transfers and Discharges**

1-d, 2-b, 3-b, 4-a, 5-d, 6-a, 7-d, 8-c, 9-b

Chapter 18, **Providing Care for People with Specific Illnesses**

1-d, 2-b, 3-b, 4-c, 5-a, 6-c, 7-c, 8-a, 9-a

Chapter 19, **Providing Care for People with Cognitive Changes and Dementia**

1-c, 2-b, 3-a, 4-c, 5-a, 6-d, 7-a, 8-d, 9-b, 10-c, 11-c, 12-b

Chapter 20, **Providing Care for People at the End of Life**

1-a, 2-c, 3-c, 4-b, 5-a, 6-c, 7-b, 8-b, 9-b, 10-b

Chapter 21, **Providing Care to Infants and Children**

1-b, 2-c, 3-d, 4-a, 5-a, 6-b, 7-d, 8-b, 9-d

Chapter 22, **Providing Care for People In Their Homes**

1-b, 2-c, 3-a, 4-c, 5-d, 6-d, 7-b, 8-a, 9-c

Chapter 23, **Entering the Workforce**

1-c, 2-c, 3-b, 4-c, 5-b, 6-a, 7-c

Chapter 24, **Enjoying Professional Success**

1-c, 2-c, 3-a, 4-b, 5-b, 6-b, 7-a

GLOSSARY

A

abandonment: withdrawal of one's support or help from another person, despite having the responsibility to provide this support or help

abuse: the willful infliction of injury or harm on another

accreditation: official recognition by a professional association or non-government agency that the facility provides care to a certain standard

acquired immunodeficiency syndrome (AIDS): a condition caused by the human immunodeficiency virus (HIV) that results in a breakdown of the body's defense systems

activities of daily living (ADLs): routine tasks of everyday life, essential for meeting a person's basic physical needs

acute care setting: a health care setting that specializes in providing care to people who become sick or injured suddenly, or who have other conditions that require short-term health care

acute condition: an illness or injury that develops rapidly and usually resolves completely, after a period of time, with treatment

acute pain: pain that occurs suddenly with injury, with illness or from surgery; lasts less than 6 months and lessens as tissue heals

admission: a person's formal entry into the health care setting

advance directive: a legal document stating how the person wants health decisions made if he or she is unable to make or communicate these decisions independently in the future

age-related memory impairment: difficulties remembering or recalling information, or learning new information, that occur with normal aging and do not impair a person's ability to carry out normal routines and activities

agnosia: the inability to interpret sensory input to recognize familiar things or people

alignment: correct positioning of body parts relative to each other to maintain good posture

ambulation: the medical term for walking

amnesia: memory loss

angina: chest pain that occurs because the heart is not getting enough oxygen

anorexia: loss of appetite

anxiety: a feeling of unease, dread or worry

aphasia: problems with communication resulting from damage to the brain

appetite: desire for food

apraxia: the inability to plan and perform purposeful motor movements to complete a task despite having the ability and the desire to perform the task

arthritis: a condition that causes joints to become inflamed, swollen, stiff and painful

aspiration: inhalation of fluids or other foreign materials into the lungs

aspiration pneumonia: pneumonia that occurs when foreign material (such as food or vomit) is inhaled into the lungs

assault: an action that causes a person to fear being touched in a harmful or unwelcome way

assertive: adjective used to describe a person who is able to state his or her feelings and needs in a direct way, while still respecting the feelings and needs of others

assisted-living facility: a long-term care facility that provides limited assistance with selected tasks; residents are more independent than the residents of nursing homes

asthma: an illness in which certain substances or conditions, called "triggers," cause inflammation and construction of the airways, making breathing difficult

atraumatic care: a philosophy of caring for ill or injured children that focuses on reducing the negative effects associated with illness and injury by minimizing the physical and emotional stress the child and family members experience

atrophy: loss of muscle mass

automated external defibrillator (AED): a device that delivers a defibrillation shock automatically or with the push of a button to help the heart restore an effective pumping rhythm

B

balance: stability achieved through the even distribution of weight

baseline: initial measurements that are taken to be compared with measurements taken later on

battery: touching another person in a harmful or unwelcome way

benign: noncancerous

bereavement care: care that is provided for people who are grieving after a loved one dies

bisexual: word used to describe a person who is attracted to people of both sexes

bloodborne pathogen: a disease-causing microbe that is transmitted through contact with an infected person's blood

body fluids: liquid or semiliquid substances produced by and released from the body, such as blood, urine, feces, saliva, mucus, vomit, semen, vaginal secretions, breast milk, wound drainage and sweat

body mechanics: using the body in a safe and efficient way to avoid placing unnecessary strain on muscles and joints

bony prominence: parts of the body where there is only a thin layer of fat and muscle between the skin and the underlying bone or cartilage

C

calorie: the unit of measure used to describe the amount of energy a food supplies

cancer: the abnormal growth of new cells that crowd out or destroy other body tissues

cardiopulmonary resuscitation (CPR): a technique used to sustain breathing and circulation for a person who has gone into cardiac arrest

care plan: a document that details the care the person requires, as well as the methods, equipment and frequency for providing that care

catastrophic reaction: an intense emotional and behavioral outburst over a seemingly small event, seen in people with dementia

cerebrovascular accident: a disorder that occurs when blood flow to part of the brain is blocked, causing the brain cells to die; also called a "stroke"

chain of infection: the six requirements that must be met before an infection can pass from one person to another

chemotherapy: the use of drugs to stop or slow the growth of cancer cells

chronic condition: an illness or injury that is ongoing and usually requires continuous treatment to manage

chronic heart failure: a condition that occurs when the heart is damaged or weak and is unable to effectively pump blood throughout the body

chronic obstructive pulmonary disease (COPD): a term used to describe lung disorders that make it difficult for air to enter or leave the lungs

chronic pain: pain that lasts longer than 6 months

circumcision: surgical removal of the foreskin of the penis

client: a person who receives care in his or her home

closed bed: a bed where the bedspread is pulled up to cover the linens

cognition: thinking processes, which include memory, reasoning, judgment and language

cognitive impairment: problems with thinking processes involving memory, reasoning, judgment and language

comfort (supportive) care: care that makes the person more comfortable but does not prolong the person's life, such as oxygen therapy, the administration of pain medications and personal care

compassion: the quality of recognizing another person's hardship, accompanied by a desire to help relieve that hardship

communication: the process of giving and receiving information

condom catheter: a condom-like device that is placed over a man's penis and is connected by tubing to a drainage bag to collect urine; used in the management of incontinence

constipation: difficult elimination of dry, hard feces

contaminated: soiled with pathogens

contracture: a condition that results when a joint is held in one position for too long, causing the tendons to shorten and become stiff, resulting in loss of motion in the joint

coordination: the use of direction and force for purposeful action

cover letter: a brief letter to a potential employer explaining why you are interested in the job and the organization, and summarizing the qualifications and experience you have that makes you an appropriate candidate for the job

culture: a shared set of beliefs, values, customs and practices that characterizes a group of people or a society

cuticle: the skin along the edge of the nail

D

defecation: the elimination of solid waste from the body

dehydration: too little fluid in the body

delegation: the process of giving another person the authority and responsibility to complete a task on one's behalf

delirium: a rapid change in cognition that is related to chemical changes in the body

delusion: a fixed, false belief

dementia: a term used to describe a cluster of symptoms involving progressive decline in memory and thinking abilities, such as the use of language and the ability to reason and make judgments

depilatory: a chemical cream or powder that is applied to the skin to dissolve and remove hair

depression: a mental health disorder characterized by a persistent feeling of sadness

diabetes: a disorder characterized by the body's inability to process glucose (sugar) in the bloodstream

dialysis: a treatment that replaces the function of the kidneys by removing waste products and excess fluid from the body

diarrhea: the frequent passage of loose, watery feces

diet: the food and beverages a person consumes

dietitian: a health care professional who has specialized knowledge and training in the field of nutrition

disaster: a severe event that causes widespread damage and destruction, affecting many people and disrupting normal functioning of the community

discharge: a person's formal release from the health care setting where he or she is currently receiving care

discharge planning: a process that involves identifying the person's ongoing care needs and making arrangements to have those needs met after the person leaves the facility

disinfectant: a chemical solution used to kill microbes on an object or surface

do-not-resuscitate (DNR) order: an order to withhold cardiopulmonary resuscitation (CPR) in the event of cardiopulmonary arrest

durable power of attorney for health care: a legal document that gives the responsibility for making health care decisions on the person's behalf to someone else in case the person becomes unable to make these decisions on his or her own behalf

dyspnea: labored, difficult breathing

E

edema: too much fluid in the body

emergency: a situation that arises suddenly and requires immediate action to keep a person safe

empathy: the quality of seeking to understand another person's situation, point of view or feelings

employee orientation: an informational session conducted with new employees within the first few days of employment, during which the employee is given information about the organization's policies and procedures and the benefits employees are entitled to receive

enema: the introduction of fluid into the bowel through the anus to remove feces from the bowel

entrapment: an injury that occurs when a person's head or other body part becomes trapped between, under, or on the side rails, or between the mattress and the side rail

epilepsy: a chronic seizure condition

erection: stiffening of the penis

ethical dilemma: a situation where there may be more than one good or moral solution, depending on one's point of view

ethics: moral principles or standards that we use to decide the correct action to take

ethics committee: a group of people representing many different areas of expertise and with an in-depth knowledge of ethical principles that is brought together to help resolve ethical dilemmas

expressive aphasia: the inability to use language to express oneself, verbally or in writing (or both)

F

family-centered care: a philosophy of caring for injured or ill children that emphasizes an open, working relationship among health care providers, the child and family members

fecal impaction: a serious form of constipation that occurs when constipation is not relieved and feces build up in the bowel until the bowel is almost completely blocked

feces: solid body waste

fever: a temperature that is higher than the normal range

fiber: a substance found in foods that helps the digestive tract function properly and lowers the risk for conditions such as heart disease and diabetes

first aid: care that is provided to an injured or ill person while waiting for more advanced help to arrive

Fowler's position: a variation of supine position where the head of the bed is raised 45 degrees

fraud: lying to gain profit or advantage

friction: rubbing of two surfaces against each other

G

gender identity: a person's inner sense of being male or female

glucose: the body's most basic source of energy

graduate: a pitcher-like device used for measuring fluids

grief: intense sadness that occurs as a result of loss

H

hallucination: seeing, hearing, tasting, smelling or feeling something that does not exist

hangnail: ragged and torn cuticle

harassment: ongoing behavior that causes significant distress to another person

health care–associated infection: an infection that a person gets while receiving care in a health care facility

health care team: a group of people with specialized knowledge and skills who work together to provide personalized quality care that meets the person's physical, emotional, social and spiritual needs

hemiparesis: weakness on one side

hemiplegia: paralysis on one side

hepatitis: inflammation of the liver

heterosexual: word used to describe a person who is attracted to people of the opposite sex

high-efficiency particulate air filter (HEPA) mask: a special type of mask that filters out very small droplets suspended in the air (aerosols)

high Fowler's position: a variation of Fowler's position where the head of the bed is raised 90 degrees

homebound: adjective used to describe a person who is unable to leave his or her home without assistance

homosexual: word used to describe a person who is attracted to people of the same sex

hospice: a model of care that focuses on providing supportive care to people who are dying, and on supporting their families, during the end-of-life period

human development: social, emotional and cognitive changes that a person experiences as he or she grows older

human growth: physical changes that a person experiences as he or she grows older

human immunodeficiency virus (HIV): a bloodborne pathogen that invades and destroys the cells that help to fight infections

hyperglycemia: excessively high blood-glucose levels

hypertension: (1) high blood pressure; (2) a disorder characterized by chronically high blood pressure

hypoglycemia: excessively low blood-glucose levels

hypotension: low blood pressure

hypothermia: a temperature that is lower than the normal range

I

immobility: the state of not moving

incident: anything unusual that happens to a person receiving care, a staff member or a visitor to the facility and has the potential to cause harm

incontinence: the inability to control the release of urine or feces

indwelling urinary catheter: a small tube inserted through the urethra into the bladder that is left in place to drain urine from the bladder on a continuous basis

infection: a disease caused by the growth of pathogens in the body

infection control: actions taken to control the spread of microbes that can cause disease

influenza: a highly contagious viral infection that affects the respiratory tract

informed consent: permission given by a patient, resident or client (or the person authorized to make decisions on the patient's, resident's or client's behalf) to go ahead with a treatment or procedure

ingrown toenail: a condition that occurs when the toenail is trimmed too short and the edge curls down and grows into the neighboring skin

inpatient care: care that is provided in a hospital or other acute care setting that requires at least one overnight stay

in-service training: additional training offered by an employer to employees, designed to teach new skills and knowledge or keep existing skills and knowledge current

insulin: a hormone that causes glucose to be moved from the bloodstream into the cells

intimacy: the need and ability to feel emotional closeness to another person and to have that closeness returned

J

job application: a form that employers use to collect basic information about a job applicant, such as the person's contact information, employment history, educational history, additional experience and skills, the hours the person is available to work, and the names and contact information of references

job interview: a meeting between a job candidate and an employer that allows both parties to find out more about each other

K

kidney (renal) failure: the inability of the kidneys to filter waste products

L

larceny: theft

laws: rules established by a governing authority to protect people from harm and provide a framework for resolving conflicts

life-sustaining treatments: treatments that will prolong life, such as cardiopulmonary resuscitation (CPR) or mechanical ventilation

living will: a legal document that gives specific directions about what steps the health care team should or should not take to prolong the person's life when death seems near

logrolling: a method used to turn a person onto his or her side in bed when the person's spine must be kept in alignment throughout the move

long-term care setting: health care facilities that provide residents with ongoing assistance with meeting medical, personal and social needs

long-term memory: memory of the past

low Fowler's position: a variation of Fowler's position where the head of the bed is raised 30 degrees

M

malignant: cancerous

malnutrition: failure to take in enough of the right kinds of nutrients to stay healthy

masturbation: touching or rubbing one's own genitals for sexual release or pleasure

Medicaid: an insurance program for people with low incomes, jointly funded by federal and state governments

medical record: a legal document that details the person's condition, the measures taken by the health care team to diagnose and manage the condition, and the person's response to the care provided

Medicare: a federally funded insurance program for people who are 65 years and older

metastasize: the spreading of cancerous cells to other parts of the body other than where the cancer originated

microbe (microorganism): a tiny living thing that can be seen only through the magnification of a microscope

mild cognitive impairment: problems with memory, language or thinking processes that are noticeable to other people, but do not interfere with the person's ability to live a normal life

miter: a folding technique that creates a neat, tight corner and holds the sheet securely to the mattress

modified side-lying position: the person is positioned on his or her side and leaning slightly toward the back to relieve pressure on the hip

mucous membranes: sticky, moist membranes that line the respiratory, genitourinary and digestive tracts

multiple sclerosis (MS): a chronic neurologic disorder that gradually destroys the protective coating on the nerves in the brain and spinal cord

myocardial infarction: a condition that results when blood flow to part of the heart muscle (the myocardium) is blocked, causing the cells in that area to die; also called a "heart attack"

N

nausea: a sick feeling in the stomach often accompanied by the urge to vomit

nonverbal communication: communication through body language, including gestures, facial expressions, tone of voice, and body position and movement

nursing home: a long-term care facility that provides nursing care and supervision for residents who require a high level of care

nursing team: staff members with specialized knowledge and training in the delivery of nursing care; consists of, at minimum, a nurse and a nurse assistant

nutrients: substances that the body needs to grow, maintain itself and stay healthy

nutrition: the process of taking in and using nutrients

O

Occupational Safety and Health Administration (OSHA): a government agency that was established to help protect workers in all industries (not just health care) from on-the-job injuries

ombudsmen: volunteers who advocate for (act on the behalf of) nursing home residents and their family members to resolve problems related to quality of care

Omnibus Budget Reconciliation Act of 1987 (OBRA): legislation that emphasizes the responsibility of nursing homes to provide residents with a comfortable and fulfilling lifestyle and to promote their physical, mental, emotional and spiritual well-being to the highest degree possible

occupational exposure: exposure to disease in the workplace

open bed: a bed where the bedspread, blanket and top sheet have been folded back to the bottom of the bed

osteoporosis: a disease in which loss of bone tissue causes the bones to become very fragile and prone to breaking

ostomy appliance: a pouch worn on the outside of the body, over a stoma, to collect feces or urine

outpatient care: care that is provided in a hospital or other acute care setting that does not require an overnight stay

P

pain: an unpleasant sensation that signals actual or potential damage to the body

pain threshold: the point at which the person becomes aware of experiencing pain

pain tolerance: the highest level of pain that a person is willing to experience before taking action to relieve it

palliative treatments: treatments provided to relieve uncomfortable symptoms without actually curing the disease that is causing the symptoms

paralysis: the loss of movement and sensation

paranoia: excessive suspicion without cause

paraplegia: paralysis that affects both legs and the lower trunk

Parkinson's disease: a neurologic disorder characterized by muscle tremors and difficulty with movement as a result of insufficient amounts of dopamine

pathogen: a microorganism that causes disease

patient: a person who receives care in a hospital or other acute care setting

perineal care: cleansing of the area between the legs, including the genitals and the anus

personal protective equipment: protective gear worn to prevent microbes from contaminating your uniform, skin or mucous membranes; includes gloves, gowns, masks and protective eyewear

pneumonia: inflammation of the lungs

podiatrist: health care provider who specializes in care of the feet

postmortem care: care that is provided for a person's body after death

pre-placement health evaluation: health screening tests done after a job offer is made to ensure that a new employee is physically and emotionally capable of meeting the job requirements, and to identify any accommodations that may need to be made so that the employee can perform the job competently and safely

pressure ulcer: a sore that develops when part of a person's body presses against a hard surface for a long period of time; also called a decubitus ulcer

prioritize: to list items or tasks in order of importance

probationary period: a period of time during which the employer closely evaluates the job performance and potential of a new employee to ensure that the employee is performing the job to expectations

prone position: the person is positioned on his or her stomach

pulse oximetry: a technique used to measure the oxygen levels in a person's blood

Q

quadriplegia: paralysis that affects both arms, the trunk and both legs

R

radiation: the use of high-energy x-rays to destroy cancer cells

range-of-motion exercises: exercises that help to keep joints functional by moving them in a systematic way

receptive aphasia: the inability to understand communication from others

recording (documenting): the written exchange of information between members of the health care team

reference list: a document providing the contact information for three to five people who know you well enough in a professional capacity to speak to a potential employer about your experience and suitability for a job

regression: a return to a previous stage of development

reporting: the verbal exchange of information among members of the health care team

resident: a person who receives care in a long-term care setting

restorative care (rehabilitation nursing): nursing care that helps people maintain abilities that they still have and helps regain, to the greatest extent possible, abilities that they have lost

restraint: any device that inhibits a person's freedom of movement; may be physical or chemical

resume: a document summarizing your contact information, education and previous experience

rigor mortis: stiffening of the muscles of the body after death

S

schedule: a written plan that lists the time and order of several tasks

scope of practice: the range of tasks that a health care worker is legally allowed to do

seizure: involuntary changes in body movement, function, sensation, awareness or behavior as a result of abnormal electrical activity in the brain

separation anxiety: anxiety that is experienced when the child is away from his or her parents or other primary caregivers

sexual behaviors: physical activities, such as sexual intercourse and masturbation, related to obtaining sexual pleasure and reproduction

sexual identity: a person's sexual orientation and preferences with regard to sexual partners

sexuality: how we perceive of ourselves and express ourselves sexually

sharps container: a sturdy, puncture-proof plastic box with a tight-fitting lid used for the disposal of sharp objects such as needles or razors

shearing: one surface moves in the opposite way against another surface that offers resistance, creating a dragging effect

shock: a condition in which the circulatory system fails to deliver enough oxygen-rich blood to the body's tissues and vital organs

short-term memory: memory of recent events

shroud: a cloth covering placed around the body of a deceased person

side-lying (lateral) position: the person is positioned on his or her side

Sims' position: the person is positioned on his or her side, leaning very far forward

skin breakdown: loss of healthy, intact skin

spirituality: a belief in something greater than oneself that helps the person assign meaning and purpose to life

standard precautions: practices used by caregivers when providing care to a person, regardless of the person's condition or injury, to minimize the spread of pathogens carried in body fluids

sterilization: a technique that uses gas, liquid, dry heat or pressurized steam to destroy all microbes on an object or surface

stethoscope: a piece of equipment that is used to listen to sounds produced inside the body

stoma: a surgically created opening made in the abdominal wall to allow the elimination of waste

sub-acute care setting: a special unit of a hospital or nursing home or a separate facility that specializes in providing care to patients who are well enough to leave the hospital but still require treatments that can only be provided by health care professionals

suicide: the act of deliberately taking one's own life

supine position: the person is positioned flat on his or her back

surgical bed: a bed where the bedspread, blanket and top sheet have been folded to the side of the bed

T

terminal illness: an illness for which there is no treatment and that is ultimately expected to lead to the person's death

therapeutic diet: a special diet ordered to help a person regain or maintain health

transfer: a move from one part of a facility to another

transfer (gait) belt: a wide, webbed belt that is placed around a person's waist to provide a safe place to grasp when helping a person to stand, walk or transfer

transgender: word used to describe a person who feels that his or her gender does not match the physical body he or she was born with

transmission-based precautions: practices used by caregivers to minimize the spread of microbes when the person has a disease known to be transmitted in a specific way; includes airborne precautions, droplet precautions and contact precautions

transsexual: word used to describe a person who alters his or her physical appearance to more closely match the gender he or she most strongly identifies with

tuberculosis: a bacterial infection of the lungs that is spread through the air from one person to another

tumor: a solid mass of tissue

U

urination: the elimination of liquid waste from the body

urine: liquid body waste

V

validation therapy: a technique for working with those with cognitive impairment or dementia that shows respect for the person's thoughts and feelings and validates (acknowledges) what the person believes, regardless of the actual truth

verbal communication: communication using spoken, written or American Sign Language

vital signs: measurements that give us basic information about how a person's body is functioning, including temperature, pulse, respirations and blood pressure

RESOURCES

CHAPTER 1: **BEING A NURSE ASSISTANT**

Nurse Assistant Training and Education

U.S. Department of Health and Human Services (DHHS). Office of the Inspector General: Nurse Aide Training. November 2002.

CHAPTER 2: **WORKING IN THE HEALTH CARE SYSTEM**

Resident Rights

State of Wisconsin Board on Aging and Long-Term Care. Ombudsman Program: Residents' Rights. http://www.dhs.wisconsin.gov/bqaconsumer/nursinghomes/resRightsNHs.pdf. Accessed June 20, 2012.

Protecting Health Care Workers

Occupational Safety and Health Administration.

http://www.osha.gov/. Accessed June 20, 2012.

CHAPTER 3: **UNDERSTANDING LEGAL AND ETHICAL ASPECTS OF HEALTH CARE**

General

Nursing Assistant Resources on the Web. Legal Issues for CNAs. http://www.nursingassistants.net/educational-articles/legal-issues-for-cnas/. Accessed June 20, 2012.

Abuse

Agency for Healthcare Research and Quality. Elder Abuse Prevention. http://guideline.gov/content.aspx?id=34018&search=elder+abuse. Accessed June 20, 2012.

CHAPTER 4: **UNDERSTANDING THE PEOPLE IN OUR CARE**

Older Adults

Healthy People. 2020 Topics and Objectives: Older Adults. http://www.healthypeople.gov/2020/topicsobjectives2020/overview.aspx?topicid=31. Accessed June 20, 2012.

CHAPTER 6: **CONTROLLING THE SPREAD OF INFECTION**

General

The Society for Healthcare Epidemiology of America and the Association for Professionals in Infection Control. SHEA/APIC Guideline: Infection Prevention and Control in the Long-Term Care Facility, 2008. http://premierinc.com/safety/topics/guidelines/surveil.jsp. Accessed June 20, 2012.

Office of Health and Safety, Centers for Disease Control and Prevention. Guidelines for Laundry in Health Care Facilities. http://www.pandemicreferenceguides.com/pdfFiles/InfectionControl/GuidelinesforLaundry.htm. Accessed June 20, 2012.

Health Care–Associated Infections

Association for Professionals in Infection Control and Epidemiology, Inc. Practice Guidance for Infection Control. http://www.apic.org/Professional-Practice/Overview. Accessed June 20, 2012.

Centers for Disease Control and Prevention. Antibiotic/Antimicrobial Resistance. http://www.cdc.gov/drugresistance/index.html. Accessed June 20, 2012.

Centers for Disease Control and Prevention. Healthcare-Associated Infections. http://www.cdc.gov/hai/. Accessed June 20, 2012.

Handwashing

Centers for Disease Control and Prevention. Hand Hygiene in Healthcare Settings. http://www.cdc.gov/handhygiene/index.html. Accessed June 20, 2012.

World Health Organization. WHO Guidelines on Hand Hygiene in Health Care. http://whqlibdoc.who.int/publications/2009/9789241597906_eng.pdf. Accessed June 20, 2012.

Disinfection and Sterilization

Centers for Disease Control and Prevention. Guideline for Disinfection and Sterilization in Healthcare Facilities, 2008. http://www.cdc.gov/hicpac/Disinfection_Sterilization/3_4surfaceDisinfection.html. Accessed June 20, 2012.

Centers for Disease Control and Prevention. Healthcare Infection Control Practices Advisory Committee (HICPAC). General Guidelines. http://www.cdc.gov/hicpac/pubs.html. Accessed June 20, 2012.

Personal Protective Equipment

U.S. Food and Drug Administration. Personal Protective Equipment. http://www.fda.gov/MedicalDevices/ProductsandMedicalProcedures/GeneralHospitalDevicesandSupplies/PersonalProtectiveEquipment/default.htm. Accessed June 20, 2012.

Bloodborne Pathogens

Centers for Disease Control and Prevention. Bloodborne Infectious Diseases: HIV/AIDS, Hepatitis B, Hepatitis C. http://www.cdc.gov/niosh/topics/bbp/guidelines.html. Accessed June 20, 2012.

Occupational Safety and Health Administration. OSHA's Bloodborne Pathogens Standard. http://www.osha.gov/OshDoc/data_BloodborneFacts/bbfact01.pdf. Accessed June 20, 2012.

Transmission-Based Precautions

Centers for Disease Control and Prevention. Cover Your Cough. http://www.cdc.gov/flu/protect/covercough.htm. Accessed June 20, 2012.

Centers for Disease Control and Prevention. Tuberculosis. http://www.cdc.gov/tb/topic/basics/default.htm. Accessed June 20, 2012.

Siegel, J.D.; Rhinehart, E.; Jackson, M.; Chiarello, L.; and the Healthcare Infection Control Practices Advisory Committee. 2007 Guideline for Isolation Precautions: Preventing Transmission of Infectious Agents in Healthcare Settings. http://www.cdc.gov/hicpac/pdf/isolation/Isolation2007.pdf. Accessed June 20, 2012.

Safe Use of Bleach

California Department of Public Health. California Work-Related Asthma Prevention Program: Cleaning Products and Work-Related Asthma. http://www.cdph.ca.gov/programs/ohsep/documents/wra-cleaningprod.pdf. Accessed June 20, 2012.

San Francisco Asthma Task Force. Bleach Exposure in Child Care Settings: Strategies for Elimination or Reduction. http://www.sfgov3.org/Modules/ShowDocument.aspx?documentid=665. Accessed June 20, 2012.

CHAPTER 7: **PREVENTING INJURIES**

General

The Joint Commission. Patient Safety. http://www.jointcommission.org/. Accessed June 20, 2012.

Safe Patient Handling and No-Lift Policies

Occupational Safety and Health Administration. Ergonomics: Guidelines for Nursing Homes. http://www.osha.gov/ergonomics/guidelines/nursinghome/. Accessed June 20, 2012.

Occupational Safety and Health Administration. Healthcare-Wide Hazards: Ergonomics. http://www.osha.gov/SLTC/etools/hospital/hazards/ergo/ergo.html. Accessed June 20, 2012.

Body Positioning

Occupational Safety and Health Administration. Good Working Positions. http://www.osha.gov/SLTC/etools/computerworkstations/positions.html. Accessed June 20, 2012.

Fall Prevention

Agency for Healthcare Research and Quality. Falls Management Program. http://www.ahrq.gov/research/ltc/fallspx/fallspxman1.htm. Accessed June 20, 2012.

Bednar, Joseph. "Falling Statistics: Hospitals Implement Policies to Cut Down on Patient Falls." *Healthcare News* (May 2007). http://healthcarenews.com/article.asp?id=1584. Accessed June 20, 2012.

Centers for Disease Control and Prevention. Falls in Nursing Homes. http://www.cdc.gov/HomeandRecreationalSafety/Falls/nursing.html. Accessed June 20, 2012.

Centers for Disease Control and Prevention. Falls—Older Adults. http://www.cdc.gov/HomeandRecreationalSafety/Falls/index.html. Accessed June 20, 2012.

Cochrane Summaries. Interventions for Preventing Falls in Older People in Nursing Care Facilities and Hospitals. http://summaries.cochrane.org/CD005465/interventions-for-preventing-falls-in-older-people-in-nursing-care-facilities-and-hospitals. Accessed June 20, 2012.

Currie, Leanne. "Chapter 10: Fall and Injury Prevention." *Patient Safety and Quality: An Evidence-Based Handbook for Nurses.* Agency for Healthcare Research and Quality. 2007. http://www.ahrq.gov/qual/nurseshdbk/docs/CurrieL_FIP.pdf. Accessed June 20, 2012.

Hartford Institute for Geriatric Nursing. Nursing Standard of Practice Protocol: Fall Prevention. http://consultgerirn.org/topics/falls/want_to_know_more. Accessed June 20, 2012.

Health Care Association of New Jersey. Fall Management Guideline. March 2007. http://www.hcanj.org/docs/hcanjbp_fallmgmt6.pdf. Accessed June 20, 2012.

Hitcho, E.B., et al. "Characteristics and Circumstances of Falls in a Hospital Setting: A Prospective Analysis." *Journal of General Internal Medicine* (July 2004); 19(7): 732-739. http://www.ncbi.nlm.nih.gov/pmc/articles/PMC1492485/. Accessed June 20, 2012.

Ohio Health Care Association. Falls Workgroup. Fall Reduction and Injury Mitigation: A Systematic Approach. 2007.

Rask, K., et al. "Implementation and Evaluation of a Nursing Home Fall Management Program." *Journal of American Geriatric Society* (March 2007); 55(3): 342-349.

Shanley, Chris. *Putting Your Best Foot Forward: Preventing and Managing Falls in Aged Care Facilities.* http://www.cera.usyd.edu.au/manual_extract/putting_extract.pdf. Accessed June 20, 2012.

State Operations Manual. Appendix PP—Guidance to Surveyors for Long-Term Care Facilities. CMS. Rev. 70, January 2011. http://www.cms.gov/manuals/Downloads/som107ap_pp_guidelines_ltcf.pdf. Accessed June 20, 2012.

Texas Department of Aging and Disability Services. Fall Prevention and Management for Nursing Homes. February 2012. http://www.dads.state.tx.us/qualitymatters/qcp/fall/nf.html. Accessed June 20, 2012.

Restraints

Advancing Excellence in America's Nursing Homes. Reducing Restraint Use. http://www.nhqualitycampaign.org/files/factsheets/Staff%20Fact%20Sheet%20-%20Reducing%20Restraint.pdf. Accessed June 20, 2012.

Appleby, J., and Gillum, J. "Fewer Care Facilities Use Restraints for Elderly Residents." *USA Today* (February 2009). http://www.usatoday.com/news/nation/2009-02-16-nursing-home-restraints_N.htm. Accessed June 20, 2012.

Evans, L., and Cotter, V. "Avoiding Restraints in Patients with Dementia." *AJN* (March 2008); 108(3): 40-49. http://www.nursingcenter.com/pdf.asp?AID=775972. Accessed June 20, 2012.

Gastmans, C., and Milisen, K. Use of Physical Restraint in Nursing Homes: Clinical-Ethical Considerations. *Journal of Medical Ethics* (March 2006); 32(3): 148-152. http://www.ncbi.nlm.nih.gov/pmc/articles/PMC2564468/. Accessed June 20, 2012.

Haut, A., et al. "Evaluation of an Evidence-Based Guidance on the Reduction of Physical Restraints in Nursing Homes: A Cluster-Randomised Controlled Trial." *BMC Geriatrics 2009,* 9:42; doi: 10.1186/1471-2318-9-42. http://www.biomedcentral.com/1471-2318/9/42. Accessed June 20, 2012.

Information and Quality Healthcare. Physical Restraints: Overview. http://iqh.org/index.php?option=com_content&view=article&id=137:physical-restraints-overview&catid=84:articles&Itemid=230. Accessed June 20, 2012.

Laurin, D., et al. "Physical Restraint Use Among Nursing Home Residents: A Comparison of Two Data Collection Methods." *BMC Nursing 2004*, 3:5. http://www.biomedcentral.com/1472-6955/3/5. Accessed June 20, 2012.

Minnesota Department of Health. Safety Without Restraints: A New Practice Standard for Safe Care. http://www.health.state.mn.us/divs/fpc/safety.htm. Accessed June 20, 2012.

National Institute of Nursing Research (NINR). Problems Associated with the Use of Physical Restraints. October 2006. http://www.ninr.nih.gov/NR/rdonlyres/87C83B44-6FC6-4183-96FE-67E00623ACE0/4769/Restraints.pdf. Accessed June 20, 2012.

Nursing Home Ombudsman Agency of the Bluegrass, Inc. Guidelines on Use of Physical Restraints in Nursing Homes. 2000. http://www.ombuddy.org/InfoSheet/restraints.htm. Accessed June 20, 2012.

State Operations Manual Appendix PP – Guidance to Surveyors for Long Term Care Facilities. CMS. Rev. 70, January 2011. http://www.cms.gov/manuals/Downloads/som107ap_pp_guidelines_ltcf.pdf. Accessed June 20, 2012.

CHAPTER 8: **RESPONDING TO EMERGENCIES**

First Aid

American Red Cross. *First Aid/CPR/AED Participant's Manual.* StayWell Health and Safety Solutions. 2011.

Disaster Preparedness

American Red Cross. Preparedness Fast Facts. http://www.redcross.org. Accessed June 20, 2012.

CHAPTER 12: **ASSISTING WITH POSITIONING AND TRANSFERRING**

Pressure Ulcer Prevention

Agency for Healthcare Research and Quality. Preventing Pressure Ulcers in Hospitals: A Toolkit for Improving Quality of Care. http://www.ahrq.gov/research/ltc/pressureulcertoolkit/. Accessed June 20, 2012.

Cochrane Summaries. Can Pressure Ulcers Be Prevented by Using Different Support Surfaces? April 2011. http://summaries.cochrane.org/CD001735/can-pressure-ulcers-be-prevented-by-using-different-support-surfaces. Accessed June 20, 2012.

National Pressure Ulcer Advisory Panel. *Pressure Ulcer Prevention.* http://www.npuap.org/Final_Quick_Prevention_for_web_2010.pdf. Accessed June 20, 2012.

National Pressure Ulcer Advisory Panel. Pressure Ulcer Stages. http://www.npuap.org. Accessed June 20, 2012.

CHAPTER 13: **ASSISTING WITH PERSONAL CLEANLINESS AND GROOMING**

Mouth Care

American Dental Association. How to Brush Your Teeth. http://www.ada.org

Centers for Disease Control and Prevention. Oral Health for Older Americans. http://www.cdc.gov/oralhealth/publications/factsheets/adult_older.htm. Accessed June 20, 2012.

Felton, D., et al. "Evidence-Based Guidelines for the Care and Maintenance of Complete Dentures." *Journal of the American Dental Association* (February 2011). http://jada.ada.org/content/142/suppl_1/1S.full. Accessed June 20, 2012.

CHAPTER 14: **ASSISTING WITH MEALS AND FLUIDS**

General

Pioneer Network: New Dining Practice Standards. August 2011. http://www.pioneernetwork.net/Latest/Detail.aspx?id=294. Accessed June 20, 2012.

State Operations Manual. F325 – Nutrition Guidelines (Rev. 36, Issued: 08-01-08, Effective: 08-01-08 Implementation: 08-01-08).

U.S. Department of Agriculture (USDA). Selecting Healthy Food Choices from the Five Food Groups. http://www.choosemyplate.gov/. Accessed June 20, 2012.

Problems with Nutrition and Hydration in the Elderly

Agency for Healthcare Research and Quality. Mealtime Difficulties. In: Evidence-Based Geriatric Nursing Protocols for Best Practice. http://guideline.gov/content.aspx?id=12267&search=dysphagia. Accessed June 20, 2012.

Hartford Institute for Geriatric Nursing. Mealtime Difficulties. Nursing Standard of Practice Protocol: Assessment and Management of Mealtime Difficulties. http://consultgerirn.org/topics/mealtime_difficulties/want_to_know_more. Accessed June 20, 2012.

Illinois Council on Long-Term Care. Water: The Fountain of Life. http://www.nursinghome.org/fam.html. Accessed June 20, 2012.

Pirlich, M., and Lochs, H. "Nutrition in the Elderly." *Best Practice & Research Clinical Gastroenterology.* December 2001; 15(6): 869–884.

Liberalized Diets in Long-Term Care

Nutrition 411. Liberalized Diets. *http://www.rd411.com/nutrition-management/clinical-inservices/item/236-liberalized-diets.* Accessed June 20, 2012.

CHAPTER 15: **ASSISTING WITH ELIMINATION**

Urinary Tract Infection Prevention

Centers for Disease Control and Prevention. CAUTI Guideline Fast Facts. http://www.cdc.gov/hicpac/CAUTI_fastFacts.html#1. Accessed June 20, 2012.

CHAPTER 16: **PROMOTING COMFORT AND REST**

AGS Panel on Persistent Pain in Older Persons. The Management of Persistent Pain in Older Persons. *Journal of the American Geriatric Society.* 2002; 6(Suppl): S205-24.

American Geriatrics Society. American Geriatrics Society Announces New Guidelines to Improve Pain Management, Quality of Life, and Quality of Care For Older Patients. *Medical News Today.* May 2009. Retrieved from http:www.medicalnewstodaycom/releases/148692.php.

International Association for the Study of Pain. Facts on Pain in Older Persons. http://www.iasp-pain.org/Content/NavigationMenu/GlobalYearAgainstPain/GlobalYearAgainstHeadache/default.htm. Accessed June 20, 2012.

Gibson, S.J. "Older People's Pain." *Pain: Clinical Updates* (2006); 14:1-4.

Goldman, L.; Hines, T.; and Kopits, I. "Common Complaints in the Elderly." *Reichel's Care of the Elderly.* 6th ed. New York: Cambridge University Press, 2009; pp. 41-42.

Hadjistavropoulos, T. Pain Assessment Among Older Persons with Dementia. http://www.iasp-pain.org/AM/AMTemplate.cfm?Section=Home&CONTENTID=5473&TEMPLATE=/CM/ContentDisplay.cfm. Accessed June 20, 2012.

Hadjistavropoulos, T. "Assessing Pain in Older Persons with Severe Limitations in Ability to Communicate." *Pain in the Elderly.* Edited by Gibson, S.J , and Weiner, D. Seattle, Washington: IASP Press, 2005: 135-15.

CHAPTER 17: **ASSISTING WITH ADMISSIONS, TRANSFERS AND DISCHARGES**

Advancing Excellence in America's Nursing Homes. Improving Resident/Family Satisfaction. http://www.nhqualitycampaign.org/files/factsheets/Staff%20Fact%20Sheet%20-%20Resident%20Satisfaction.pdf. Accessed June 20, 2012.

CHAPTER 18: **PROVIDING CARE FOR PEOPLE WITH SPECIFIC ILLNESSES**

Parkinson's Disease

Fok, P.; Farrell, M.; McMeeken, J.; and Kuo, Y. "The Effects of Verbal Instructions on Gait in People with Parkinson's Disease: A Systematic Review of Randomized and Non-Randomized Trials." *Clinical Rehabilitation* (May 2011); 25(5): 396-407.

Miller, N.; Noble, E.; Jones, D.; and Burn, D. "Hard to Swallow: Dysphagia in Parkinson's Disease." *Age Ageing* (November 2006); 35(6): 614-618.

Parkinson's Disease Foundation. Understanding Parkinson's. http://www.pdf.org/en/understanding_pd. Accessed June 20, 2012.

Parkinson's Disease Foundation. Understanding Parkinson's: Falls Prevention. http://www.pdf.org/pdf/fs_falls_prevention_10.pdf. Accessed June 20, 2012.

Cancer

Coppola, C. Today's Caregiver. Tips for Keeping Safe at Home with Chemotherapy. http://caregiver.com/channels/cancer/articles/keeping_safe_at_home.htm. Accessed June 20, 2012.

Occupational Safety and Health Administration (OSHA). Controlling Occupational Exposure to Hazardous Drugs. http://www.osha.gov/dts/osta/otm/otm_vi/otm_vi_2.html. Accessed June 20, 2012.

CHAPTER 19: **PROVIDING CARE FOR PEOPLE WITH COGNITIVE CHANGES AND DEMENTIA**

Alzheimer's Association. 2012 Alzheimer's Disease Facts and Figures. www.alz.org/downloads/facts_figures_2012.pdf. Accessed June 20, 2012.

Alzheimer's Association. Frontotemporal Dementia. www.alz.org/alzheimers_disease_frontotemporal_dementia.asp. Accessed June 20, 2012.

Alzheimer's Association. Vascular Dementia. www.alz.org/alzheimers_disease_vascular_dementia.asp. Accessed June 20, 2012.

Association for Frontotemporal Degeneration. Fast Facts About Frontotemporal Degeneration (2011). www.theaftd.org/wp-content/uploads/2009/02/Fast-Facts-Final-6-11.pdf. Accessed June 20, 2012.

Association for Frontotemporal Degeneration. FTD vs. Alzheimer's Disease. www.theaftd.org/frontotemporal-degeneration/diagnosis. Accessed June 20, 2012.

Byrd, L. "Caregiver Survival 101: Strategies to Manage Problematic Behaviors Presented in Individuals with Dementia." Eau Claire, Wisconsin: PHC Publishing Group, 2011.

Collins, L.; Rovner, B.; and Marenberg, M. "Evaluation and Treatment of Dementia." *Reichel's Care of the Elderly.* 6th ed. New York: Cambridge University Press, 2009; pp. 176-187.

Lewy Body Dementia Association. Lewy Body Dementia Symptoms and Diagnostic Criteria. www.lbda.org/node/14. Accessed June 20, 2012.

Lewy Body Dementia Association. What Is LBD? www.lbda.org/category/3437/what-is-lbd.htm. Accessed June 20, 2012.

Mayo Clinic. Vascular Dementia. April 30, 2011. www.mayoclinic.com/health/vascular-dementia/DS00934. Accessed June 20, 2012.

National Institute of Neurological Disorders and Stroke. NINDS Alzheimer's Disease Information Page. www.ninds.nih.gov/disorders/alzheimersdisease/alzheimersdisease.htm?css=print. Accessed June 20, 2012.

National Institute on Aging. Alzheimer's Disease Fact Sheet. www.nia.nih.gov/print/alzheimers/publication/alzheimers-disease-fact-sheet. Accessed June 20, 2012.

National Institute on Aging. What Are the Signs of Alzheimer's Disease? www.nia.nih.gov/print/alzheimers/publication/understanding-alzheimers-disease/what-are-signs-alzheimers-disease. Accessed June 20, 2012.

Parks, S., and Winter, L. "The Elderly, Their Families, and Their Caregivers." *Reichel's Care of the Elderly.* 6th ed. New York: Cambridge University Press, 2009; pp. 572-576.

CHAPTER 20: **PROVIDING CARE FOR PEOPLE AT THE END OF LIFE**

Grief

Hospice Foundation of America. An Introduction to Grieving. http://www.hospicefoundation.org/pages/page.asp?page_id=171387. Accessed June 20, 2012.

Role of the Nurse Assistant

Hospice and Palliative Nurses Association. HPNA Position Statement: The Value of the Nursing Assistant in End of Life Care. http://www.hpna.org/pdf/PositionStatement_ValueOfNAs.pdf. Accessed June 20, 2012.

Signs of Approaching Death

National Cancer Institute at the National Institutes of Health. End-of-Life Care for People Who Have Cancer. http://www.cancer.gov/cancertopics/factsheet/Support/end-of-life-care. Accessed June 20, 2012.

CHAPTER 22: **PROVIDING CARE FOR PEOPLE IN THEIR HOMES**

U.S. Department of Agriculture (USDA). Basics for Handling Food Safely. http://www.fsis.usda.gov/Fact_Sheets/Basics_for_Handling_Food_Safely/. Accessed June 20, 2012.

CHAPTER 23: **ENTERING THE WORKFORCE**

Preparing a Resume

LeClaire, J. Monster.com. Resume Tips to Help Nursing Assistants Get Noticed. http://nursinglink.monster.com/topics/10449-resume-tips-to-help-nursing-assistants-get-noticed/posts. Accessed June 20, 2012.

CHAPTER 24: **ENJOYING PROFESSIONAL SUCCESS**

Workplace Violence Prevention Programs

Occupational Safety and Health Administration (OSHA): Workplace Violence. http://www.osha.gov/SLTC/etools/hospital/hazards/workplaceviolence/viol.html. Accessed June 20, 2012.

Workers Compensation Board of British Columbia. Preventing Violence in Health Care: Five Steps to an Effective Program. http://www.worksafebc.com/publications/health_and_safety/by_topic/assets/pdf/violhealthcare.pdf. Accessed June 20, 2012.

Professional Development

Nursing Assistant Resources on the Web. Ten Tips for Writing Great Resumes. http://www.nursingassistants.net. Accessed June 20, 2012.

E

F

G

H

T

U

V

T

U

V

Q

R

S